W9-AOV-988

# PELVIC AND ACETABULAR FRACTURES

## AUTHORS

Dana C. Mears,
BM, BCh, PhD, MRCP, FRCS(C), FACS
Associate Professor of Orthopaedic Surgery
University of Pittsburgh
Staff, Presbyterian University Hospital,
Children's Hospital, Pittsburgh
Fellow, American Academy of Orthopaedic Surgeons

Harry E. Rubash, MD
Assistant Professor of Orthopaedic Surgery
University of Pittsburgh
Staff, Presbyterian University Hospital,
Children's Hospital, Pittsburgh
Consultant, Veterans Administration Hospital, Pittsburgh

## CONTRIBUTORS

Claude L. Martimbeau, MD, FRCS(C)
Assistant Clinical Professor of Orthopedic Surgery
Loma Linda (California) University

Joel M. Matta, MD
Assistant Professor of Orthopaedic Surgery
University of Southern California, Los Angeles

Jill D. Smith Forster, MD
Research Fellow, Department of Orthopaedic Surgery
Duke University, Durham, North Carolina

# PELVIC AND ACETABULAR FRACTURES

DANA C. MEARS
HARRY E. RUBASH

SLACK Incorporated, 6900 Grove Road, Thorofare, New Jersey 08086.

Printed in the United States of America

Library of Congress Catalog Card Number: 83-50280

ISBN: 0-943432-07-3

Published by: SLACK Incorporated
6900 Grove Road
Thorofare, NJ 08086

Last digit is print number: 8 7 6 5 4 3 2 1

# CONTENTS

# PREFACE

More than ten years ago, during my first month of clinical practice, a young woman was referred to me with an infected nonunion of the pelvis and massive associated open wounds. After a careful clinical examination and reflection upon my limited knowledge of major pelvic trauma, I sought the assistance of my orthopaedic and general surgical colleagues, who clearly possessed an equally meager understanding of the pelvis. In a subsequent review of the available literature, the limited experience with the use of external pelvic fixation reported by Slatis in Helsinki and Tile in Toronto was encouraging. At that time a local implant manufacturer, the Sampson Company, fabricated an external frame that functioned extremely well, particularly in light of its somewhat primitive design.

This experience provided an incentive to initiate a biomechanical and clinical study of external pelvic fixation, particularly for application to an acute pelvic injury. The early results were notable for a striking arrest of profuse retroperitoneal hemorrhage and alleviation of the severe pelvic pain. Upon a review of the postoperative radiographs, many examples of persistent malalignment were evident. The potential role for a supplementary open reduction and internal fixation as a means of providing a more accurate reduction with rigid stability was questioned. During the following years, as the striking biomechanical and clinical attributes of internal fixation were confirmed, our referral pattern showed a progressive evolution. Instead of an acute referral of a local trauma victim who possessed a simple unstable pelvic ring disruption amenable to a relatively simple technique of external pelvic fixation, increasingly the referrals to Pittsburgh comprised more comminuted injuries, especially with multiple sites of pelvic disruption and acetabular involvement. The impetus for biomechanical, anatomical, and clinical investigations of the acetabulum was created, along with a need for a precise three-dimensional appreciation of the complex cases. By a collaborative project with our radiologists, especially Larry Burk, along with the General Electric Co., a routine clinical service for the provision of three-dimensional reformated images was established.

Pelvic reconstruction requires detailed knowledge of the relevant surgical anatomy, patterns of injury, diverse surgical approaches to the pelvis, and techniques of reduction and stabilization. In this volume these topics are reviewed systematically, along with an analysis of the clinical results of acute, subacute, and late presentations. With the currently available armamentarium of techniques of external and internal fixation, highly satisfactory techniques appear to be available to reconstruct almost all types of acute pelvic ring disruptions and most acetabular fractures. The authors hope that publication of these methods will provide a firm basis for more widespread application of the techniques, and a stimulus for further basic research and clinical innovations.

Dana C. Mears

# ACKNOWLEDGEMENTS

This volume would not have materialized without the contributions and encouragement provided by many individuals, to whom I am most grateful. In addition to the invaluable assistance of my collaborative authors, my professional colleagues and members of the orthopaedic staff have referred the extraordinary cases that provided the clinical basis for the study. Jeff Mast provided a detailed account of the surgical anatomy of the pelvis based upon his study under Professor Arthur von Hockhstetter of Basel, Switzerland. Many orthopaedic residents at the University of Pittsburgh gave freely of their time and effort in the research laboratory, the operating room, and on the wards, especially Freddie Fu, Patrick Stone, Dirk Nelson, and J.C. Harvell. Takeshi Sawaguchi and Tom Brown undertook most of the biomechanical studies, with the proficient technical assistance of Warren Thompson. Allan Grossman assisted with the clinical documentation and medical illustrations. Larry Burk and Larry Cooperstein of the Department of Radiology, along with Bruce Teeter of General Electric Company, and Gabor Herman of the University of Pennsylvania, provided the radiological expertise for the three-dimensional reformated imaging. The superb medical illustrations were prepared by Jon Coulter of Pittsburgh, with the assistance of Hoyt Smith, from Tulsa, Oklahoma. Douglas Sellers and his associates at the Department of Medical Photography, Montefiore Hospital, were responsible for the excellent photographic reproductions. Harold Miller and his colleagues at Slack, Incorporated, displayed extraordinary patience and cooperation as the magnitude of the project progressively increased, with corresponding deferrals of the projected date of completion.

Janice Westwood served as my administrative assistant, to direct the organization and type and review the manuscript amidst a hectic clinical and research environment. Her meticulous attention to the plethora of tedious allied chores was instrumental in the completion of the project.

# DEDICATION

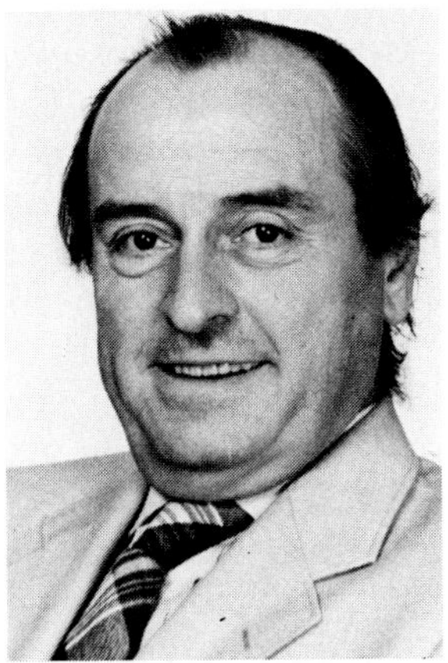

To Emile Letournel
Professor of the Hospital of Paris
Chief, Department of Orthopaedic Surgery
Centre Medico-Chirurgical de la Porte de Choisy

It is my pleasure to honor Emile Letournel for his pioneering efforts in the management of pelvic and acetabular fractures.

He was born on the St. Pierre et Miquelon Islands, a territory of France located about 50 miles from Newfoundland, Canada. He attended high school and medical school in Paris. Afterwards, he undertook his training in orthopaedic surgery with Robert Judet, whose fertile mind stimulated Emile to explore uncharted ground, such as fractures of the pelvis and os calcis.

On one occasion the master surgeon and his prize pupil undertook a posterior approach to an acetabular fracture. When the exposure of the pelvis was completed, the fracture was not visible! As Judet apologized to his senior resident about his premature departure from the operating room to attend a meeting in London, Emile closed the wound, repositioned the patient, and successfully visualized the fracture through an anterior approach. With the limitations of the available radiographic views so starkly illustrated, Letournel was encouraged to undertake his pioneering investigations in the radiology of the pelvis with the application of lead wires to a cadaveric bone. By careful scrutiny of three radiographic views, he was able to identify all of the principle pelvic landmarks and to characterize the standard patterns of acetabular disruption. Once an acetabular fracture was defined according to the region and extent of involvement, novel surgical exposures and techniques of reduction and stabilization inevitably followed. Rigorous documentation of the results of hundreds of cases in which the improved methods were employed amply confirmed the valuable role of meticulous reconstruction of a displaced acetabular fracture. Despite the publication of the classic book by Letournel and Judet, *Fractures of the Acetabulum*, and the pilgrimage of numerous surgeons to Paris to observe the new surgical methods, the complexity of the cases stifled the widespread dissemination of the techniques.

Several years ago, Letournel came to Pittsburgh to help us with a few cases. With his lucid instruction and deft surgical technique, precise anatomical reconstructions of diverse patterns of complex acetabular fractures were reproducibly achieved. Moreover, Letournel readily acknowledged the shortcomings of his methods and defined the technical hurdles that remained to be overcome. Under his impetus we were encouraged to extend our investigations on the biomechanics and reconstruction of the pelvis to the acetabulum. Periodically the informative discussions with Emile have continued at meetings, and more productively, on Alpine ski slopes and tennis courts.

In the preparation of this volume, three other students of Emile—Joel Matta, Claude Martimbeau, and Jeff Mast—have provided able assistance. As a token of gratitude for his pioneering spirit and skillful guidance, we have prepared this book in the hope that other surgeons will be enticed to meticulously reassemble the pelvis and to devise superior methods of treatment for the future.

# PELVIC AND ACETABULAR FRACTURES

# CHAPTER 1

# Introduction

Fractures of the pelvis constitute a diverse group of skeletal injuries that often result from major traumatic impact. Motor vehicular accidents, industrial trauma and falls from heights are the most important sources of these injuries. Pelvic disruptions can be classified as fractures of individual bones with minimal displacement, acetabular fractures, and pelvic ring fractures.

Fractures of individual bones in the pelvic ring without a break in the continuity of the ring account for approximately one-third of all pelvic fractures, and are subdivided into avulsion fractures (e.g. ischial tuberosity, iliac spine), fractures of a single pubic ramus, and isolated minimally displaced fractures of the iliac wing, sacrum or coccyx. Most of these injuries heal uneventfully when nonoperative therapeutic methods such as bed rest are applied. These minor fractures of individual pelvic bones are mentioned for completeness, but will not be discussed further.

Many authors choose to include single breaks in the pelvic ring as a second category of pelvic fracture. These fractures generally are documented in close proximity to either the symphysis pubis or the sacroiliac joint. In fact, isolated breaks in the pelvic ring probably do not occur. If the pelvis of such a patient is studied by the use of a technetium diphosphonate bone scan performed about three weeks after the time of the injury, a second area of increased uptake in the scan is visualized, which confirms the presence of a second minimally displaced fracture of the pelvic ring.[1] Nevertheless, such injuries heal predictably with minimal morbidity when a course of bed rest and subsequent limitation of activity is followed for three to six weeks. Serial radiographic assessment is performed, however, to ensure that such a presumed second fracture in the pelvic ring does not undergo late progressive displacement.

Disruption of the pelvic ring requires at least two sites of injury, typically at a sacroiliac joint or at the adjacent ilium or sacrum, and at the symphysis pubis or at the adjacent rami. With the immense amount of force needed to provoke disruption of the pelvic ring, it is not surprising that a patient who sustains such an insult frequently presents with other serious or life-threatening injuries. Most often the musculoskeletal (85%) and respiratory (60%) systems are involved. These associated injuries are followed in frequency by disruption of the central nervous system (40%), gastrointestinal system (30%), urogenital system (12%), and cardiovascular system (6%).[2] The management of a pelvic ring fracture, therefore, requires concomitant treatment of the musculoskeletal and other systemic injuries.

Historically, the management of a patient with a pelvic ring fracture has focused upon the emergency care of the associated injuries, with primary neglect of the osseous disruption. Usually, the immobilization of the pelvic fracture was accomplished by the application of bed rest, a pelvic sling, skeletal traction, or a hip spica cast. The pelvic sling was extremely uncomfortable, and frequently painful for the patient. Apart from its application to certain patients who had sustained anteroposterior compression "open book" injuries, it rarely provided an accurate reduction. Often its use was associated with the complications of prolonged enforced recumbency, including urinary retention, urinary tract infections, pulmonary emboli and infections, decubitus ulcers, and actual sloughing of soft tissues under the sling itself.[3,4]

Historically, the bilateral hip spica cast was described by Watson-Jones.[5] It possessed a limited application for use in a patient who sustained an "open book" type of anteroposterior compression fracture. This technique, with and without ancillary external fixation, was employed by Tile and Pennal.[6] While this method remains in widespread use for the management of a child with a pelvic ring fracture, the principal liabilities associated with the use of the hip spica for an adult include the previously mentioned complications associated with absolute recumbency and difficulties encountered with attempts to improve the initial reduction of the fracture. Skeletal traction (Figure 1-1) has also been described as a mode of treatment for a pelvic ring fracture, especially for a vertical shear injury associated with a substantial superior migration of a hemipelvis. Frequently, the reduction achieved by the use of skeletal traction has been unsatisfactory, with a predilection for a symptomatic pelvic malunion or nonunion.[7,8] Likewise, skeletal traction has been associated with the pulmonary, gastrointestinal and urologic complications of prolonged recumbency. Thus, historically, it was not surprising that the mortalities for patients who underwent treatment for a closed pelvic ring fracture ranged from 10% to 40%.[9,10] With the limitations associated with the earlier methods of pelvic stabilization, most traumatologists attempted to minimize definitive immobilization by reacting to problems that arose during or after a period of enforced recumbency rather than anticipating the need for surgical intervention by the presence of crucial radiological and supplementary clinical findings. This reactionary format has characterized the whole management protocol for pelvic trauma including the investigative procedures. In the past decade, McMurtry,[2] Tile,[6] and Letournel and Judet[11] have emphasized the need for a thorough diagnostic scrutiny in virtually all pelvic and acetabular fracture patients so that the associated injuries and the detailed nature of the pelvic osseous disruption are accurately documented. Algorithms for the resuscitative protocol and for restoration of adequate pelvic stability have been devised that employ the observations gleaned from the diagnostic procedures.

There is a widespread erroneous opinion among traumatologists that most pelvic fracture victims who survive their injuries sustain few major late problems. These surgeons contend that the principal role of the management protocol is referable to survival. Recently, Tile[12] has reviewed the retrospective results of treatment for several series of pelvic fracture patients in various European and North American trauma centers, as well as the outcome of a prospective series in 100 consecutive cases managed at his unit in Toronto. While several of the series did not report the incidence of late sequelae, those that did acknowledged a substantial likelihood for late problems. Huittinen and Slatis[13] reported the largest series to that date, 407 consecutive cases of which 65 patients sustained a double vertical unstable pelvic fracture. Of those 65 patients, 21 (32%) had significant gait abnormalities and 11 (17%) had pelvic pain, generally at one or both sites of posterior disruption. Holdsworth[14] reported 50 pelvic fractures managed by a pelvic sling or traction. Of the 27 patients with a sacroiliac dislocation, 12 were able to do heavy work and 15 were precluded from work by severe sacroiliac pain. Of the 15 additional patients with a posterior fracture, 13 were able to undertake a laboring job while two were wholly disabled by their pelvic pain. In the retrospective and prospective series reported by Tile,[12] 37 of 148 (25%) and 35 of 100 (35%) of the patients in the two series had unsatisfactory results. The principal problem was persistent pelvic pain, although other complications included an apparent leg length discrepancy of greater than 2cm, nonunion, permanent nerve damage and urethral symptoms. Both the mortality and morbidity correlated with energy dissipation at the time of injury. The unstable pelvic fractures had the highest incidence of mortality and other problems including pelvic deformity, nonunion, and permanent nerve or genitourinary damage. The patients who had a proper reduction and stabilization of the pelvic ring had much better results than those in whom the pelvis was left unreduced.

For about twenty years, sporadic attempts have been made to employ external fixation for immobilization of a pelvic ring fracture. Initially, as Tile has reported,[15] Pennal employed a Roger-Anderson apparatus supplemented by a double hip spica cast. The external fixation device facilitated a more accurate closed reduction of the fracture, although the associated application of the large cast compromised the assets associated with the use solely of rigid external fixation including mobility of the patient and access to his lower abdomen and thighs.

In 1973, Carabalona et al[16] and Connes[17] reported their first experience with external pelvic fixation. These authors used various types of frame configurations attached to the anterior iliac crests by a series of pins. Either a single transverse connecting bar or double bars mounted as a quadrilateral frame (Figure 1-2) were employed. By adjustment of the threaded connecting bars, the two ilia could be compressed together. When compression was applied, it was imposed primarily upon the anterior part of the pelvic ring. Despite the difficulties encountered with the external pelvic frames, these authors stimulated widespread interest in the development of satisfactory methods to stabilize pelvic fractures.

During the past decade, Gunterberg et al[18] and Slatis and his colleagues[19] have popularized the use of a simple trapezoidal external frame configuration (Figure 1-3). The external frame was attached to the iliac crests by three 4mm half pins. Laboratory tests suggested that mounting the compression frame as a trapezoid at a 70° inclination to the long axis of the body permitted the application of compression across the posterior disruption. Subsequent testing of the frame's stability in biomechanical loading experiments suggested that the load tolerance of the frame was closely related to the type of pelvic injury. For the stabilization of a patient with an anterior and a posterior vertical disruption by the application of a trapezoidal frame, Slatis recommended deferral of weight bearing for three weeks after the injury. For a double posterior vertical fracture with an accompanying anterior disruption, marked instability of the external fixation necessitated enforced recumbency of the patient for four to six weeks.

In a small series of patients who had sustained a pelvic ring fracture, J. Muller[20] and K. Muller[21] reported successful application of an anterior compression frame erected from the Wagner device or the AO tubular system. In a somewhat similar way, Grosse[7] applied a trapezoidal frame to a series of patients who had sustained a central acetabular fracture. While additional case reports of the successful management of pelvic ring fractures by the use of external fixation appeared in the literature,[22] increasingly the inability to attain or maintain a satisfactory pelvic reduction with a simple two-dimensional pelvic frame was acknowledged.[23] Biomechanical studies on a cadaveric pelvic fracture model were undertaken by Brown, Rubash, Mears et al[24,25] to define the parameters for an external frame that could provide effective stability for most unstable pelvic fractures. Ultimately, a triangular frame configuration was devised that fulfilled the biomechanical criteria.

Recently, internal fixation applied to various types of displaced pelvic ring fractures has been reported by Judet and Letournel,[26] Tile,[12] and Mears et al.[27,28] Internal fixation provides an opportunity for accurate open realignment of the pelvic ring, rigid stabilization, and osseous union. In the past, for the reduction and immobilization of an "open book" type of fracture, many workers employed 18-gauge wires, which were inserted around the rami or through the obturator foramina to provide compression at the symphysis pubis (Figure 1-4).[29] Frequently, prior to healing of the fracture, the wires would break or erode through the rami. Other workers applied a single plate and screws to compress a diastasis of the symphysis pubis.[30] A high incidence of premature loss of fixation was observed. As primary methods of management, however, these techniques were widely discouraged. They were associated with difficulties in surgical exposure, major intraoperative hemorrhage, inability to achieve adequate fixation, and pelvic infection (Figure 1-5).

Theoretically, however, open reduction and internal fixation do possess several major advantages. With operative exposure, an accurate reduction may be obtained, whereas with the use of a closed reduction

Figure 1-1A,B. Anteroposterior and inlet radiographs of the pelvis following the application of skeletal traction anchored with threaded bolts. Marked malalignment with superior migration of the right hemipelvis and instability of both sacroiliac joints is evident.

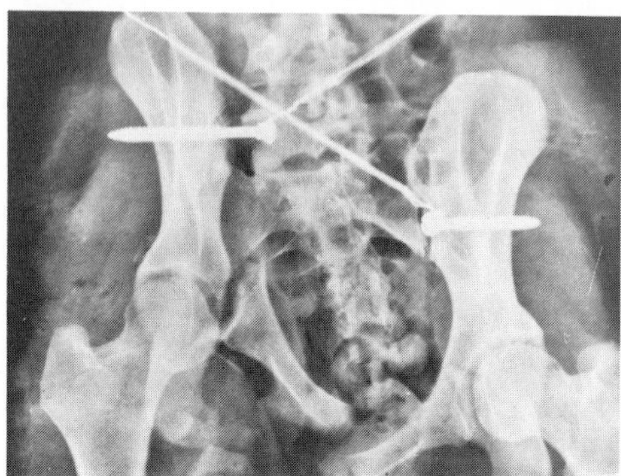

Figure 1-1A.

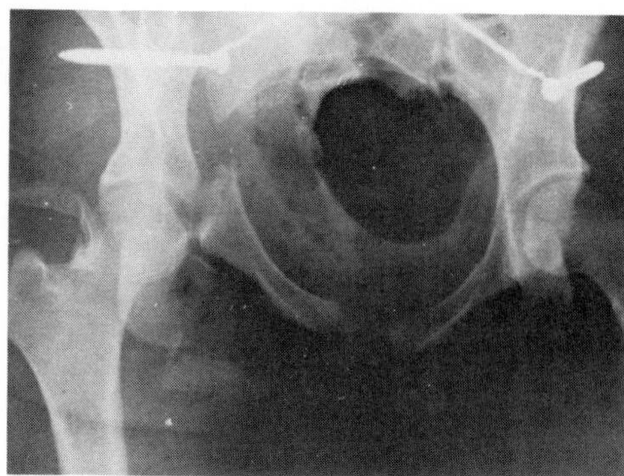

Figure 1-1B.

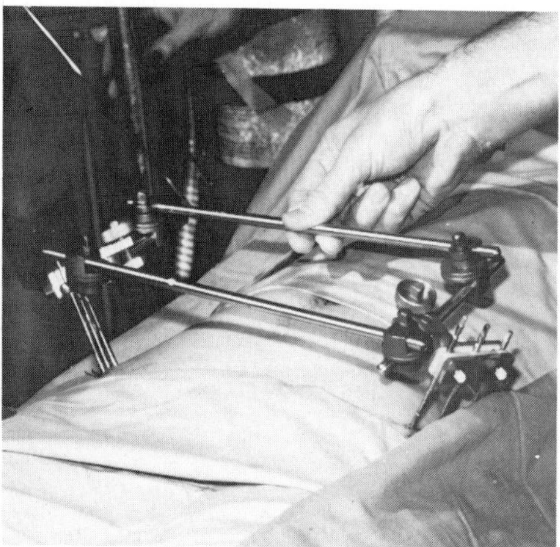

Figure 1-2. A quadrilateral frame.

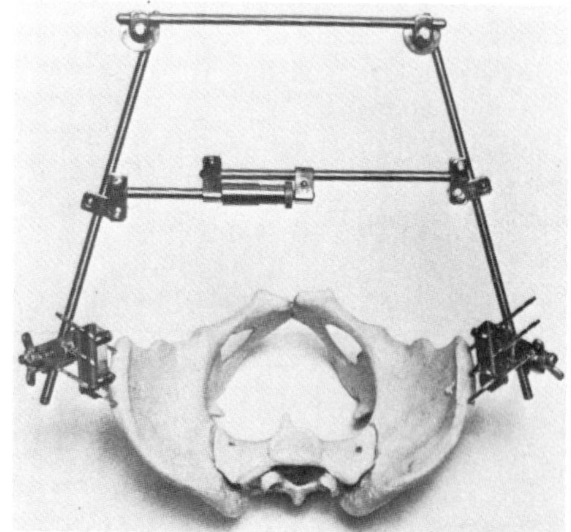

Figure 1-3. The Slatis frame.

Figure 1-4A,B. Anteroposterior radiographs present bilateral sacroiliac subluxations and a diastasis taken before and after fixation with wire. In the latter view taken two months after injury, the wire has failed prematurely.

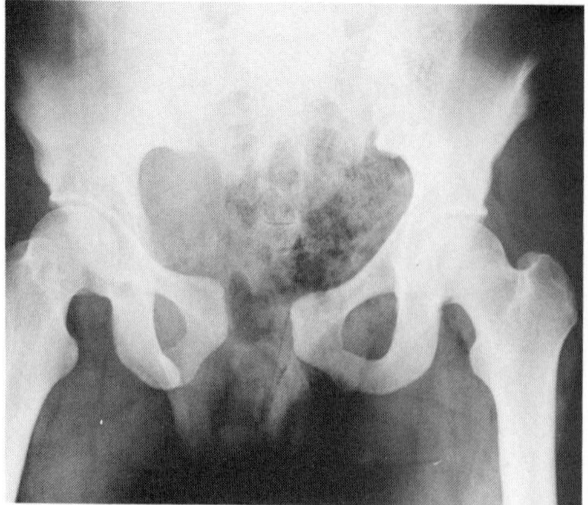

Figure 1-4A.

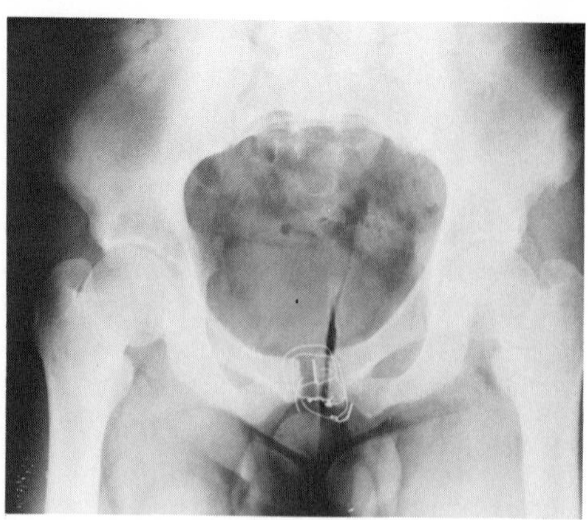

Figure 1-4B.

Figure 1-5. Anteroposterior pelvic radiographs illustrate bilateral sacroiliac dislocations and a diastasis initially managed with screws and wire fixation of the symphysis. Figure 1-5A was taken six months afterwards when the fixation had failed with a massive wound infection, exposure of the bladder and marked instability of both hemipelves. In Figure 1-5B, the pelvis has been reduced and stabilized with external fixation.

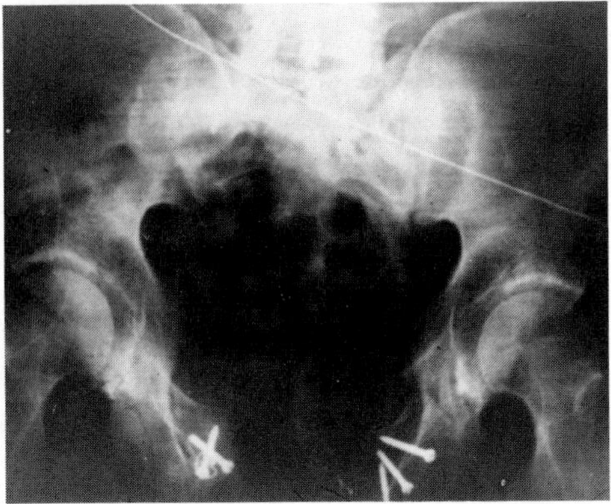

Figure 1-5A.

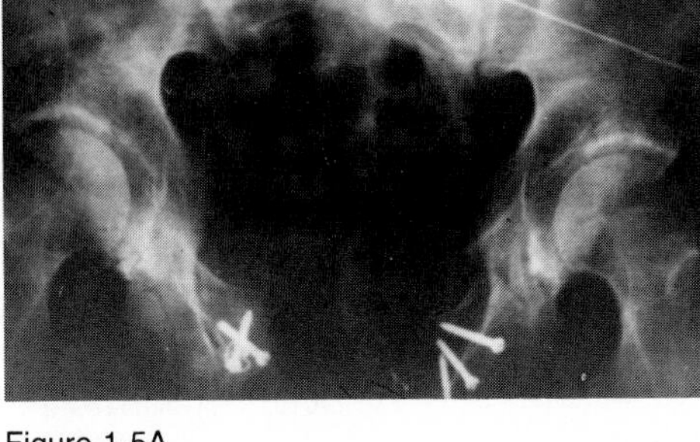

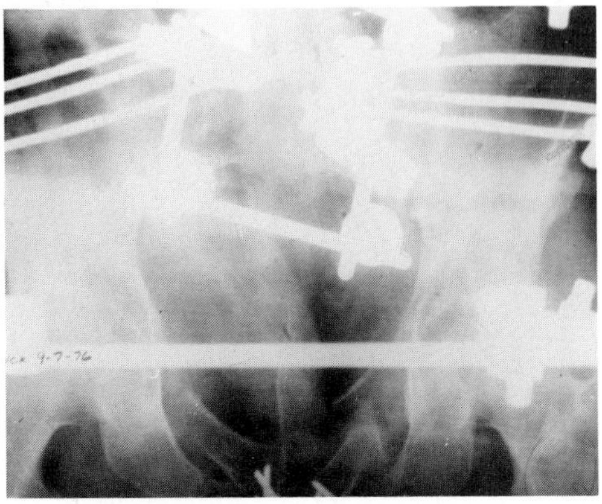

Figure 1-5B.

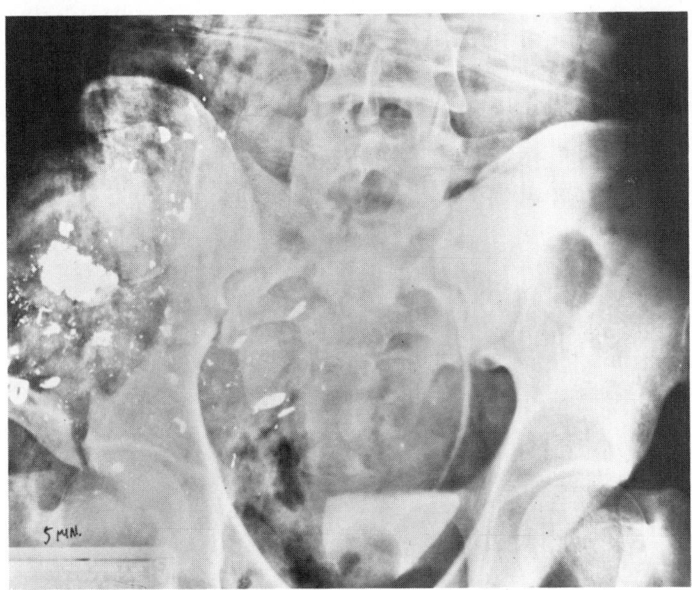


Figure 1-6. A radiograph of a shotgun blast with a pelvic fracture and a massive open wound.

and external pelvic fixation, a moderate to marked residual displacement of the fracture may ensue. This displacement provides a predisposition for a late pelvic nonunion or malunion possibly with an apparent limb length discrepancy, posttraumatic sacroiliac arthritis, and symptoms related to a malaligned bony prominence. Internal fixation provides a greater degree of mechanical rigidity to ensure maintenance of an accurate open reduction. The improved stability encourages the formation of a stable osseous union rather than a potentially unstable and painful fibrous union. The protocol for nursing care and wound toilet are greatly simplified. In addition, internal fixation is essential for the stabilization of a pelvic nonunion or major malunion. In such cases excision of the fibrous union, or osteotomy of the malaligned pelvic ring, is followed by the application of specialized techniques of internal fixation.

The open pelvic fracture has formed a unique subgroup. Open pelvic fracture was associated with a mortality of greater than 50% and significant morbidity.[31] Such an injury possesses a direct communication between the fracture site and a vaginal, rectal, perineal or a cutaneous laceration. The fracture may acquire bacterial contamination from the gastrointestinal or genitourinary tract or from the exterior. Pedestrian and motorcycle accidents account for the majority of the open pelvic fractures. Infrequently, the open injuries complicate blunt pelvic injuries, shotgun blasts (Figure 1-6) and penetrating abdominal or pelvic trauma. The disparity between the mortality for open pelvic fractures and for similar closed fractures is due to a higher incidence of profuse hemorrhage, sepsis, renal failure and complications related to the fracture management. With these problems in mind, a treatment protocol for the patient who sustains an open pelvic fracture was needed that would focus particular attention on the control of massive hemorrhage and the prevention of infection at the fracture site.[32]

Since Callisen[33] first described a central acetabular fracture in 1788, the optimal form of management of this intraarticular disruption has remained controversial. Admittedly, there is a consensus that a minimally displaced acetabular fracture without dislocation of the femoral head has an excellent prognosis when it is managed nonoperatively by bed rest or by a short period of traction followed by a variable period of a partial weightbearing gait.[34,35] To attain reproducibly good results in the management of most intraarticular fractures, it is generally agreed that perfect restoration of the alignment of the articular surfaces is highly desirable, if not essential. While this principle is rigorously accepted for most intraarticular fractures, it remains controversial in the case of the displaced acetabular fracture. At first glance this exception is nonsensical. A review of the proponents of the nonoperative and the operative schools, however, provides an explanation for this controversy.

## Conservative Treatment of Acetabular Fractures

It is solely of historical interest that some workers[36] espoused hip spica cast immobilization for variable periods in the range of several weeks as a suitable form of management.[37] Without provision for accurate reduction of a displaced acetabular fracture or for early posttraumatic restoration of joint mobility, cast immobilization is recognized as a wholly unsuitable technique.

Cutaneous or skeletal traction[38,39] remains widely employed to the present time.[34,35,40] Multiple traction pins can be inserted into the greater trochanter and the distal femur or the proximal tibia. In this way, the principal vector of the distraction can be directed to correct proximal and medial displacement of the femoral head and acetabulum respectively. Early active motion exercises of the hip joint can be undertaken and continued for the variable period of distraction, frequently for nine to twelve weeks. Many authors suggested that under the influence both of skeletal traction applied to the femur and of the presumably intact capsule of the hip joint, the acetabular fragments are realigned reproducibly in an anatomical configuration. This concept of "ligamentotaxis" as defined by Vidal[41] may apply to minimally displaced and minimally comminuted fractures. For the more comminuted and displaced acetabular insults, however, skeletal traction permits only moderate realignment of the femoral head but not accurate reapproximation of the comminuted acetabular fragments. Frequently, many of the comminuted fragments, especially in the dome region, undergo marked rotational displacement. A critical assessment of follow-up radiographs indicates that the acetabular fragments tend to unite in their malaligned configuration with the formation of a fibrous or fibrocartilaginous lining. Subsequently, when full weight bearing ultimately is restored, this pseudarticular fibrocartilaginous surface generally undergoes rapid deterioration (Figure 1-7).[11]

Some authors[36] have acknowledged that while significant displacement of the superior or weightbearing portion of the acetabulum fails to respond satisfactorily to skeletal traction, comparable displacement of the residual portions of the acetabulum is favorably influenced by this technique. While successful results following skeletal traction applied to uncomminuted fractures of the medial wall with modest displacement have been documented, more recent reports have indicated a substantial incidence of failure with late traumatic arthritis when many other fracture patterns with residual acetabular displacement are uncorrected.[36,42]

Upon a careful study of the paper by Rowe and Lowell,[36] the results of operative versus nonoperative treatment by the use of skeletal traction were observed to correlate with the displacement of the femoral head and the

Figure 1-7. An anteroposterior pelvic radiograph (A) taken one year after a posterior column fracture was managed with skeletal traction. The residual subluxation of the femoral head and displacement of the ischial fragment is evident. This painful hip required a total hip joint replacement. Pelvic radiographs (B-E) present a "T" fracture managed by skeletal traction.

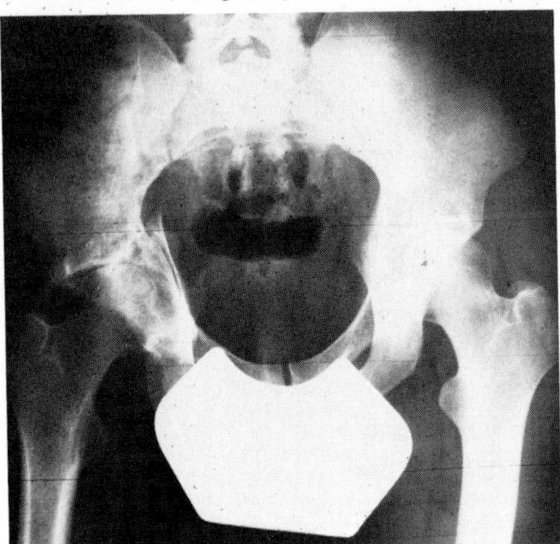

Figure 1-7A.

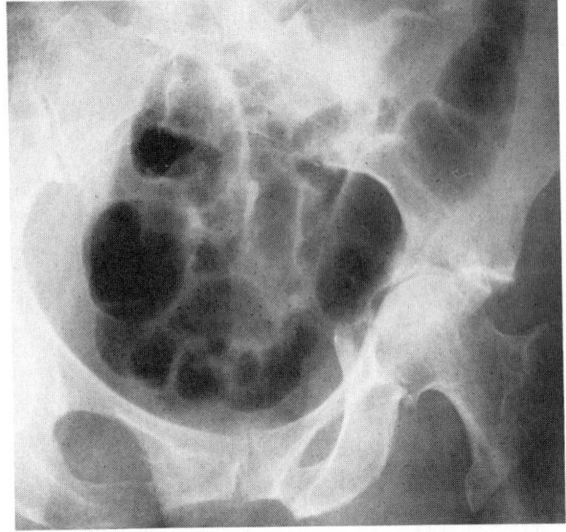

Figure 1-7B. Initial anteroposterior view.

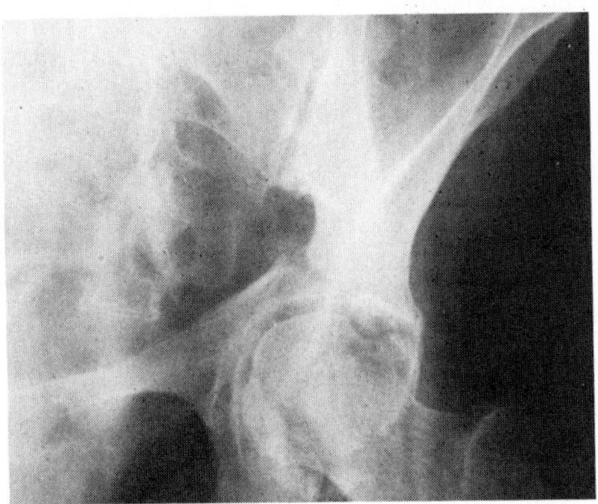

Figure 1-7C. Obturator oblique view taken after the application of skeletal traction.

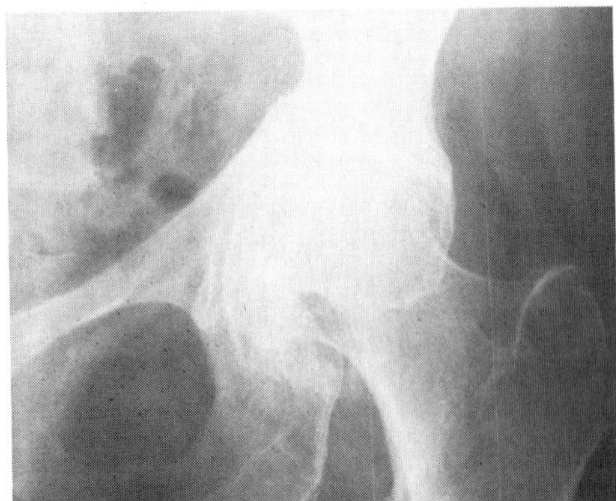

Figure 1-7D. Eight months later, posttraumatic arthritis ensues, with persistent posterior displacement of the posterior column fragment and femoral head.

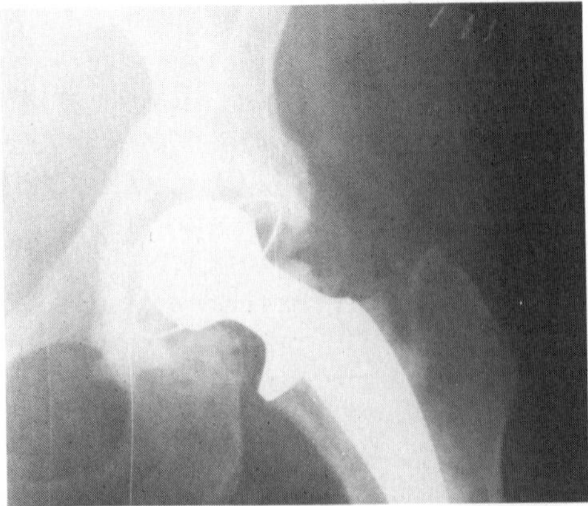

Figure 1-7E. After total hip joint replacement.

acetabular fragments. Favorable results were documented for linear, simple fracture patterns with minimal displacement. The fractures associated with a posterior dislocation and instability of the hip had poor results after closed reduction and a greater number of satisfactory results after open reduction and internal fixation. In the cases with involvement of the superior weightbearing dome, an anatomical reduction of the dome culminated in greater than 80% satisfactory results; in the cases where the dome was not reduced all of them had poor results. In the presence of a fracture of the medial wall, if congruity was achieved by resort to a closed reduction and was maintained by skeletal traction, satisfactory results were achieved in 90% of the cases.

Recently, other workers observed that acetabular malalignment secondary to a "step-off" of greater than 2-3mm, a loss of sphericity, or segmental impaction in any portion of the acetabulum all contributed heavily to the onset of late traumatic arthritis.[11,43] Two other patterns of acetabular fracture were widely recognized for their failure to respond to nonoperative management. In the presence of a loose osteochondral fragment interposed between the traumatized acetabulum and the femoral head, rapid onset and progression of traumatic arthritis can be anticipated.[44] Also, in the presence of a displaced acetabular fracture with a concomitant displaced pelvic ring fracture, nonunion and/or malunion of both the acetabular and pelvic ring disruptions is likely to follow (Figure 1-8).[45]

## Surgical Treatment of Acetabular Fractures

In 1912, Vaughn[39] provided the first American report of a central acetabular fracture managed by open reduction. In 1943, Levine[46] heralded the use of open reduction and internal fixation for the treatment of a central acetabular fracture. In 1948, Armstrong[47] suggested that certain markedly displaced and comminuted central acetabular fractures possessed such a high rate of anticipated failure after resort to the available methods of treatment that primary arthrodesis was advised. In 1954, Westerborn[48] documented such equally unsatisfactory results following the use of conservative therapy for the reconstruction of a central acetabular fracture/dislocation that he recommended a primary cup arthroplasty. In the ensuing years several authors, such as Pennal,[42] reported the use of open reduction and internal fixation. Levine,[46] Urist,[49] Elliott,[50] and Judet and Letournel[51] recorded the use of various modes of fixation including screws, plates, and Hagie pins. While isolated cases of successful surgical intervention were reported, there was a general dissatisfaction with operative management. As Letournel acknowledged in 1961,[52] given the available radiological views of the pelvis, surgeons could not identify the disrupted segment of the acetabulum. Even when the fracture was visualized, with the then available techniques of reduction and stabilization, failures to achieve and maintain a satisfactory congruent reduction were exceedingly common (Figure 1-9). This environment provided the stimulus to initiate basic studies on acetabular disruption. Okelberry[53] and Knight and Smith[54] described the mechanisms of acetabular disruption and provided a practical classification of central acetabular fractures. These workers studied anteroposterior radiographs of acetabular fractures and attempted to correlate specific fracture lines with the radiological findings.

Meanwhile, Judet and Letournel[11,51] initiated their pioneering efforts on the pelvis. For his dissertation,[52] Letournel applied lead wires to a cadaveric pelvis and undertook various radiological views to characterize the specific anatomical features of the pelvis. To supplement the conventional anteroposterior view, the French school introduced two novel oblique radiological views to facilitate identification of the anatomical origins of displaced fracture fragments. These workers extended their acetabular studies with an assessment of various surgical approaches. With the application of a posterior and/or anterior exposure they were able to visualize virtually all types of fracture patterns. They devised special bone holding forceps and curved bone plates that greatly facilitated the reduction and immobilization of acetabular fragments. As a culmination of their extraordinarily productive research on the acetabulum, by 1964 Judet and Letournel[51] recommended open reduction and internal fixation for all displaced acetabular disruptions. In 1981, these authors reported 568 cases of acetabular fractures that were managed by open reduction.[11] In their follow-up of two to 21 years, 74% of the cases showed very good results with a normal hip, 6% of the results were good, and 5% were fair. In this series a perfect initial postoperative radiographic reduction was consistent with an 85% very good result and a 7.6% good clinical result. Thus, late follow-up of acetabular disruptions treated by open reduction and internal fixation supported the contention that a satisfactory outcome can be anticipated if the initial fracture reduction is perfect. The converse, however, is also true. If the initial postoperative reduction is imperfect, symptomatic traumatic arthritis can be anticipated.[11,43]

Figure 1-8A,B. Anteroposterior and inlet views of a young woman taken one year after sacral and ipsilateral acetabular fractures were managed with skeletal traction. Minor external rotation of the ilial and ischial fragments accompanies the protrusio and the displaced posterior wall fragment.

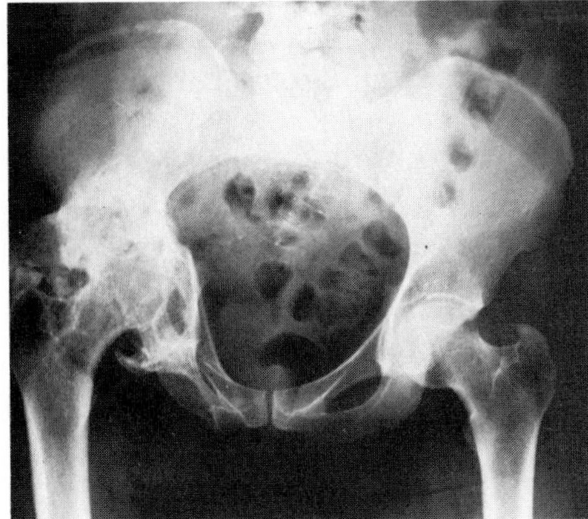

Figure 1-8A.

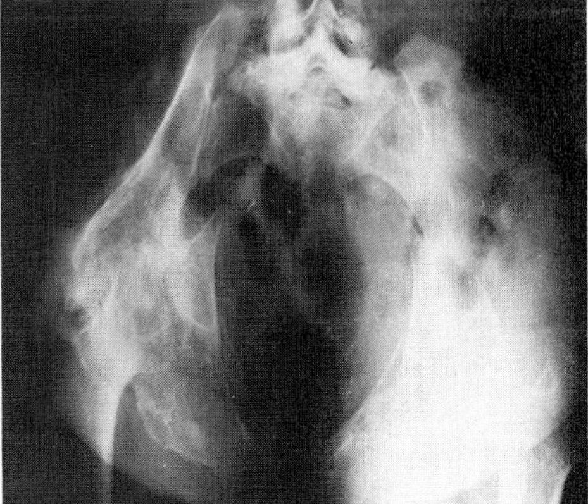

Figure 1-8B.

Figure 1-9A,B. Anteroposterior radiographs illustrate a posterior wall and posterior column fracture taken before and one year after open reduction and fixation with two screws. In Figure 1-9B, loss of fixation and the acetabular reduction with displacement of the femoral head is evident.

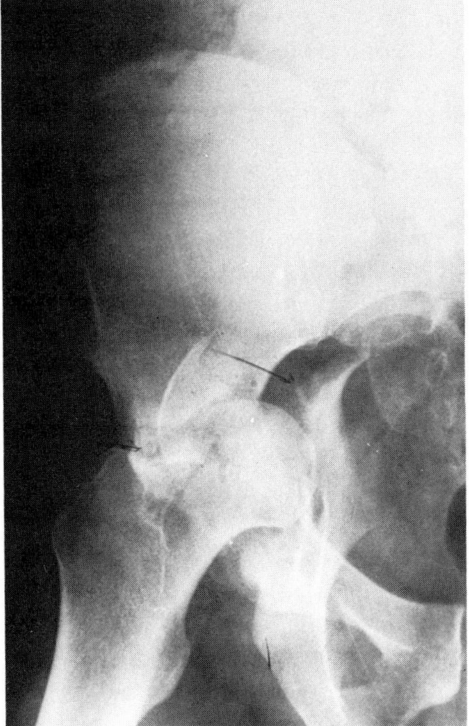

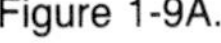

Figure 1-9A.

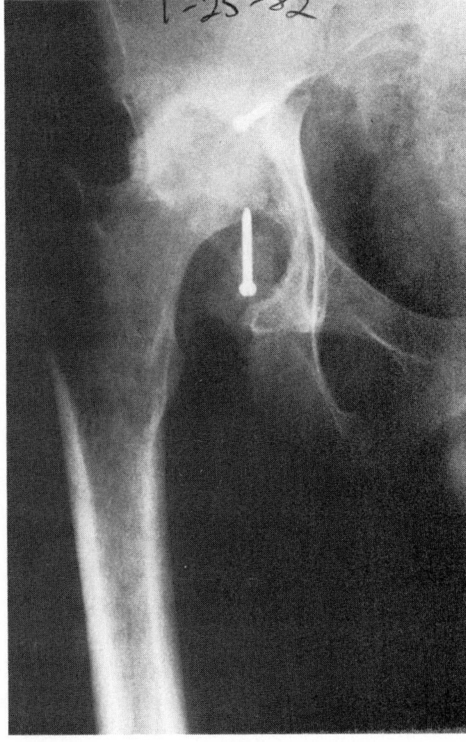

Figure 1-9B.

In the past decade Pennal,[38] Tile,[55] and other workers confirmed certain of the observations documented by Judet and Letournel.[11] They acknowledged that a successful open reduction and stabilization of a displaced acetabular fracture generally culminated in a very good late result. Many of these workers were troubled by the complexities of the exposure, reduction and stabilization of the various comminuted acetabular fractures or even of the transverse fracture patterns. These surgeons cautiously recommended open reduction for a limited variety of simple acetabular fractures. For the more complex variants with the anticipated technical complexities, they recommended consideration for skeletal traction.

By 1980, most surgeons in the United States agreed that the prognosis for a particular acetabular disruption correlated with: **1)** the nature of the injury, especially the magnitude of displacement and comminution and the involvement of the weightbearing dome and the femoral head; **2)** aspects of the closed or open management including the accuracy of the reduction and the method of stabilization; and **3)** the presence of postoperative complications such as avascular necrosis of the femoral head, heterotopic ossification, a wound infection, or a sciatic nerve palsy.

This knowledge provided a dilemma for the rational management of a displaced acetabular fracture. Nonoperative methods were advised for minimally displaced fractures or for complex comminuted and displaced injuries. Operative treatment was advised only for relatively simple but displaced fractures that failed to undergo an adequate reduction under the influence of skeletal traction. The crux of the optional form of management rested upon a preoperative assessment of the technical feasibility of a surgical procedure. Several surgeons studied simpler methods to expose, reduce and stabilize these complex acetabular reduction. Ruedi,[56] Letournel,[57] Senegas,[58] and Mears and Rubash[59] devised extensile surgical exposures. Superior reduction forceps and the availability of more malleable plates further simplified the surgical procedure. On this basis, Mears and Rubash[59] reaffirmed the observation of Letournel et al[11] that operative methods were preferred for application to virtually all displaced acetabular fractures.

Before acetabular and pelvic reconstruction would achieve widespread application with the provision for reproducible clinical results, several aspects of knowledge about the pelvis would require organization and dissemination: a detailed radiological characterization of acetabular disruptions; the surgical anatomy and principles of surgical approach; the techniques of open reduction; and the biomechanics of internal and external fixation. The rationale for the preparation of this manuscript arose from these considerations.

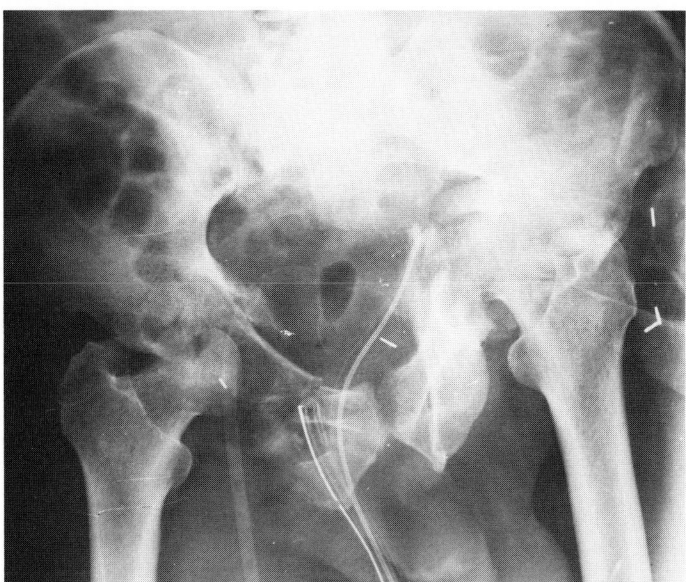

Figure 1-10. An anteroposterior pelvic radiograph taken six months after an associated "T" fracture with an ipsilateral sacroiliac dislocation was managed with nonoperative methods. By this time a formidable procedure is needed to reconstruct the left hip.

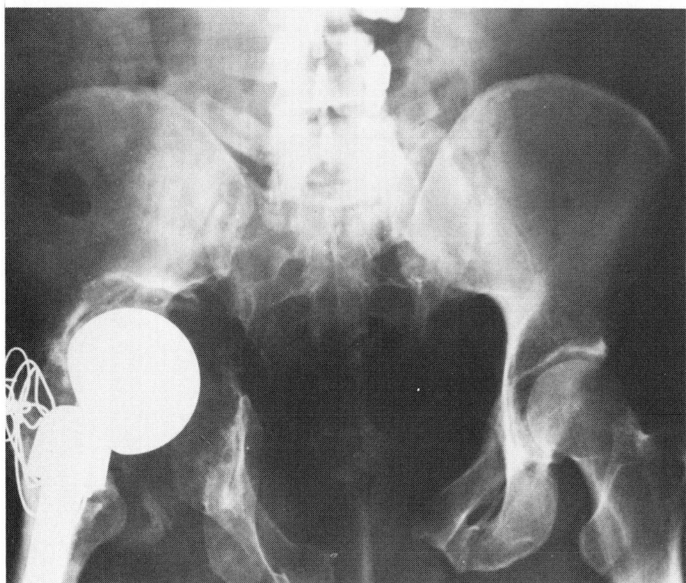

Figure 1-11. An unsuccessful attempt to reconstruct a pelvic nonunion/malunion with a failed hip joint following a "T" fracture, a diastasis of the symphysis, and an unstable ipsilateral sacroiliac joint managed by the use of a bipolar prosthesis. The foremost objective, to reconstruct the pelvic ring with open reduction and stable internal fixation, was not recognized by the surgical team.

In the presence of marked pelvic and acetabular malalignment that is uncorrected by the application of closed or open methods of treatment, a formidable reconstructive problem ensues. Subsequently, when a patient presents with a painful pelvic or acetabular nonunion or malunion, or traumatic arthritis of the hip, a late surgical solution is immeasurably more difficult to undertake than an appropriate reconstruction procedure undertaken within a few days after the time of injury (Figure 1-10). While pelvic nonunions were previously perceived as excessively uncommon, Pennal and Messiah documented 42 symptomatic patients from Southern Ontario. The principal complaint was pelvic pain, although a limp, instability, and clinical deformity were associated features. Letournel,[11,60] Tile,[12] and Mears and Rubash[61] have confirmed the more widespread presence of symptomatic pelvic nonunions and malunions and attempted to develop reconstructive surgical solutions. All of these surgeons agree that the principal solution to this problem is prevention. For the acute pelvic and acetabular fracture with marked displacement and instability, appropriate radiographic documentation and surgical management is essential. If a patient does present with pelvic pain or other late symptoms, then rigorous radiological evaluation is needed to identify the origin of the problem. The surgical management of a pelvic and acetabular nonunion or malunion remains in its infancy (Figure 1-11). Apart from anecdotal reports no systematic evaluation of a management protocol has been undertaken. Undoubtedly this problem will receive much greater scrutiny by future investigators.

## References

1. Gertzbein SD, Chenoweth DR: Occult injuries of the pelvic ring. Clin Orthop 128:202, 1977.
2. McMurtry R, Walton D, Dickinson D, Kellam J, Tile M: Pelvic disruption in the polytraumatized patient: A management protocol. Clin Orthop 151:22, 1980.
3. Dunn W, Morris HO: Fractures and dislocations of the pelvis. J Bone Joint Surg 50A:1634, 1968.
4. Noland L, Conwell HE: Acute fractures of the pelvis. JAMA 94:174, 1930.
5. Watson-Jones R: Dislocations and fracture/dislocations of the pelvis. Brit J Surg 25:773-781, 1938.
6. Tile M, Pennal G: Pelvic disruption: Principles of management. Clin Orthop 151:56, 1980.
7. Grosse A: Stabilization of pelvic fractures with Hoffmann external fixation: The French experience, in: External Fixation: The Current State of the Art. Baltimore, Williams and Wilkins, 1979, p 10.
8. Hundley JM: Ununited unstable fractures of the pelvis. J Bone Joint Surg 48A:1025, 1966.
9. Conolly WB, Hedberg EA: Observations on fractures of the pelvis. J Trauma 9:104, 1969.
10. Kane WJ: Fractures of the pelvis, in Rockwood CA Jr, Green DP (eds): Fractures in Adults. Philadelphia, Lippincott, 1984, vol 2, p 1093.

11. Letournel E, Judet R: Fractures of the Acetabulum. New York, Springer Verlag, 1981, p 13.
12. Tile M: Fractures of the Pelvis and Acetabulum. Baltimore, Williams and Wilkins, 1984, p 56.
13. Huittinen VM, Slatis P: Fractures of the pelvis, trauma mechanism, types of injury and principles of treatment. Acta Chir Scand 138:563, 1972.
14. Holdsworth FW: Dislocation and fracture dislocation of the pelvis. J Bone Joint Surg 30B:461, 1948.
15. Tile M: Fractures of the acetabulum. Orthop Clin North Am 11:3:481, 1980.
16. Carabalona P, Rabichong P, Bonnel F, Perruchon E, Pugurat F: Apports-du fixateur externe dans les dislocations du pubis et de l'articulation sacro-iliaque. Montpell Chir 19:61, 1973.
17. Connes H: Hoffmann's Double Frame External Anchorage. Paris, GEAD, 1973, p 97.
18. Gunterberg B, Goldie I, Slatis P: Fixation of pelvic fractures and dislocations: An experimental study on the loading of pelvic fractures and sacroiliac dislocations after external compression fixation. Acta Orthop Scand 49:278, 1978.
19. Slatis P, Karaharju E: External fixation of unstable pelvic fractures: Experience in 22 patients treated with a trapezoid compression frame. Clin Orthop 151:73, 1980.
20. Muller J, Bachmann B, Berg H: Malgaigne fracture of the pelvis: Treatment with percutaneous pin fixation. J Bone Joint Surg 60A:992, 1978.
21. Muller KH, Muller-Farber J: Die Osteosynthese mit dem Fixateur Externe am Becken. Arch Orthop Traumat Surg 92:273, 1978.
22. Mears DC: Clinical techniques in the pelvis, in: External Skeletal Fixation. Baltimore, Williams and Wilkins, 1983, p 339.
23. Slatis P: External fixation of pelvic fractures, in Johnston RM (ed): Advances in External Fixation. Chicago, Year Book Medical Publishers, 1980, p 77.
24. Brown TD, Stone JP, Schuster JH, Mears DC: External fixation of unstable pelvic ring fractures: Comparative rigidity of some current frame configurations. Med Biol Eng Comput 20:727, 1982.
25. Rubash HE, Brown TD, Nelson DD, Mears DC: Comparative mechanical performance of some new devices for fixation of unstable pelvic ring fractures. Med Biol Eng Comput 21:657, 1983.
26. Judet R, Judet J, Letournel E: Fractures of the acetabulum: Classification and surgical approaches for open reduction. J Bone Joint Surg 45A:1615, 1964.
27. Mears DC, Fu F: External fixation in pelvic fractures. Orthop Clin North Am 11:3:465, 1980.
28. Mears DC, Rubash HE: External and internal fixation of the pelvic ring. AAOS Instructional Course Lectures. St. Louis, Mosby, 1984, vol 33, p 144.
29. Whiston G: Internal fixation for fractures and dislocations of the pelvis. J Bone Joint Surg 45A:701, 1953.
30. Sharp I: Plate fixation of disrupted symphysis pubis. J Bone Joint Surg 55B:618, 1973.
31. Perry JF: Pelvic open fractures. Clin Orthop 151:40, 1980.

32. Rubash H, Steed D, Mears DC: Fractures of the pelvic ring. Surg Rounds 5:8, 16, 1982.
33. Lansinger O: Fractures of the acetabulum: A clinical, radiological and experimental study. Acta Orthop Scand suppl 165, 97, 1977.
34. Carnesale PG, Stewart MJ, Barnes SN: Acetabular disruptions and central fracture-dislocations of the hip. J Bone Joint Surg 57A:1054, 1975.
35. Tipton WW, D'Ambrosia RD, Garrett RP: Nonoperative management of central fracture-dislocations of the hip. J Bone Joint Surg 57A:888, 1975.
36. Rowe CR, Lowell JD: Prognosis of fractures of the acetabulum. J Bone Joint Surg 43A:30, 1961.
37. Peet MM: Fractures of the acetabulum with intrapelvic displacement of the femoral head. Ann Surg 70:296, 1919.
38. Pennal GF, Massiah KA: Nonunion and delayed union of fractures of the pelvis. Clin Orthop 151:124, 1980.
39. Vaughn GT: Central dislocations of the femur. Surg Gynecol Obstet 15:249, 1912.
40. Pearson JR, Hargodon EJ: Fractures of the pelvis involving the floor of the acetabulum. J Bone Joint Surg 44B:550, 1962.
41. Vidal J, Adrey J, Connes H, Buscayret C: A biomechanical study and clinical application of the use of Hoffmann's external fixator, in Brooker AF, Edwards CC (eds) External Fixation: The Current State of the Art. Baltimore, Williams and Wilkins, 1979, p 327.
42. Pennal GF, Davidson J, Garside H, Plewes J: Results of treatment of acetabular fractures. Clin Orthop 151:115, 1980.
43. Matta J: Fractures of the acetabulum: Results of a prospective series. AAOS 50th annual meeting, Anaheim, 1983.
44. Epstein HC: Posterior fracture-dislocations of the hip. J Bone Joint Surg 56A:1103, 1974.
45. Rubash HE, Mears DC: Fractures of the acetabulum. AAOS 50th annual meeting, Anaheim, 1983.
46. Levine MA: A treatment of central fractures of the acetabulum. J Bone Joint Surg 25:902, 1943.
47. Armstrong JR: Traumatic dislocations of the hip joint: Review of one hundred and one dislocations. J Bone Joint Surg 30B:430, 1948.
48. Westerborn A: Central dislocations of the femoral head treated with mold arthroplasty. J Bone Joint Surg 36A:307, 1954.
49. Urist MR: Fractures of the acetabulum. Ann Surg 127:1150, 1948.
50. Elliott RB: Central fractures of the acetabulum. Clin Orthop 7:189, 1956.
51. Judet R, Judet J, Letournel E: Fractures of the acetabulum: Classification and surgical approaches for open reduction. J Bone Joint Surg 46A:1615, 1964.
52. Letournel E: Les fractures du cotyle: Etude d'une serie de 75 cas. Thesis, Paris, 1961, p 11.
53. Okelberry AM: Fractures of the floor of the acetabulum. J Bone Joint Surg 38A:441, 1956.
54. Knight RA, Smith H: Central fractures of the acetabulum. J Bone Joint Surg 40A:1, 1958.

55. Tile M: Pelvic fractures: Operative versus nonoperative treatment. Orthop Clin North Am 11(3): 423, 1980.
56. Ruedi T: Personal communication, 1981.
57. Letournel E: Acetabular fractures: Classification and management. Clin Orthop 151:81, 1980.
58. Senegas J, Yates M: Complex acetabular fractures: A transtrochanteric lateral approach. Clin Orthop 151:107, 1980.
59. Mears DC, Rubash HE: Extensile exposure of the pelvis. Contemp Orthop 6:21, 1983.
60. Letournel E: Nonunions and malunions of the pelvis and acetabulum. First International Symposium on Fractures of the Acetabulum and Pelvis, Paris, 1984.
61. Mears DC, Rubash HE: Surgical management of pelvic and acetabular nonunions and malunions. AAOS 50th annual meeting, Anaheim, 1983.

# CHAPTER 2

# Anatomy of the Pelvis and Acetabulum

## Introduction

Undoubtedly, one of the explanations for the reluctance of trauma surgeons to undertake open reduction and internal fixation of pelvic and acetabular disruptions is the limited exposure of most orthopaedic residents to the relevant anatomy. With their inadequate anatomical knowledge of the pelvis, such surgeons are understandably reluctant to enter a region notable for the presence of numerous large nerves, vessels and viscera situated within a highly irregular bony ring. A detailed descriptive account of the pelvic anatomy is available in numerous standard anatomical references[1-4] and in a recent review by Kane.[5] This chapter focuses upon the surgical or applied anatomy of the pelvis referable to pelvic trauma and reconstruction.

## Superficial Landmarks

Upon inspection of the front of the pelvis and torso, the most prominent features are the symmetrical iliac crests, anterosuperior iliac spines, and the symphysis pubis. In a lean individual the inguinal ligament visibly spans from either anterosuperior iliac spine to the ipsilateral pubic tubercle in a cord-like fashion. If the iliac crest is traced posteriorly, the palpating finger courses from the crest to the posterosuperior iliac spine and continues obliquely in a medial and distal fashion to the tip of the sacrum and coccyx. Anterior or posterior scrutiny of the torso is notable for the lateral prominences of the greater trochanter and abductor musculatures. Large muscles are evident in a symmetrical distribution coursing from the spine to the bony pelvis and from the pelvis to the lower extremity. Upon initial inspection of the patient who has sustained a major disruption of the pelvic ring or an acetabular fracture, a careful scrutiny and palpation of these bony landmarks may indicate an asymmetrical disposition, instability, or other abnormality.

## Bony Pelvis

The pelvic girdle is a ring-like structure comprising two innominate bones, which articulate anteriorly in a direct fashion at the symphysis pubis and posteriorly by an interposed sacrum (Figure 2-1). In turn the sacrum articulates superiorly with the lumbar spine and inferiorly with the coccyx. The pelvic ring is subdivided into an upper or false pelvis, a clinical extension of the abdomen, and an inferior or true pelvis. The dividing line, the pelvic inlet is an oblique plane that passes through the upper symphysis pubis, and the iliopectineal and arcuate lines to the promontory of the sacrum (Figure 2-2). In the erect posture the plane of the pelvic inlet is directed at 55° with respect to a horizontal plane. The true pelvis contains the organs of reproduction, portions of the urinary and digestive systems, and major neurovascular structures coursing to the lower extremities. In an erect posture, weightbearing forces are transmitted from the spinal column through the sacrum and sacroiliac joints, along the thick sections of ilia to the acetabulae and, thereby, to the proximal femora. While this femorosacral arch is crucial for weight transmission in an erect posture in a sitting position, weightbearing forces pass through the sacroiliac joints into the ilia to the ischial tuberosities via the ischiosacral arch. To a lesser degree, weight-bearing forces are transmitted around the anterior portions of the pelvic ring. With the limited mobility of the pelvic articulations at the sacroiliac and sacrococcygeal joints and symphysis pubis, the muscles originating on the pelvis provide locomotion for the lower extremities or postural support for the torso (Figure 2-3). Each innominate bone is derived embryologically from three separate bones, the ilium, ischium, and pubis, which fuse at the acetabulum upon skeletal maturity.

Judet and Letournel[6] have re-examined the innominate bone to characterize the structural support of the

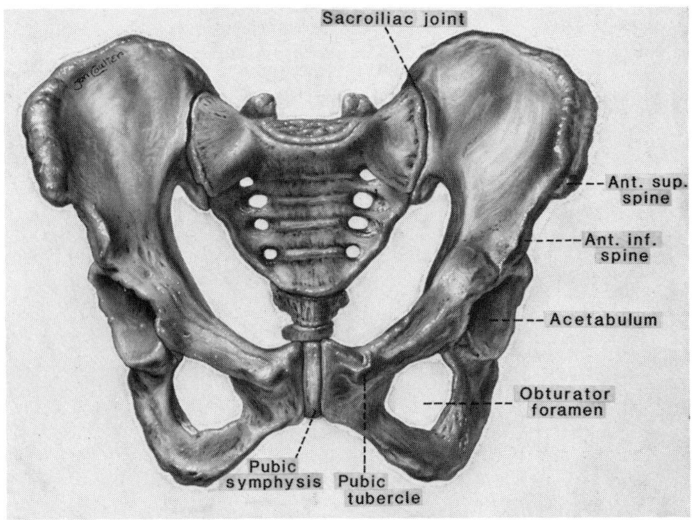


Figure 2-1. Anterior view of the pelvis.

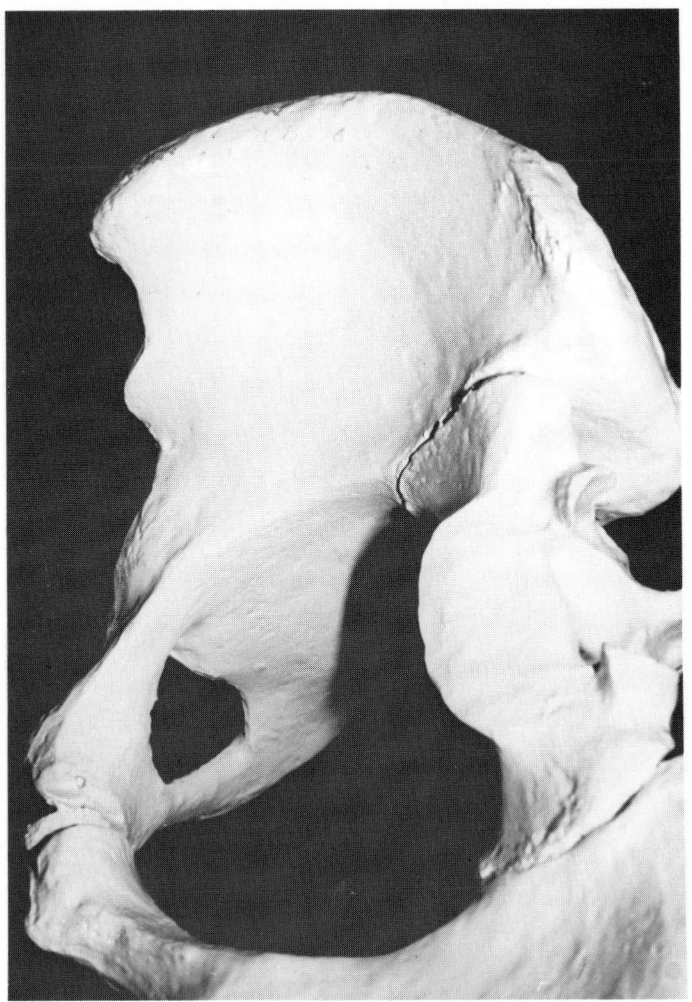

Figure 2-2. Oblique pelvic view to show features of the true and false pelvis.

Figure 2-3. The muscular attachments to a right hemipelvis.

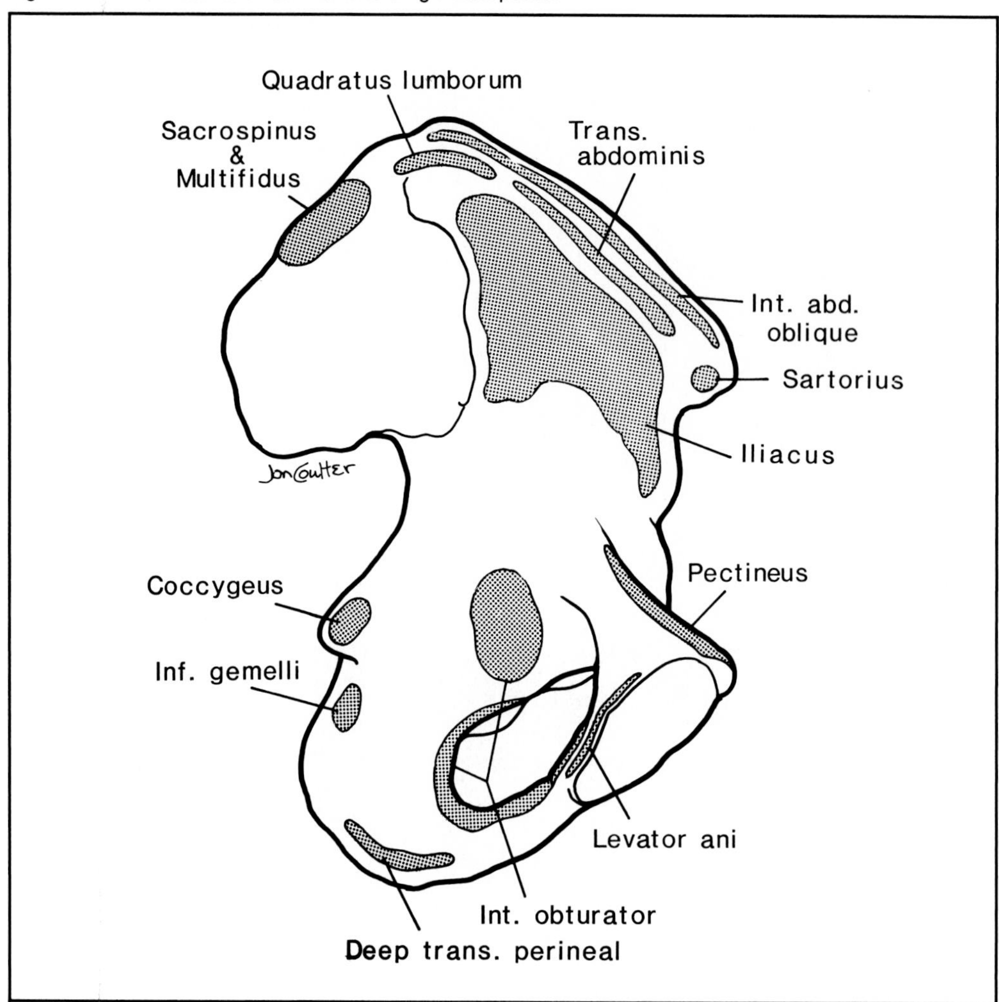


Figure 2-3A. Inner pelvic view.

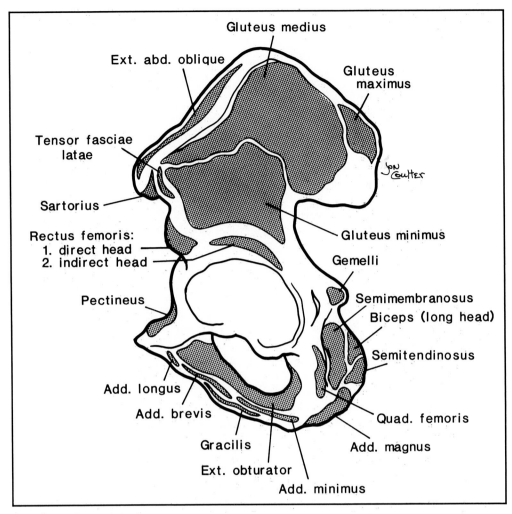

Figure 2-3B. Outer pelvic view.

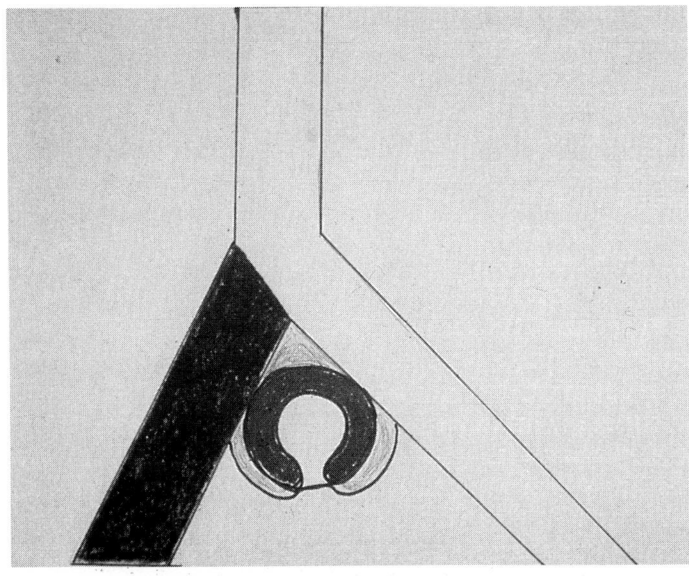

Figure 2-4. Schematic view of the innominate bone and acetabulum as perceived by Judet and Letournel.[6] The anterior column is white and the posterior column is gray.

acetabulum. Their description of the bone employs the concept of two columns or supportive elements. The acetabulum is regarded as a socket contained within two arms of an inverted "Y" formed by a posterior column, the ilioischial component, and a longer anterior column, which extends from the anterior extension of the superior iliac crest to the pubic symphysis (Figure 2-4). The upper end of the posterior column is attached directly to the posterior aspect of the anterior column (Figure 2-5). Since the nomenclature of Judet and Letournel will be employed, their observations are presented in some detail.

## Posterior Column

This ilioischial column extends from the superior ilium to the inferior ischium (Figure 2-6). It is a thick supportive element highly suitable for the application of internal fixation. Its triangular cross-section provides internal, posterior and anterolateral surfaces. The internal surface comprises the quadrilateral surface on the inner aspect of the body of the ischium. It extends posteriorly to the spine of the ischium. The posterior surface extends superiorly from the posterior wall of the acetabulum to the ischial spine and ultimately to the ischial tuberosity. The anterolateral surface includes the posterior portion of the articular surface of the acetabulum. The region is bounded by the projecting inferior acetabular horn, which also forms the edge of the subcotyloid groove a concavity for the tendon of the obturator externus. More inferiorly, the anterolateral surface continues as the body of the ischium. The posterior border of the ilioischial column is formed superiorly by the ilium and inferiorly by the greater and lesser sciatic notches, separated by the spine of the ischium.

## Anterior Column

This iliopubic column extends from the anterior portion of the iliac crest to the pubic symphysis (Figure 2-7). It is notable for a concavity both anteriorly and medially, the latter of which is bridged by the inguinal ligament. It is subdivided into iliac, acetabular and pubic segments. The iliac segment or anterior portion of the iliac wing possesses a concave inner or pelvic surface that extends to the iliopectineal line. Its outer or external surface is notable for a thick, roughened anterior pillar or gluteal ridge that extends superiorly from the roof of the acetabulum to the gluteus medius tubercle. Its anterior border possesses two thick projections, the anterior superior and anterior inferior iliac spines, separated by the interspinous notch. The anterior inferior spine is continuous with the acetabular margin. The acetabular segment possesses a triangular prismatic configuration with three surfaces. The posterolateral

Figure 2-5. Columns of the acetabulum.

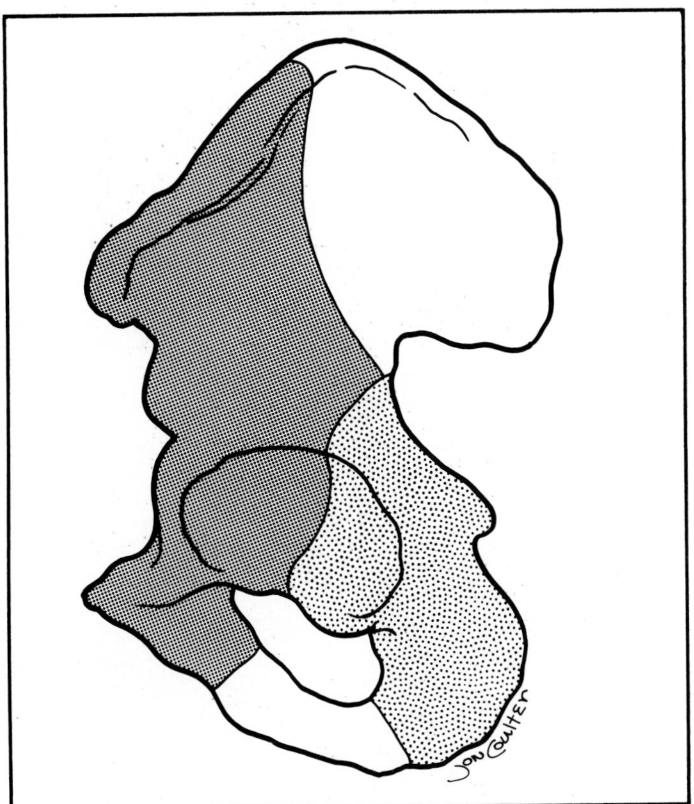


Figure 2-5A. Outer aspect.

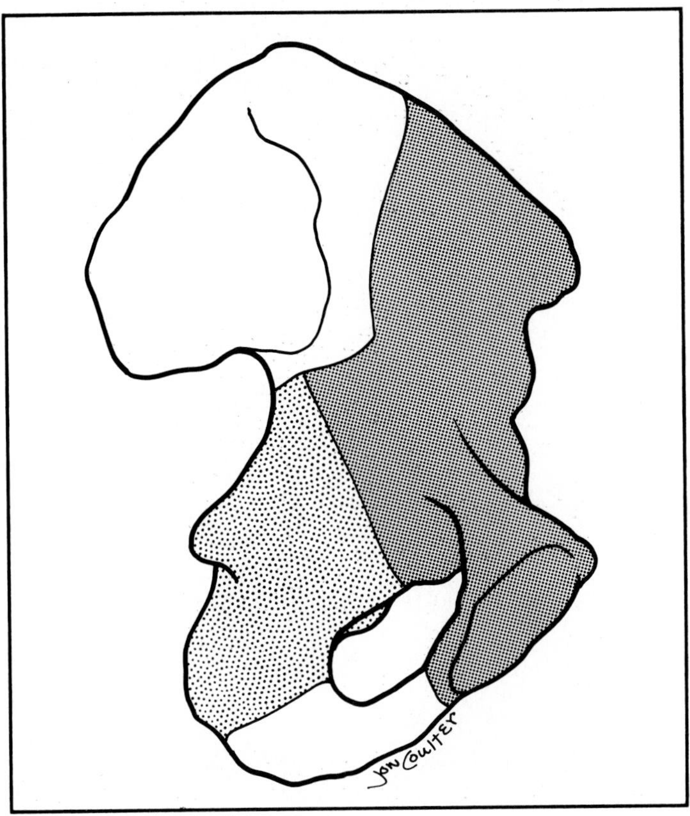


Figure 2-5B. Inner aspect.

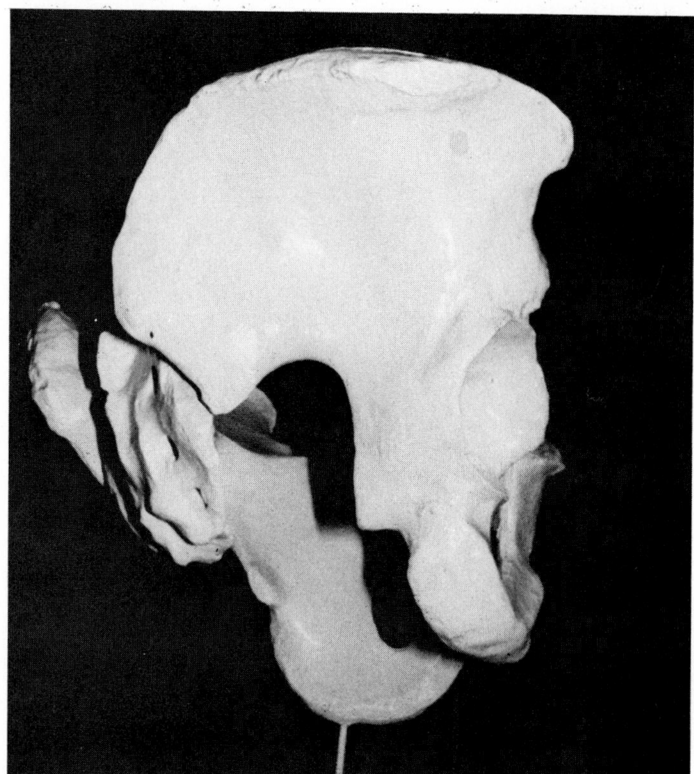

Figure 2-6. An iliac oblique view of the outer pelvis highlights the posterior column.

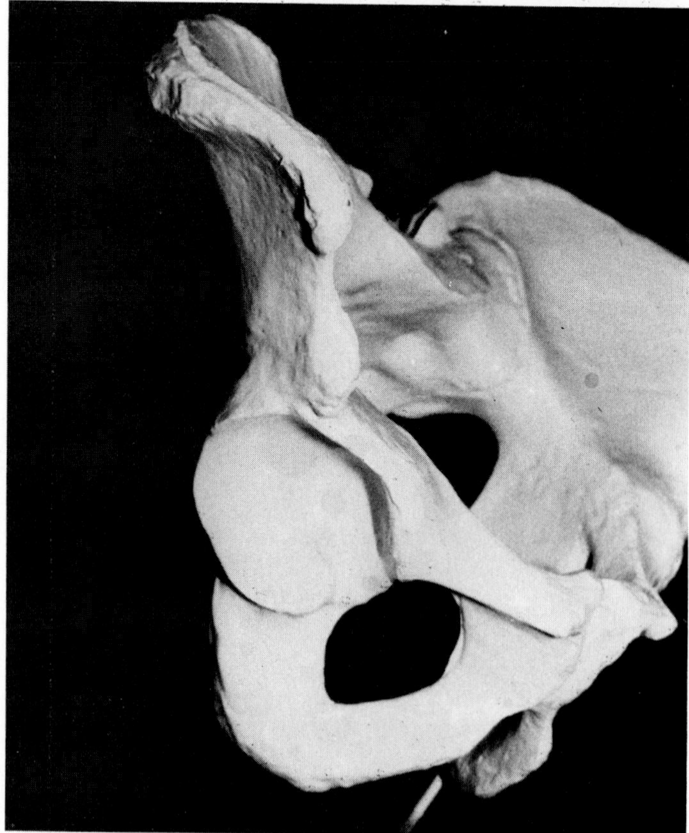

Figure 2-7. An obturator oblique view of the outer pelvis highlights the anterior column.

surface buttresses the anterior articular segment of the acetabulum and the frontal portion of the cotyloid fossa. The anterior acetabular horn is situated about 1cm superior to the level of the upper border of the obturator foramen. The concave inner surface extends from the anterior part of the quadrilateral surface to the obturator canal. It is limited anteriorly and superiorly by the iliopectineal line. Immediately below the anterior inferior iliac spine and the iliopectineal eminence, the anterosuperior surface possesses a superior gutter for the iliopsoas tendon. It continues as the inner wall of the anterior acetabulum and is limited internally by the iliopectineal line. With further scrutiny the inferior extension of the iliopectineal eminence extends more inferiorly than the anterior horn of the acetabulum. The most inferior portion of the anterior column, the pubic segment, constitutes the superior pubic ramus. This, the slenderest portion of the column and its most forward and medial extension, possesses a triangular cross-section. Its anterosuperior surface provides an insertional site for the pectineus muscle. A plate applied to it for internal fixation requires a three-dimensional contour with a twist to accurately approximate its spiral configuration. The area extends posteriorly to the site of attachment of the pectineal arch of the inguinal ligament and terminates at the pubic spine. The concave internal surface is directed almost medially. It continues with its posterosuperior inclination as the pelvic surface of the body of the pubis. The inferior surface constitutes the bony roof of the obturator foramen and is directed inferiorly and increasingly anteriorly as it approaches the body of the pubis.

To assess the continuity of the intricate anterior column, the main attention is focused upon the iliopectineal line as a reinforcing arch that buttresses the anterosuperior portion of the acetabulum. A disruption of the iliopectineal line is indicative of a fracture of the anterior column. Immediately superior to the midportion of the anterior column is the common origin of the anterior and posterior columns (Figure 2-8). They unite with an inclination of about 60°. The acetabulum itself subtends the angle, with a superior keystone of compact bone constituting its roof. The anatomical roof corresponds to a segment of articular surface that subtends an angle of 45° to 60°, housed between the anterior inferior iliac spine and the ilioischial notch of the acetabular margin. The anatomical roof extends medially to a distinct plate of compact bone situated on the superior border of the cotyloid fossa. The anterior and posterior columns are continuous with the auricular surface of the sacroiliac joint in the form of a dense sciatic buttress described by Rouviere.[7] This sciatic

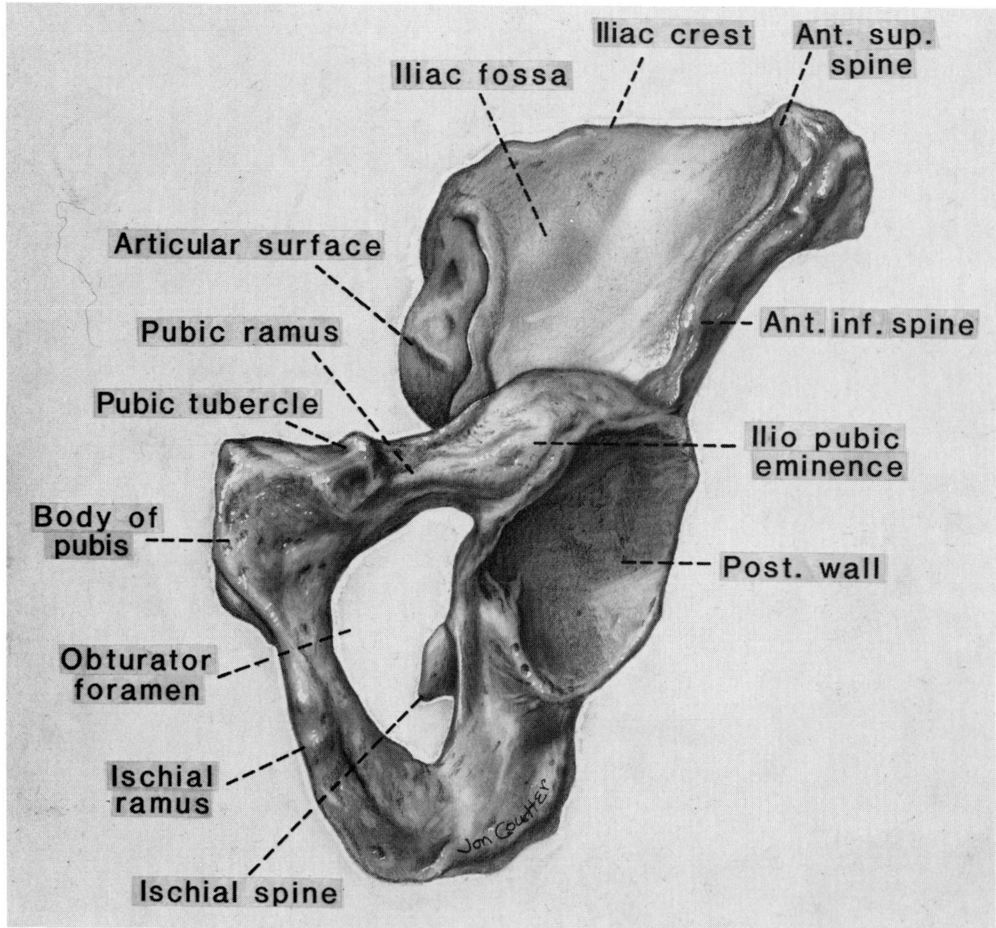


Figure 2-8. A lateral view of the outer pelvis highlights the articular surface of the acetabulum.

buttress and its superior extension of ilium are directed at 90° with respect to the inferiorly situated rami. The obliquity of the upper versus the lower half of the innominate bone accounts for the need for special oblique radiological views to highlight specific anatomical features and to characterize the various fracture patterns.

## The Sacrum

The sacrum is a large irregular truncated pyramid with five surfaces. Its embryological origin is five fused vertebrae of diminishing size from superior to inferior. The principal component, the first sacral vertebra, is tilted forward in the erect posture at an angle of about 30° to 40°. The slightly convex posterior surface possesses a thickened medial crest as a modification of the spinous processes (Figure 2-9). The slightly concave anterior surface forms the posterior wall of the pelvis. Four pairs of sacral foramina are evident on both the anterior and posterior surfaces. A lateral mass of bone, the ala, possesses dense cancellous bone as a highly suitable

Figure 2-9. The outer surface of the sacrum and adjacent ilia.

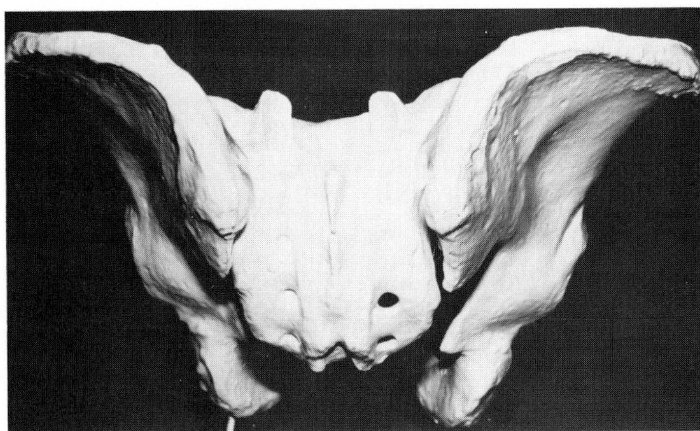

Figure 2-9A. Posterior view.

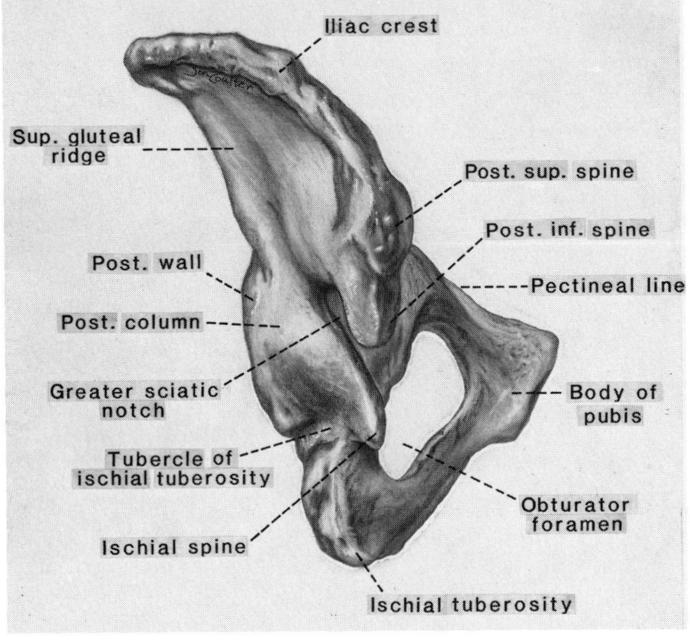


Figure 2-9B. Oblique view.

site for lag screw fixation. The sacrum is positioned about 3cm anterior to the posterior iliac crests. A posterior surgical approach to a sacroiliac joint, with its recessed position, provides a marginal view so that the accuracy of an open reduction is difficult to ascertain.

## Principal Structural Supports of the Innominate Bone

The shape and internal configuration of the innominate bone reflect the forces that are transmitted from the vertebral column to the femoral head. Thickened condensations of bone with corresponding trabecular systems were described in the early observations by Rouviere (Figures 2-10 and 2-11). A sciatic buttress passes from the auricular surface of the ilium adjacent to the sacroiliac joint and extends immediately superior to the roof of the greater sciatic notch, where it bifurcates. A superior continuation progresses to the posterosuperior part of the acetabulum en route to the anterior column. A second inferior continuation is directed toward the ischial tuberosity to buttress the posterior column. Campanacci[8] has characterized these trabecular systems as sacroacetabular, sacropubic, and sacroischial supports. These massive thickenings afford a relative protection from fracture in comparison with the more attenuated portions of the acetabulum. Inevitably these buttresses provide attractive sites for the application of internal fixation to the innominate bone.

## Joints and Ligaments

### Sacroiliac Joints

The adjacent surfaces of the ilium and sacrum possess inferior articular surfaces and superior tuberosities. The articular surface of the sacrum with its hyaline cartilaginous bearing surface impinges upon the fibrocartilaginous covering of the adjacent ilium. Movement of the articulation is markedly restricted by dense ligaments, especially the interosseous ligaments that unite the tuberosities of the ilium and sacrum to confer enormous stability upon the posterior sacroiliac complex (Figure 2-12). A supplementary posterior sacroiliac ligament extends obliquely from the tubercle or ridge of the sacrum to the posterior superior and posterior inferior spine of the ilium. This so-called short posterior sacroiliac ligament is supplemented by lengthy longitudinal fibers that run from the posterior superior iliac spine to the lateral portion of the sacrum. The anterior sacroiliac ligaments, which pass from the anterior surface of the sacrum to the adjacent surface of the anterior ilium, are relatively weak and serve primarily as a joint capsule.

Two crucial supplementary ligaments afford rotational stability to the hemipelvis (Figure 2-13). The sacrotuberous ligament is an exceptionally strong, fan-shaped band extending from the lateral portion of the entire dorsum of the sacrum and the adjacent posterior surfaces of the posterior superior and inferior iliac spines to the ischial tuberosity. Some portions of the ligament cover while others are contiguous with the sacrospinous ligaments. Laterally at its superior origin it provides an attachment for the gluteus maximus. A supplementary

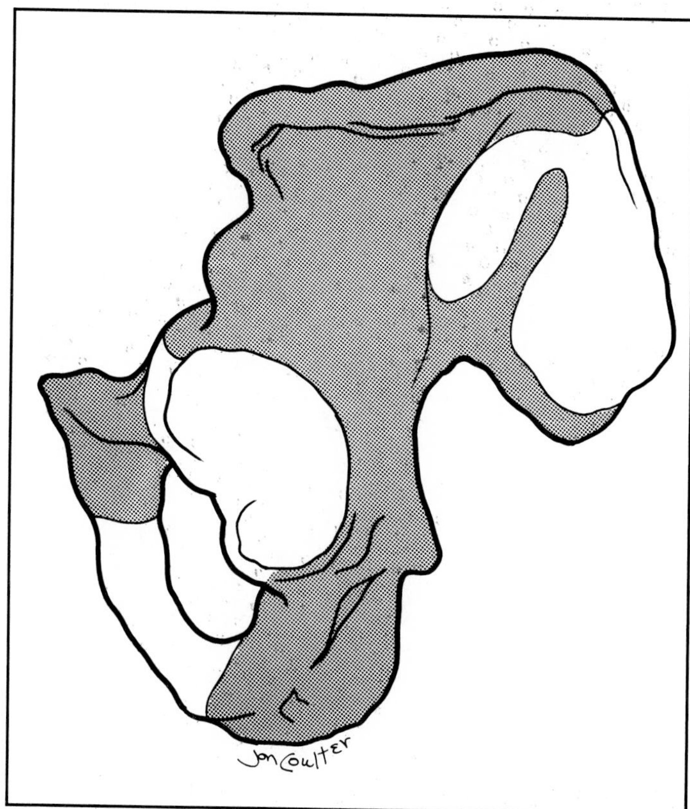


Figure 2-10. Schematic view to illustrate the thickened condensations of cancellous bone. The iliac fossa possesses thin bicortical tables of bone.

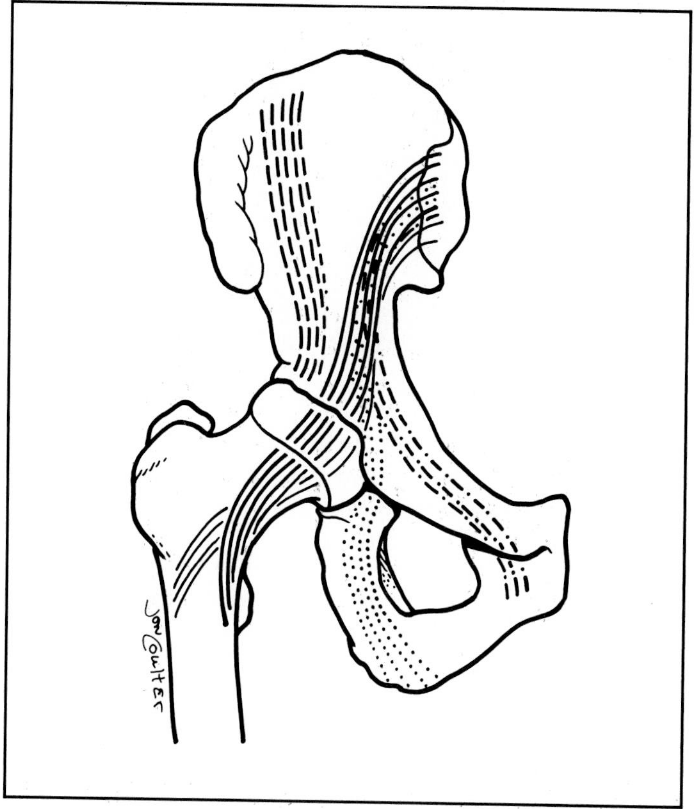


Figure 2-11. Schematic diagrams of the trabecular systems characterized by Campanacci.[8] The lighter solid lines represent the posterior sacroacetabular; heavier solid lines, the anterior sacro-acetabular; dot-and-dash lines, the sacropubic; dotted lines, the sacroischial; and dashed lines, the ilioacetabular.

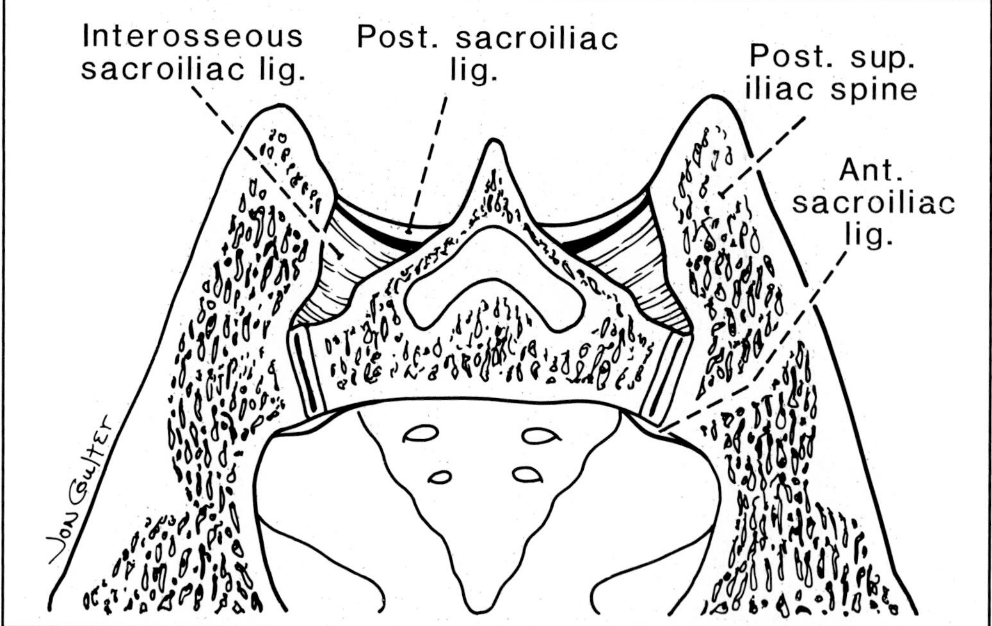


Figure 2-12. A schematic cross-sectional view of the sacroiliac joints shows the principal anterior and posterior ligaments.

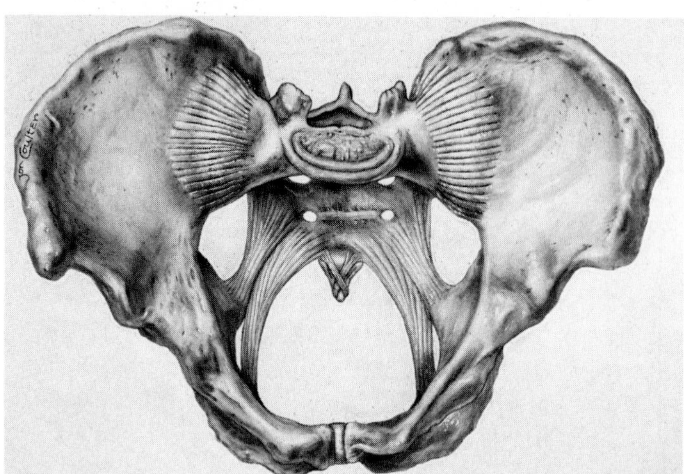

Figure 2-13. A schematic inlet view illustrates the sacrospinous and sacrotuberous ligaments.

sacrospinous ligament is a strong triangular sheet deep to the sacrotuberous ligament, which arises from the lateral margin of the sacrum and the coccyx and inserts on the ischial spine. It divides the ischial area into the greater sciatic notch and the lesser sciatic foramen.

### Iliolumbar Ligaments

At the lumbosacral articulation, iliolumbar ligaments covering the quadratus lumborum secure the axial skeleton to the pelvis and supplement the strong intervertebral disc. At their periphery the iliolumbar ligaments attach the tip of the fifth lumbar transverse process to the iliac crest. Supplementary lateral lumbosacral ligaments continue from the fifth lumbar transverse process to the ala of the sacrum. All of these posteriorly placed ligaments, including the sacrotuberous and sacrospinous ligaments, selectively constitute the posterior tension band of the pelvis, which resists rotational deforming forces as well as longitudinal shearing forces. With its wedge-shaped configuration the sacrum is suspended by the ligaments as a self-locking system.

### Symphysis Pubis

At the anterior interface of the opposing innominate bones, the opposing pubic rami are covered with hyaline cartilage and united by layers of fibrocartilage and fibrous tissue. Superiorly and anteriorly dense ligamentous fibers augment the fibrocartilage while inferiorly the symphysis is reinforced by a more independent buttress, the inferior pubic or arcuate ligament.

### The Floor of the True Pelvis

The true pelvis is the basin deep to the pelvic brim. Its lateral wall is composed of the pubis and ischium with a small triangular portion of the ilium anteriorly to supplement the rami. The obturator foramen separates the pubic from the ischial ramus. The foramen is covered by a membrane deficient superiorly to permit the passage of the obturator vessels and nerve. These neurovascular structures are vulnerable to disruption with pelvic trauma. Below the obturator foramen the lateral wall of the pelvis is lined with the obturator internus muscle and fascia, which exit the pelvis through the lesser sciatic foramen. The piriformis muscle arises from the lateral mass and the anterior surface of the sacrum, and leaves the pelvis through the greater sciatic notch. The muscle defines the position of the sciatic nerve, which generally exits the pelvis inferior to it. Rarely, the peroneal division of the nerve penetrates the piriformis or exits above it. The pelvic organs are supported by a musculature floor consisting of the levator ani and the coccygeus muscles. This floor or diaphragm is perforated by the urethra, the rectum, and the vagina.

## Blood Vessels

A knowledge of the vascular supply in and around the pelvis is crucial both for the recognition of sites of potentially massive hemorrhage accompanying pelvic disruption and for the nutrition of the pelvis following reconstructive surgery.

In instances of pelvic trauma, the most important vessel is the internal iliac artery, which arises from the common iliac vessel in the false pelvis (Figure 2-14). The internal iliac artery courses to the pelvic brim, where it divides into anterior and posterior divisions. During its course it is situated medial to the external iliac vein, the psoas muscle and the obturator nerve. Anteriorly resides the ureter, and posteriorly, its accompanying vein. With severe pelvic trauma the internal iliac artery, or rarely the common iliac artery, can be disrupted; urgent surgical repair provides the only likelihood for survival. Its posterior division is particularly vulnerable to severe pelvic trauma with posterior displacement. Generally, the superior gluteal, the iliolumbar, and the lateral sacral arteries arise from the posterior division. The superior gluteal artery, the largest branch, courses across the sacroiliac joint to the greater sciatic notch where it is positioned on the ilium. It makes a U-turn around the notch into the gluteal region along with its accompanying nerve and vein. With pelvic trauma it may be divided to provoke massive hemorrhage or rarely a traumatic aneurysm. Also, it may be occluded, jeopardizing the nutrition of the gluteus medius and minimus muscles if the origins and insertions of these principal hip abductors are divided as part of an extensile surgical exposure. The iliolumbar artery is a small somatic artery of the fifth lumbar segment, which ascends across the ala of the sacrum where it is vulnerable to injury. The lateral sacral artery descends lateral to the anterior sacral foramina and in front of the sacral complex. The anterior division of the internal iliac artery possesses visceral branches that supply the bladder, genitalia and a portion of the rectum. The internal pudendal artery, another branch, descends anterior to the sacral plexus and passes between the borders of the piriformis and coccygeus and into the gluteal region. A third branch, the inferior gluteal artery, passes between the first, second or third sacral nerves and exits from the pelvis inferior to the piriformis to supply the gluteus maximus. The internal pudendal artery crosses the ischial spine and re-enters the pelvis through the lesser sciatic foramen along with its nerve, which is particularly vulnerable to trauma with displacement of the pelvis at the greater sciatic notch. The obturator artery courses along the side wall of the pelvis to the obturator foramen where it is positioned between its nerve and vein. As it exits the pelvis through the superior defect in the obturator membrane it is vulnerable to injury with displacement of a pubic ramus fracture. An extensive venous plexus accompanies the principal arteries within the true pelvis. Most of the veins drain into the internal iliac vein with supplementary outflow into the superior rectal system, which courses via the inferior mesenteric to the portal vein. Profuse hemorrhage from the venous plexus may follow pelvic trauma.

At the time of pelvic recontruction with open reduction and internal fixation, preservation of the blood supply to each major bony fragment is crucial to permit satisfactory healing of the bone and resistance to infection. The blood supply of the bone is profuse with vessels provided through broad areas of musculature that attach as supplements to nutrient arteries. On the inner surface of the bone the anterior ilium and iliac crest is nourished by the deep circumflex iliac artery, which arises from the external iliac artery. A still larger nutrient foramina is situated in the iliac fossa 1cm anterior to the auricular surface of the sacroiliac joint and 1cm superior to the iliopectineal line, where it receives a branch from the iliolumbar artery. Other smaller nutrient foramina are located below the iliopectineal line and anterior to the greater sciatic notch, as well as in the roof of the obturator canal where they are supplied by branches from the obturator artery. Still others, observed on the inner surface of the ischial ramus are supplied by the internal pudendal artery. Posterior to the auricular surface of the sacroiliac joint the bone is nourished by branches of the iliolumbar artery. On the external surface of the bone a large nutrient foramen is observed in the middle of the gluteal area of the wing of the ilium, which receives a branch from the superior gluteal artery. Supplementary supplies include multiple nutrient vessels around the margin of the acetabulum, which form a complete vascular circle arising from the obturator artery and the inferior and superior gluteal arteries. The cotyloid fossa is perforated by small vessels from the acetabular branch of the obturator artery. The body of the pubis is supplied by multiple small branches of the obturator artery. The sciatic buttress receives numerous branches from the superior gluteal artery. Judet and Letournel[6] have examined the interosseous arterial supply by the use of arteriography. They demonstrated the presence of numerous anastomotic vessels coursing within the trabecular bone.

## Nerves

Virtually all portions of the lumbosacral and coccygeal nerve plexuses may be injured by pelvic trauma. Recently, Tile[9] has succinctly outlined the principal types of injuries to nerves that accompany pelvic fractures. The lumbosacral and coccygeal nerve plexuses are derived from the anterior rami of the T-12 to S-4 spinal nerves (Figure 2-15). The L-4 to S-1 segments are particularly

Figure 2-14. The principal blood vessels including the vascular supply to the innominate bone.

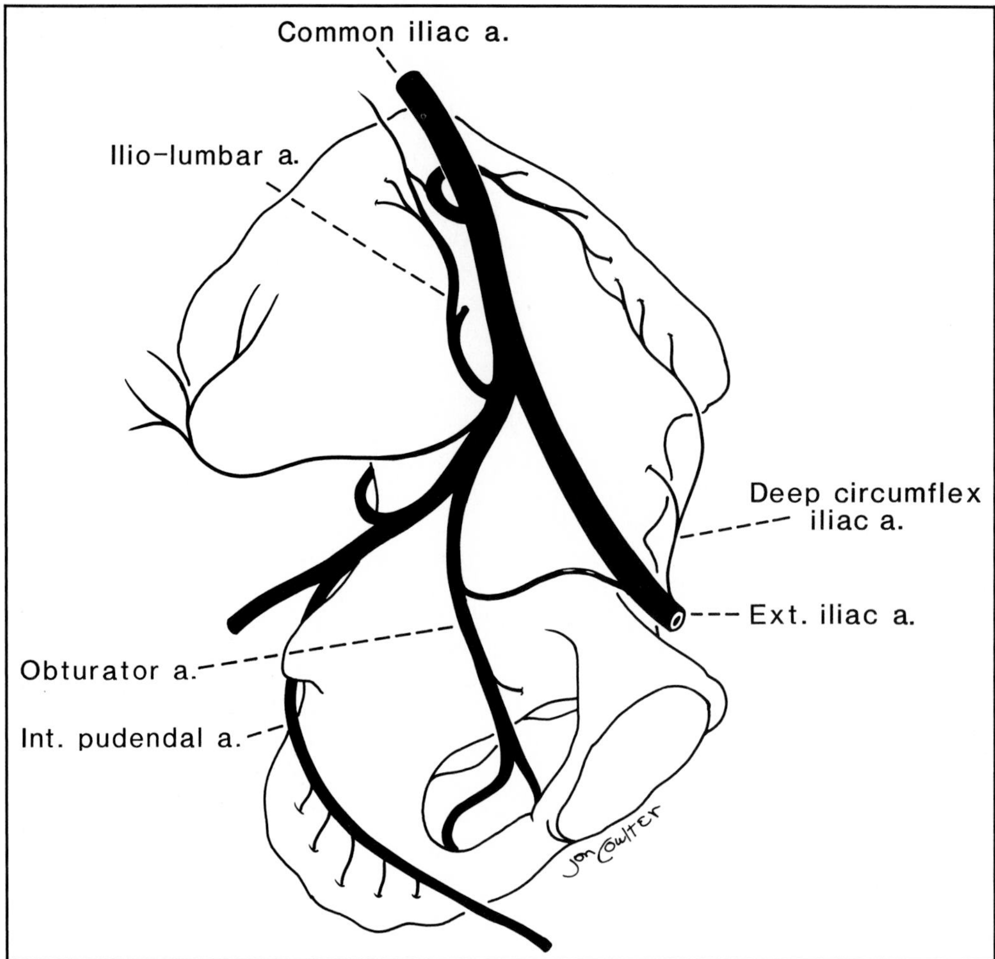


Figure 2-14A. Inner aspect.

prone to injury including the femoral nerve. The pelvic splanchnic nerves, the nervi erigentes, arise from the anterior rami of S-2, S-3, and S-4. The most superior contributing branch of the lumbosacral plexus arises from the L-4 root which crosses the fifth lumbar transverse process. The L-5 root crosses and indents the ala of the sacrum where it joins with L-4 to form the lumbosacral trunk. The upper four anterior sacral rami exit from sacral foramina that groove the ala of the sacrum. The lumbosacral trunk and the first sacral root unite anterior to the sacroiliac joint, which in turn joins with S-2, S-3, and S-4 anterior to the piriformis. The common outflow divides into two terminal branches, the sciatic and pudendal nerves, and supplementary collateral branches including the superior and inferior gluteal nerves. Muscular branches from the roots of the plexus innervate the piriformis, levator ani and

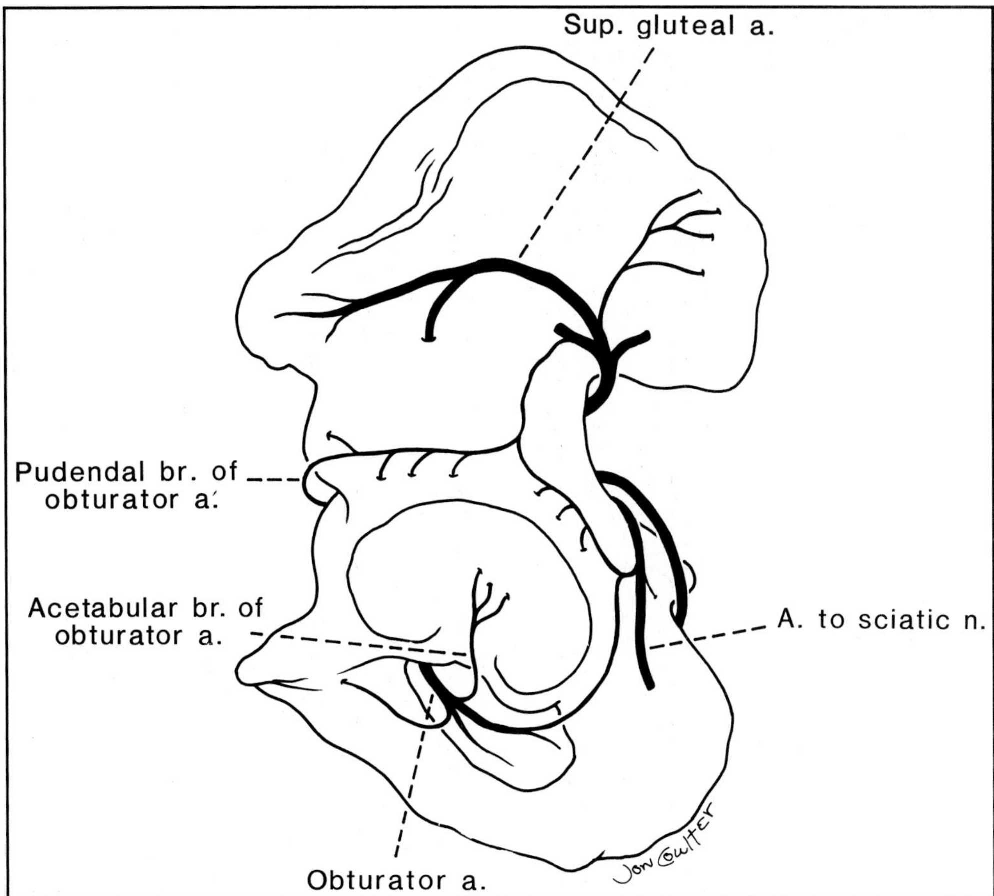


Figure 2-14B. Outer aspect.

coccygeus, and supply the pelvic splenic nerve. Many of the branches pass through the greater sciatic notch, notably the sciatic nerve, which forms the largest branch of the sacral plexus. The sciatic nerve exits the pelvis between the inferior border of the piriformis and the ischial border of the greater sciatic notch. It possesses two divisions, the tibial and peroneal, which are loosely bound together. The nerve is vulnerable to pelvic trauma especially with a posterior dislocation of the hip or a posterior acetabular fracture. The peroneal division is particularly susceptible to injury and less likely to recover. The principal L-5 root contribution to the peroneal division of the sciatic nerve is subject to injury at the root level, where it passes through the greater sciatic notch and behind the hip joint. Frequently it is difficult to distinguish the site of such an injury. The pudendal nerve (S-2 to S-4) exits between the piriformis and the

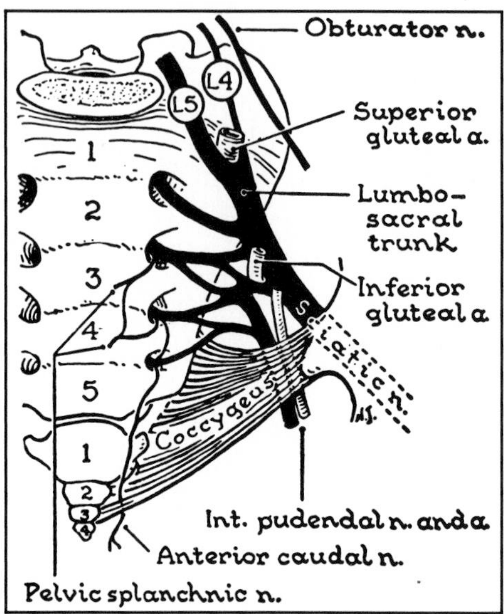


Figure 2-15. The lumbosacral plexus (from M Tile[9]).

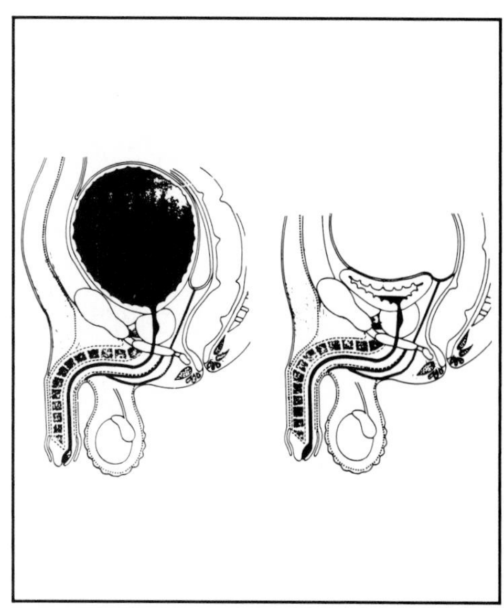

Figure 2-16. Sagittal sections of the male pelvis to show the positions of the full and empty bladder. The full bladder displaces the peritoneal reflection from the anterior abdominal wall so that a suprapubic catheter can be inserted extraperitoneally (left). The empty bladder resides retropubically (right) (from WJ Kane[5]).

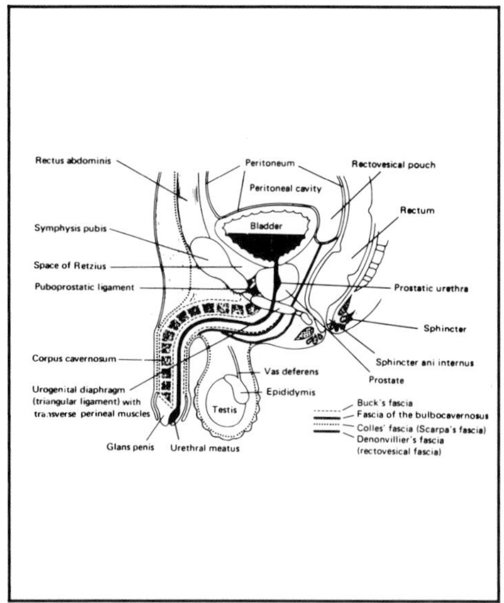


Figure 2-17. Sagittal section of the lower pelvic anatomy and male genitalia. The urethra is divided into prostatic, membranous and cavernous portions (from WJ Kane[5]).

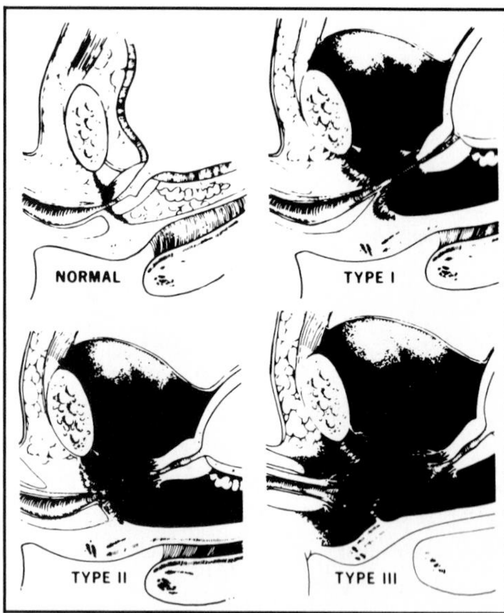


Figure 2-18. Classification of urethral tears. Normal: the prostate and urogenital diaphragm are continuous as a single functional unit. Type I: While clinical findings may suggest a complete rupture, the urethra is intact although attenuated. Type II: the classic supradiaphragmatic injury. Type III: Sub-diaphragmatic rupture as a complete or incomplete disruption. In this common pattern, a retrograde urethrogram shows perineal extravasation (from V Colapinto[10]).

coccygeus medial to the sciatic nerve. The latter nerve arises from the plexus to innervate the superior gluteal, the inferior gluteal, the obturator internus (L-5 to S-2), and quadratus femorus (L-4 and L-5), along with the posterior cutaneous nerve of the thigh (S-1 to S-3).

The superior gluteal nerve (L-4 to S-1) with its accompanying artery and vein exits from the pelvis circuitously around the greater sciatic notch. While traumatic injury to the artery is common, associated injury to the nerve is uncommon. With posterior surgical approaches to the hip joint or acetabular reconstruction, a traction injury to the nerve may follow excessive retraction or the application of a lengthy posterior plate. The inferior gluteal nerve (L-5 to S-2) exits from the pelvis inferior to the piriformis and posterior to the sciatic nerve, where it supplies the gluteus maximus.

The coccygeal plexus provides terminal branches as the perforating cutaneous branch of S-2 and S-3 and the peroneal branch of S-4. These nerves descend anteriorly to the coccygeus muscle, where they become cutaneous to supply the skin of the buttock and perineum. The anterior coccygeal plexus is formed by the anterior rami of S-5 and C-1. The plexus culminates in the anterior caudal nerve, a sensory nerve that supplies the coccygeal area.

## The Lower Urinary Tract

The bladder is positioned posterior to the symphysis pubis and the two pubic bones. In infancy the bladder is an intraabdominal organ which does not attain its pelvic position until adulthood. A greater proportion of the infantile bladder is covered with peritoneum. The infantile bladder appears to be particularly susceptible to injury in association with pelvic trauma. In the adult the peritoneum is reflected from the anterior abdominal wall across the dome of the bladder to extend posteriorly to the bladder neck. If the bladder is emptied the peritoneum extends to the symphysis. The distended bladder rises above the symphysis to contact the abdominal wall so that a suprapubic catheter can be inserted extraperitoneally (Figure 2-16). At the site of origin of the urethra, the bladder neck is attached to the pelvis with a ligamentous support. In men, the neck of the bladder is in close contact with the prostate gland, which surrounds the proximal portion of the urethra. In women, the neck of the bladder is in greater contact with the pubococcygeal portions of the levator ani muscles beneath it. The lateral ligamentous extensions of the bladder are augmented by the neurovascular pedicle of the bladder, and in men, the vas deferens.

The male urethra is conceptually divided into three portions (Figure 2-17). A pelvic portion 2cm in length passes vertically downward within the surrounding prostate gland. Inferior to this prostatic portion, the urethra passes through the urogenital diaphragm or pelvic floor, where it is called the membranous urethra. The urogenital diaphragm is perceived as two separate fascial layers spanning the pubic arch with intervening skeletal muscle. More recent anatomical observations by Colapinto[10] conclude that the prostate and urogenital diaphragm are a single functional unit. Smooth muscle surrounds the membranous urethra and extends into the prostatic urethra. The muscle ends abruptly at the inferior surface of the diaphragm at the start of the bulbous urethra. This attenuated portion of the urethra accounts for the characteristic sites of rupture in the bulbous urethra. If the prostate or the urogenital diaphragm is displaced precipitously the membranous urethra is ruptured at the lateral plane of weakness between the apex of the prostate and the superior surface of the diaphragmatic fascia. Colapinto and McCallum[11] have classified the urethral tears into three patterns (Figure 2-18). Type I presents with an intact although attenuated urethra. Type II is the classic supra-diaphragmatic injury, while Type III is a sub-diaphragmatic rupture. The third and most commonly encountered disruption can be partial or complete. In these patients a retrograde urethrogram is notable for peritoneal extravasation. In the cases with intrapelvic extravasation of urine following a rupture of the urethra or bladder, generally the extravasation is extraperitoneal. With a rupture of the dome of the bladder, however, intraperitoneal extravasation can occur.

In a woman the urethra is 3cm to 5cm in length. It is relatively immobilized by its lengthy attachment to the anterior vaginal wall and to the urogenital diaphragm. It achieves a greater mobility with the relatively poor development of the diaphragm which is perforated not only by the urethra but also by the vagina. In the presence of a pelvic fracture, the female urethra is less subject to secondary injury than its male counterpart in view of its short length, the absence of the prostate, and the greater mobility of the female urogenital diaphragm.

## References

1. Brach JC: Cunningham's Textbook of Anatomy. London, Oxford Press, 1951, p 875.
2. Hollinshead WH: Anatomy for Surgeons: The Thorax, Abdomen & Pelvis. New York, Hoeber, 1956, vol 2, p 574.
3. Breatnach AS: Frazer's Anatomy of the Human Skeleton. Boston, Little, Brown, 1965, p 106.
4. Hoppenfeld S, deBoer P: Surgical Exposures in

Orthopaedics: The Anatomic Approach. Philadelphia, Lippincott, 1984, p 301.

5. Kane WJ: Fractures of the pelvis, in Rockwood CA Jr, Green DP (eds): Fractures in Adults. Philadelphia, Lippincott, 1984, p 1094.
6. Letournel E, Judet R: Fractures of the Acetabulum. New York, Springer-Verlag, 1981, p 1.
7. Rouviere H (ed): Traite' d'Anatomie Humaine. Masson, Paris, 1940, p 57.
8. Campanacci M: Lesioni traumatiche del bacino, in Gaggi A (ed): Proceedings of 52nd Congress of the Societa Italiana di Ortopedia, Rome, 13-15 October, 1967. Bologna, Stanya Artie, 1967.
9. Tile M: Fractures of the Pelvis and Acetabulum. Baltimore, Williams and Wilkins, 1984, p 17.
10. Colapinto V: Trauma to the pelvis: Urethral injury. Clin Orthop 151:46, 1980.
11. Colapinto V, McCallum RW: Injury to the male posterior urethra in fractured pelvis: A new classification. J Urol 118:575, 1977.

# CHAPTER 3

# Biomechanics of the Pelvis and Pelvic Fixation

## Biomechanics of the Pelvis

While the anatomical features of the pelvic ring are closely correlated with their functional attributes, initially it appears contradictory that the bony constituents of the pelvis, which afford protection for the lower abdominal viscera and undergo transference of load between the trunk and lower limbs, possess little if any inherent stability. If the osseous pelvis is stripped of its soft tissue supportive elements, it separates spontaneously into the two innominate bones and the sacrum. The crucial ligamentous support is provided by the posterior sacroiliac ligamentous complex, which prevents inferior migration and forward rotation of the sacrum. If a cross-section of the sacrum and adjacent ilia is examined, it becomes evident that the posterior ligamentous structures form a tension band to support the posterior portion of the pelvic ring. Tile[1] has likened this structure to a suspension bridge, in which the posterior superior iliac spines serve as pillars while the interosseous sacroiliac ligaments are the suspension bars and the sacrum is the bridge. Further support is afforded by the iliolumbar ligaments, which anchor the transverse processes of L-5 to the iliac crest, supplemented by the intervening transverse fibers of the interosseous sacroiliac ligaments. The role of the posterior sacroiliac ligamentous complex is to prevent posterior displacement of the pelvic ring on the sacrum or likewise anterior displacement of the sacrum and the axial skeleton on the pelvis during weight bearing. With locomotion a small degree of rotatory motion is permitted at the sacroiliac joints. While the superior part of the posterior pelvic ring is stabilized primarily by the posterior sacroiliac ligaments, the inferior portion is augmented by the sacrospinous and sacrotuberous ligaments (Figures 2-12 and 2-13). The former join the sacrum to the ischial spines to resist external rotational forces while the latter join the sacrum to the ischial tuberosity to resist shearing and rotational forces. These two supplementary ligaments, the sacrospinous and sacrotuberous ligaments, are positioned at right angles to one another. This orientation augments their capability to resist the major rotational and shearing forces that act upon the pelvis.

The remainder of the pelvic ligaments provide modest supplementary stabilizing influences. The weak attenuated anterior sacroiliac ligaments serve primarily as a joint capsule to separate the sacroiliac joint from the pelvic cavity. An anterior sacrococcygeal ligament is a continuation of the anterior longitudinal ligament of the vertebral column. The anterior pubic rami with the intervening symphysis pubis afford little stability to the pelvic ring. They do complete the birth canal and provide origins for various muscle groups. However, even when the anterior structures are absent or displaced secondary to congenital or traumatic alteration, the stability of the pelvic ring is minimally compromised, provided that the posterior ligamentous structures are intact. Apart from one exception, child birth, the pelvic ring is notable for its extraordinary stability to afford only minor rotational movement at the sacroiliac joints and symphysis pubis. Under hormonal impetus during pregnancy and labor, the symphysis pubis widens temporarily to a limited degree while the sacrospinous and anterior and posterior sacroiliac joints remain relatively undisplaced.

If the symphysis pubis is experimentally divided, it yawns apart by less than 2.5cm[1] (Figure 3-1). Despite further external rotational force applied to the two hemipelves, further displacement is prevented by the intact sacrospinous ligaments. If the sacrospinous and anterior sacroiliac ligaments also are divided under the impetus of continued external rotational force, the symphysis widens progressively until the posterior superior spines impinge upon the sacrum. No vertical or rotational malalignment ensues, however. If the sacrotuberous and ipsilateral posterior iliac ligamentous complex are divided, complete instability of a hemipelvis results so that displacement occurs in the vertical and rotational planes. If the sacrotuberous and posterior sacroiliac ligaments are divided on both sides of the pelvis, complete disruption of the pelvic ring accompanies the loss of a stable connection between the spine and the lower extremities.

With its ring-like nature, distortion of the ring occurs only when two discrete sites are damaged. This observation was reported by Gertzbein and Chenoweth[2] in a series of patients who sustained a so-called undisplaced pelvic ring disruption accompanied by a minimally displaced ramus fracture or another comparable anterior injury. In each case a positive technetium polyphosphate uptake in the posterior sacroiliac complex was documented, providing an indication of a minimally displaced posterior lesion. Recent postmortem observations by Bucholz[3] confirmed the presence of a posterior lesion in every specimen where a so-called straddle fracture of all four rami had been detected in posttraumatic radiographs.

## Mechanisms of Pelvic Disruption

With the immense amount of force required to disrupt the pelvic ring, it is not surprising that distinct patterns of injury arise when the direction of the provocative force is altered. Previous studies undertaken by Pennal and his associates[4] characterized a distinct correlation between the patterns of pelvic injury and the vector of the provocative force. These workers devised a classification of pelvic injuries based upon the direction of the traumatic force. Pennal undertook a biomechanical assessment supplemented by clinical observations on 359 patients who sustained a pelvic fracture. As the Toronto school recognized, usually the direction of the provocative force is oblique to the pelvis of the trauma victim so that clinically an almost infinitely broad spectrum of injury patterns is documented. Nevertheless, the Pennal classification scheme provides such extraordinary insight into the mechanisms of pelvic injury and a guideline to therapeutic management that it merits detailed scrutiny.

### *Anteroposterior or External Rotational Force*

If an anteroposterior force is applied either to the symphysis or to a posterior iliac spine, external rotation of one or both hemipelves may follow to create a separation at the symphysis pubis (Figure 3-2). Previously a blow to the front of the pelvis was felt to be the principal source of this pattern of injury. More recently Tile[1] has attributed it either to force imposed upon a posterior superior iliac spine or an external rotational force applied to both femora. Despite the relatively low magnitude of

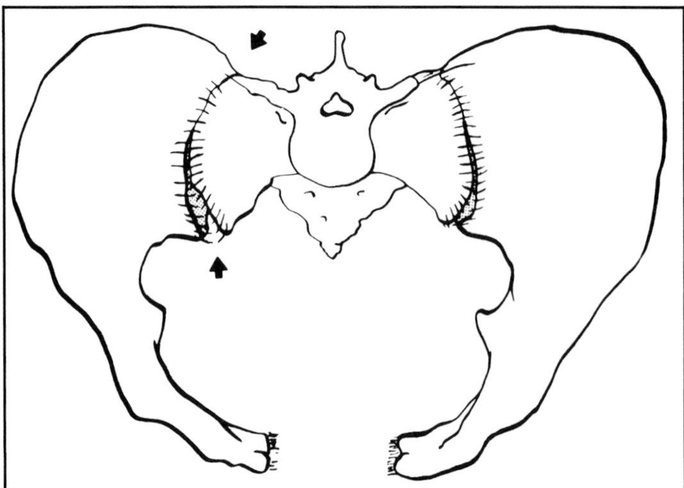

Figure 3-1. Schematic diagram of an anteroposterior compression or external rotation injury.

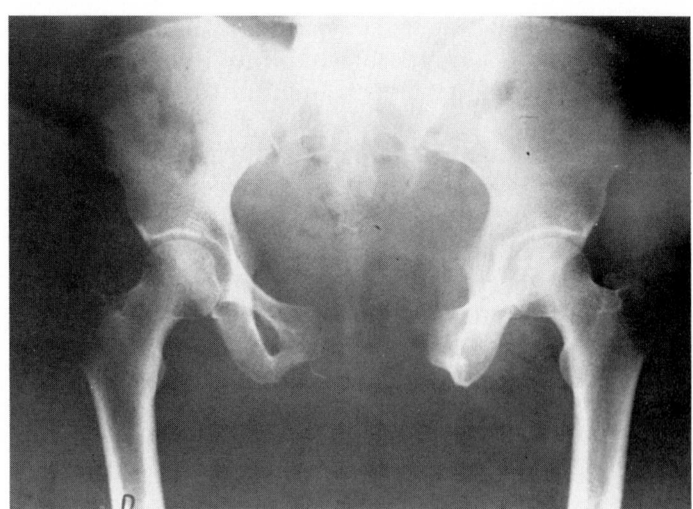

Figure 3-2. Anteroposterior radiograph of an anteroposterior compression injury.

energy dissipation, the symphysis undergoes a temporary diastasis that spontaneously returns to an anatomical configuration. With the application of greater force, the anterior sacroiliac and sacrospinous ligaments are ruptured, whereupon a diastasis of the symphysis pubis is documented radiologically. In the vast majority of patients, however, the posterior sacroiliac ligamentous complex remains intact and further displacement is precluded, especially in a vertical plane. Probably in less than 10% of cases in which a particularly wide diastasis of the symphysis is documented, the posterior ligamentous complex is disrupted to create a wholly unstable hemipelvis.

### *Lateral Compression Injuries*

Undoubtedly the most frequent source of pelvic injuries is the imposition of a laterally disposed force upon the pelvis. If a direct lateral force is applied to the iliac crest and adjacent ilium, it is likely to provoke a crushing insult to the sacrum through its weakest point, the foramina. Since the sacral bony trabeculae course parallel to the vector of the lateral compressive force, a stable crushing injury ensues. Generally, the adjacent ligamentous structures are spared. If a progressively greater traumatic force is applied to the ilium, then ipsilateral or contralateral rami fractures or disruption of all four pubic rami as a so-called straddle fracture or a diastasis of the symphysis may occur. Various combinations of these anterior injuries also are documented.

If the lateral compressive force impinges upon the greater trochanter with transmission of the force across the hip joint, then an acetabular fracture, with or without a concomitant pelvic ring disruption, may follow. The medial displacement of the acetabulum is greatest immediately after the moment of impact. A certain degree of elastic recoil spontaneously provides a partial reduction so that the original radiographs do not indicate the magnitude of the initial deformity.

### *Unstable Lateral Compression Injuries*

Many of the commonly encountered lateral compression injuries arise from either an anterolateral or less frequently a posterolateral insult (Figure 3-3). Particularly in the former case, internal rotation of the affected hemipelvis is likely to follow. The anterior portion of the sacrum is crushed at the sacroiliac joint as rotation of the hemipelvis progresses. The ipsilateral or contralateral rami are fractured and migrate through a variable but substantial distance. With the sharp spike of mobile ramus, impalement of the bowel or bladder is likely to occur. Ultimately with substantial rotation of the hemipelvis, the posterior sacroiliac ligaments are disrupted to create an unstable hemipelvis. If the traumatic force follows an oblique vector with a somewhat superior direction, the mobile hemipelvis rotates to produce a displacement that may be misinterpreted on an anteroposterior radiograph as the superior migration documented with a vertical shear fracture.

### *Vertical Shear Fracture*

In unusual situations a vertical shearing force is applied to one or both sacroiliac joints. This situation arises when an individual falls from a great height to land on one or occasionally both feet, when a heavy weight strikes the shoulder of an upright individual, or when a reclining motorcyclist with extended hips and knees strikes a motionless object or an oncoming vehicle. All of the principal ligamentous structures on the anterior and

Figure 3-3. Lateral compression injuries. A: Schematic diagram with ipsilateral ramus fractures. B: Typical radiograph of a similar ipsilateral pattern with malrotation deformity of the right hemipelvis. C: Schematic diagram with contralateral ramus fractures. D: Radiograph of similar contralateral pattern and extravasation of contrast medium consistent with a ruptured bladder. E: Pelvic outlet view of bilateral ramus fractures.

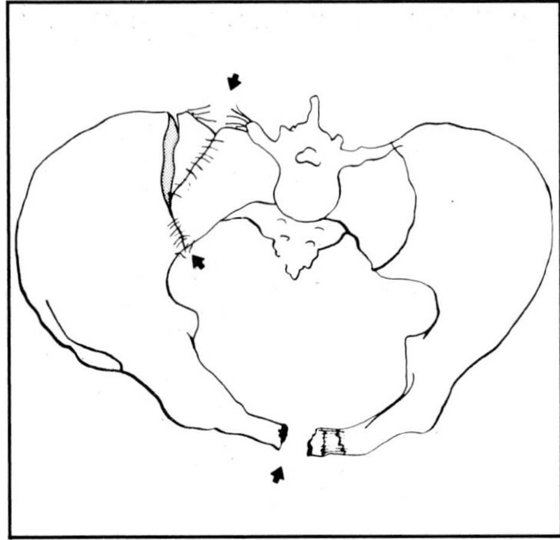

Figure 3-3A.

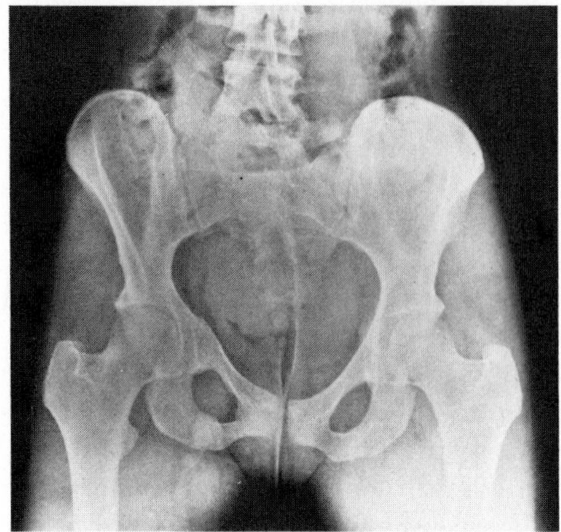

Figure 3-3B.

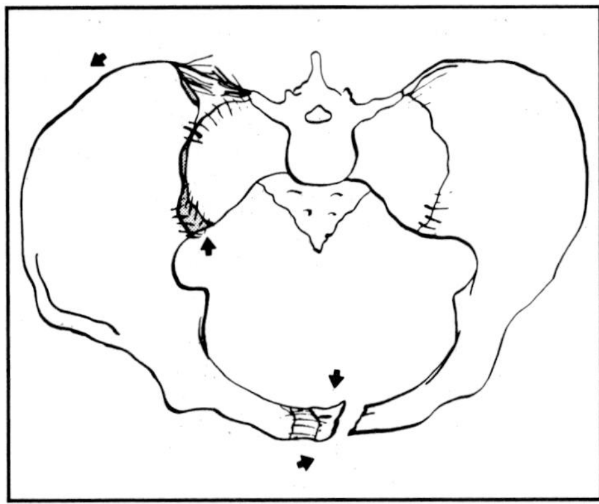

Figure 3-3C.

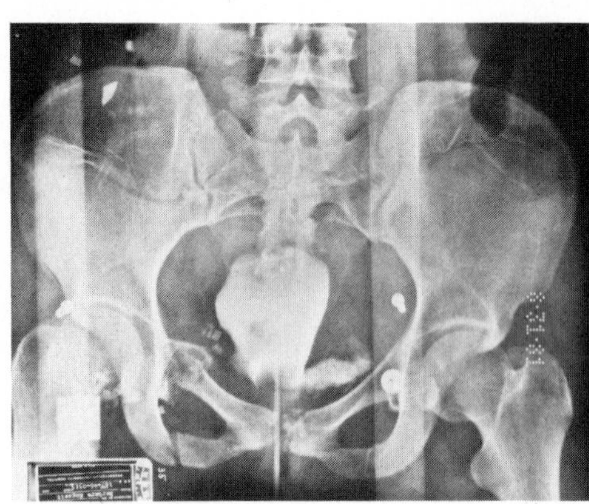

Figure 3-3D.

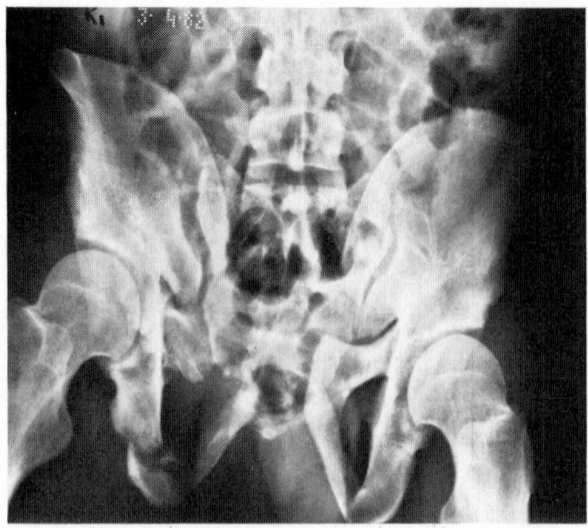

Figure 3-3E.

Figure 3-4. Vertical shear injury. A: Schematic AP view. B: Schematic inlet view illustrates the frequent accompanying posterior migration of a hemipelvis. C: A radiograph of a healed malreduced vertical shear injury reveals the vertical migration of the left hemipelvis with apparent limb length discrepancy and a symptomatic nonunion/malunion of the left sacroiliac fracture dislocation.

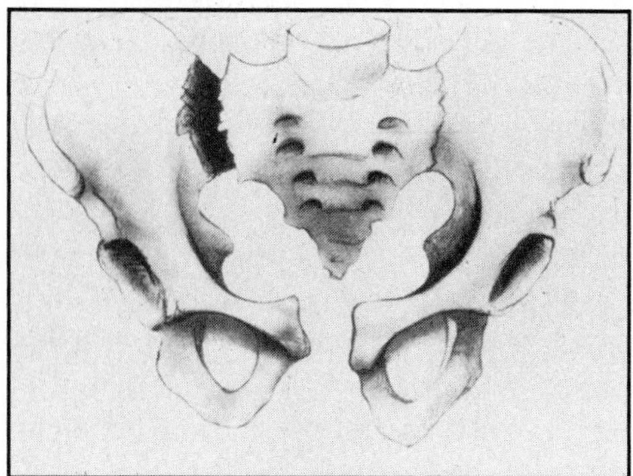

Figure 3-4A.

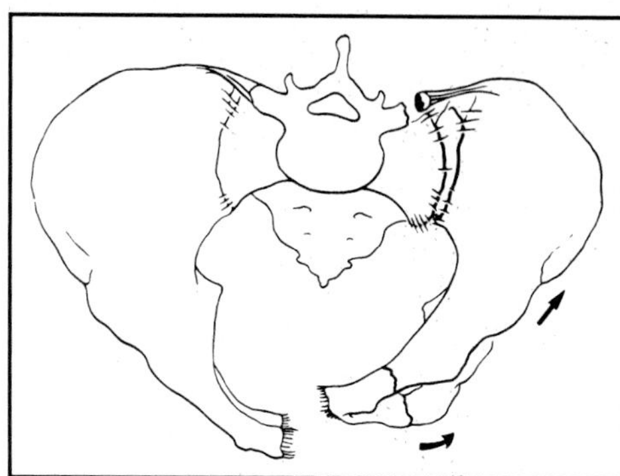

Figure 3-4B.

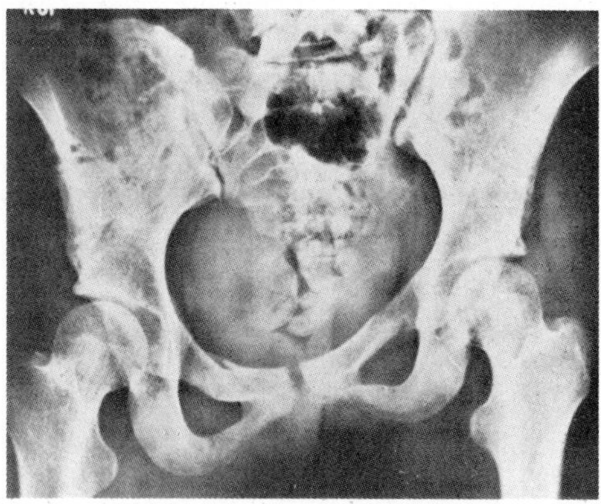

Figure 3-4C.

posterior aspects of the pelvic ring are disrupted with marked displacement of the innominate bone (Figure 3-4).

In most traumatic situations, combinations of the anterior, posterior, lateral and vertical forces are encountered to create a great variety of injury patterns. Another frequently encountered combination is posterior migration of one hemipelvis with a variable degree of rotation. Other contributing factors include the magnitude of the force and the degree of osteoporosis of the bone.

The specific sites in the pelvic ring where mechanical failure is most likely to occur reflect not only the vector and magnitude of the provocative force but also the mechanical properties of the bone or ligamentous supports. The reproducibility of the sites documented in pelvic trauma victims has provided the basis for the alternative classification schemes of pelvic disruption.[3,5] Fractures of the pelvic ring usually violate the rami, the sacrum through the ipsilateral neural foramina, or the attenuated lateral ilium. Vertical and/or horizontal fractures of the lateral ilium extend across the thin and weak portion of the bone. Fracture dislocations of the sacroiliac joint that propagate from the joint into the adjacent ilium or sacrum are more frequently encountered than a pure sacroiliac dislocation. Disruption of the symphysis pubis is documented as frequently as multiple ramus fractures.

In an attempt to identify the optimal sites for insertion of pelvic pins for use in halo-pelvic stabilization, O'Brien[6] critically examined isolated cadaveric pelves. The thickest portions of bone were documented in the roof of the acetabulum from the anterior inferior spine to the roof of the greater sciatic notch, followed by the iliac crest. White and Hirsch[7] examined segments of iliac crest in an attempt to identify the segments that would provide the optimal resistance to deformation under compressive loads encountered clinically when iliac crest bone grafts are employed for spinal reconstruction. The gluteal tubercle was observed to be the strongest part of the iliac crest. Incidentally, these limited observations are indicative of the relative dearth of knowledge of the fracture analysis and allied biomechanics of the pelvic ring.

## Pelvic Stability

Previously, the degree of posttraumatic instability of the pelvis had been ascertained by a combination of clinical and radiographic features. Errors in the assessment of pelvic stability are a notorious problem when conventional radiographs are used as the sole method of evaluation, particularly if a single anteroposterior view is used.[3] Many clinical cases of pelvic trauma with a perfectly aligned pelvis documented in an initial posttraumatic anteroposterior radiograph have culminated in a late pelvic nonunion or malunion with marked pelvic displacement, even when such patients have been managed with bedrest for periods of one to two months.[5] Pelvic stability is a crucial guideline for the selection of an appropriate therapeutic method. Presumably if an accurate assessment of pelvic stability could be reproducibly ascertained in the clinical setting, a detailed algorithm of the most suitable type of nonoperative or operative treatment for virtually every pattern of pelvic disruption could be characterized.

Walheim[8] and his associates have attempted to employ biomechanical techniques to document the motion at the symphysis pubis in patients who were assessed for pelvic hypermobility and in pelvic trauma victims who were managed with a trapezoidal type of external fixation frame. One threaded pin was inserted into either superior pubic ramus. Transducers were mounted on the two pins. With appropriate electromechanical instrumentation, motion at the symphysis was recorded in three planes when the patients undertook various movements. An attempt was made to correlate the mechanical data with stereoradiographs. While the technique as presently available is not perfected for use on acute trauma victims, it does provide insight into the type of biomechanical analysis that is needed for the future. Currently available methods to estimate pelvic stability remain imperfect; nevertheless, certain general principles are now available as useful therapeutic guidelines.

### *Assessment of Pelvic Stability*

With an anteroposterior compression injury and separation of the symphysis pubis by less than 2cm, usually substantial pelvic ligamentous integrity prevails so that spontaneous recovery without any supplementary immobilization is needed. In the more typical case where a diastasis of between 2.5cm and 6cm is documented, the crucial posterior sacroiliac ligamentous complex is spared and rotational stability is preserved.[1,3] Limited fixation of the symphysis by resort to a plate or a simple external frame affords adequate stability to permit a reliable recovery with an anatomically realigned pelvis. Once the diastasis is more than 8cm, there is a considerable likelihood that the posterior ligamentous complex has been violated or that there is a fracture of the adjacent sacrum or ilium, creating an equivalent degree of pelvic instability. Rigorous scrutiny of the posterior portion of the pelvic ring by resort to a computed scan is crucial to document the degree of instability and, thereby, the appropriate therapeutic protocol (Figure 3-5). If a computed scan through the sacroiliac joint shows evidence of separation of the front of the sacroiliac joint but apposition of the back of the joint, the posterior sacroiliac ligaments are intact. If a gap is visualized at the back of the sacroiliac joint or if there is an anteroposterior or rotational displacement of the ilium referable to the adjacent sacrum, complete instability is documented. In the latter instance, much more rigorous stabilization of the relevant hemipelvis is required. In many of these wholly unstable instances on clinical examination, the presence of excessive mobility of the hemipelvis is confirmed.

In the lateral compression injuries with rotation of a hemipelvis, clinical and conventional radiographs are notoriously misleading to ascertain the degree of pelvic instability. Telltale signs include avulsion fractures of the ischial spines or the opposing portions of the sacrum as indices of sacrospinous ligamentous disruption

Figure 3-5. Computed pelvic scans with examples of unilateral sacroiliac disruptions. A: Unstable dislocation of left sacroiliac joint. B: Unstable right fracture dislocation involving posterior ilium and sacrum. C: Unstable fracture dislocation involving right sacroiliac joint and adjacent sacrum.

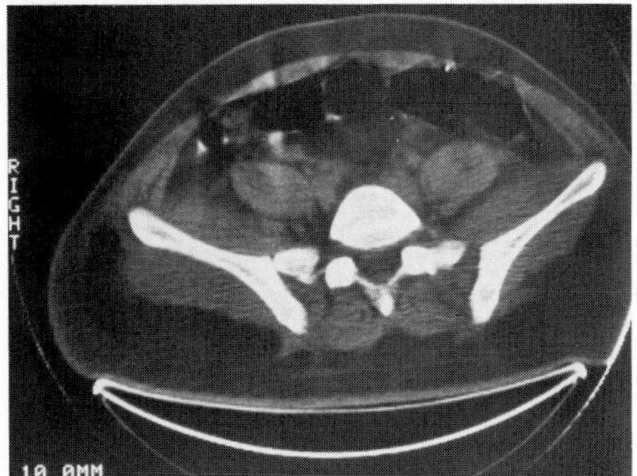


Figure 3-5A.

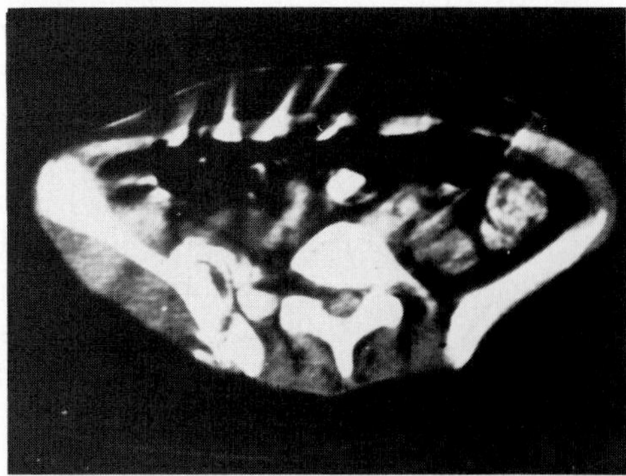

Figure 3-5B.

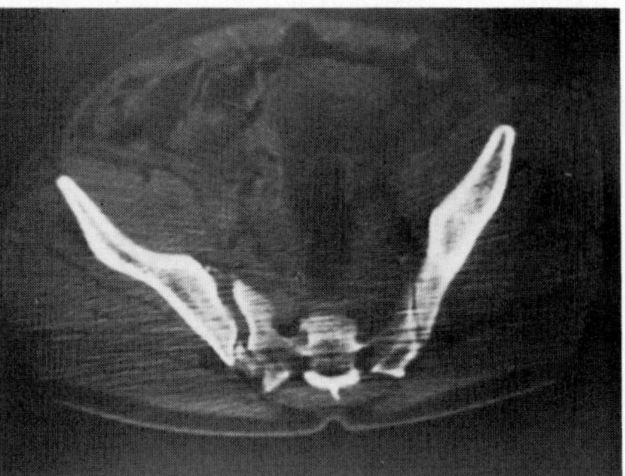

Figure 3-5C.

(Figure 3-6). At present, however, a computed scan of the posterior pelvis is the only reproducible way to confirm the degree of pelvic instability. In the presence of a vertical shearing injury, vertical or posterior displacement of a hemipelvis by more than 1cm indicates complete disruption of the ligamentous structures. Meticulous examination of the conventional radiographs is required; otherwise a vertical migration of the hemipelvis is readily confused with a rotational displacement of the pelvis about the anteroposterior plane (Figure 3-3B). Whenever there is radiological suspicion of a vertical shearing injury, a computed scan of the pelvis is strongly recommended.

## Mechanisms of Acetabular Disruption

Fractures of the acetabulum arise indirectly from an excessive force applied across the hip joint. The provocative force can be imposed upon the greater trochanter, the knee or the foot.[9] Rarely, the provocative force is applied in a reverse fashion, to the back of the pelvis. Fractures of the acetabulum are notorious for

Figure 3-6. Computed scans with examples of bilateral sacroiliac disruptions. A: Bilateral disruptions with stable subluxation on right and unstable dislocation on left. B: Unstable bilateral injuries with right sacroiliac dislocation and fracture dislocation involving the left side of the sacrum.

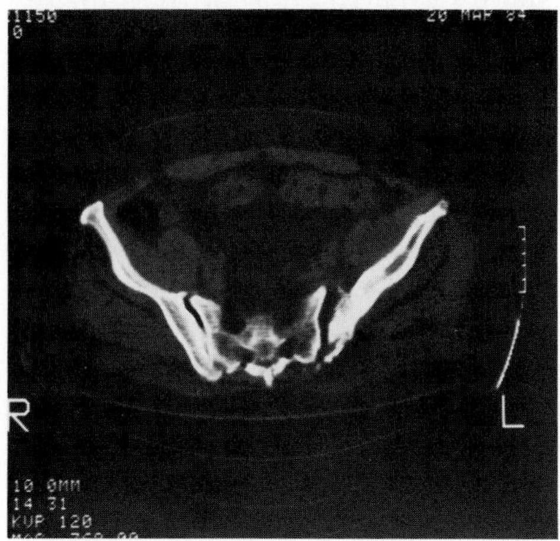


Figure 3-6A.

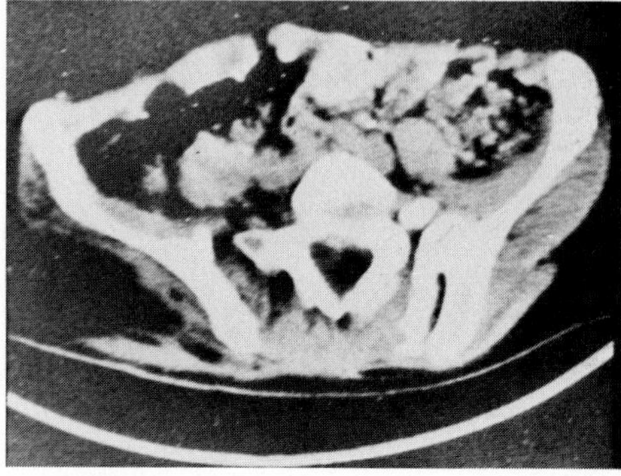

Figure 3-6B.

Figure 3-7. Schematic diagrams of the hip in coronal and horizontal sections. A: Coronal section in 20° internal rotation shows the sites of acetabular impact with variation in abduction-adduction (a—20° adduction of lower limb; b—neutral abduction of femoral neck or 60° abduction of lower limb; c—50° abduction of femoral neck). B: Horizontal section shows the sites of acetabular impact with variation in internal and external rotation (a—25° external rotation provokes an anterior column fracture; b—20° internal rotation provokes a transverse or a both column fracture; c—maximum 50° internal rotation provokes a transverse and posterior wall fracture).

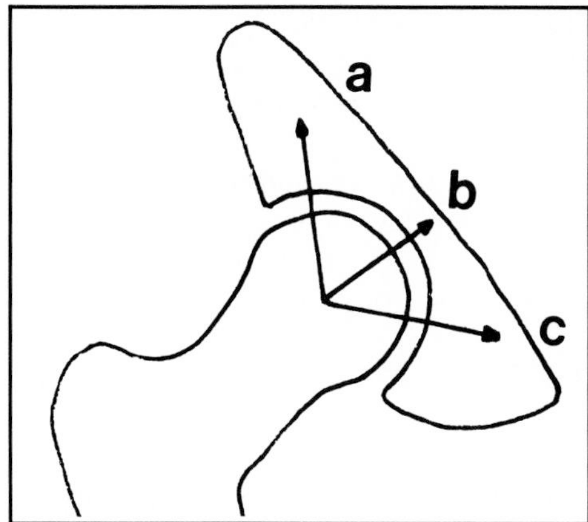


Figure 3-7A.

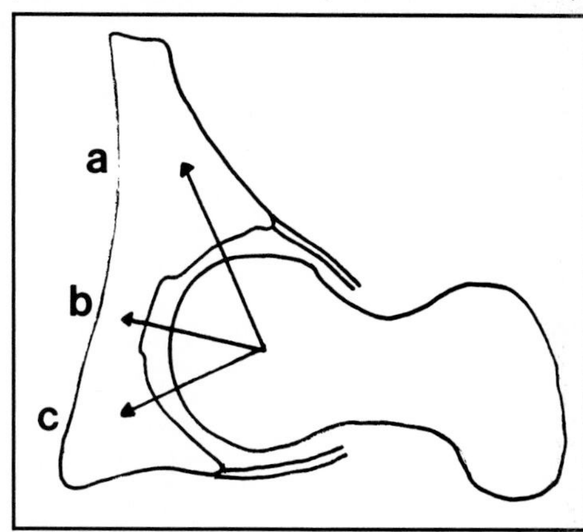


Figure 3-7B.

the great variety of patterns of injury. This variety is related to the vector of the provocative force and the position of the hip at the moment of impact, as well as the magnitude of the force and probably its rate of application. Most of the fractures arise from forces applied directly to the greater trochanter along the axis of the femoral neck. The point of impact of the femoral head against the acetabulum is determined largely by the degree of abduction or rotation of the femur and minimally by the degree of flexion (Figure 3-7). In a clinical study,[9] Letournel has examined the correlation between the range of external and internal rotation of the hip with neutral abduction-adduction. Throughout the range of external-internal rotation of the hip, the site of impact resides along the line of latitude of 30° to 40°. The specific site is determined by the direction of the femoral neck and is largely referrable to the degree of femoral anteversion. In neutral rotation given a normal degree of femoral anteversion, the force is transmitted to the region between the cotyloid fossa and the anterior horn of the acetabulum. The fracture site focuses upon the center of the acetabulum and the anterior column. When the hip is positioned with about 25° of external rotation, the impact impinges upon the anterior column. With extreme external rotation of 40° to 50°, the force is dissipated along the anterior acetabular wall. With internal rotation progressing to about 20°, the site of principal impact is shared by both columns to create a simple transverse fracture, a "T" fracture, or a both-column fracture. With extreme internal rotation of 50° the impact focuses upon the junction between the cotyloid fossa and a posterior articular horn. A posterior column fracture ensues that is associated with a partial or complete transverse fracture.

Letournel[10] extended this thesis to account for positions of abduction and adduction of the hip. With a position of 20° of internal rotation and neutral abduction-adduction, the focus of the impact is the inner margin of the acetabular roof to provoke a transverse or "T" fracture or a both-column fracture. As the degree of adduction increases, the impact primarily affects the roof of the acetabulum to create a transverse fracture. With a position of abduction the site of impact shifts progressively more inferior to provoke a transverse fracture below the articular margin of the roof with a horizontal inclination. Inevitably, various combinations of rotation and adduction/abduction could create virtually an infinite array of fracture patterns.

If a force is sustained by the front of the flexed knee, and the hip is also flexed at 90°, the acetabulum may be fractured indirectly. The position of flexion/extension and abduction/adduction largely determines the site of principal impact, although the degree of femoral rotation is relatively noncontributory. In neutral abduction, the posterior wall of the acetabulum receives the principal impact. It is subject to fracture at the time of posterior dislocation of the hip. With about 15° of abduction, the posterior column is the site of injury, whereas with 50° of abduction the posteromedial segment is damaged to create a posterior column fracture with likely extension as a transverse fracture. If the femur is adducted, the posterior margin of the acetabulum is the principal site of impact, creating a posterior dislocation with or without a wall fracture.

As the degree of hip flexion increases, the inferior portion of the posterior wall is fractured with or without extension to the upper pole of the ischial tuberosity. As the degree of hip flexion drops below 90°, the posterosuperior portion of the acetabulum is affected.

Frequently, another mechanism of injury is encountered during a frontal collision of a car, when the provocative force is transmitted through the brake pedal to the foot, across the extended knee, to the hip joint. If the hip is in neutral or slight adduction, a posterosuperior wall fracture ensues, with or without a supplementary transverse component.

More recently, Lansinger has undertaken a biomechanical study[11] as a fracture analysis on 24 isolated cadaveric pelves subjected to a force directed towards the greater trochanter. The orientation and magnitude of the force were correlated with the pattern of the acetabular fracture in 44 specimens. While some experimental difficulties were encountered, when a force greater than 480Nm was applied either a transverse or a "T" fracture was produced. The results appear to confirm the clinically derived observations of Letournel. In a somewhat similar way, Waller produced posterior acetabular fractures on a cadaveric model.

### *Acetabular Impaction*

In addition to the degree of comminution and displacement, another variable feature of an acetabular injury is impaction of the articular surface into the underlying cancellous bone.[9] This mechanism of injury may accompany a posterior wall fracture or a central acetabular disruption. Presumably the propensity for impaction correlates with the degree of osteoporosis of the subchondral bone. The zone of impaction is readily perceived on a computed scan, although it is easily overlooked during the scrutiny of a conventional radiograph. Displacement of the fracture fragment can exist immediately adjacent to a zone of marginal impaction. Clearly a substantially different technique is required to reduce the impacted articular zone as opposed to the technique for reduction of a displaced fragment. At the moment of impact as the femoral head strikes the acetabulum, it also is liable to deformation by impaction. In the current absence of an effective technique to restore the sphericity of the femoral head, the prognosis for the hip joint is markedly compromised.

## Biomechanics of Pelvic Fixation

During the past decade as the restoration of pelvic stability by resort to internal and external fixation has surged in popularity, an increasing need has arisen for biomechanical observations to confirm the degree to which pelvic stability can be restored by the application of various therapeutic methods. Particularly with the several versatile external skeletal fixation systems, numerous different configurations of frame can be assembled with widely differing capabilities to restore pelvic stability. A similar problem also has arisen with respect to various techniques of internal fixation. For applications of internal and external fixation to long bones the main structural parameters have been examined meticulously by many investigators. In 1978, Gunterberg et al[12] published cadaveric biomechanical tests that assessed the optimal stability that could be achieved by the use of the Slatis pelvic frame. Shortly afterwards in Pittsburgh a biomechanical evaluation of pelvic stability achieved by the application of techniques of external and internal fixation was initiated.[13,14] The biomechanical analysis was complemented by a clinical program that confirmed the underlying hypotheses and the validity of the novel therapeutic methods.[15,16] More recently, McBroom and Tile[17] undertook comparable experiments in Toronto that largely confirmed the results accrued in Pittsburgh. The underlying biomechanical studies referable to external and subsequent internal fixation of the pelvis are now described.

## External Fixation

The classic biomechanical characterization of certain parameters of external fixation for application to long bones was undertaken by Vidal,[18] Chao,[19] and Boltze et al.[20] Subsequently, Carabalona et al[21] employed a somewhat similar experimental protocol to assess the stability of a pelvic ring immobilized by a variety of single bar and quadrilateral frames. In either iliac crest of a cadaveric pelvis, a cluster of three 4mm half-pins was inserted into the bone and anchored to the external quadrilateral frame. Then the frame was manipulated to apply a compressive force upon the anterior part of the pelvic ring. Electromagnetic measurements of the compressive forces documented at the symphysis pubis and the sacroiliac joint of a simulated pelvic disruption were reported for the various configurations of external frames. In another study on a disarticulated cadaveric pelvis,[22] Gunterberg, Goldie and Slatis analyzed the amount of load imposed upon a variety of pelvic fracture-dislocations stabilized by a trapezoidal compression frame. The ischial tuberosities and the inferior pubic rami of the specimens were immobilized in two epoxy blocks with the pelvis positioned in a simulated upright stance. The maximum accepted load was recorded for a variety of fractures and compared to a hypothetical physiological load exerted upon the lumbar vertebrae in a standing position. In their experimental model with fresh male cadaveric pelves, anterior and posterior dislocations were created by transsection of the symphysis pubis and a sacroiliac joint. The two halves of the pelvis were restored with either a single transverse compression frame or a trapezoidal compression frame. The frames were inclined at 70° or 120° with respect to the long axis of the body. Compression at the sacroiliac joint and symphysis pubis was measured by the use of a mercury monometer. Inadequate stability of the pelvis was documented when a single transverse compression bar was employed. In their initial observations a trapezoidal compression frame mounted at 70° with respect to the long axis of the body afforded good stability to the cadaveric pelves. The compressive force appeared to be applied to the sacroiliac joint instead of the symphysis pubis. For a unilateral sacroiliac joint disruption with a diastasis of the symphysis pubis, stabilization with a trapezoidal frame provided adequate resistance to excessive deformation of the joints under the imposition of a load that was calculated to be twice that applied to an intact pelvis in an upright standing position. A comparable degree of stability was documented for experimental osseous disruptions of the sacrum or ilium and the ipsilateral pubic rami. The stability was greatly compromised, however, when bilateral sacral or iliac fractures or bilateral sacroiliac dislocations occurred in combination with a disruption of the symphysis pubis or two ipsilateral rami. A review of the experimental data indicated that the external trapezoidal compression frame provided adequate stability of the pelvic girdle to withstand a surprisingly large vertical load. This data pertained to the pelvic disruption when an absolutely accurate anatomical reduction was achieved prior to the application of the external frame. In clinical practice where a closed reduction of the pelvis is undertaken, an absolutely anatomical reduction of a displaced sacroiliac joint associated with a displaced lateral compression or vertical shear injury is rarely achieved.

Subsequently, Slatis[23] reported his clinical experience with 22 patients in whom a double vertical fracture of the pelvis was managed by the application of a trapezoidal frame. In each case, weight bearing was initiated three weeks after the accident and removal of the frame was undertaken six weeks after injury. No loss of reduction was observed at any time after the application of a frame. In a more recent report on the management of comparable cases, however, Slatis[24] documented a 50% incidence of migration of a hemipelvis following the initiation of weightbearing gait. Other workers[17] reported comparable unfavorable observations. A reappraisal of the biomechanics of pelvic stabilization, therefore, appeared to be needed. An appropriate laboratory biomechanical model was required that would permit accurate quantitative assessment of the degree of pelvic stabilization that had been achieved by the application of various techniques of external and internal fixation. The methods employed for the Pittsburgh study are now described.[13,14]

### Method

With the unique degree of geometrical complexity of the pelvis, and the difficulty in posing rational interface conditions at irregular disruption sites, the biomechanical study of pelvic fracture stabilization was undertaken experimentally, rather than analytically. For the injury model, a Malgaigne fracture[3] with dislocations of one sacroiliac joint and the symphysis pubis was selected. This injury was created reproducibly by means of sharp dissection in a series of 17 fresh unembalmed cadaveric pelves. The test specimens were removed from male decedents less than 65 years of age who expired from causes not affecting the skeletal system. For the experimental models all of the ligamentous structures bridging the dislocation sites were removed (Figure 3-8). After mounting in an Instron unit, a specimen was subjected to quasistatic (1.27cm/min) longitudinal compressive loading across the sacroiliac joint, supplied by constant cross-head motion. The active muscular loading of the pelvis that normally would occur in a convalescent trauma patient was not included in the model. Special fixtures were constructed to allow examination of each pelvis under support conditions characteristic of both standing and sitting postures. For the standing case (Figure 3-9), the applied load was transferred through the neutrally-extended hip joints to the proximal femora. The femora were potted in separate epoxy blocks that rested freely upon the Instron base. For the seated case, the epoxy-potted femora were flexed beyond 90°, so that the nonpotted ischial tuberosities rested directly upon the Instron base.

Load-induced shearing displacements occurring along each of the fracture sites were continuously recorded using noncontacting variable impedence transducers (Multi-VIT Model KD 2300-8C, Kaman Sciences Corp., Colorado Springs, Colorado) (Figure 3-10). At each fracture site, the element of the transducer coil was attached to one side, and the transducer target element to the other side. Malleable copper tubing was contoured so that the shearing displacements occurring at the fracture site resulted in planar axial displacements of the metallic target face relative to the coil. Bench tests

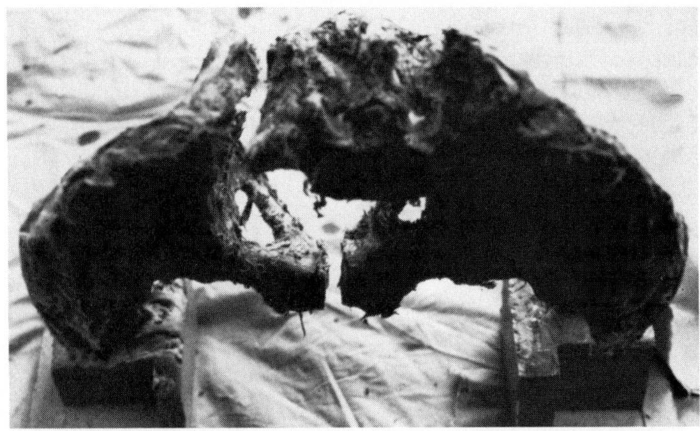

Figure 3-8. A cadaveric model of a Malgaigne fracture with a diastasis of the symphysis and a unilateral sacroiliac dislocation for biomechanical tests.

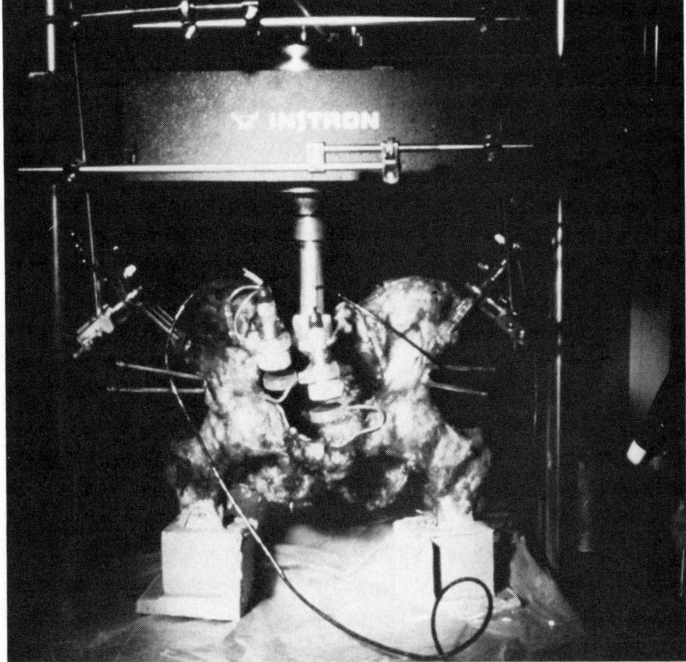


Figure 3-9. A cadaveric pelvis mounted in a standing position for biomechanical testing in an Instron unit.

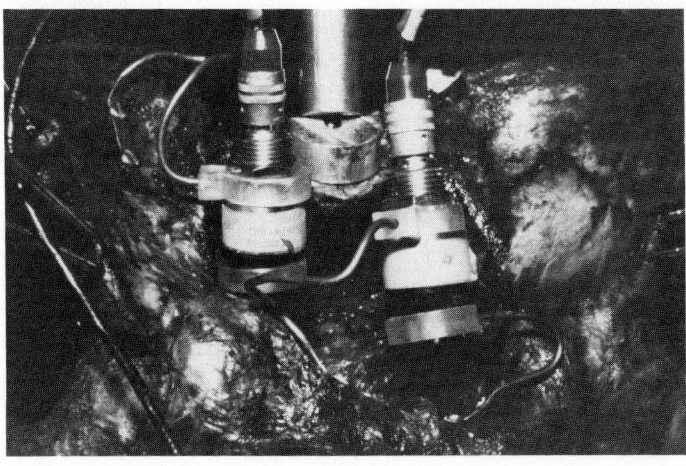

Figure 3-10. A close-up view of the pelvis and transducers.

confirmed a linear transducer output versus axial target displacements of up to 20mm. The magnitude of the output signal was imperceptibly altered for transverse target displacements of less than 8mm. Also, at the instant of peak load acceptance, the magnitude of the transverse diastasis of the symphysis pubis was measured by the use of calipers.

In the preliminary tests the load/displacement behavior of the specimens correlated closely with the frictional characteristics of the distal support interface between the pelvis and the Instron base. The results published previously for the Slatis frame mounted in a seated configuration with the ischial tuberosities potted in epoxy blocks could not be reproduced. In subsequent studies, the stability of the Slatis frame was further compromised when the unpotted tuberosities were positioned directly upon rough metal surfaces, and even more so when the supportive surface was smooth. For minimization of the frictional restraints to lateral movement between the pelvis and its base supports, multiple layers of polyurethane sheets were inserted between the pelvic model and the support. With these experimental alterations, the results reflected the stability afforded solely by the application of the frame itself. A spurious contribution afforded by friction between the potted tuberosities and the testing machine base was eliminated.

Five principal categories of external fixation devices, each with multiple subgroups, were studied. All of the frames were assembled from standard Hoffmann components (Howmedica, Inc., Rutherford, New Jersey). As an experimental control an intact pelvis was examined prior to the surgical creation of a Malgaigne injury. For the second category various frames were constructed by the use of 4mm half-pins. These frames included the conventional Slatis trapezoidal design (Figure 3-11), the Bonnel quadrilateral frame (Figure 3-12) and several novel, complex assemblies including **1)** an uncoupled double anterior frame, essentially two independent Slatis frames constructed with 12 half-pins per pelvis; **2)** a coupled double anterior frame, comprising a three-dimensional box-like assembly anchored to 12 half-pins per pelvis (Figure 3-13); **3)** two separate anterior and posterior quadrilateral frames constructed upon six anterior half-pins and four posterior half-pins; and **4)** two separate frames, as anterior and posterior quadrangular frames attached to the exposed ends of transfixing pins (Figure 3-14).

For the third major category, three frames were constructed upon 5mm half-pins. The configurations under scrutiny included a Slatis frame, a coupled double anterior frame, and a new triangular design for the

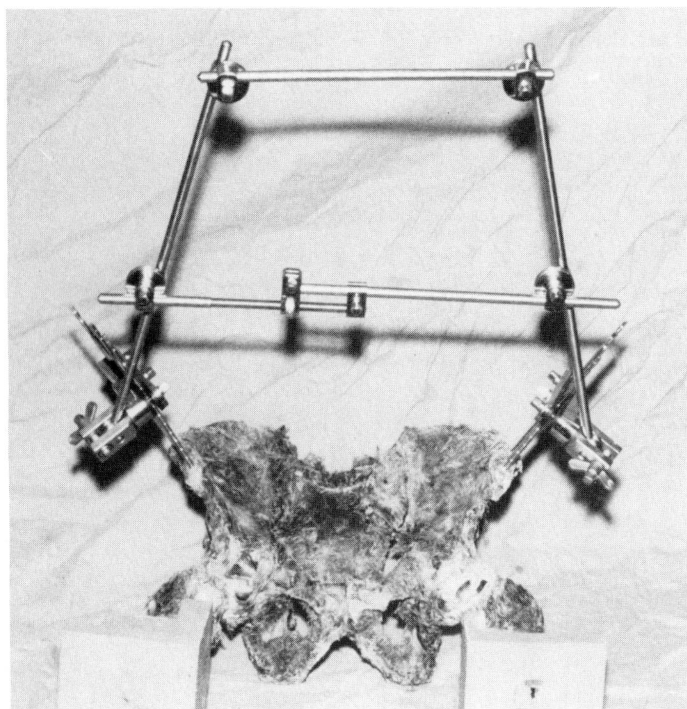

Figure 3-11. A laboratory model of a conventional Slatis frame assembled on 4mm half pins.

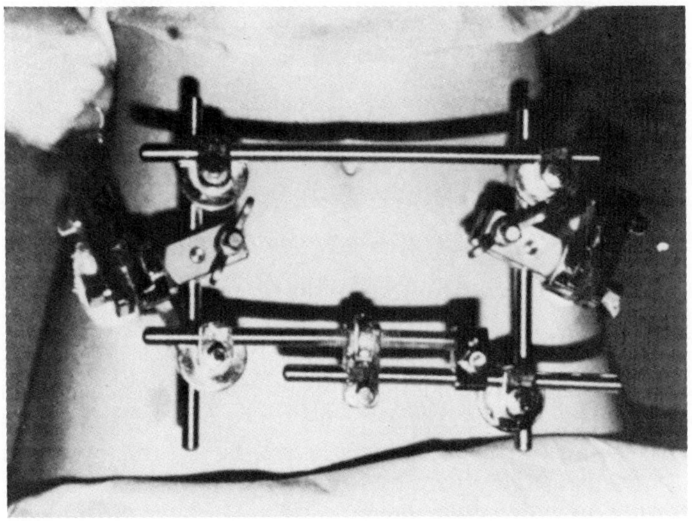

Figure 3-12. A Bonnel type frame is shown on a patient.

conventional Slatis frame. Three standard 4mm half-pins in either hemipelvis were replaced with 5mm half-pins. Likewise, the coupled anterior frame design was reassembled by the use of the larger 5mm half-pins. The stability of the coupled double anterior frame assembly with 12 standard half-pins was compared with that achieved by the use of eight per pelvis (Figure 3-15). Finally, a new assembly, designated the Pittsburgh triangular frame, was studied. The new triangular frame was a modification of the double anterior frame

Figure 3-13. A coupled double quadrilateral frame. A: Anteroposterior view on cadaveric model. B: Iliac oblique view on pelvic model (from HE Rubash and DC Mears[15]).

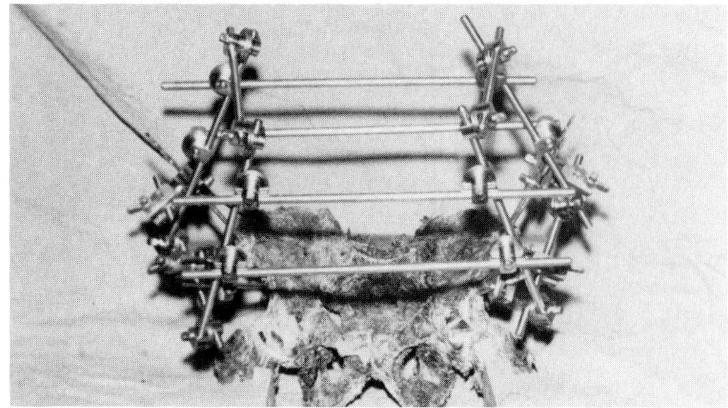

Figure 3-13A.

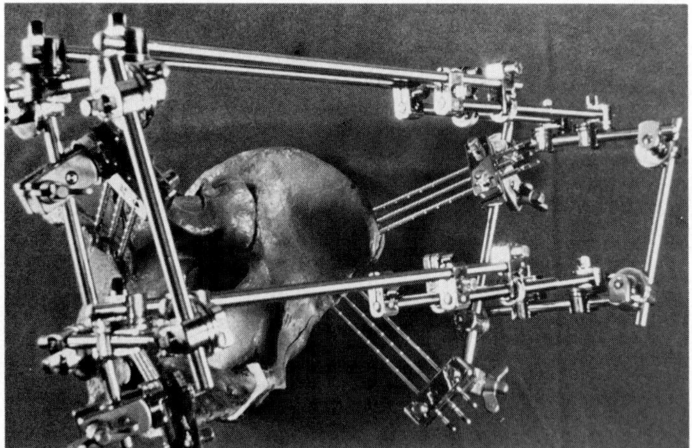

Figure 3-13B.

configuration with substantially fewer components that might provide comparable biomechanical performance (Figure 3-16).

For the fourth major category, anterior external fixation was supplemented by posterior internal fixation. In this group, all of the pelves were stabilized anteriorly by a Slatis frame constructed upon 5mm half-pins. Various types of supplementary posterior fixation were investigated. Initially a DC or a T-plate (Synthes Ltd. (USA), Wayne, Pennsylvania) (Figure 3-17) was applied across the posterior surface of the sacroiliac joint and anchored to the sacrum and ilium by the use of 6.5mm cancellous screws. The cancellous screws did not violate the sacroiliac joint. In a subsequent experiment, three 6.5mm cancellous screws inserted into the lateral ilium provided lag screw fixation of the sacroiliac joint (Figure 3-18). The screws were inserted into a three-hole plate that served as a "washer" in an attempt to augment rotational stability. In a third series of tests, posterior fixation was achieved by a unique "Double Cobra" plate

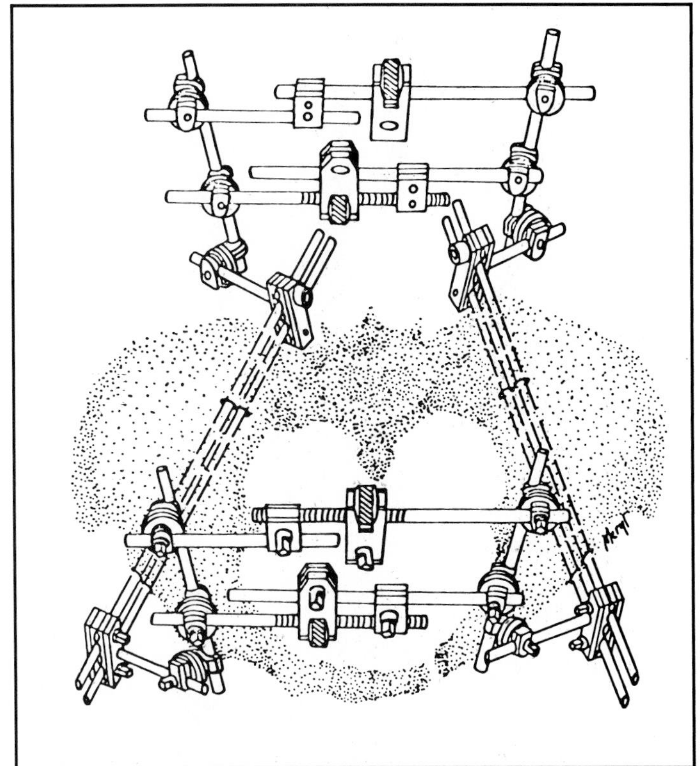

Figure 3-14. Schematic diagram of pelvic fixation achieved by the use of anterior and posterior quadrilateral frames assembled on transfixing pins (from DC Mears: *External Skeletal Fixation.* Baltimore, Williams & Wilkins, 1983).

(Howmedica, Inc., Rutherford, New Jersey), which spanned both of the sacroiliac joints and the posterior ilia (Figures 3-19 and 3-20). Cancellous screws transfixed the sacroiliac joints and supplemented screws inserted through the plate and into the sacrum or ilia. For additional experiments, bilateral sacroiliac dislocations were prepared along with a diastasis of the symphysis pubis. Anterior fixation was provided by a Slatis frame erected upon 5mm half-pins. For posterior fixation a "Double Cobra" plate was applied with cancellous lag screws across both of the sacroiliac joints.

For the fifth and final major category, internal fixation of the pelvic ring was examined. Anterior fixation of the symphysis was realized by application of two plates anchored to the superior and anterior aspects respectively of the superior pubic rami (Figure 3-21). Posterior fixation was provided by either three sacroiliac lag screws across each sacroiliac joint (Figure 3-22), bilateral sacroiliac plates, or a "Double Cobra" plate.

Several types of pelvic fixation were studied in an attempt to compare and contrast the modes of fixation and to identify the optimal methods of pelvic stabilization.

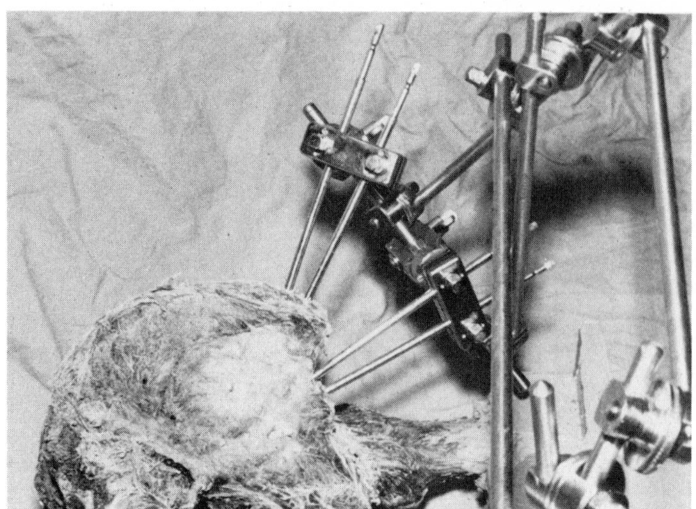

Figure 3-15. The coupled double anterior frame assembly erected on eight 5mm half-pins.

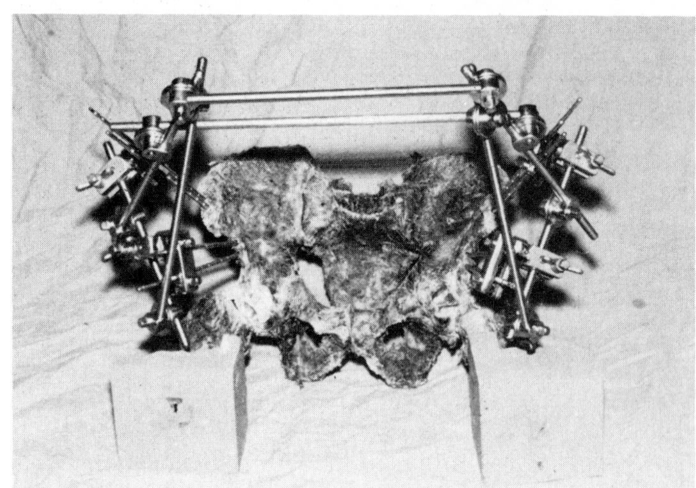

Figure 3-16. The Pittsburgh "triangular" frame.

For all of the experiments, every effort was made to obtain an accurate reduction of the pelvic ring. The two displacement transducer outputs versus the Instron load cell output were displayed on a storage oscilloscope. The data traces were photographed, stylus digitized, reduced to force versus deformation records, and then to fitted polynomial curves to facilitate statistical analysis. The entire series consisted of 1,224 individual runs.

## *Results*

The essential features of a typical load-versus-shear deformation curve are illustrated in Figure 3-23. The basic linear character observed beyond the toe region of the "pure-frame" (i.e. unreduced fracture) curve shown at the left is strongly suggestive of the small deformation bending/torsional behavior of an elastic framework. By contrast, the markedly nonlinear nature of the reduced-

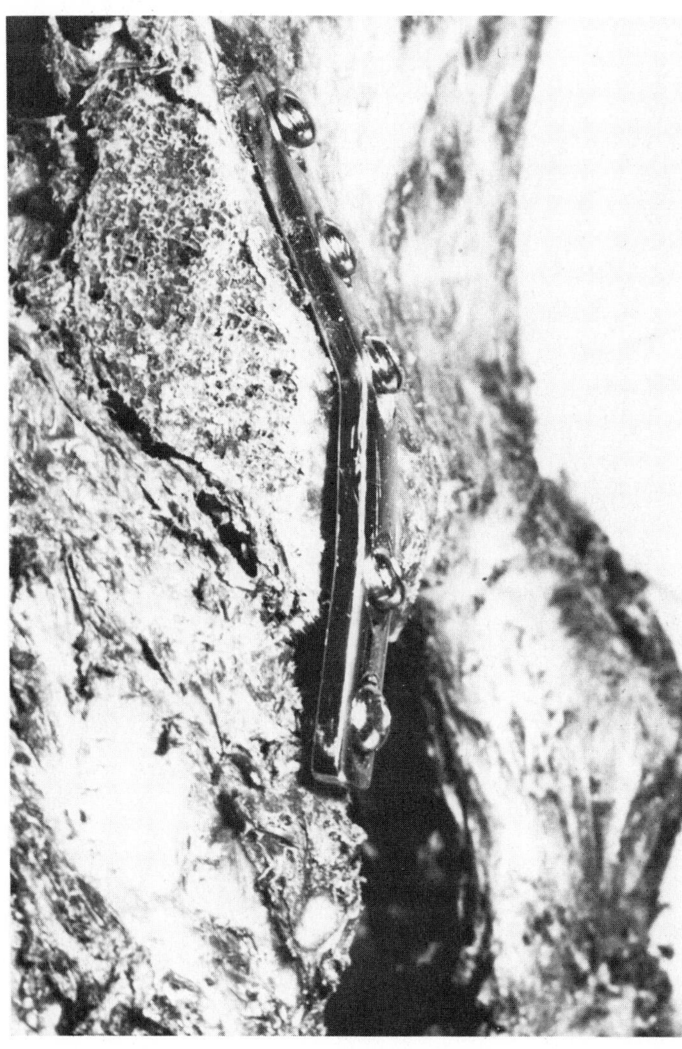

Figure 3-17. A 4.5 DC plate applied across the sacroiliac joint is shown.

fracture curve shown at the right is attributable to friction and interlock effects of the joint surfaces at the fracture sites in the initially horizontal segment. In this case the overall joint slippage was minimal and the load uptake was quite rapid. A region of rapidly and progressively reducing overall stiffness characterized by appreciable (0.5mm) slippage at the fracture site followed. In many instances, the specimens passed through a negative stiffness or "recoil" regime. In most tests, the effective stiffness diminished to a point where the specimen essentially exhibited "free-slip." Ultimately, a region of subsequent re-stiffening to levels approximately those of the corresponding unreduced-fracture case generally followed. The tests were terminated either when a near-physiological load level (800N) was developed at the sacrum, or when a clinically unacceptable degree of shear deformation (greater than 15mm) had been documented either at the symphysis pubis or, more commonly, at

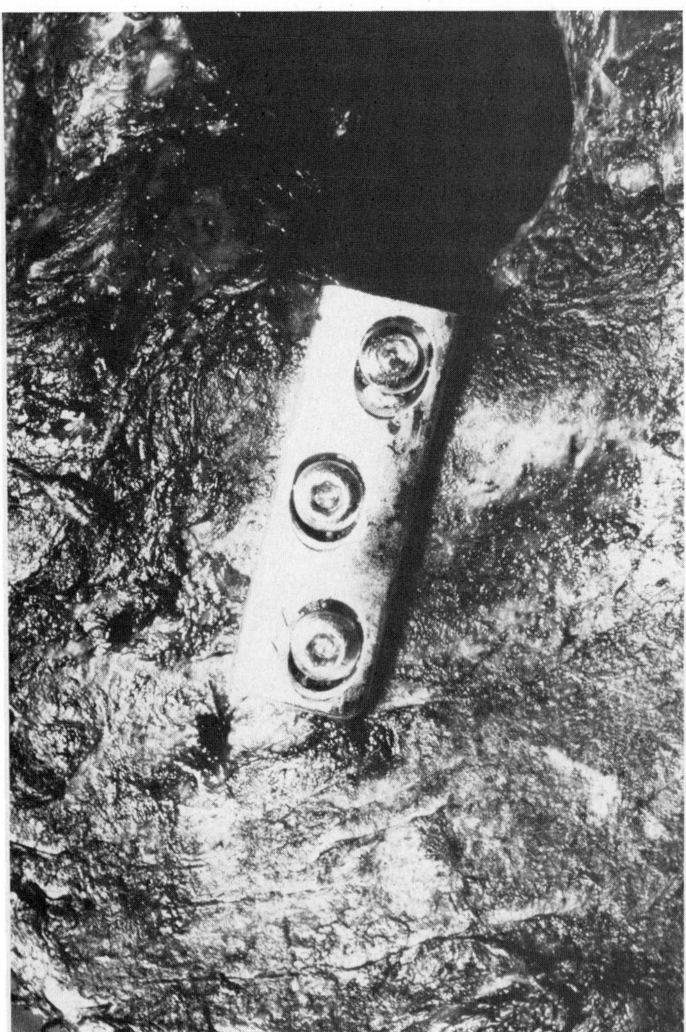

Figure 3-18. Posterior fixation with the use of three cancellous lag screws inserted through a three-hole plate, which serves as a washer.

the sacroiliac joint. The relative rigidity of fracture reduction achievable with the various frames was characterized by the load necessary to induce 0.5mm shear slippage at the dislocation sites (slip load), and by the load that provokes frank loss of reduction with greater than 15mm of shear slippage (fail load). These values are documented in Figures 3-24 to 3-30.

## Discussion

**Frames Constructed Upon 4mm Half-Pins.** Slatis and his colleagues[25,26] reported generally favorable results with adequate stabilization when their trapezoid frame design was applied to a wide variety of stable and unstable pelvic fractures. Due to their use of potted ischial tuberosities in biomechanical testing, however, their measured frame rigidity values were substantially higher and overly optimistic compared to the more clinically

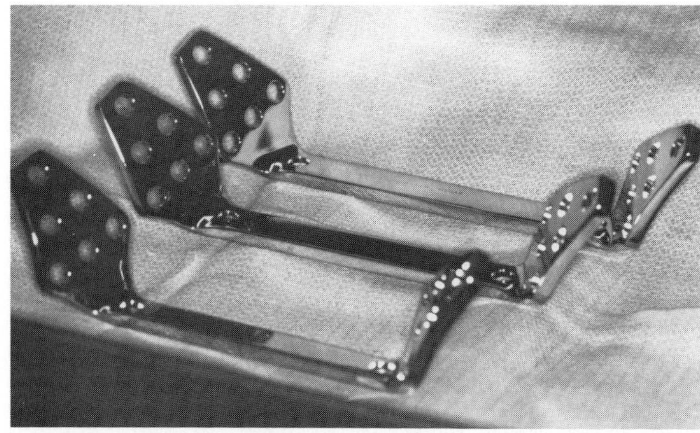

Figure 3-19. Three of the available sizes of the Double Cobra plate. (from HE Rubash and DC Mears[15]).

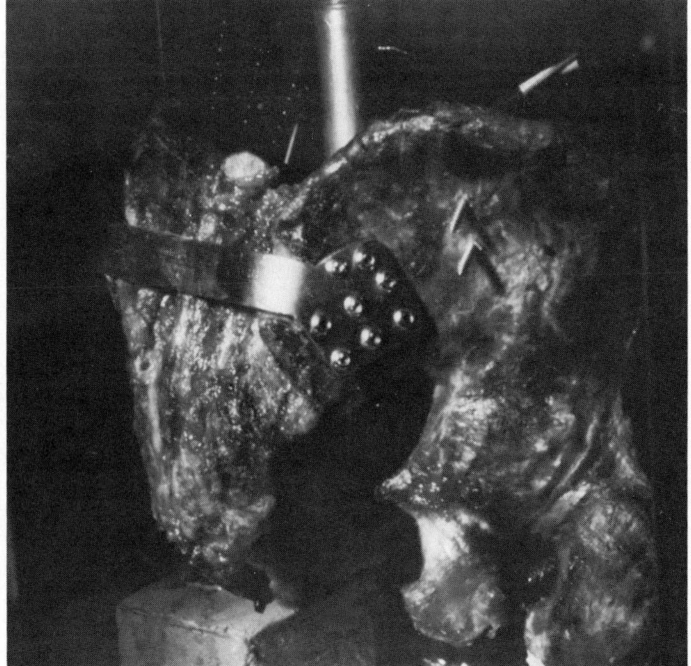

Figure 3-20. A Double Cobra plate applied to a pelvic fracture model.

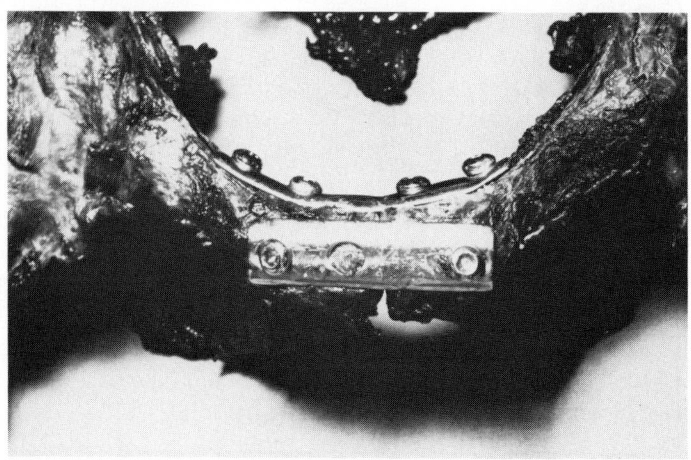

Figure 3-21. Fixation of symphysis pubis with two plates.

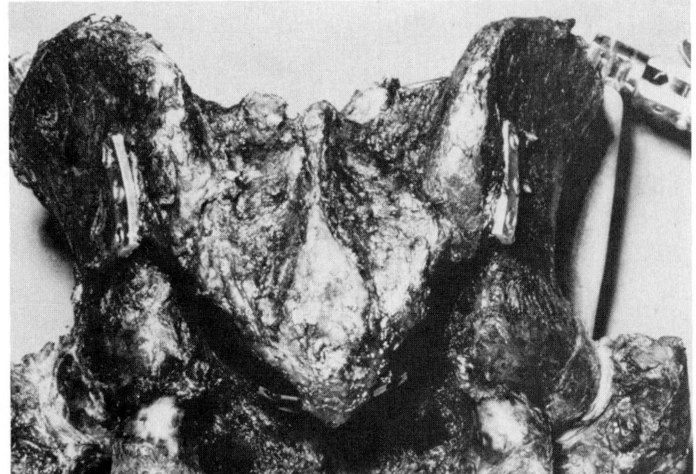

Figure 3-22. Bilateral stabilization of the sacroiliac joints with 6.5mm cancellous screws inserted through short plates serving as washers.

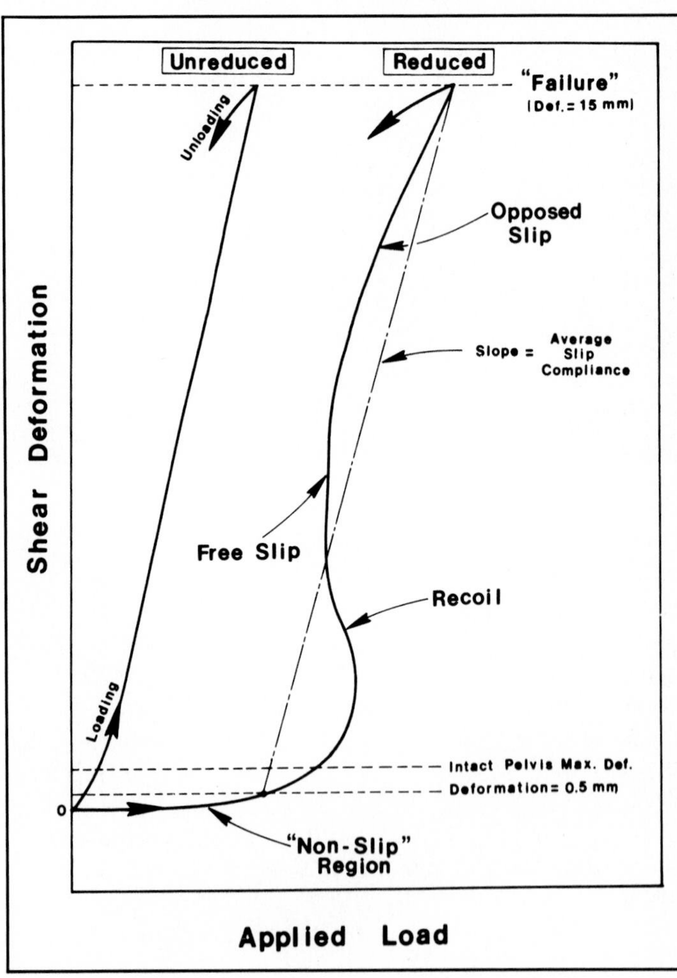


Figure 3-23. A typical load versus shear deformation curve (from TD Brown et al[13]).

Figure 3-24 A, B. Slip load versus fixation of pelves mounted in the seated and standing configurations. Initially, the sacroiliac joint usually slipped prior to the symphysis pubis. Only for combined anterior and posterior fixation methods was the difference in sacroiliac and symphysis slip loads statistically significant ($P<.001$) by the paired T-test. The results indicate three levels of pelvic stability afforded by simple and complex anterior frames and by supplementary posterior fixation respectively. The posterior fixation achieved by the use of transfixing pins, separate anterior and posterior half-pins, or posterior T-plate are about equal. (From TD Brown et al.[13])

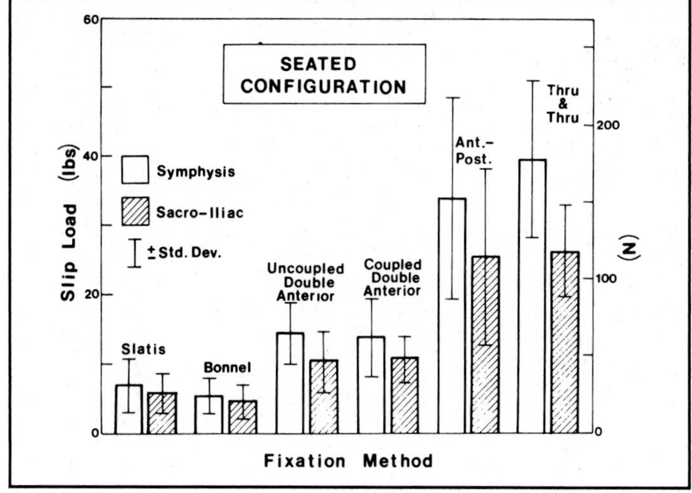


Figure 3-24A.

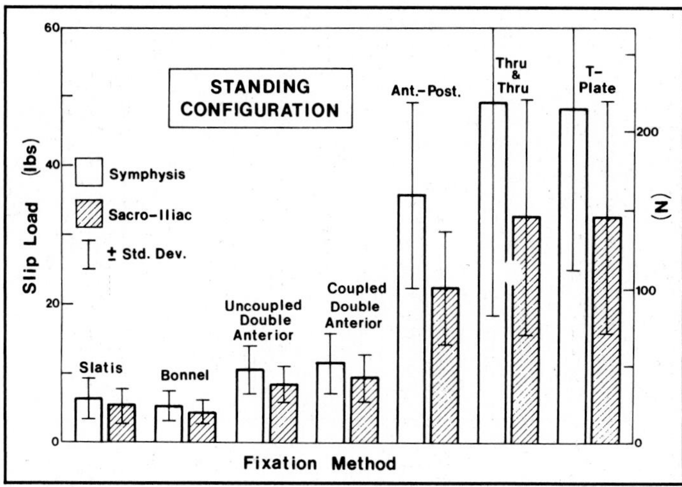


Figure 3-24B.

representative values that were recorded when the frictional effects between the test specimen and the loading machine support base were deliberately eliminated in the Pittsburgh tests.

Stability measurements of the Bonnel frame compare favorably to the loading data accrued for the Slatis frame (Figures 3-24 and 3-25). While the proponents[21,22] of various frame designs have attributed extraordinary mechanical properties to their unique geometries of

Figure 3-25 A, B. Failure load versus fixation method for the seated and standing configurations. For cases in which the failure criteria of 15mm of shearing displacement at the dislocation sites was not achieved, the failure load was defined as 800N. The variations among the four fixation groups (single anterior, double anterior, anterior and posterior frames and anterior frame with posterior plate) are all statistically significant (P<.001). (Reproduced with permission from TD Brown et al.[13])

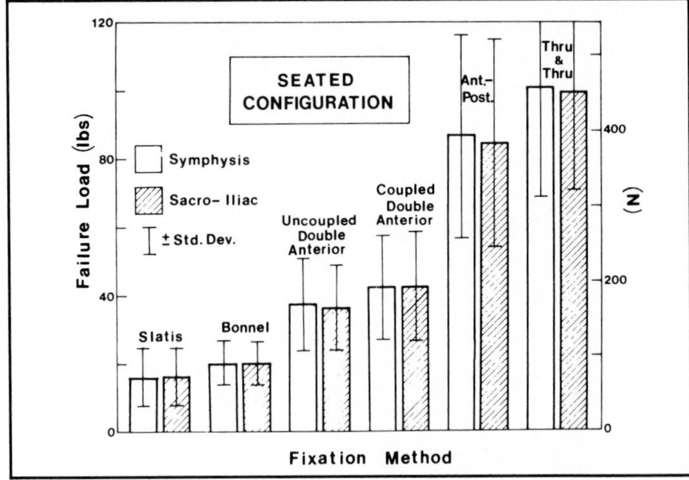


Figure 3-25A.

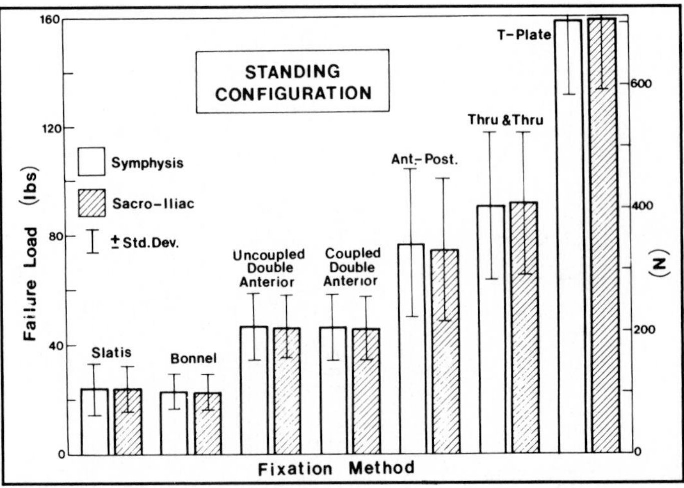


Figure 3-25B.

various frames, the recent study documented comparable low rigidity for the several designs. For a potentially improved variant of the Slatis frame in which a second Slatis frame is anchored by a second set of pins to the anterior inferior iliac spines, the mechanical rigidity afforded by this "uncoupled double anterior frame" was approximately twice that provided by a single Slatis frame. A modification of the double anterior frame was tested in which the two Slatis frames were coupled by four crossbars to create a box-like anterior frame assembly. The coupling did not augment the loading characteristics

Figure 3-26 A, B. Bar graphs to compare the slip and failure loads for the various fixation techniques.

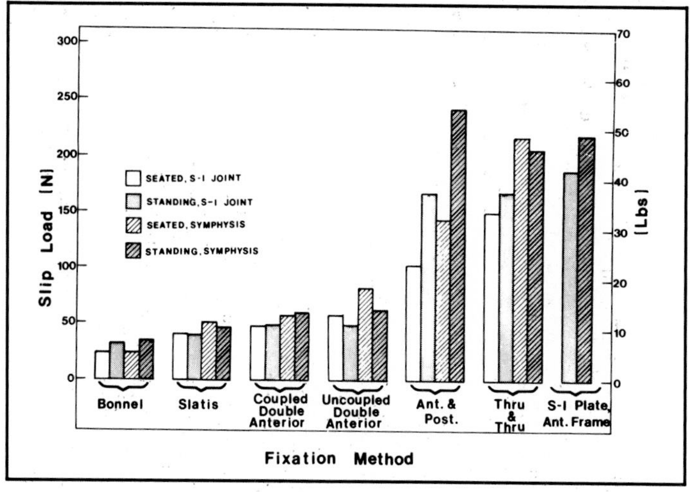


Figure 3-26A.

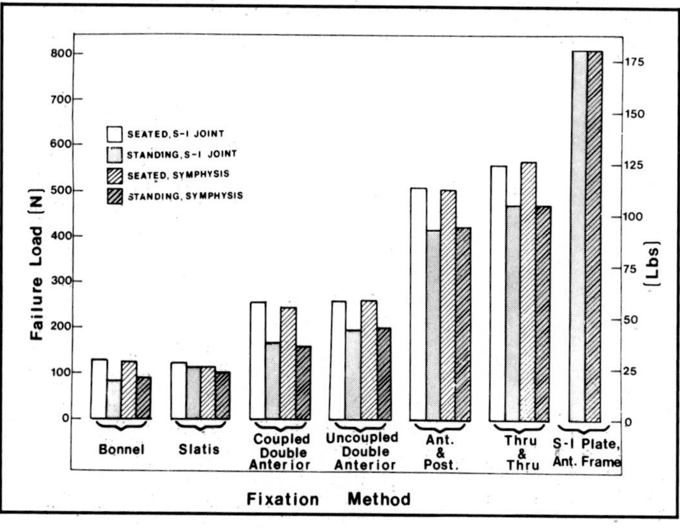


Figure 3-26B.

of the two independent Slatis frames. The initial studies confirmed the need for more radical changes in the frame configuration if a substantial improvement in pelvic stability was to be achieved.

One such modification in frame design was the use of two separate frames anchored to the anterior and posterior aspects of the pelvis, respectively. From the biomechanical data, the rigidity of the novel design was four times that achieved by the use of the original Slatis design, and twice that attained by the use of the coupled double anterior frame. Next the two separate sets of threaded half-pins were replaced by a single set of transfixing pins, and identical anterior and posterior frames were constructed. Now a pelvic stability five times that provided by the Slatis design and $2^1/_2$ times that

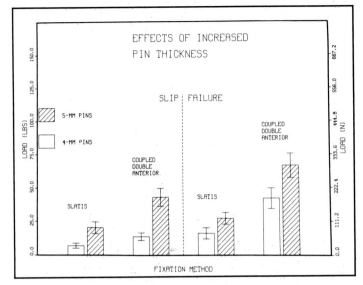

Figure 3-27. Bar graph display of the slip and failure loads for a Slatis and coupled double anterior frames erected upon 4mm and 5mm pins. The variations among the fixator groups are all statistically significant (P<.001). (From HE Rubash et al.[14])

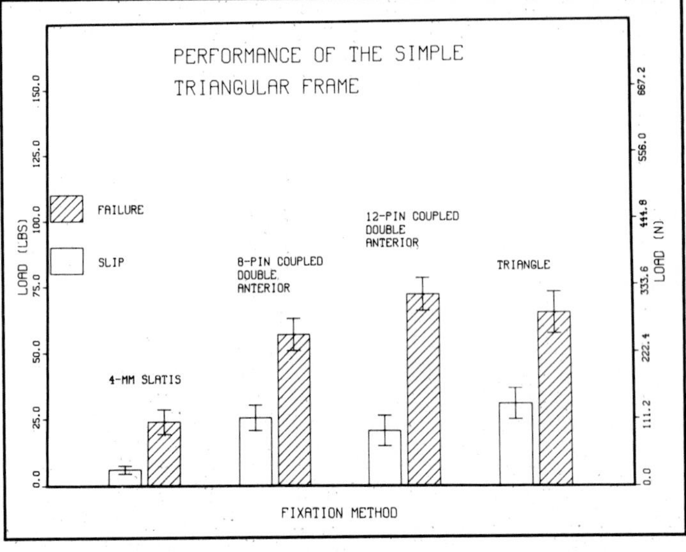


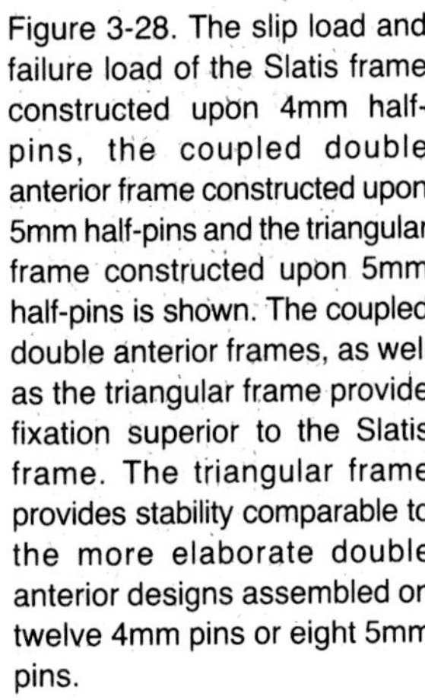

Figure 3-28. The slip load and failure load of the Slatis frame constructed upon 4mm half-pins, the coupled double anterior frame constructed upon 5mm half-pins and the triangular frame constructed upon 5mm half-pins is shown. The coupled double anterior frames, as well as the triangular frame provide fixation superior to the Slatis frame. The triangular frame provides stability comparable to the more elaborate double anterior designs assembled on twelve 4mm pins or eight 5mm pins.

of the double anterior frame was recorded. Clearly, as anticipated, supplementary posterior stabilization provided a great improvement in pelvic rigidity. In five clinical cases transfixing pins were inserted by the use of a special elaborate drill guide employed to pre-drill the pelvis accurately (Figure 3-31). While the anterior and posterior frames provided sufficient stability to maintain the reductions of unstable pelvic fractures, the use of posterior pelvic external fixation possessed substantial clinical liabilities associated with the patient discomfort of the recumbent individual and difficulties in nursing care. A special split or slotted mattress was necessary so that the patient could be turned in bed. Nevertheless the satisfactory mechanical performance

Figure 3-29, A: A comparison of the slip and failure loads of the triangular frame, T-plate with Slatis frame, and longitudinal posterior plate with an isolated Slatis frame. The posterior supplementary fixation greatly improves the optimal anterior fixation afforded by a triangular frame. B: A simplified comparison of the pelvic stability provided by a Slatis frame (S), a triangular frame (▲), and a Slatis frame with posterior lag screws (E/I) (from DC Mears[16]).

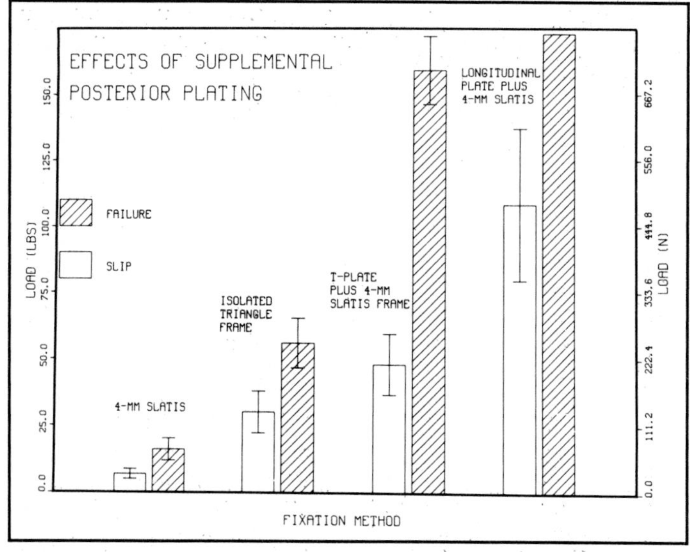


Figure 3-29A.

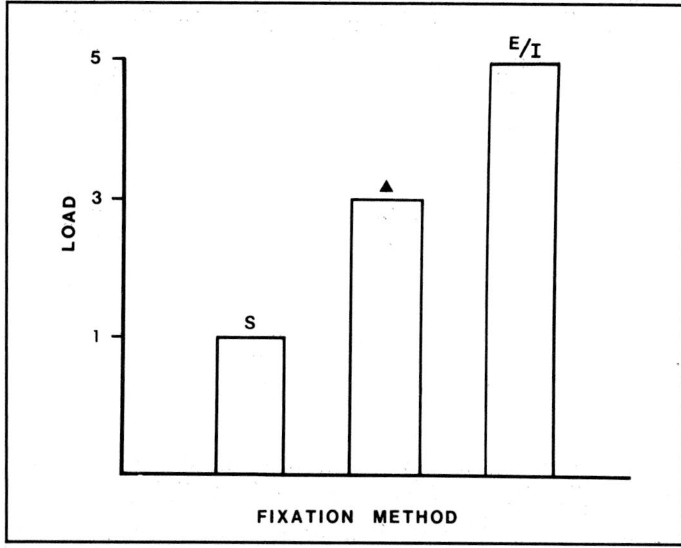


Figure 3-29B.

of this method provided insight for the subsequent investigations in the role of supplementary posterior internal fixation.

**Frames Constructed Upon 5mm Half-Pins.** In their investigations of the mechanical characteristics of external fixation applied to long bones, Chao[19] and other

Figure 3-30. A: The slip and failure loads for combinations of internal and external pelvic fixation are compared. Anterior external fixation refers to the use of a Slatis frame, whereas anterior internal fixation refers to the use of double plates. The posterior fixation was provided by lag screws or a double Cobra plate. The variations in the stability achieved by the five techniques were not statistically significant. B: A simplified comparison of the pelvic stability provided by a triangular frame (▲), a Slatis frame with posterior lag screws (E/I), anterior and posterior internal fixation (I), and the intact pelvic ring (P) (from DC Mears[16]).

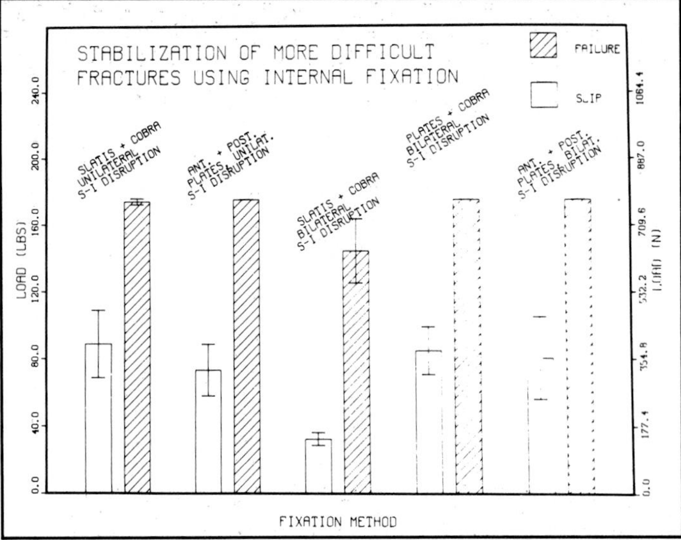


Figure 3-30A.

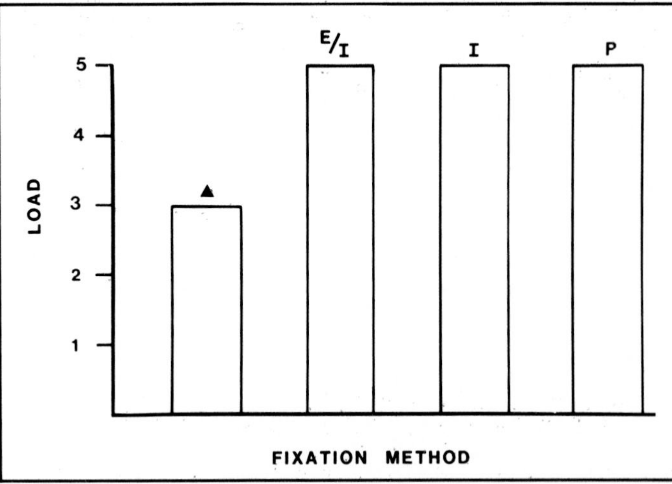


Figure 3-30B.

workers[20] characterized the attributes of the crucial pin-bone interface that provided the optimal stabilization. The degree of stability attained by an external frame correlates with the diameter and number of the fixation pins and to the spacing between the pins. As the diameter and the number of pins is increased along with the distance between adjacent pins, the stability of a frame is augmented. Pins inserted with oblique orientation

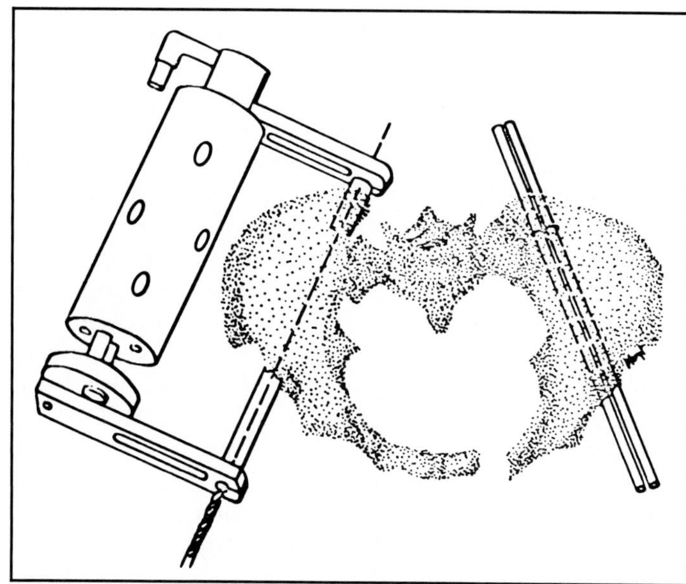

Figure 3-31. A special drill guide (Jaquet Freres, Geneva, Switzerland) used to provide a safe technique for the insertion of transfixing iliac pins (from DC Mears: *External Skeletal Fixation.* Baltimore, Williams & Wilkins, 1983).

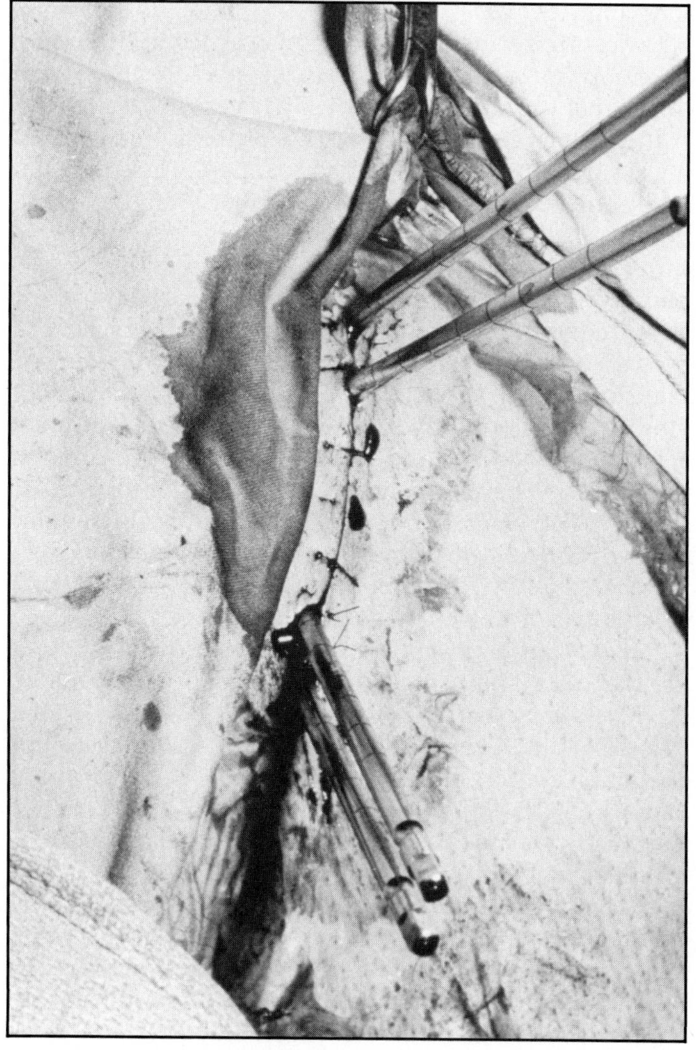

Figure 3-32. A clinical example of the four ipsilateral pelvic pins employed for a triangular frame. The wide spacing between the most superior and inferior pins is evident, along with the obliquity of the superior and inferior pin clusters. Both of these features augment the stability of the frame.

provide superior stability compared with pins inserted in parallel array.

For the Pittsburgh study, these known parameters were explored as a means to achieve superior pelvic stability. One example was the application of threaded half-pins of progressively larger diameters, up to 6mm outside diameter. In several instances, the 6mm pins rivaled the thickness of the cadaveric iliac crest, or during their insertion they cleaved the inner from the outer pelvic tables to compromise the fixation. In the typical adult, the optimal diameter of the threaded pin was 5mm, although in some small women 4mm pins were the largest that could be effectively employed. For the subsequent experiments the various frames were erected upon 5mm pins. When the original Slatis frame erected upon 4mm pins was compared with the variation based upon the 5mm half-pins, the 5mm design showed a slip load value of approximately 2.2 times that of the 4mm design, as well as a modest increase of 35% in the failure load (Figure 3-27).

The coupled anterior frame was constructed with twelve 4mm or 5mm pins. When these two designs were compared, the latter showed a slip load of 3.1 times that of the former and a failure load 1.6 times greater than the former (Figure 3-28). Clearly, substantial benefits were achieved with the use of the larger 5mm half-pins. In a comparison of the coupled double anterior frame with twelve or eight 5mm pins, the data for these two designs (Figure 3-28) showed no statistically significant advantage for the use of 12 pins. This observation is consistent with the results by Chao et al[19] who showed that the spacing of the most remote pins in a cluster of pins is far more important for the transmission of bending moments than the absolute number of pins in the cluster. The use of the anterior inferior spines for the insertion of a second set of half-pins to complement those in the anterior superior spines provided a way to increase stability by extending the space between the most superior and inferior pins (Figure 3-32).

The triangular configuration demonstrated a mechanical stability comparable to that provided by the far more complicated coupled double anterior frame (Figure 3-28). The triangular frame possessed a slip-load stabilization about 6.5 times that of the original Slatis frame, and a failure load about 2.8 times that of the Slatis frame. This substantial improvement in stability is achieved despite a marked decrease in the complexity and cost of the frame. Undoubtedly, the change in orientation of the two sets of ipsilateral pins, the rotational stability provided by the triangular configuration, and the compact nature of the final frame contributed to the improvement in stability.

**Anterior External Fixation With Posterior Internal Fixation.** In the initial attempts to provide posterior internal fixation with the use of a T-plate across the sacroiliac joint no lag screws were used (Figure 3-17). Nevertheless, by a combination of the posterior T-plate and the original anterior Slatis frame, the slip load and failure loads were increased by factors of eight and ten times, respectively, above the figures recorded for the isolated Slatis frame (Figure 3-29). When the use of the posterior T-plate and Slatis frame is compared to the isolated triangular frame applied to a comparable pelvic disruption, the former shows a slip load about 3.8 times greater than the triangular frame, and a failure load about 3.2 times greater than the triangular frame. Clearly, the supplementary posterior internal fixation provides a much greater contribution to pelvic stabilization than does the use of an isolated anterior frame of even the optimal configuration.

When a Slatis frame was combined with three 6.5mm cancellous lag screws and a posterior longitudinal plate for a "washer," the slip load approximated 300N. Even when an 800N load was applied, there was no ultimate failure of the pelvic ring (Figure 3-22). This extraordinary improvement in stability confirmed the role of a posterior plate to resist rotational motion of the screws and the importance of the cancellous lag screw technique. While the triangular frame has been confirmed by clinical assessment to possess adequate stabilization for an unstable unilateral sacroiliac disruption with an anterior disruption, nevertheless, supplementary posterior lag screw fixation provides far superior mechanical attributes.

**The Use of the Slatis Anterior Frame With a Posterior Double Cobra Plate for a Unilateral Sacroiliac Disruption.** During the development of the Double Cobra plate, cadaveric measurements indicated substantial variation in the width of the sacrum and posterior pelvis (Figure 3-19). Ultimately, the plate was fabricated in six sizes, differing in the width of the central portion. A biomechanical assessment of the plate was undertaken prior to the fabrication of the full complement of sizes. The slip loads and failure loads documented when the Double Cobra plate was used to immobilize a unilateral sacroiliac dislocation with a diastasis of the symphysis pubis approximately equaled the results obtained by the use of a Slatis frame with lag screws across the sacroiliac joint. However, superior mechanical performance of the Double Cobra plate would have been anticipated if the full complement of sizes of the plate had been available at the time of the laboratory tests (Figures 3-20 and 3-30). The Double Cobra plate was applied with use of cancellous lag screw fixation across the sacroiliac joints. Various numbers and orientations of screws were studied, ranging from two to six screws, with either parallel or oblique orientation of adjacent screws. The best results were obtained when a minimum of three screws was used with moderate obliquity between the adjacent screws. The results were not significantly improved when the number of screws was increased to six.

The Double Cobra plate provides an alternative method to achieve posterior stabilization when sacroiliac lag screws cannot be employed. One indication for the use of the Double Cobra plate is a comminuted fracture of the body of the sacrum through the foramina and the adjacent articular or alar portion of the bone. Another indication is a comminuted fracture of the posterior ilium adjacent to the sacroiliac joint. In such instances, the Double Cobra plate provides the optimal available technique to restore pelvic stability. A third indication for use of the Double Cobra plate is a bilateral sacroiliac disruption.

**Bilateral Sacroiliac Disruption.** One previously unsolved fracture problem is a bilateral sacroiliac disruption with a diastasis of the symphysis pubis or an equivalent anterior injury (Figure 3-30). Previous workers agree that conventional anterior pelvic external fixation provides inadequate fixation, since the external frame does not anchor the sacrum to the residual portions of the pelvic ring. As Slatis has suggested,[24] attempts to compress the displaced iliac wings against the sacrum are analogous to the application of a thumb and index finger to squeeze a bar of wet soap. The sacrum undergoes marked anterior displacement. Another potential solution is the application of one or two Harrington compression rods across the back of the pelvis with associated sacral hooks or bolts attached to the posterior iliac crests.[1] This method possesses two major liabilities. The posterior portions of the iliac crests consist of relatively soft bone, which is likely to permit migration of the fixation hooks or bolts. Also, the method does not provide reattachment of the sacrum to the ilia. As an attempt is made to tighten the posterior fixation by the application of compression, approximation of the ilia is accompanied by progressive anterior migration of the sacrum. Furthermore, a posterior rod does not provide any rotational stability to the reconstructed pelvis unless it is supplemented with lag screws across the sacroiliac joints. With the use of a posterior Double Cobra plate with cancellous lag screws and a Slatis anterior frame, however, our test data showed that a load of 800N could be resisted in such fractures. This combination of internal and external fixation provides a sound mechanical solution to a complex problem.

**Internal Fixation of the Pelvic Ring—Symphysis Pubis Diastasis With Unilateral Sacroiliac Disruption Treated by the Use of Two Anterior Plates and a Unilateral Sacroiliac Plate.** Various preliminary experiments were undertaken with the use of 3.5mm and 4.5mm plates applied to a disruption of the symphysis pubis (Figure 3-30). Even in skeletally immature and young adults, the rami are composed of relatively soft cancellous bone that does not provide good holding capacity for screws. In the presence of an unstable pelvic injury, a unilateral plate applied to the rami is likely to fail under the imposition of rotational forces with loosening of the screws. The application of a second plate on the superior aspect of the rami greatly reduced this tendency. Since the bone is of insufficient size to accommodate a second 4.5mm plate, a smaller 3.5mm plate is employed. In the laboratory model four screws were used in each of the six-hole plates, whereas in the clinical setting six screws have been used for each of the six-hole plates. The laboratory data showed that this combined form of internal fixation was moderately superior to the use of an anterior Slatis frame augmented by unilateral posterior lag screws. Both of these methods of treatment, however, appear to provide effective stabilization for appropriate fracture patterns in clinical situations. The double anterior plating may be preferred for use in a wide diastasis, where the plates are readily applied. This method may be used at the time of a reconstruction of a ruptured bladder or where a satisfactory reduction of the pelvic ring cannot be achieved by closed methods. In a paraplegic or quadriplegic patient with insensitive skin, anterior internal fixation is preferred to external fixation to facilitate nursing care and repositioning of the patient. When the anterior fracture violates the rami, however, the surgical exposure of the fracture may be more complicated than an approach to the symphysis. In this instance, the use of anterior external fixation is preferred, particularly since the cancellous rami usually show early callus formation and healing within three to five weeks. In cases of late presentation as delayed or frank nonunions and malunions, generally with a degree of disuse osteoporosis, internal fixation provides superior fixation to external fixation.

**Internal Fixation of the Pelvic Ring—Double Sacroiliac Disruption and a Symphysis Pubis Diastasis Immobilized by the Use of Double Anterior Plates and Bilateral Sacroiliac Lag Screws or Anterior Plates and a Double Cobra Plate.** The mechanical data for these two systems showed excellent and equivalent rigidity (Figure 3-30). Again, the mechanical stability with these reconstructions rivaled that degree observed in the intact human pelvis. The Double Cobra plate possesses certain advantages for complex fracture patterns with comminution of the sacrum or ilium adjacent to the sacroiliac joint, where the application of the unilateral posterior lag screws would be inappropriate. Where a true sacroiliac disruption is present in a bilateral configuration, however, the use of two separate lag screw fixations involves a somewhat simpler surgical technique of exposure and achieves a comparable degree of stability. When these results are compared to those of a Slatis anterior frame with a Double Cobra posterior plate, the results are equivalent. Anterior stabilization by means of internal or external fixation is equally satisfactory from the biomechanical point of view. The use of the anterior plate may be preferred for a diastasis of the symphysis and for most cases with a late presentation, whereas external fixation is preferred for rami fractures and/or when minimal surgical intervention is preferred.

## Biomechanics of Acetabular Fixation

All of the available techniques of acetabular reconstruction necessitate the insertion of screws in periarticular bone for the application of lag screw fixation or buttress plates. Most of the previous observations on the optimal clinical techniques evolved empirically. Much previous attention was focused upon the sites of available bone for application of the fixation devices. In 1967, Campanacci[27] published drawings of the internal architecture of the innominate bone with the gross trabecular systems. Letournel[9] employed these elegant analyses to plan the optimal sites for insertion of screws. Brand et al[28] and Oonishi et al[29] examined the three-dimensional periacetabular osseous architecture by the use of sections from multiple pelves in coronal, parasagittal and horizontal planes, and by a three-dimensional finite element method respectively. Maximum compressive and tensile stresses were determined by a finite element model of the acetabulum. The results showed a favorable correlation in specimens accrued from different pelves. The subchondral bone was always much thicker than the trabecular bone. From the model, correspondingly greater stresses were predicted in the subchondral bone. The magnitude of the tensile stresses exceeded that of the compressive stresses. Of the two prevalent periacetabular trabeculae, a more prominent and regular system possessed a radial orientation while a less prominent one possessed concentric spheres about the acetabulum.

None of the previous studies have reported the mechanical stabilization of acetabular disruptions afforded by various techniques of internal fixation. In previous clinical attempts to reconstruct acetabular fractures, the application of effective techniques of fixation has provided one of the foremost problems. As the complexity of the fracture increases, particularly with marked comminution, the difficulties encountered with the attempt to implement effective internal fixation by the application of multiple plates and screws mount precipitously.

Probably at least 50% of all acetabular fractures are associated patterns that involve both the anterior and posterior columns.[9] Therefore, a laboratory study on a cadaveric fracture model was undertaken to compare the mechanical rigidity that could be achieved by the use of isolated lag screws, plates, and combined techniques of fixation.[30] A transverse central acetabular fracture was adopted as a representative fracture involving both columns. The fractured pelvis was instrumented, reduced, stabilized, and loaded to compare the various types of internal fixation devices.

## Materials and Methods

Nine fresh unembalmed cadaveric pelves were obtained from males less than 70 years of age who had expired from diseases unrelated to the skeletal system. The fifth lumbar vertebra and the proximal third of both femurs were included in the specimens. Prior to the biomechanical tests the specimens were grossly cleaned of soft tissues. A transverse central acetabular fracture was created reproducibly in the cadaveric pelvis by the use of a chisel. The fracture line was prepared 1cm below the base of the anterior inferior iliac spine, passing through the highest point of the cotyloid fossa and exiting through the posterior column (Figure 3-33).

The anterior column was secured with one of the following devices: a 3.5mm Dynamic Compression Plate (D) (Synthes Ltd. (USA), Wayne, Pennsylvania); a 3.5mm Reconstruction Plate (R) (Synthes Ltd. (USA), Wayne, Pennsylvania); a Letournel Plate (L) (Howmedica, Inc., Rutherford, New Jersey); or a long (32mm) threaded 6.5mm AO cancellous screw (S) (Synthes Ltd. (USA), Wayne, Pennsylvania) (Figure 3-34). When utilized, the anterior column plate was applied from the inner surface of the ilium along the iliopectineal line to the superior surface of the superior pubic ramus (Figure 3-35). When lag screw fixation of the anterior column was employed, the screw was inserted with a washer from the outer

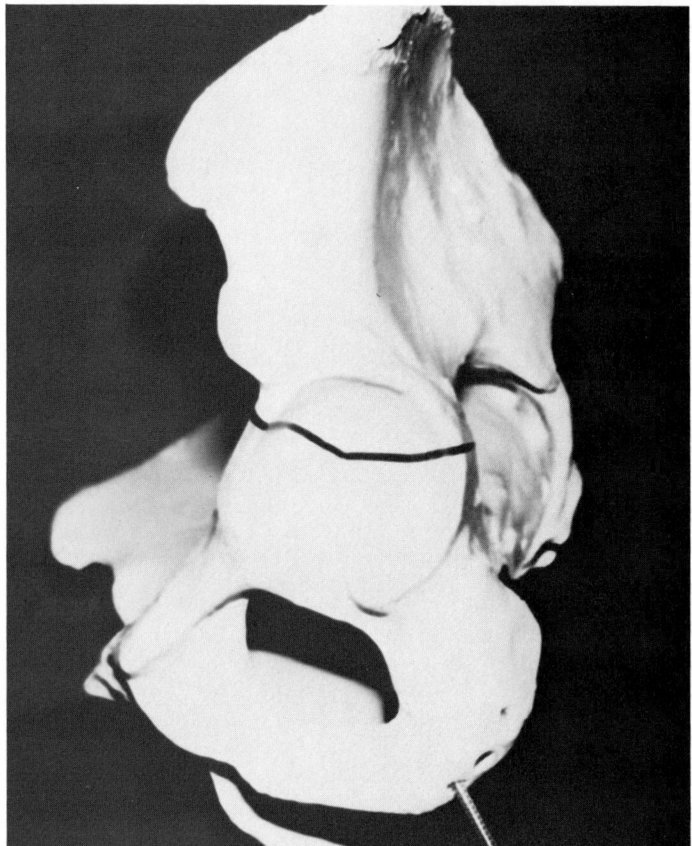

Figure 3-33. A model pelvis shows the site of the experimental transverse acetabular fracture. In the cadaveric specimen, the fracture line begins 1cm inferior to the base of the anterior inferior iliac spine and continues through the most superior point in the cotyloid fossa.

surface of the ilium across the acetabular dome into the superior pubic ramus (Figure 3-34). In all of these cases the posterior column was immobilized with a plate that extended from the outer surface of the ilium to the ischial tuberosity (Figure 3-36). All of the plates were secured with 3.5mm cortical screws (Synthes Ltd. (USA), Wayne, Pennsylvania).

For the purpose of comparison, plates and screws of identical lengths were used. For the tests that assessed a 3.5mm Dynamic Compression or a Reconstruction Plate, a seven-hole model was used for the anterior column, and an eight-hole one was used for the posterior column.

For the Letournel plate, a six hole model was used for both columns. The anterior column lag screw was a 6.5mm cancellous screw, 90mm in length (Figure 3-34). To minimize the artifactual losses in screw purchase a particular testing sequence was undertaken for each of the six different combinations of fixation under study (Figure 3-37).

Each pelvis was mounted in a standing position and supported distally by articulation with the intact femoral heads. The latter were potted in separate epoxy resin

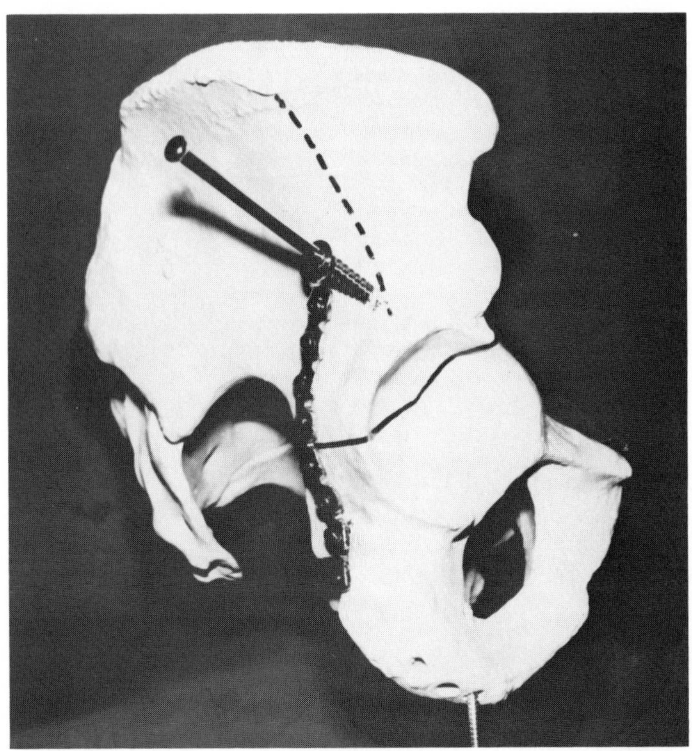

Figure 3-34. A: A model transverse acetabular fracture shows fixation with a 6.5mm cancellous lag screw across the anterior column and a 3.5mm reconstruction plate for the posterior column. B: Internal fixation devices employed in the biomechanical assessment of acetabular fixation. From above, an eight-hole Letournel plate, an eight-hole 3.5mm Reconstruction plate, an eight-hole 3.5mm Dynamic Compression plate, a seven-hole 3.5mm Dynamic Compression plate, and a 6.5mm AO cancellous screw, 90mm in length with a thread length of 32mm.

Figure 3-34A.

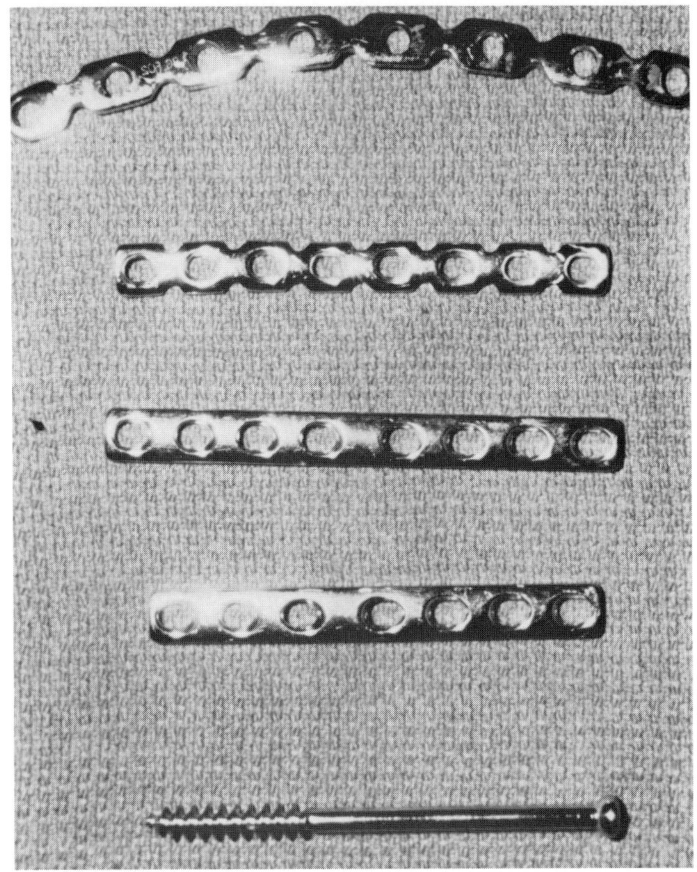

Figure 3-34B.

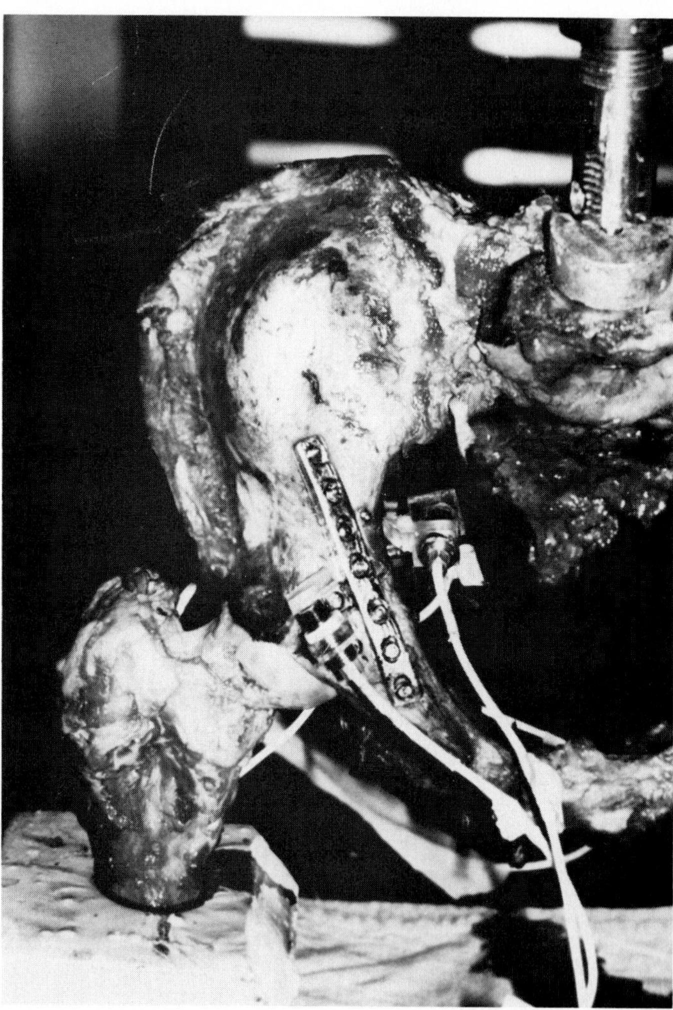

Figure 3-35. The anterior column plate is applied along the iliopectineal line from the inner surface of the ilium to the superior surface of the superior pubic ramus.

blocks. The specimens were subjected to a quasistatic (1.27cm/minute) longitudinal compressive loading of the fifth lumbar vertebral body, up to a maximum of 1334N. The loads were supplied by an Instron unit with a constant crosshead speed (Figure 3-38). Active muscular loading was not included in the model. The resultant deformation at the fracture site was measured by noncontacting variable impedence transducers (Proximity Measuring System, Model KD-2400, Kaman Sciences Corp., Colorado Springs, Colorado). The transducer coil and a circular brass target were mounted on opposing sides of each experimental fracture. The measurement of planar axial displacement of the metallic target face relative to the coil permitted an assessment of the linear fracture displacement. Bench tests showed that the transducer output varied linearly with axial target displacements of up to 1.75mm. The magnitude of the output signal was imperceptably changed for transverse target displacements of less than 1.5mm or

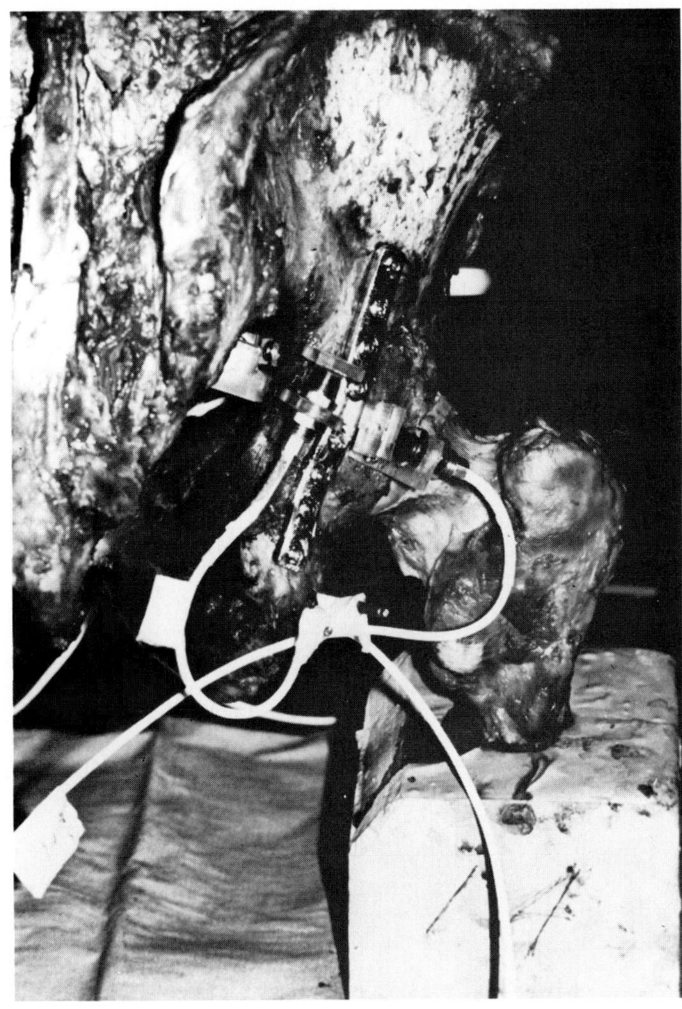

Figure 3-36. The posterior column plate is applied along the posterior column from the outer surface of the ilium to the ischial tuberosity. The strain gauges are evident at the fracture site.

for rotational target displacements of less than 15°.

The resultant deformations were measured at four sites: shear ($T_1$); along the quadrilateral area, posterior column fracture gap normal (opening or closing) movement ($T_2$); posterior column fracture shear ($T_3$); and anterior column fracture gap normal movement ($T_4$) (Figure 3-37). The four displacement transducer outputs were displayed simultaneously against the Instron load cell output on a storage oscilloscope, i.e. in the form of load-deformation curves. The data traces were photographed for subsequent analyses. Six independent tests were performed for each fixation mode.

## Results

A considerable degree of variation was documented in the configuration of the load versus deformation curves. A typical oscilloscope tracing is shown in Figure 3-39. Near linearity in the upload phase was observed in roughly half of the individual measurements, although

Figure 3-37. The transducer site displacement curves recorded for the various types of fixation. A: Shear recorded along the quadrilateral surface (Q) and gap normal movement documented at the anterior column (AC). B: Shear recorded at the posterior column (Shear PC) and gap normal movement documented at the posterior column (Gap PC) (D—3.5mm Dynamic Compression Plate; R—3.5mm Reconstruction Plate; L—Letournel Plate; S—6.5mm cancellous screw with a 32mm thread length).

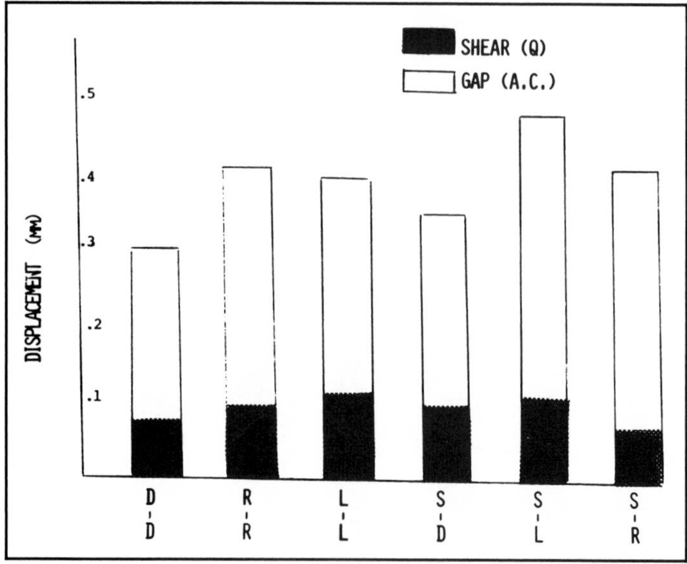


Figure 3-37A.

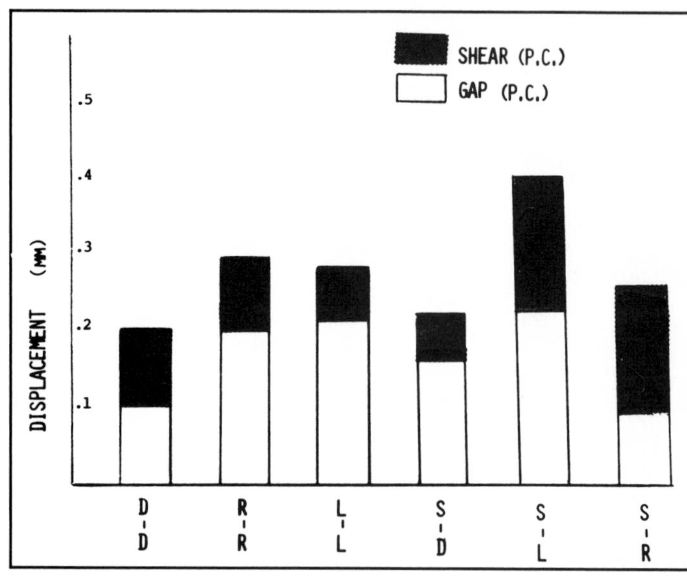


Figure 3-37B.

a substantial hysteresis effect was recorded when the load was released. When the upload curve was distinctly nonlinear, the hysteresis was almost always appreciable. These upload nonlinearities most often involved an asymptotic approach toward a limiting deformation (i.e. increasing rigidity) as peak load was approached. Despite the degree of nonlinearity or hysteresis, however, 90% or more of the observed peak deformation was recovered upon load release. Moreover, the relevant displacement magnitudes generally were quite small (series average = 0.096mm, range = 0.006—0.455mm), thereby confirming the visual observation of gross integrity of the fixation in all of the cases under study. No consistent

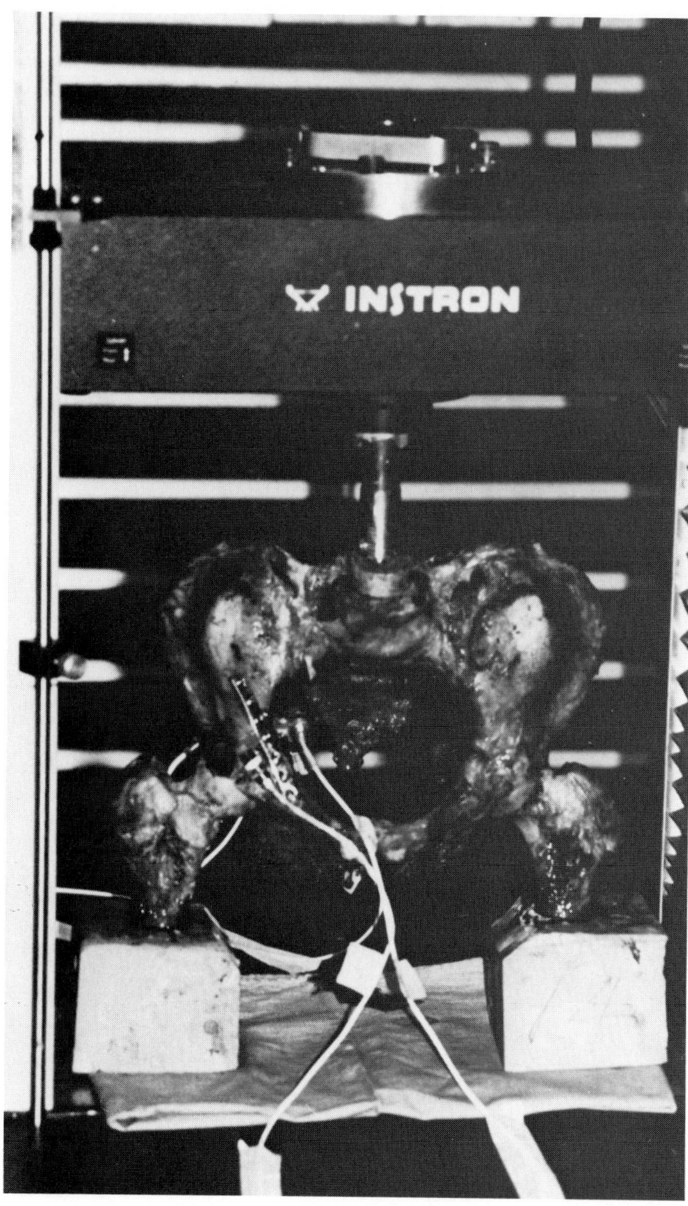


Figure 3-38. The acetabular fracture model is mounted in an Instron unit.

direction of displacement was observed for any of the transducers, irrespective of the methods of fixation. Since the degree of motion at the fracture site is a major obstacle to bony union irrespective of its direction, the largest absolute value of the fracture deformations documented during a loading cycle was the principal point of interest. The complete conspectus of the data accrued for the transducer site displacements documented with the various fixation alternatives is shown in Figure 3-37. No measurement site consistently demonstrated a larger displacement than did any other, irrespective of the type of fixation. This finding was confirmed by t-testing. More importantly, the data fail to show statistically significant

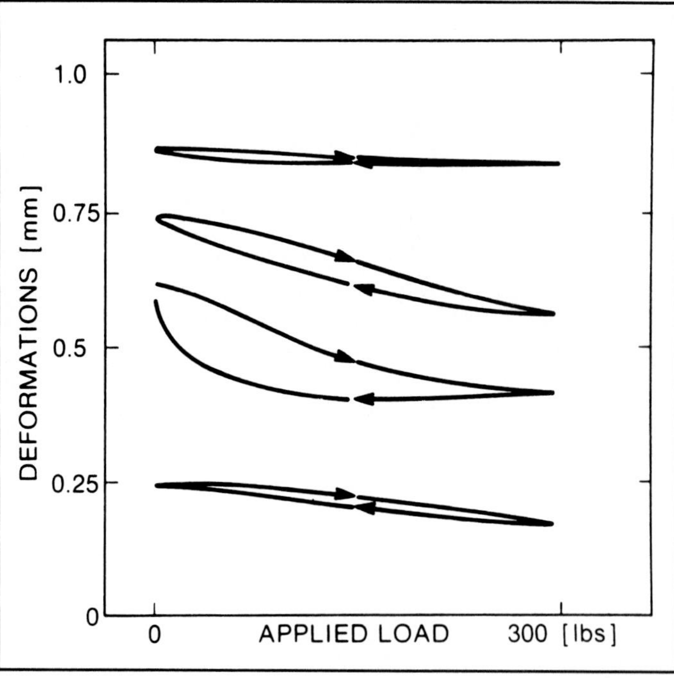


Figure 3-39. Typical features of load-deformation curve. Near-linearities in the upload phase were observed on the top and bottom curves. Upon load release a substantial hysteresis is evident. On the third curve from the top a distinct nonlinearity with appreciable hysteresis is present. This upload linearity involved an asymptotic approach toward a limiting deformation as the peak load is reached. Except on the third curve, the peak deformation was recovered upon release of the applied load.

differences ($P<.001$) between any of the fixation alternatives at any of the transducer sites.

## Discussion

Intramedullary fixation of the anterior column with a lag screw was introduced by Elliot,[31] who employed Hagie pins inserted into the anterior column to stabilize a so-called central acetabular fracture. Elliot did not use internal fixation to secure the posterior column. Senegas[32] described the insertion of a screw obliquely across the anterior column along with a plate to immobilize the posterior column. While he achieved accurate realignment of the fracture fragments, his method did not achieve widespread application. In the present biomechanical evaluation, the data clearly show that the method of anterior column lag screw fixation provides a stable mode of immobilization that can be readily undertaken with minimal stripping of soft tissues and revascularization of the inner aspect of the ilium and the superior pubic ramus. When the anterior column is secured with a plate, the inner surface of the ilium distal to the superior ramus of the pubis requires extensive exposure and a potentially hazardous elevation of the femoral nerve and the external iliac vessels. Frequently concomitant stripping of the outer pelvic wall is necessary to achieve an accurate articular reduction so that the vascularity of the bone is severely compromised. To insert an anterior column lag screw, the exposure is limited to the fracture site generally adjacent to the anterior inferior iliac spine.

While the data showed no significant difference in the rigidity afforded by the three plates under study, the crucial problem of contouring the plates to replicate precisely the intricate and irregular three-dimensional periacetabular bony structure is greatly reduced by the use of a 3.5mm Reconstruction Plate. This plate is rapidly and accurately shaped by the use of its special contouring device and bending irons. When the other less malleable plates are inaccurately contoured and applied to a fracture site, they provoke a loss of reduction and malalignment as the fragments approximate the erroneously contoured plate. Even a somewhat imperfectly contoured Reconstruction Plate attached to the pelvis by screws inserted sequentially from one end of the plate readily undergoes plastic deformation to fit closely to the reduced fracture.

While the load imposed upon the lumbar spine during unsupported sitting is about 1.4 times body weight, it is reduced by supported sitting.[33] The displacement magnitudes at fracture sites were quite small, and permanent deformations seldom occurred when a load of 1334N (roughly two times the body weight of a 70kg person) was applied. This result confirms the adequacy of a Reconstruction Plate with a supplementary lag screw for acetabular immobilization without jeopardizing the reduction and fixation, even when a patient becomes seated in the early postoperative period. A partial weightbearing gait attaining 50% of body weight can also be undertaken in the early postoperative period. Despite the apparent equivalent stability of lag screw and plate fixation documented in this study, the absence of active muscular deforming forces provides an obvious potential source for experimental error. Nevertheless, the results appear to provide a legitimate comparison of the relative mechanical effectiveness of an anterior column lag screw fixation and a plate fixation of the posterior column that is relevant for the clinical situation.

In the extensive clinical series reported by Letournel and Judet,[9] involvement of two columns was documented in 59% of the acetabular fractures (i.e. transverse fractures, 9%; "T" fractures, 6%; transverse and posterior wall fractures, 20%; associated anterior and posterior hemitransverse fractures, 4%; both column fractures, 18%). Most of these complex fracture patterns can be satisfactorily immobilized by the use of an anterior column screw fixation and a supplementary posterior column plate. While a posterior column lag screw can be employed instead of a posterior column plate, such a screw requires a carefully planned orientation or it does not secure the fracture. In many instances it cannot be inserted unless substantial soft tissue stripping is performed. If the fracture is comminuted, isolated lag screw fixation rarely provides adequate fixation.

Since the laboratory study reported here was limited to a relatively simple transverse fracture model, the optimal stabilization techniques for complex fractures have been characterized solely by clinical experience. For a comminuted posterior column fracture, a 3.5mm or 4.5mm Recontruction Plate or a 4.5mm Letournel Plate is applied to buttress the posterior column. With comminution of the adjacent acetabular rim or wall, the fragments are immobilized with a supplementary 3.5mm Reconstruction Plate. In the presence of a comminuted anterior column fracture, the use of a single anterior column lag screw is precluded. Alternatively, a 3.5mm Reconstruction Plate or a Letournel Plate is applied along the iliopectineal line, from the inner table of the ilium to the medial end of the superior pubic ramus. For the comminuted fracture variants, frequently, the rigidity of the fixation is greatly augmented if the larger fragments are repaired with 3.5mm lag screws, which supplement the buttress plate.

## Conclusions

For a variety of simple fractures, such as a transverse pattern and certain complex variants, lag screw fixation of the anterior column with a supplementary plate fixation of the posterior column affords a degree of stability equal to that provided by other techniques that necessitate greater exposure and more devascularization of the bone.

For immobilization of a simple fracture the 3.5mm Reconstruction Plate provides stability comparable to a 3.5mm Dynamic Compression Plate or a Letournel Plate. The former is more readily contoured than the latter two. In the presence of marked comminution or osteoporosis, the larger 4.5mm Reconstruction or Letournel Plates are preferred to buttress the bone effectively.

Under the imposition of approximately physiological loads in a recumbent or seated position, the displacements documented at the experimental fracture sites were quite small and recoverable upon removal of the load. Early postoperative mobilization of a patient with up to 50% weight bearing could be undertaken without jeopardizing the acetabular fixation.

While this laboratory study examined one pattern of acetabular fracture with anatomical specimens that were selected for relatively dense bone, certain practical situations complicated by comminution or osteoporosis necessitate the use of the buttress concept of fixation to prevent the loss of fixation and alignment. In this instance, a rigid supportive plate is applied to the bony surface and anchored by the use of the larger 4.5mm or even 6.5mm screws. When a more rigid plate is employed, however, it must be perfectly contoured to the anatomically restored surface of the bone or approximation of the plate to the bone will provoke malalignment of the fracture fragments. With this substantial limitation, the more rigid plates are recommended solely for those comminuted and/or osteoporotic fractures where buttressing is crucial to maintain fixation and alignment until union of the fracture has occurred. In these more complex situations, combinations of buttressing and posterior and anterior column lag screws frequently afford optimal stability.

## References

1. Tile M: Fractures of the Pelvis and Acetabulum. Baltimore, Williams and Wilkins, 1984, p 24.
2. Gertzbein SD, Chenoweth DR: Occult injuries of the pelvic ring. Clin Orthop 128:202, 1977.
3. Bucholz RW: The pathological anatomy of Malgaigne fracture-dislocations of the pelvis. J Bone Joint Surg 63A:400, 1981.
4. Pennal GF, Tile M, Waddell JP, Garside H: Pelvic disruption: Assessment and classification. Clin Orthop 151:12, 1980.
5. Letournel E: Fractures of the acetabulum and pelvis. Paris, First Symposium and Workshop, 1984.
6. O'Brien JP: The Halo pelvic apparatus: A clinical bio-engineering and anatomical study. Acta Orthop Scand suppl 163, 1975.
7. White AA, Hirsch C: An experimental study of the immediate load-bearing capacity of some commonly used iliac bone grafts. Acta Orthop Scand 42:482, 1971.
8. Walheim G: Pelvic instability, in: Aspects on Diagnosis and Treatement. Stockholm, Kongl Carolinska Medico Chirurgiska Institutet, 1983, p 6.
9. Letournel E, Judet R: Fractures of the Acetabulum. New York, Springer-Verlag, 1981, p 7.
10. Letournel E: Les Fractures du Cotyle. Paris, Libraire Arnette, 1961, p 28.
11. Lansinger O: Fractures of the acetabulum: A clinical, radiological and experimental study. Acta Orthop Scand suppl 165, 1977.
12. Gunterberg B, Goldie I, Slatis P: Fixation of pelvic fractures and dislocations: An experimental study on the loading of pelvic fractures and sacroiliac dislocations after external compression fixation. Acta Orthop Scand 49:278, 1978.
13. Brown TD, Stone JP, Schuster JH, Mears DC: External fixation of unstable pelvic ring fractures: omparative rigidity of some current frame configurations. Med Biolog Eng Comput 20:727, 1982.
14. Rubash HE, Brown TD, Nelson DD, Mears DC: Comparative mechanical performance of some new devices for fixation of unstable pelvic ring fractures. Med Biol Eng Comput 21:657, 1983.
15. Rubash HE, Mears DC: External fixation of the pelvis, in:

AAOS Instructional Course Lectures. St. Louis, Mosby, 1983, 32:329.

16. Mears DC, Rubash HE: External and internal fixation of the pelvic ring, in: AAOS Instructional Course Lectures. St. Louis, Mosby, 1984, 33:144.
17. McBroom R, Tile M: Disruption of the pelvic ring. presented at Canadian Orthopaedic Research Society Convention, Kingston, Ontario, June 1982.
18. Vidal J, Adrey J, Connes H, Buscayet C: A biomechanical study and clinical application of the use of Hoffmann's external fixator, in Brooker AF, Edwards CC (eds): External Fixation: The Current State of the Art. Baltimore, Williams and Wilkins, 1979, p 327.
19. Chao EYS, Briggs T, McCoy MT: Theoretical and experimental analyses of Hoffmann-Vidal external fixation system, in Brooker AF, Edwards CC (eds): External Fixation: The Current State of the Art. Baltimore, Williams and Wilkins, 1979, p 133.
20. Boltze WH, Chiquet C, Niederer PG: Der Fixateur externe (Rohrystem) Stabulitats sprufung. AO Bulletin 1978.
21. Carabalona P, Rabichong P, Bonnel F, Perruchon E, Pugurat F: Apports-du fixateur externe dans les dislocations du pubis et de l'articulation sacro-iliaque. Montpell Chir 19:61, 1973.
22. Gunterberg B, Goldie I, Slatis P: Fixation of pelvic fractures and dislocations: An experimental study on the loading of pelvic fractures and sacroiliac dislocations after external compression fixation. Acta Orthop Scand 49:278, 1978.
23. Slatis P, Karaharju E: External fixation of unstable pelvic fractures: Experience in 22 patients treated with a trapezoid compression frame. Clin Orthop 151:73, 1980.
24. Slatis P, personal communication, 1981.
25. Karaharju E, Slatis P: External fixation of double vertical fractures with a trapezoidal compression frame. Injury 142, 1978.
26. Slatis P, Karaharju E: External fixation of the pelvic girdle with a trapezoid compression frame. Injury 7:53, 1973.
27. Campanacci M: Lesioni traumatiche del bacino, in: Proceedings of 52nd Congress of the Societa Italiana di Ortopedia, Rome 13-15, October, 1967. Bologna, Stanya Artie, 1967.
28. Brand RA, Crowninshield RD, Pedersen DR: Architecture of the periacetabular trabecular bone. Orthopedics 5:299, 1982.
29. Oonishi H, Isha H, Hasegawa T: Mechanical analysis of the human pelvis and its application to the artificial hip joint by means of the three-dimensional finite element method. J Biomech 16:427, 1983.
30. Sawaguchi T, Brown TD, Rubash HE, Mears DC: Stability of acetabular fractures after internal fixation, a cadaveric study. Acta Orthop Scand in press, 1985.
31. Elliot RB: Central fractures of the acetabulum. Clin Orthop 7:189, 1956.
32. Senegas J, Yates M: Complex acetabular fractures: A transtrochanteric lateral approach. Clin Orthop 151:107, 1980.
33. Nachemson A: Toward better understanding of low back pain: A review of the mechanics of the lumbar disc. Rheumat Rehabil 14:129, 1975.

# CHAPTER 4

# Assessment and Classification of Injuries

## Assessment

Prior to the initiation of definitive treatment of a pelvic or acetabular fracture the injury is rigorously classified by its clinical and radiological features. From the history obtainable from an alert patient, as well as from inspection for sites of contussion or ecchymosis, the direction of the provocative force may be determined. With such information a trauma surgeon can anticipate certain likely patterns of injury that correlate with various mechanisms of injury. The age of the patient will indicate one of three groups. For the children discussed in Chapter 14, the mortality and morbidity of those who survive to present in the emergency room appears to be quite low. The young adults generally present with traumatic forces of high energy following motor vehicular trauma, industrial accidents and falls from great heights. The elderly may present with motor vehicular trauma or following simple falls in the home. With the predilection of the elderly for osteoporosis, their radiographs may illustrate a substantial degree of displacement and comminution that would be documented only in those younger adults who sustained injuries following high energy dissipation. The hemodynamic mechanisms available in the elderly to compensate for hypotension and shock are less effective than in younger adults. More aggressive medical management is generally necessary in the elderly to prevent serious and potentially fatal complications of posttraumatic hemorrhage. In the male pelvic trauma victim, associated urethral injuries should be anticipated along with the potential for impotence. While urethral injuries are uncommon in women who sustain a pelvic disruption, an associated vaginal laceration converts it into an occult open injury with a high morbidity and mortality. From the history the considerable potential for associated injuries to other organ systems is carefully reviewed. An estimate of the force of the accident provides insight into the gravity of the pelvic trauma and the potential for concomitant injuries.

The physical examination includes an inspection for pelvic asymmetry, which focuses upon the positions of the anterior and posterior iliac crests and the greater trochanters, and a search for apparent limb length discrepancy. Sites of ecchymosis, contusions, and abrasions may be indicative of the vector of the traumatic force and the likelihood for a particular injury pattern with a corresponding degree of pelvic instability. A careful scrutiny is made for open wounds especially in the groin, scrotum or perineal region, as well as in the vagina and rectum which would be indicative of an open pelvic fracture. In a man, blood escaping from the urethral meatus is suspicious of a urethral rupture. In a woman the presence of bloody discharge from the urethra or vagina is suggestive of an occult open pelvic fracture. Apparent deformities of the lower extremities, in the absence of a fracture in the lower limb, may indicate the type of pelvic fracture (Figure 4-1). If a lower extremity is foreshortened with excessive internal rotation and palpable displacement of an excessively prominent posterior iliac spine, a lateral compression injury can be anticipated. If a lower extremity is foreshortened with excessive external rotation, a highly unstable vertical shear fracture is the most likely diagnosis.

By palpation, tenderness and crepitus or abnormal mobility of an iliac crest or a ramus fracture is indicative of pelvic instability (Figure 4-2). By direct palpation of the symphysis or adjacent superior pubic ramus or the lateral ilium, a demonstrable gap may indicate an associated disruption. Excessive prominence of a tender superior ramus may indicate the presence of a marked rotational deviation of the bone. Abnormal mobility of a hemipelvis may be documented by a manual attempt to approximate the two iliac crests or to internally or externally rotate the femora. Palpation of the greater trochanter and lateral thigh may reveal medial displacement of the proximal femur associated with a

Figure 4-1. Anteroposterior radiographs of two pelvic fractures with apparent limb length discrepancy. A: Vertical shear injury with external rotational deformity of the right lower limb. B: Fracture/dislocation of the left hip as a "T" fracture and posterior wall fragment with internal rotational deformity of the left lower limb.

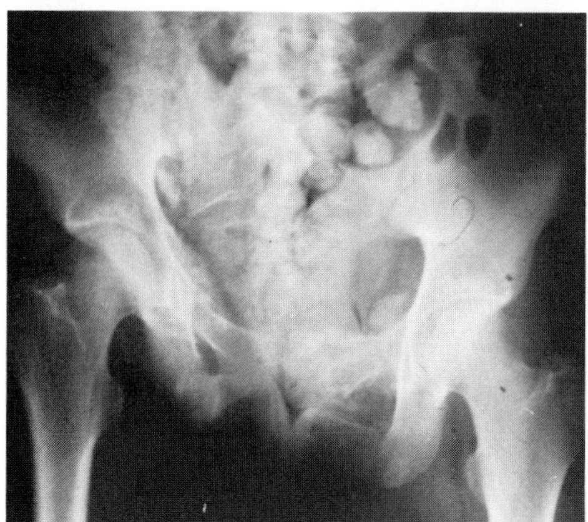

Figure 4-1A.

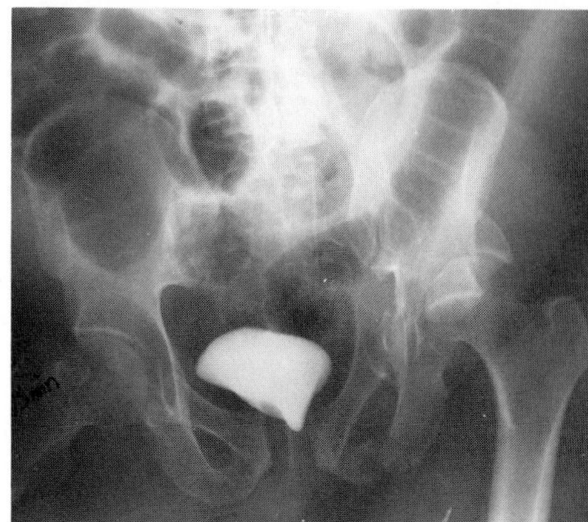

Figure 4-1B.

Figure 4-2. Pelvic radiographs with associated palpable defects. A: Diastasis of the symphysis pubis. B: Comminuted displaced iliac crest fracture.

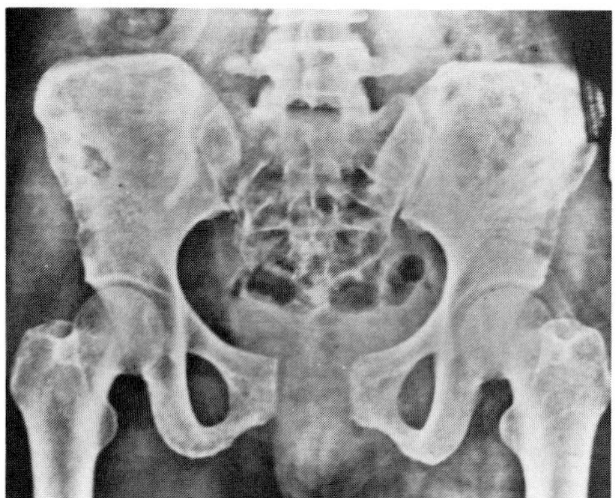

Figure 4-2A.

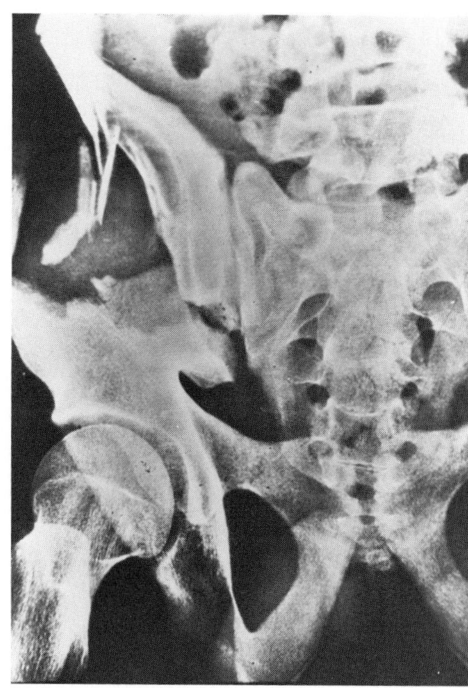

Figure 4-2B.

traumatic protrussio secondary to a acetabular fracture. With a posterior dislocation or fracture-dislocation of the hip, the femoral head may be palpated in the posterolateral thigh and accompany an internally rotated and apparently foreshortened lower extremity. Traction on a lower extremity may indicate the presence of marked pelvic instability or of an irreducible pelvic deformity accompanying an impacted fracture. The lower

Figure 4-3. Examples of the inadequacies of the anteroposterior pelvic radiograph for accurate characterization of a pelvic injury. A: Grade II lateral compression injury with rotational deformity of right hemipelvis. The magnitude and direction of the rotational deformity is not readily appreciated here. B: Anteroposterior and inlet views of a lateral compression injury of the left hemipelvis. While the AP view reveals a considerable deformity of the left ilium only the inlet view (C) permits recognition of the marked displacement at the symphysis with allied marked instability. D: This anteroposterior view of a left acetabular "T" fracture with an ipsilateral sacroiliac injury and central displacement of the femoral head does not provide insight into the anteroposterior element of the pelvic deformity.

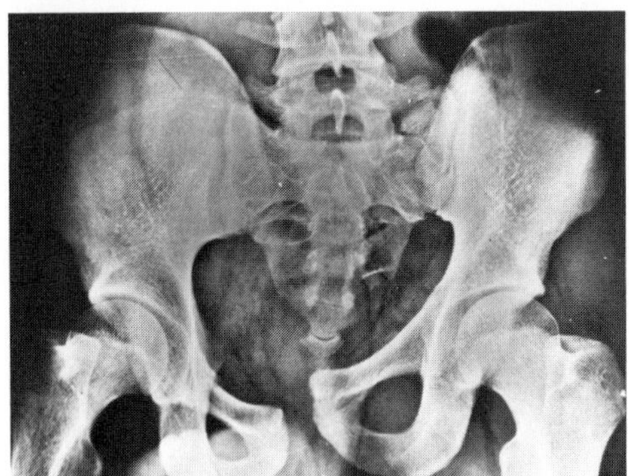

Figure 4-3A.

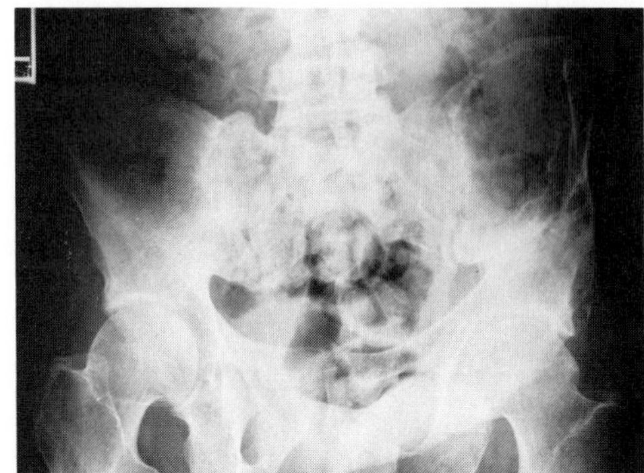

Figure 4-3B.

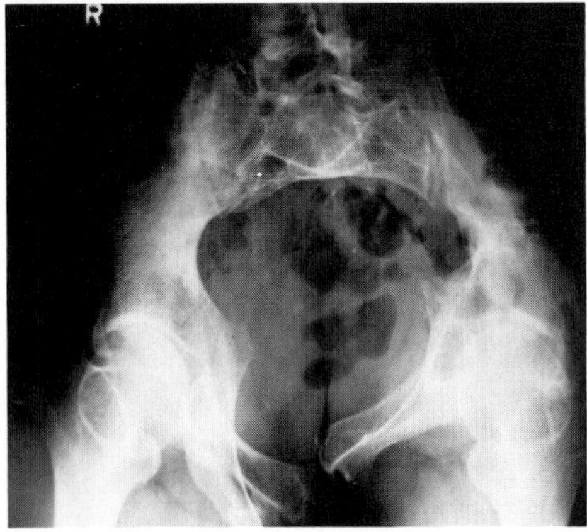


Figure 4-3C.

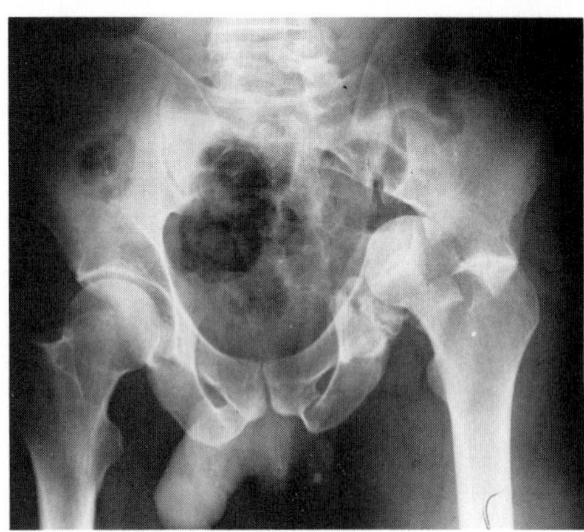

Figure 4-3D.

extremities are examined for evidence of neurological deficit consistent with a lumbosacral root or sciatic nerve injury. Most of the nerve injuries accompany marked pelvic displacement with associated instability or traumatic migration of the femoral head.

Probably the most widespread shortcoming of current routine clinical management of pelvic trauma is inadequate initial radiographic documentation solely with an anteroposterior pelvic radiograph (Figure 4-3). This view does not provide any direct evidence of anterior or posterior displacement of a pelvic fracture or the adjacent proximal femur. In the presence of a comminuted pelvic or acetabular fracture with marked displacement in multiple planes, a precise

Figure 4-4. Pelvic radiographs and a computed scan of a 15-year-old girl.

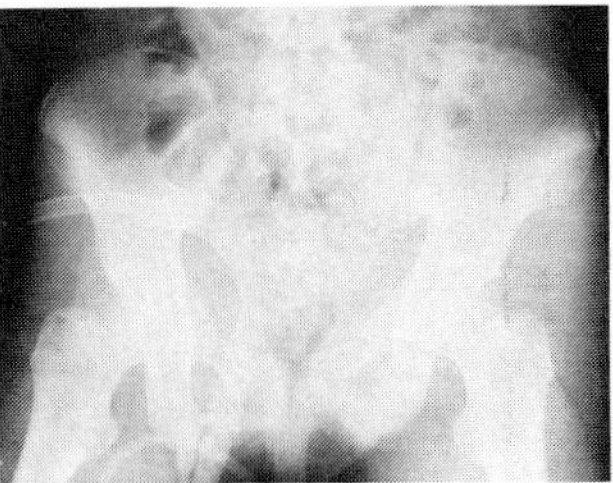

Figure 4-4A. Initial anteroposterior radiograph indicates a minimally displaced fracture dislocation of the left sacroiliac joint with bilateral ramus fractures. At first, bed rest was employed for immobilization.

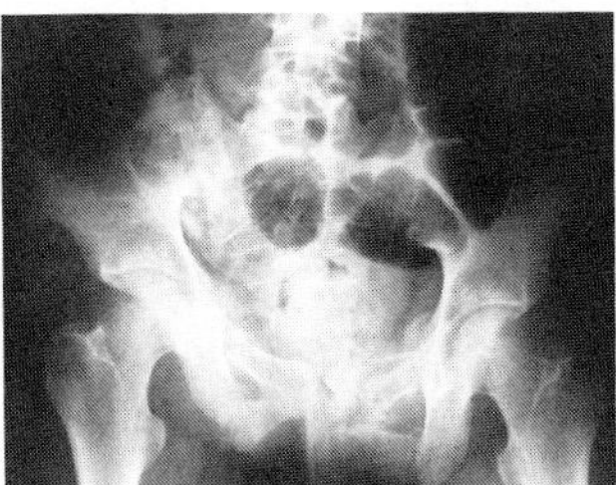

Figure 4-4B. Three weeks later, marked displacement of the right hemipelvis was detected, along with a previously unrecognized injury of the right sacroiliac joint.

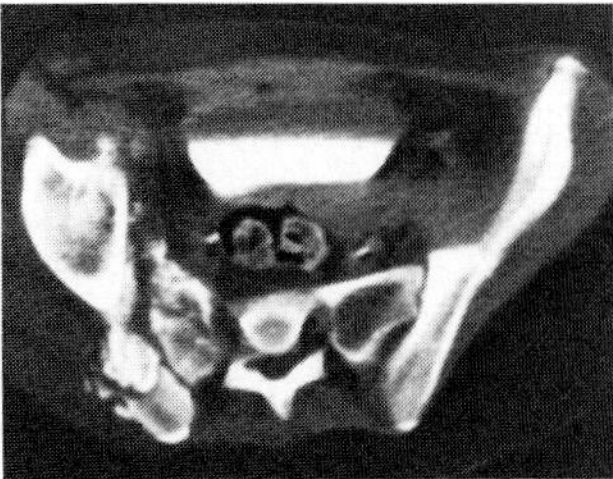

Figure 4-4D.

Figures 4-4C and 4-4D. Computed scans confirm the presence of a malaligned comminuted fracture dislocation of the right sacroiliac joint and right ramus fractures.

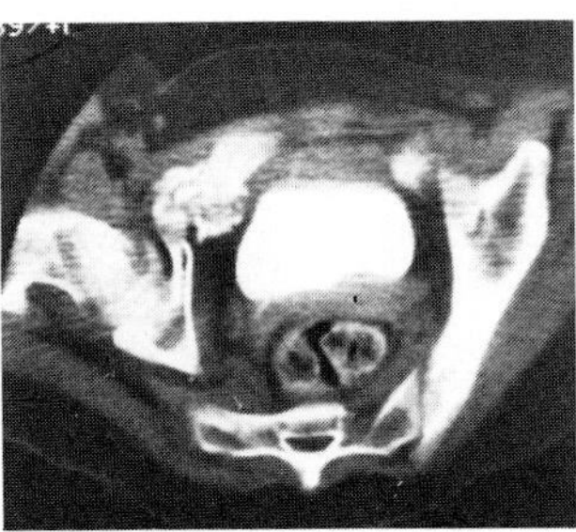

Figure 4-4D.

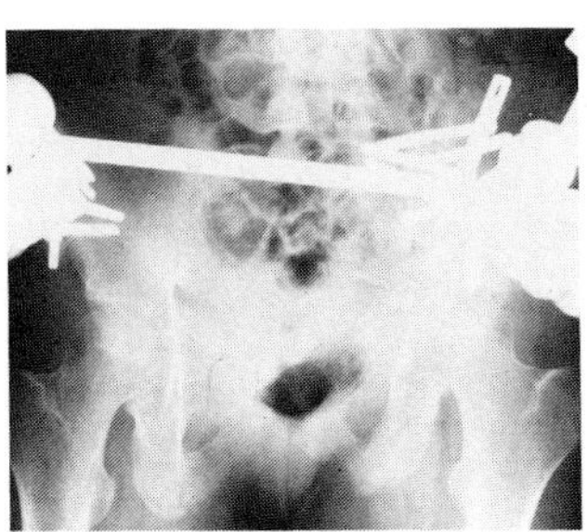

Figure 4-4E. Initial postoperative view after internal and external pelvic fixation.

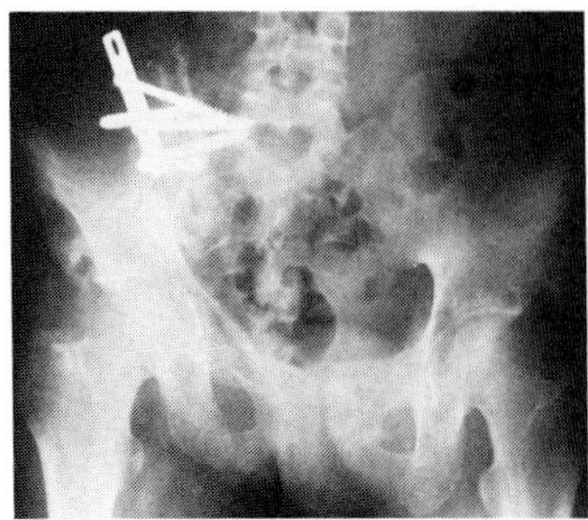

Figure 4-4F. Three months later, the patient is asymptomatic, although the final reduction is imperfect. If the initial documentation had included the computed scan, this formidable late problem would have been avoided.

characterization of the injury by analysis of a single anteroposterior radiograph is impossible.

With the complex three-dimensional anatomical configuration of the pelvic ring and innominate bone, accurate radiologic interpretation of a pelvic or acetabular fracture necessitates the application of a series of special radiologic views, preferably supplemented by computerized axial tomography (Figure 4-4).

The challenging step for the clinician is to analyze the multiple views and, thereby, to perceive a precise three-dimensional replica of the fracture pattern. To assist in this exacting preparatory step the fracture lines are drawn on the radiographs and transferred to a life-sized pelvic model. This detailed assessment characterizes the configuration of the fracture with the specific anatomical sites of disruption, the orientation and magnitude of displacement, the degree of comminution and the extent

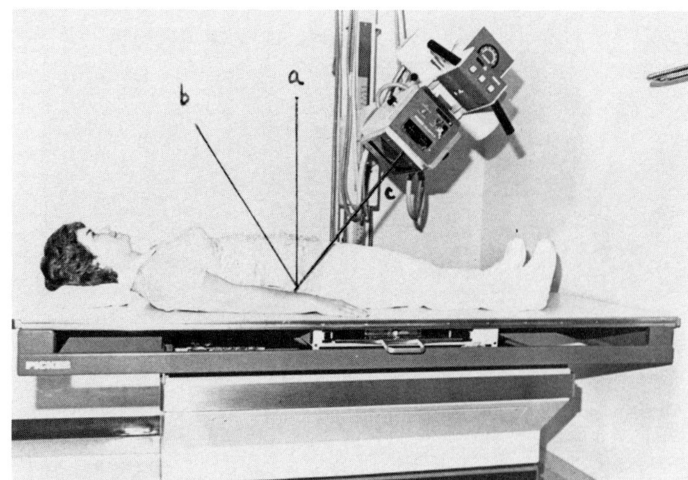


Figure 4-5. The technique for preparation of the standard pelvic radiographs. The letters A-C refer to the position of the beam for anteroposterior, inlet and outlet views respectively.

of pelvic instability. When the acetabulum is involved, the presence of free intraarticular osteochondral fragments, and subluxation or fracture of the femoral head also is noted. Admittedly, in some pelvic fracture victims, especially those with life-threatening injuries to other organ-systems, the prompt initiation of resuscitative measures may preclude a complete radiographic assessment of the pelvis until hemodynamic stability and possibly other urgent goals have been achieved. In such cases, a single anteroposterior view of the pelvis provisionally suffices to document major sites of pelvic disruption, the predilection for associated hemorrhage, especially with posterior pelvic instability, and the feasibility for emergency stabilization of the pelvis by resort to external fixation, or occasionally, limited internal fixation. Once the general stability of the patient has been documented, the definitive radiographic study of the pelvis is completed. In most cases where the general condition of the patient is stable within a brief period after his presentation, the complete radiographic protocol is undertaken in the emergency room. Currently, many trauma patients undergo a computed scan for investigation of a concomitant head, chest or abdominal injury. The additional time required to prepare two to five computed views of the pelvis is inconsequential, whereas the data are exceedingly valuable. In the typical pelvic fracture victim, inefficient utilization of time during the initial evaluation in the emergency room greatly prolongs the screening process despite an inadequate characterization of the pelvic fracture and associated injuries. If a complete investigative protocol is organized by the general, urological, neurological, and orthopaedic surgeons, with appropriate contributions from maxillofacial surgeons and others, a thorough diagnostic plan can be completed promptly within a realistic period of one to three hours that documents virtually all of the principal patterns of multiple trauma. With this information a suitable therapeutic protocol can be prepared to establish the priorities in assessment and manage all of the different combinations of injuries.

The anteroposterior view of the pelvis is taken with the patient positioned supine on the x-ray table (Figure 4-5). The beam is directed perpendicular to the midpelvis and the radiographic plate. The anteroposterior radiograph is oblique to the pelvic brim (Figure 4-6A). Anatomically, the plane of the pelvic brim subtends an angle of 45° to 60° with respect to the axis of the trunk. Scrutiny of the anteroposterior film permits ready documentation of anterior lesions, including a symphysis disruption and unilateral or bilateral rami fractures. Posterior lesions including the sacroiliac joint as pure dislocations or fracture-dislocations violating a portion of the adjacent ilium or sacrum are visible. Sacral fractures are easily overlooked, especially the typical pattern through the weakest area, the sacral foramina, particularly when gas shadows in the bowel obscure the sacrum. Appreciable displacement of a hemipelvis may indicate the presence of marked instability. Other telltale features of pelvic instability include an avulsion fracture of the tip of the transverse process of the fifth lumbar vertebra and a displaced fracture fragment on either end of the sacrospinous ligament. The fragment may originate as a displaced ischial spine or as an avulsed portion of adjacent sacrum.

Supplementary inlet and outlet views of the pelvis, devised by Pennal and Sutherland[1,2] are needed to assess the pelvic ring (Figures 4-6B and 4-6C). To obtain an inlet view of a supine patient, the beam is directed from the head to the midpelvis at an angle of about 60° with respect to the radiographic table, or 30° from the vertical reference axis. Such a projection is perpendicular to the pelvic brim and illustrates the true pelvic inlet. To obtain an outlet projection of a supine patient, the beam is directed from the foot to the pubic symphysis at an angle of 45° with respect to the radiographic plate. The inlet projection highlights anterior and posterior displacement of a pelvic ring or an acetabular fracture. An avulsion fracture of the ischial spine also is evident. The outlet projection discloses superior displacement of the posterior half of the pelvis and either superior or inferior displacement of the anterior portion of the pelvis. Apparent limb length discrepancy originating from elevation of the hip joint is documented, along with avulsion fractures of the transverse processes of the lower lumbar vertebrae or the distal part of the sacrum.

Special oblique radiographs of the sacrum and sacroiliac joints (Figure 4-7) have been devised to

Figure 4-6.Standard pelvic radiographic views.

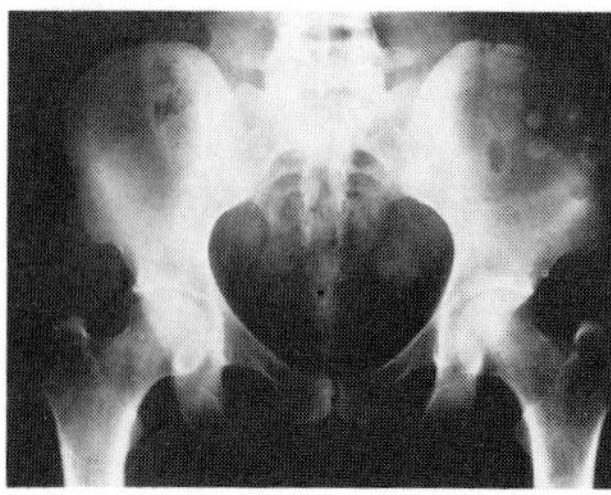

Figure 4-6A. An anteroposterior radiograph.

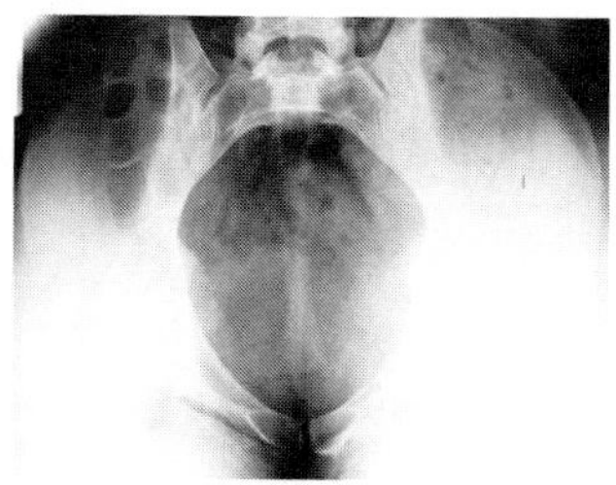

Figure 4-6B. A pelvic inlet radiograph.

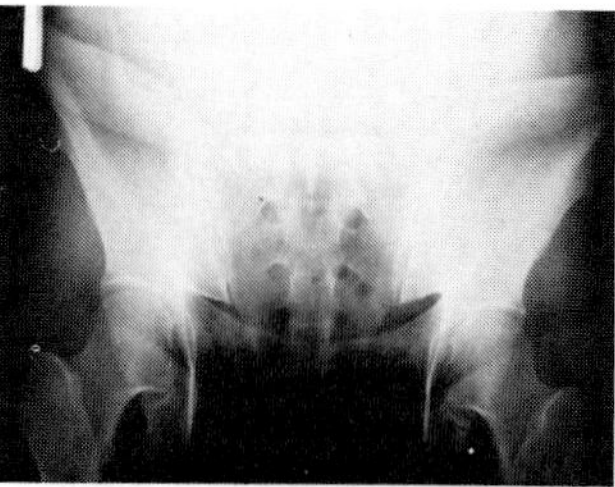

Figure 4-6C. A pelvic outlet radiograph.

Figure 4-7. A: A special oblique radiographic view of the pelvis provides a cross-section of the sacroiliac joint. B: A Fergusson tangential view of the posterior pelvis highlights posterior migration of a displaced sacral fracture or sacroiliac disruption.

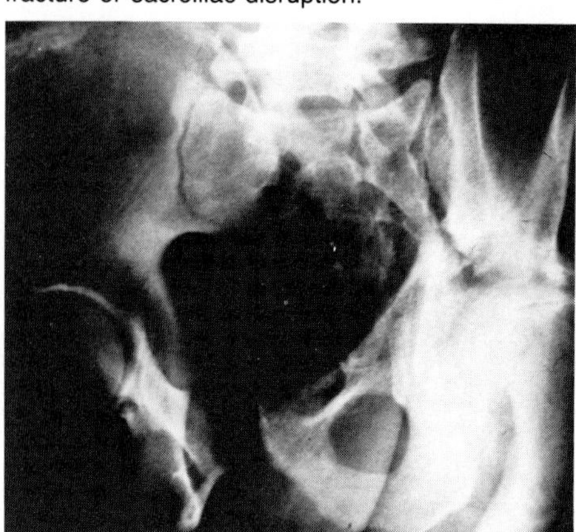

Figure 4-7A.

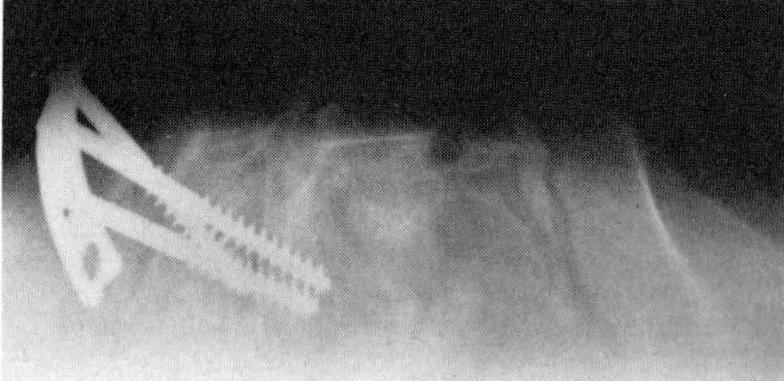

Figure 4-7B.

highlight many obscure disruptions, especially a fracture through the ipsilateral sacral foramina. Another so-called Fergusson view provides an obliquity of the posterior pelvis comparable to an inlet view. It permits recognition of posterior displacement and other disruptions that violate the dorsal surface of the sacrum and adjacent posterior ilia.

To visualize the acetabulum, the anteroposterior view provides a projection of the entire supportive elements or columns (Figure 4-8). The anteroposterior view illustrates some specific landmarks, such as the ilioischial line, the tear drop, and the pelvic brim. If the contour of the innominate bone is perceived as a propeller, then the considerable limitations of the anteroposterior view become evident. When the iliac wing is positioned in a sagittal plane, then the transverse axis of the acetabulum is directed 50° frontward and inward while the position of the obturator ring is oriented perpendicular to the plane of the wing. Despite these shortcomings, the anteroposterior view permits a recognition of the borders of the anterior and posterior walls of the acetabulum, the roof, the tear drop, the ilioischial line, and the pelvic inlet or brim of the true pelvis.

Special oblique views have been devised by Letournel and Judet[3] that provide a profile of the parts of the columns parallel to the film and section of the parts perpendicular to it. The iliac oblique view (Figure 4-9) clearly exposes the entire surface of the iliac wing along with the inner and outer surfaces of the bony ring that surrounds the obturator foramen. The other so-called obturator oblique view (Figure 4-10) displays a section of the iliac wing with superimposed anterior and posterior iliac spines, and presents an outline of the obturator ring around the obturator foramen. The two views are obtained by rolling the injured patient carefully from one side to the other to provide a transverse axis of the pelvis of 45° relative to the x-ray table (Figures 4-9 and 4-10). During the exposure of the films, the patient is supported on suitable cushions. As Letournel has outlined, for the iliac oblique view the injuried part rests on the table while the uninjured hip is elevated. The beam is directed 1cm below the level of the anterosuperior iliac spine of the injured side, and at the midportion of a line from the spine to the midline. For the obturator oblique view, the injured hip is raised and the beam is directed 1cm below and medial to the ipsilateral anterosuperior iliac spine. The entire hemipelvis, or ideally the whole pelvis, is visualized on the radiograph. To view the anterior column, its upper part, the iliac wing, is clearly visualized on the iliac oblique view. The magnitude of the displacement of an anterior column disruption is better appreciated on the obturator oblique view. The principal landmark of the anterior column, the pelvic brim, is best seen in the obturator oblique view, whereas the posterior column including any displacement is well displayed on the iliac oblique view in which its principal landmark, the posterior border of the bone, is entirely visible. The inferior half of the posterior column and the ischium are better seen in the obturator oblique view, along with the posterior border of the acetabular articular surface.

## Radiographic Distortion

The complex geometry of the pelvis and the application of oblique views provide sources of radiographic distortion (Figure 4-11). One source of distortion is the different degrees of radiographic magnification of osseous structures that approximate or depart from the x-ray tube. For the supine patient, anterior enlargement of the pelvic structures is much more significant than for posterior pelvic structures. The magnitude of displacement of an anterior fracture versus a posterior

Figure 4-8. An anteroposterior radiograph of the pelvis and acetabulum (A), with a color-coded projection of the pelvis (B). Red—posterior acetabular rim; orange—ilioischial line; yellow—tear drop; pale green—anterior acetabular rim; dark green—iliopectineal line; blue—acetabular roof.

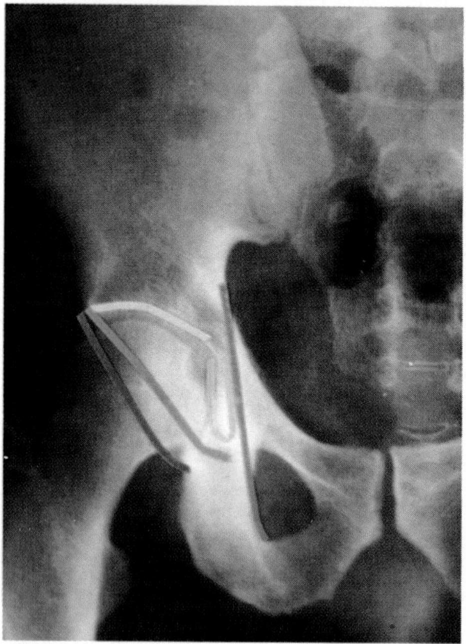

Figure 4-8A.

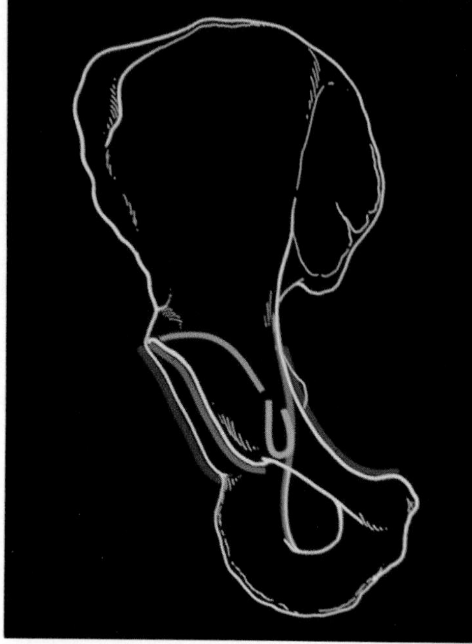

Figure 4-8B.

Figure 4-9. An iliac oblique radiograph (A), with a color-coded projection of the pelvis (B). Red—anterior acetabular rim; yellow—acetabular roof and medial wall; green—anterior superior and inferior spines; blue—medial border of posterior column with greater sciatic notch, ischial spine and tuberosity.

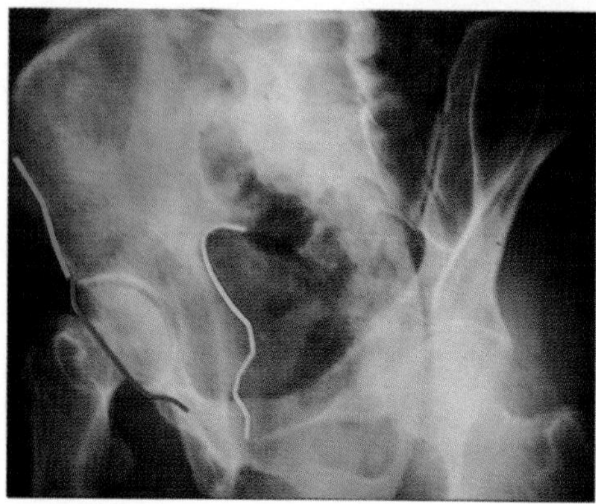

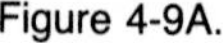

Figure 4-9A.

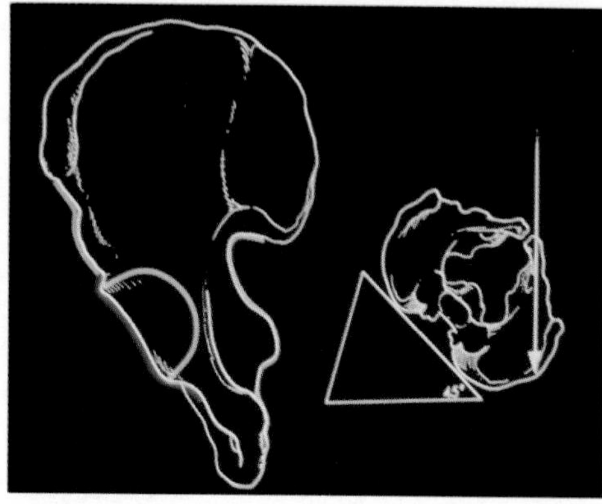

Figure 4-9B.

one is influenced in the same way. The magnitude of apparent displacement of a fracture is markedly influenced by the orientation of the radiograph. If the fracture is displaced parallel to the x-ray beam and perpendicular to the film, it will appear to have a negligible displacement in the anteroposterior view and considerable displacement in an oblique view. If the displacement of the fracture is oblique at 45° to the frontal or coronal plane, it will appear to be of moderate

Figure 4-10. An obturator oblique radiograph (A), with a color-coded projection of the pelvis (B). Red—iliopectineal line; green—superior border of obturator foramen; Blue—posterior acetabular rim.

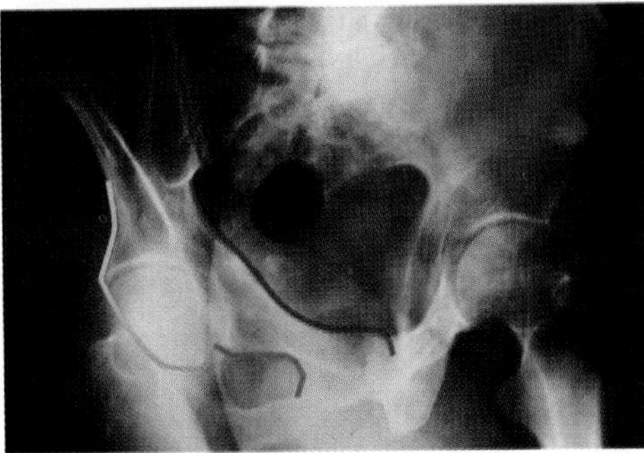
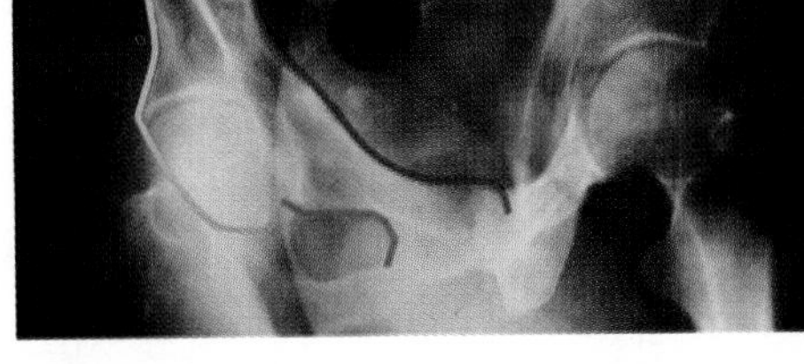

Figure 4-10A.

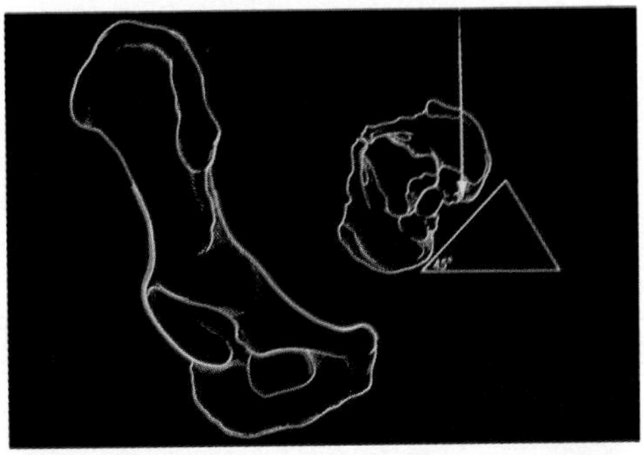

Figure 4-10B.

Figure 4-11. Examples of radiographic distortion of the pelvis. In an outlet view (A), apparent anterior enlargement of the rami with respect to corresponding posterior structures is evident in a comparison with the model pelvis (B).

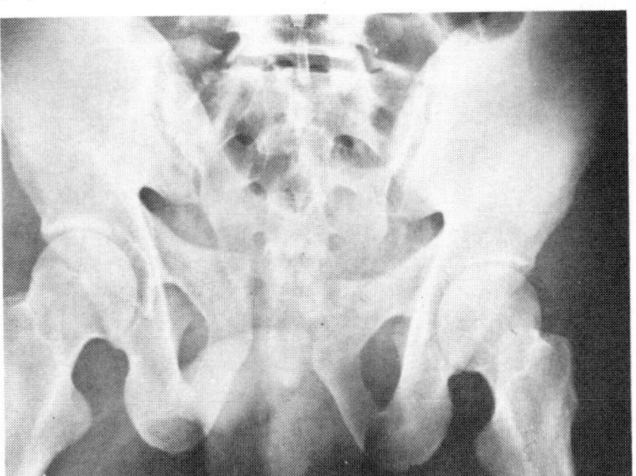

Figure 4-11A.

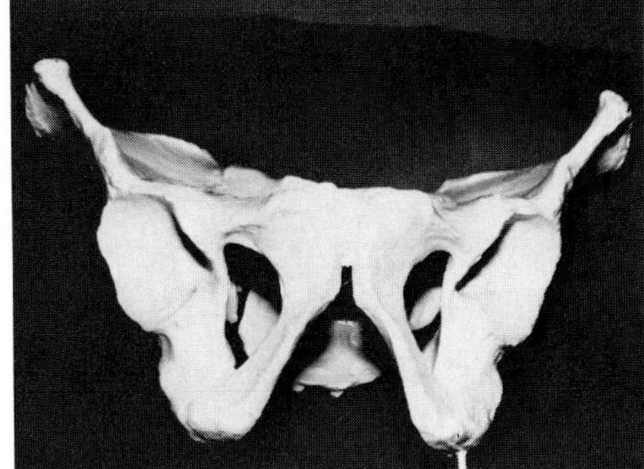

Figure 4-11B.

magnitude on the anteroposterior view, maximum on one oblique view and negligible on the other oblique view. With the 90° difference in the rotation of the two oblique views, a fracture line cannot be labeled undisplaced unless this visualization is confirmed in at least two of the three views. The linear image produced by the alignment of the x-ray beam tangential to a surface, such as the ilioischial line seen in the anteroposterior view, appears only in a single view. If an 8° to 10° rotation of the part presented to the x-ray beam occurs, its appearance is markedly altered. The ilioischial line completely vanishes. While tomography theoretically can largely eliminate these sources of error, overall it has a limited role as a source of improved resolution for the pelvis and acetabulum. In the presence of an acetabular fracture, it can permit the recognition of a loose osteochondral fragment or of a malrotated dome fragment. This method has been largely superceded by the widespread availability of computerized axial tomography.

Figures 4-12 to 4-17. A series of radiographs, schematic diagrams and computed scans present cross-sections of the pelvis. The view at the level of the anterior inferior spines is not part of the conventional series. (Reproduced with permission from Mears DC: External Skeletal Fixation, Baltimore, Williams and Wilkins, 1983.)

Figure 4-12 A-D. View at the level of the anterior superior spine.

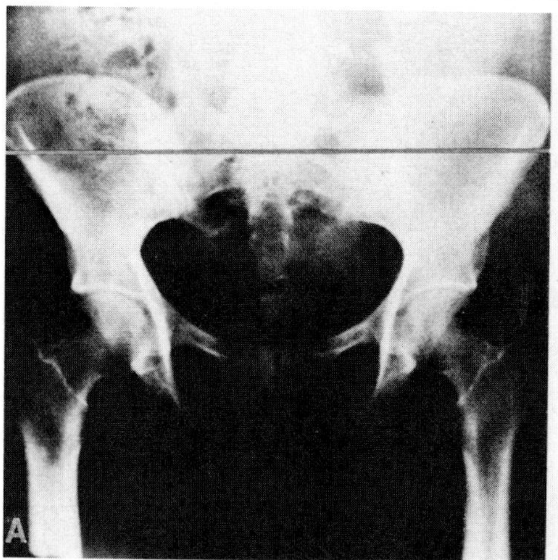


Figure 4-12A.

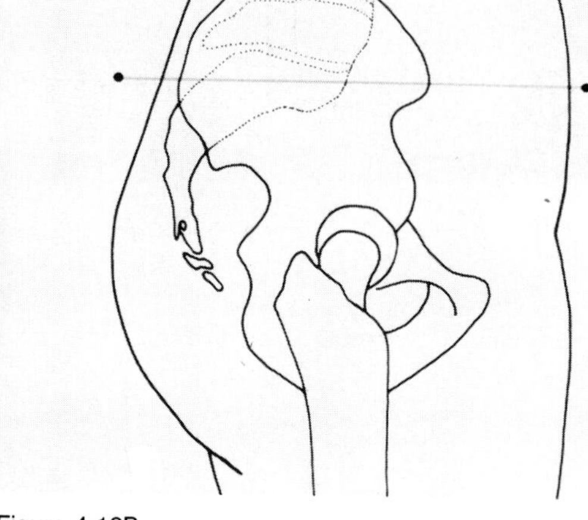

Figure 4-12B.

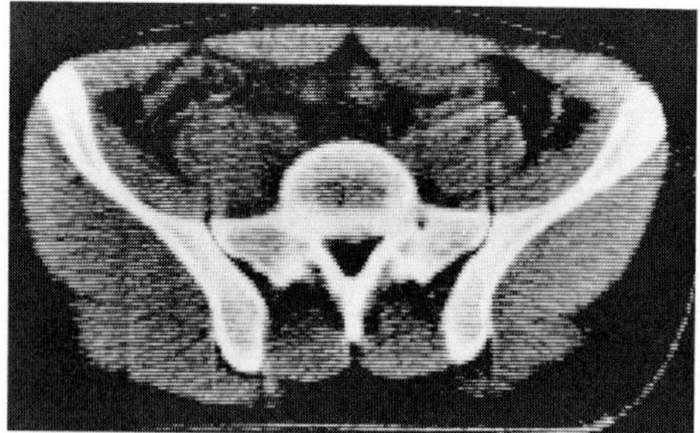

Figure 4-12C.

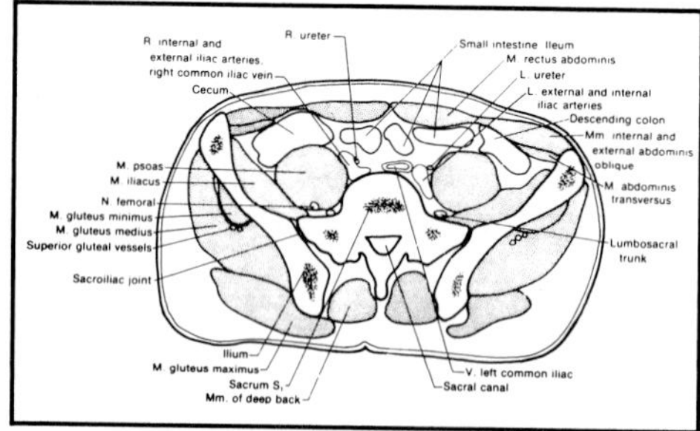


Figure 4-12D.

Computed tomography has become almost indispensible to document sites of pelvic and acetabular disruption, displacement and comminution. Its foremost role is clarification of the posterior disruption of a pelvic ring fracture. A sacral fracture that is virtually invisible in plain radiographs is readily documented by a computed scan. The stable compressive insults through the sacral foramina can be distinguished from the displaced unstable injuries. Posterior iliac or sacral fractures that extend into a displaced sacroiliac joint are easily documented by a computed scan. The degree of separation and instability of a sacroiliac joint can be ascertained. Five standard coronal sections are employed[4] (Figures 4-12 to 4-17). The most superior section demonstrates the iliac wings and the adjacent sacroiliac joints. A second section, taken about 2cm inferior to

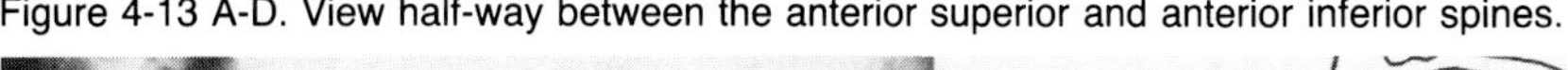
Figure 4-13 A-D. View half-way between the anterior superior and anterior inferior spines.

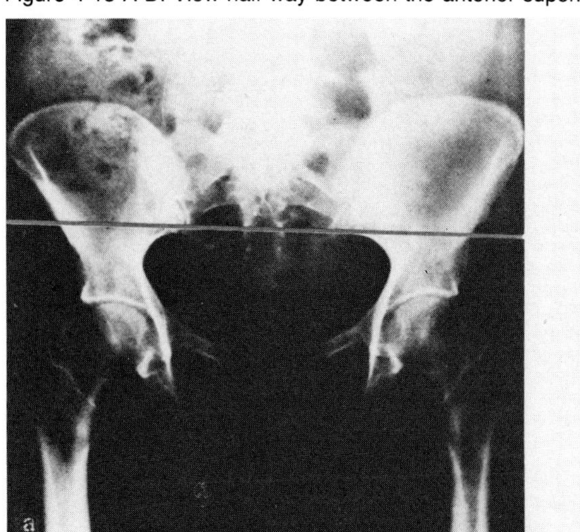

Figure 4-13A.

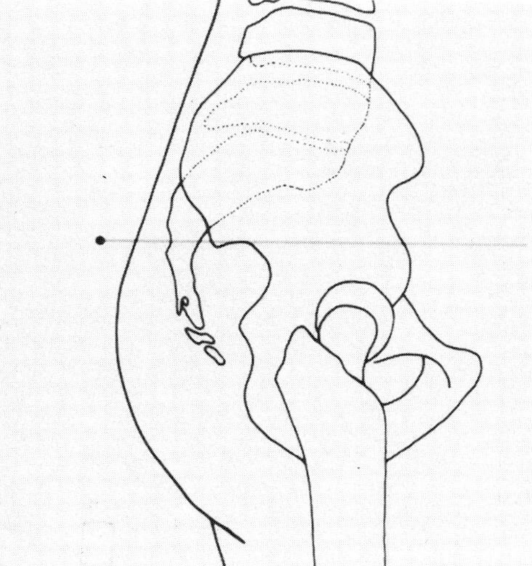
Figure 4-13B.

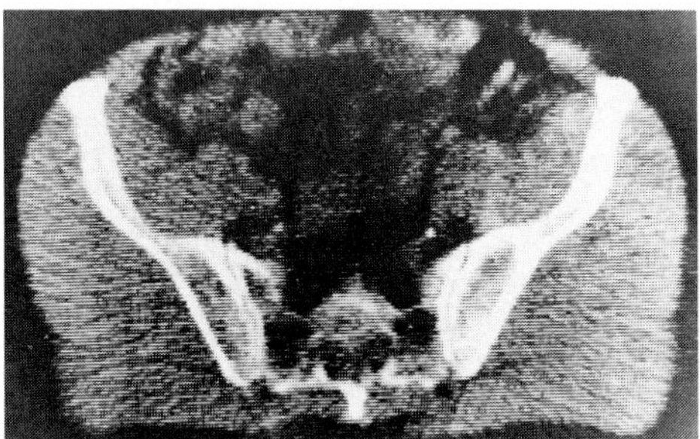
Figure 4-13C.

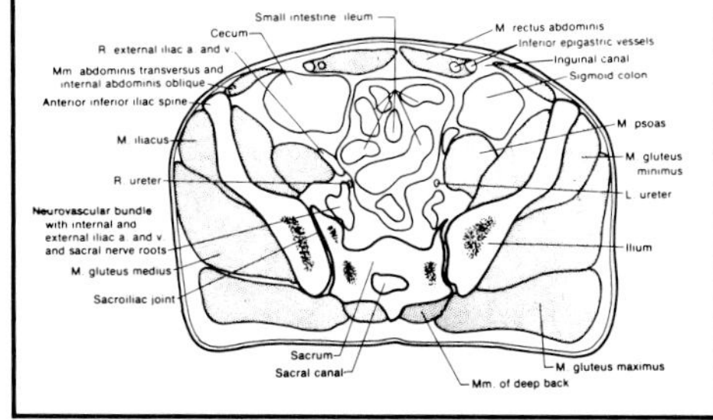

Figure 4-13D.

the first shows the principal part of the sacrum and the adjacent sacroiliac joints. A third section, prepared 1cm distal to the second, shows the dome of the acetabulum with a circular cross-section. A fourth section prepared 1.5cm distal to the third, transsects the midacetabular region where the femoral head opposes the anterior and posterior column and the site of insertion of the ligamentum teres. The most inferior section reveals the inferior pubic ramus and the ischial tuberosity, as well as the proximal femur at the level of the greater trochanter.

Conventional computed scans are hampered by their obliquity of section through the pelvis of a recumbent patient. With this obliquity the interpretation of the orientation of a fracture line through the acetabulum and the pattern of injury is difficult to characterize.[5,6] When a pelvic ring, delayed union or nonunion is assessed, a scrutiny of the partially healed ilium does not permit an accurate distinction of a partial union from an unstable nonunion.

Figure 4-14 A-D. View at the level of the anterior inferior spine.

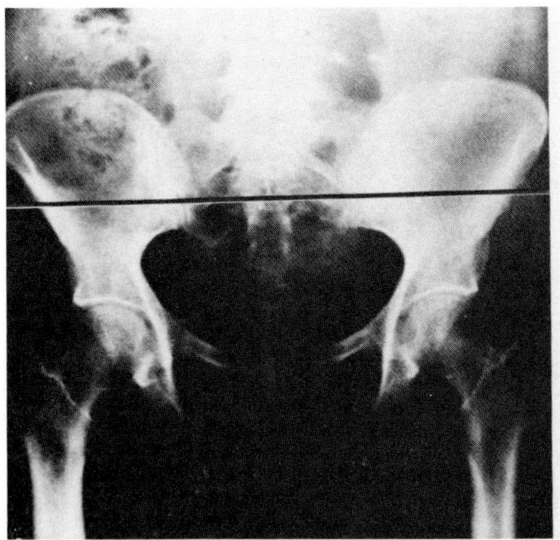

Figure 4-14A.

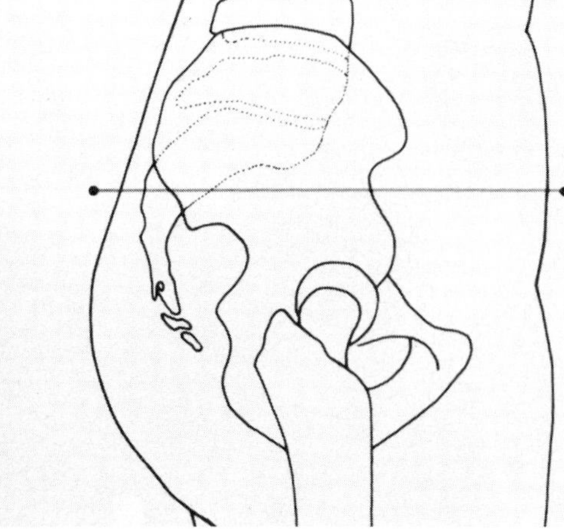

Figure 4-14B.

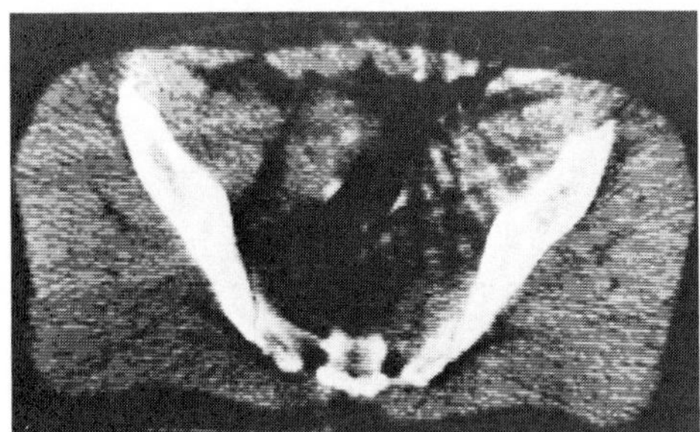

Figure 4-14C.

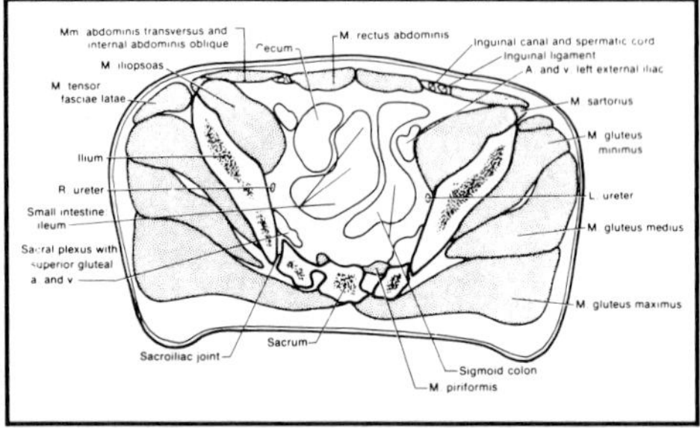


Figure 4-14D.

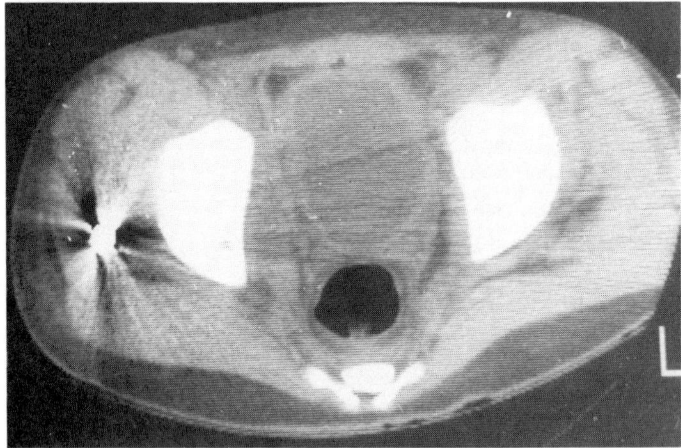

Figure 4-15. View at the acetabular dome.

In an attempt to irradicate or minimize these shortcomings, angled computed scanning techniques for the pelvis and acetabulum were developed[7] in which both the gantry of the GE 9800 scanning unit and the radiographic table were tilted by about 20° (Figure 4-

Figure 4-16 A-D. View at the horizontal equator of the femoral head.

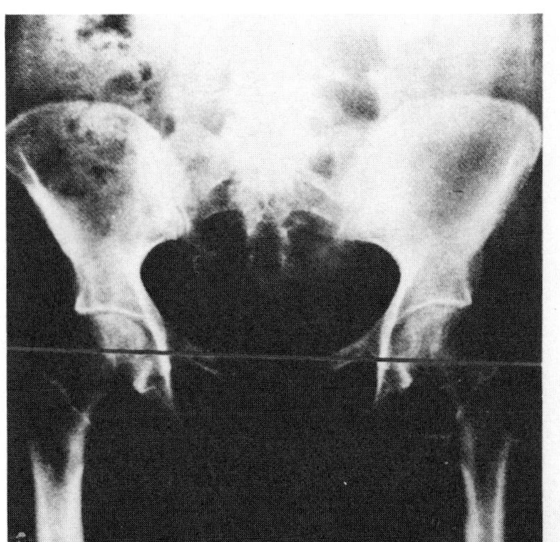

Figure 4-16A.

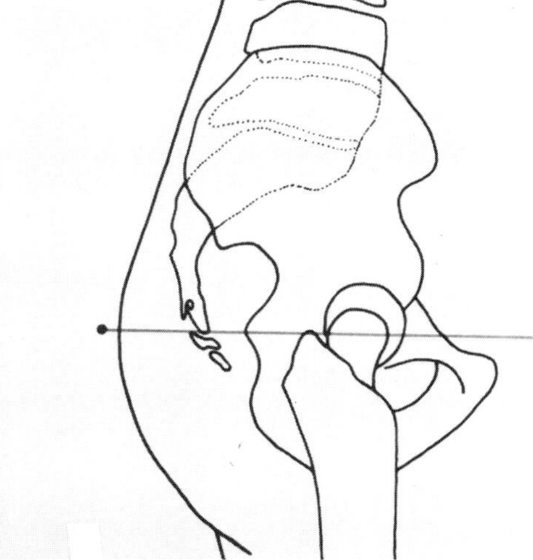

Figure 4-16B.

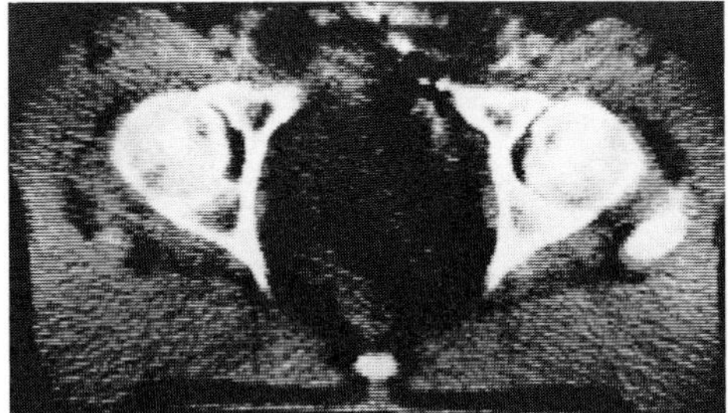

Figure 4-16C.

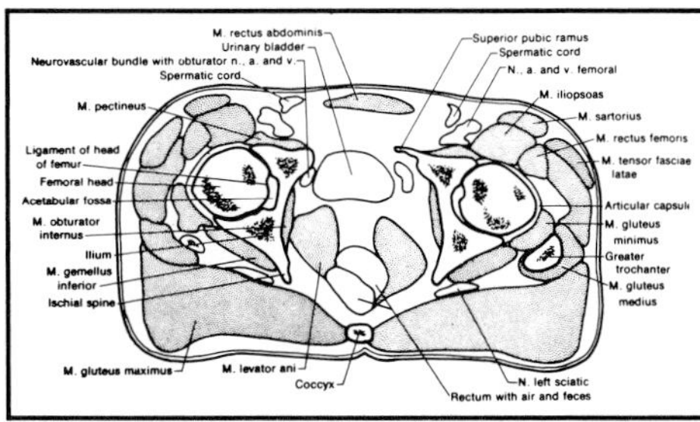


Figure 4-16D.

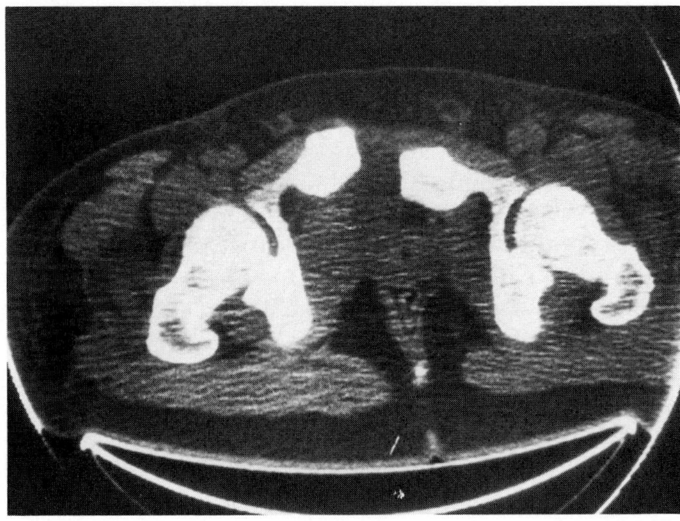

Figure 4-17. View at the superior pubic rami and symphysis.

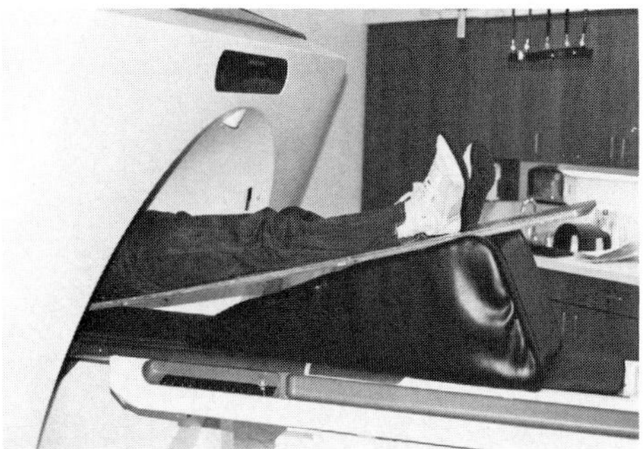

Figure 4-18. Computed scanning technique to prepare orthogonal pelvic views by the use of a GE 9800 scanning unit. Both the gantry and the radiographic table are tilted by about 20°.

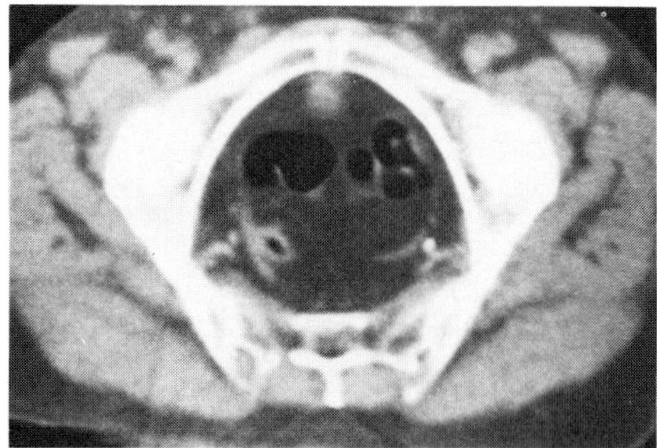

Figure 4-19. A reformatted image of a normal pelvis through the sacroiliac joints and acetabular dome.

Figure 4-20. Anteroposterior and inlet radiographs (A, B) and reformated images (C-E) of a transverse acetabular fracture with a posterior wall fragment.

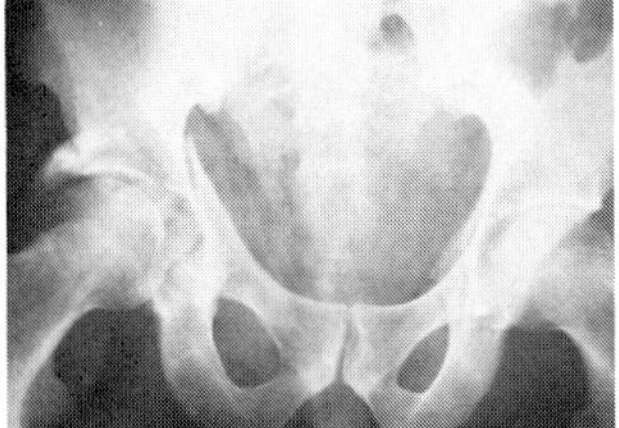

Figure 4-20A.

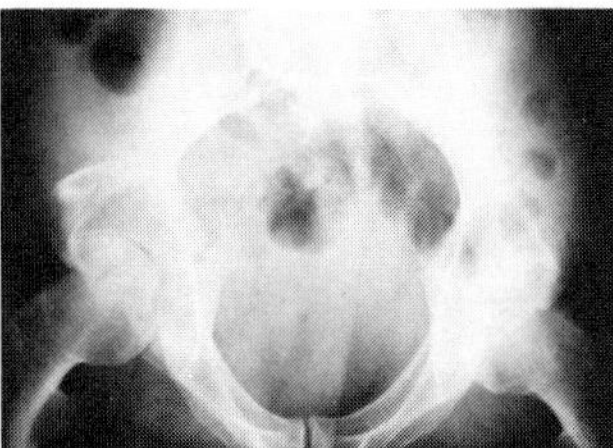

Figure 4-20B.

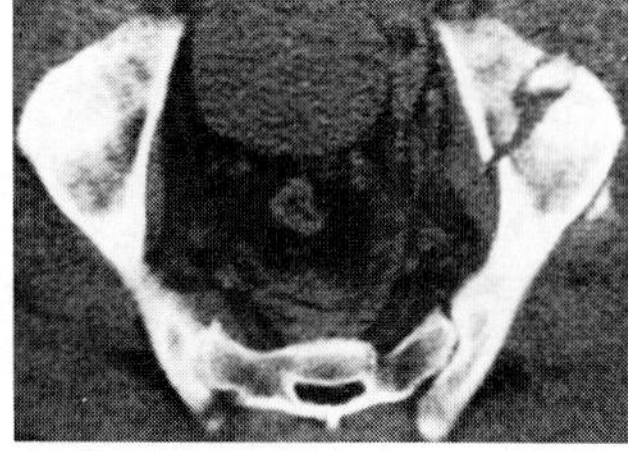

Figure 4-20C.

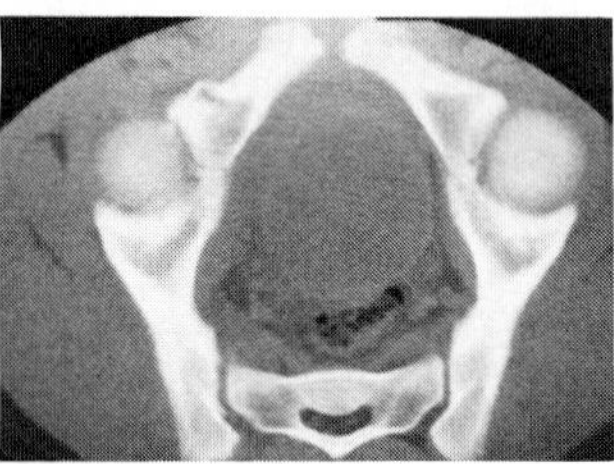

Figure 4-20D.

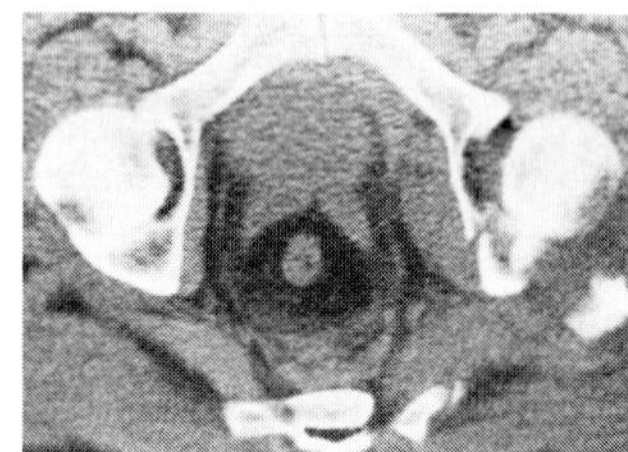

Figure 4-20E.

18). Subsequently, coronal and sagittal reformatted images were employed that also provided an image of the pelvis as a continuous ring (Figures 4-19 and 4-20). The total number of contiguous scans obtained at 10mm increments can be decreased from approximately 25 to 15 since the angled orientation of the scans more closely conforms to the configuration of the pelvis. Fifteen patients with various pelvic and acetabular disruptions were scanned with the angled technique. The principal limitations were encountered in greatly obese patients due to the inadequate size of the gantry aperture and the relative increase in thickness of the pelvis in the

Figure 4-21. Anteroposterior, iliac, and obturator oblique views (A-C), a conventional computed scan (D), and sagittal reformated images (E, F) of an associated, anterior column, posterior hemitransverse acetabular fracture.

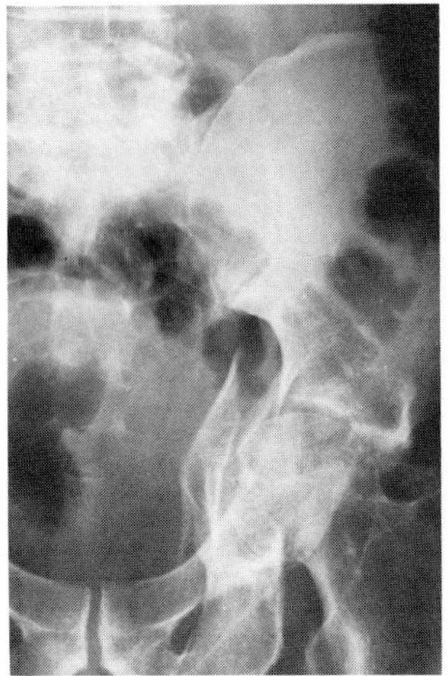

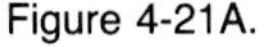

Figure 4-21A.

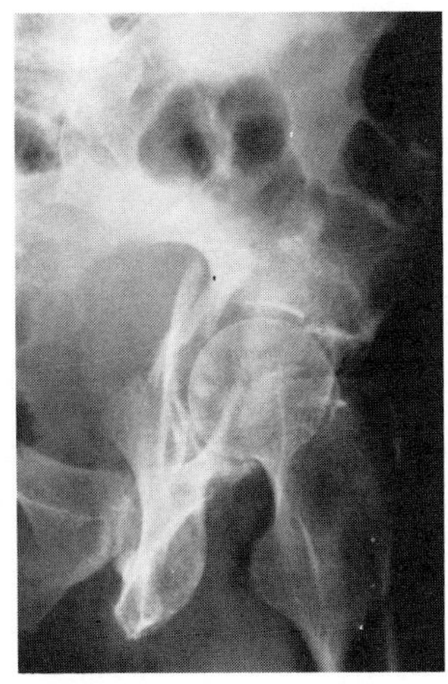

Figure 4-21B.

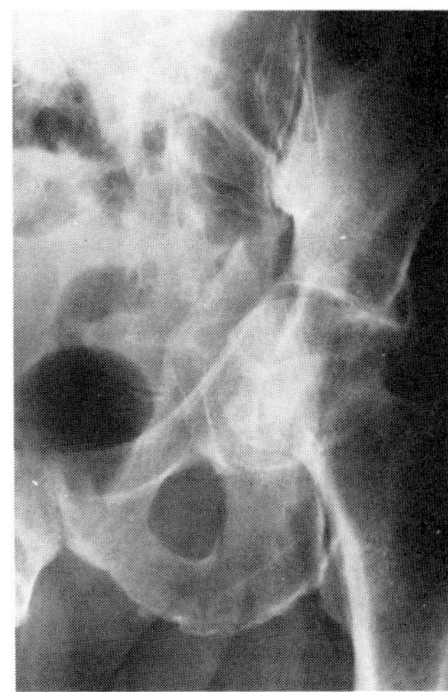

Figure 4-21C.

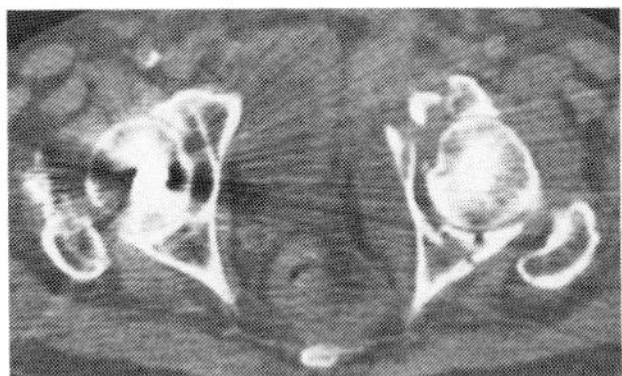

Figure 4-21D.

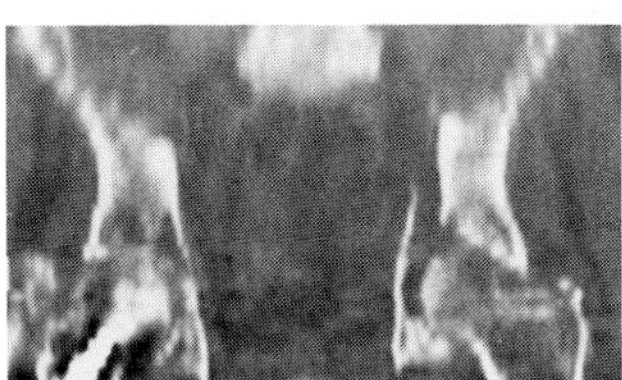

Figure 4-21E.

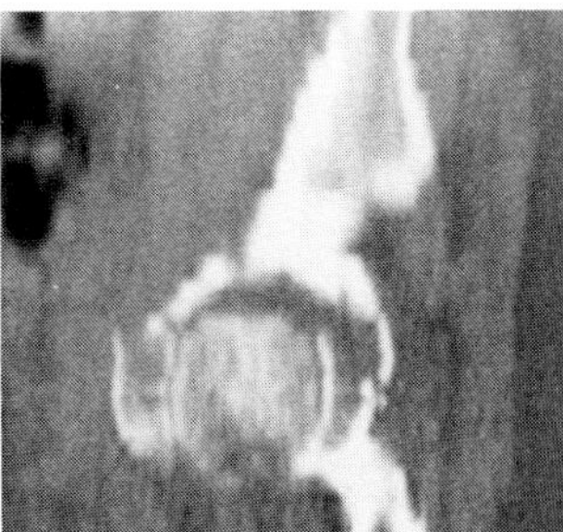

Figure 4-21F.

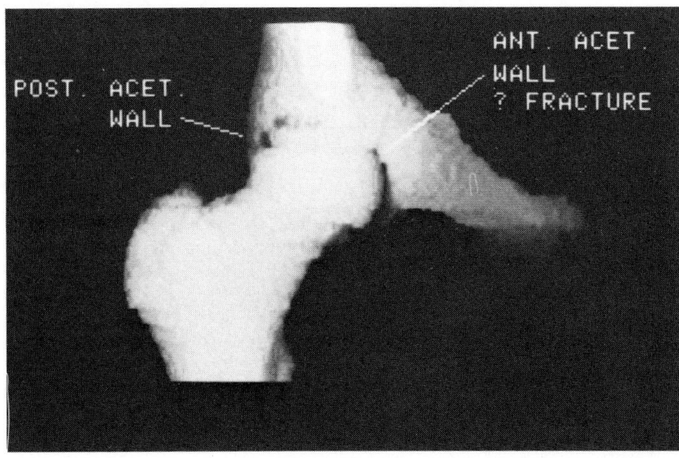


Figure 4-22. Three-dimensional surface reconstruction of the pelvis and acetabulum. This minimally displaced transverse fracture illustrates the optimal resolution (1mm to 2mm) of the method.

oblique scanning plane. Despite these advances, extensive mental integration of multiple images was required to provide an overall perspective of the complex three-dimensional bony pelvis (Figure 4-21).

Using specially designed software in conjunction with a three-dimensional reformation program developed and written by Gabor T. Herman[8] of the University of Pennsylvania, a three-dimensional surface reconstruction technique[9] was developed in collaboration with General Electric Medical Systems. The program uses data from the G.E. CT 8800 computed tomography scanner as input and runs on the associated computer. The system requires no hardware beyond the computed scanner itself. The program can produce views from virtually every vantage point. Reconstructions can be performed almost as rapidly as the raw scanning data can be cut from the CT scanner disc storage. The scans have been prepared from 2mm, 5mm and 10mm sections, as well as from combinations of these. For fine acetabular detail 2mm sections are preferred, while 10mm sections are adequate for most of the residual pelvic ring. The theoretical optimal resolution of 1mm to 2mm has been confirmed in our evaluation (Figure 4-22). The images are dimensionally accurate and, thereby, eliminate the substantial artifacts that are inevitable with conventional pelvic radiographs. Most of the stair-stepping or aliasing artifact that is present in standard plain or reconstructions is eliminated. Figure 4-23 is a representative example of a complex both-column acetabular fracture. The technique has been employed on 45 patients with a variety of acetabular and pelvic ring fractures, malunions and nonunions.[10] Many of the unique views illustrate perspectives unattainable by conventional radiography.

By the recent application of more sophisticated computerized manipulation of the data with software developed by the group at the University of Pennsylvania, subtraction of the femoral head or the acetabulum has become possible (Figure 4-24). The acetabular surface can be examined for the presence of loose interposed osteochondral fragments, impacted osteochondral fragments, large clefts, supplementary comminution, and displacement. With the three-dimensional computed scanning an accurate perception of the disrupted acetabulum and adjacent hemipelvis can be rigorously characterized to a resolution of about 1.5mm. This technology represents a major advance in diagnostic radiology for elucidation of specific patterns of pelvic and acetabular disruption. This knowledge permits a surgeon to identify the type of fracture and to plan the optimal technique of surgical approach and open reduction.

Figure 4-23. Conventional pelvic radiographs (A, B), computed scan (C, D), and a three-dimensional computed scan (E-I) of a both-column fracture of the acetabulum.

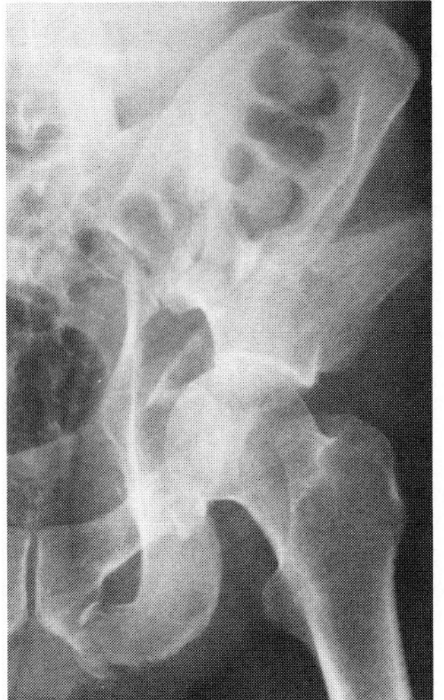

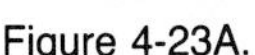

Figure 4-23A.

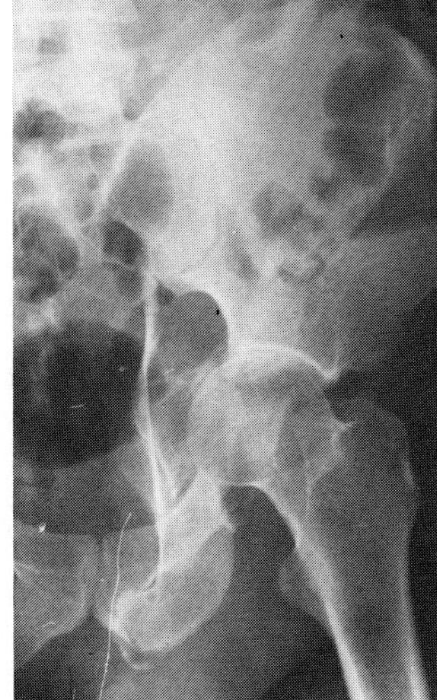

Figure 4-23B.

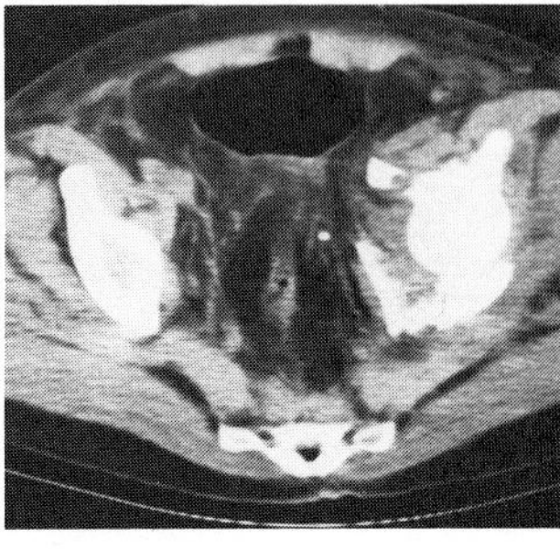

Figure 4-23C.

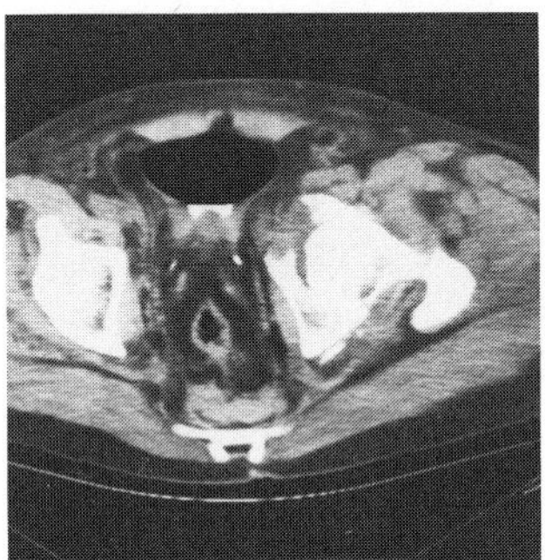

Figure 4-23D.

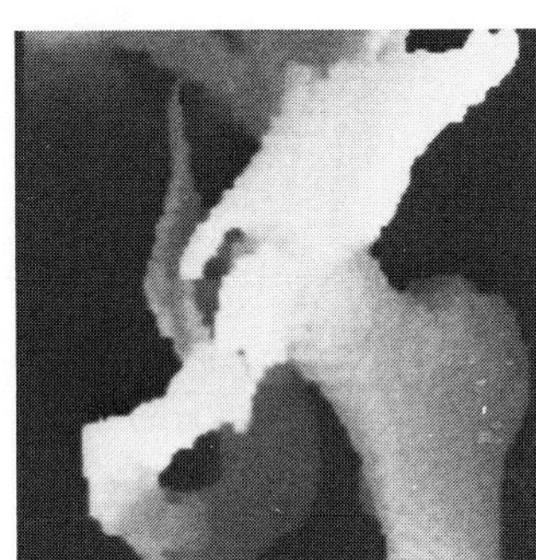

Figure 4-23E.

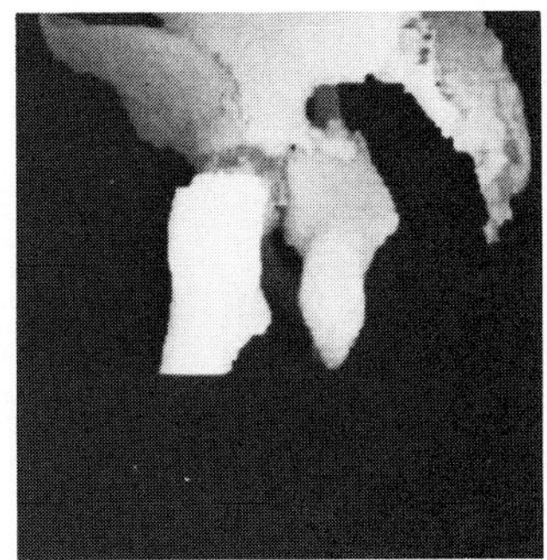

Figure 4-23F.

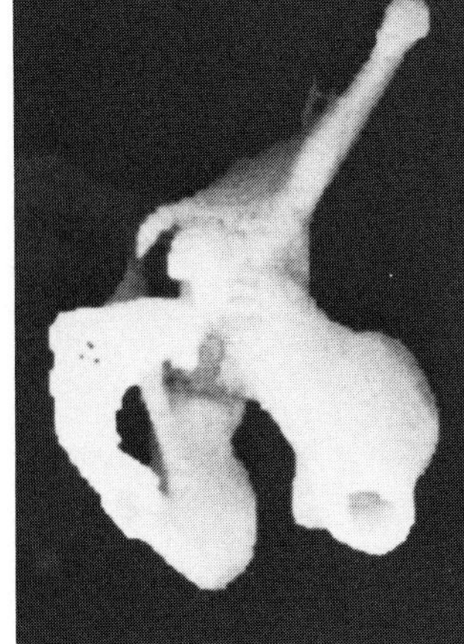

Figure 4-23G.

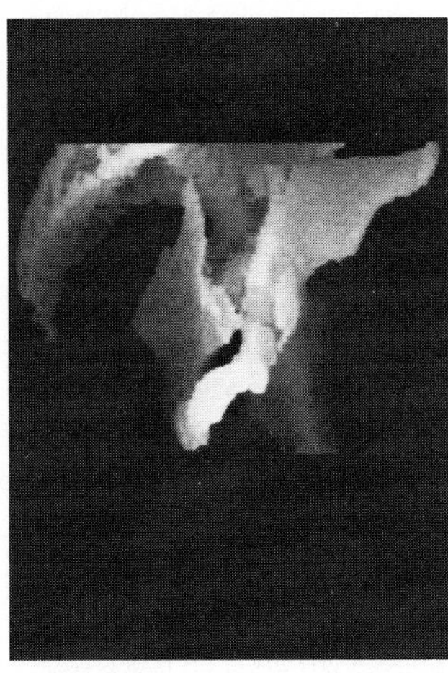

Figure 4-23H.

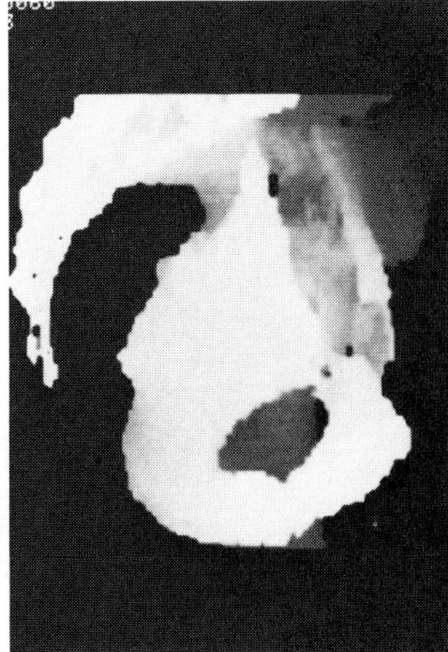

Figure 4-23I.

Figure 4-24. Computed subtraction of the femoral head (A-C) and of the acetabulum (D) permits a careful preoperative examination of the acetabular articular surface for loose interposed fragments (A), comminution (B), impaction and large gaps (C). Impacted segments of the femoral head can also be identified.

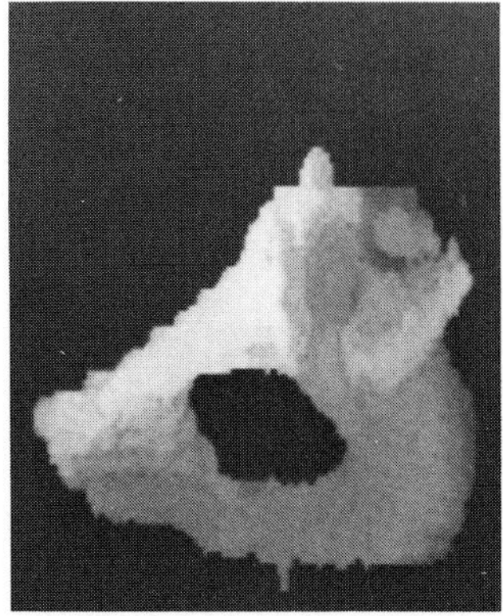

Figure 4-24A.

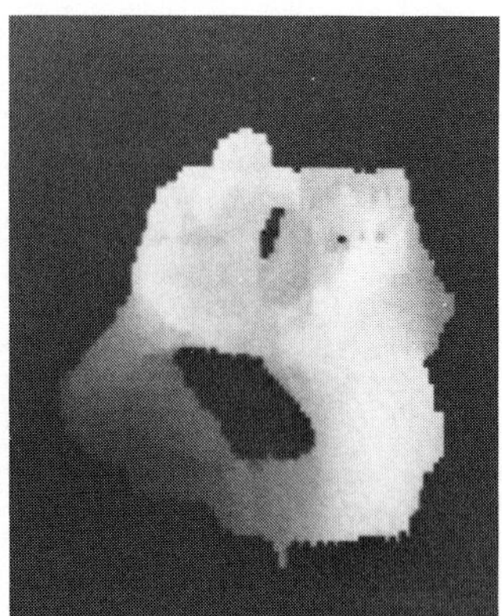

Figure 4-24B.

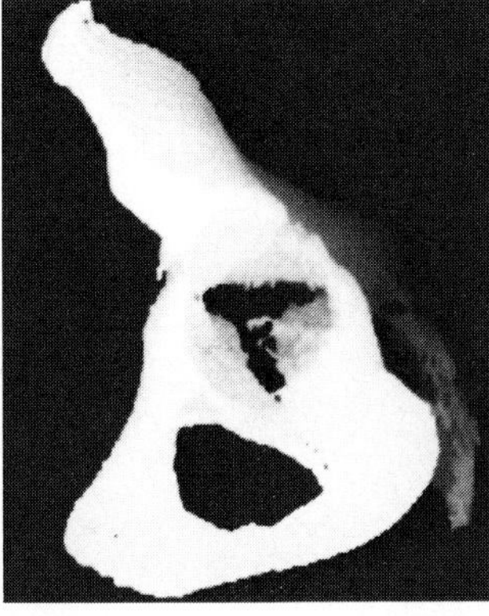

Figure 4-24C.

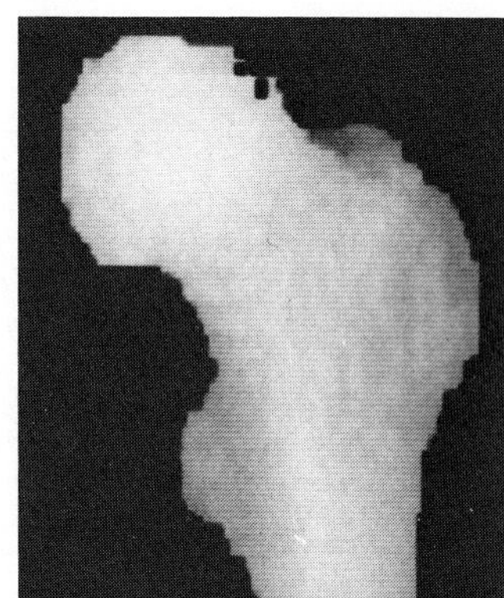

Figure 4-24D.

# Classification Schemes for Pelvic and Acetabular Fractures

With the broad spectrum of injury patterns that is documented for pelvic and acetabular disruptions, it is not surprising that numerous classification systems have evolved. Features of the different classification schemes include the number and sites of injury, the mechanism of injury, and the degree of pelvic instability. The classification systems are reviewed for the pelvis and acetabulum, respectively.

## Classification of Pelvic Ring Disruptions

Certain minor pelvic fractures arise as avulsion injuries of muscular origin. Other simple and minimally displaced fractures of the iliac wing and rami also respond to management by simple bed rest and analgesia until weight bearing can be resumed. These relatively minor

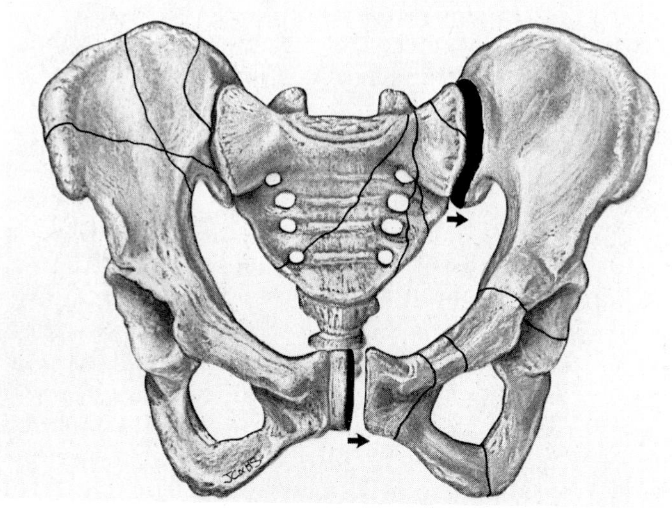

Figure 4-25. Classification scheme for pelvic ring fractures by the site of injury (after Letournel).

injuries will not be further considered under classification or treatment. To classify the principal pelvic ring disruptions, Pennal and Tile[2] devised a scheme based upon the direction of the provocative force. Injuries were categorized as anteroposterior compression, lateral compression, or vertical shear. The asset of this format is the presentation of distinct categories both in regard to the nature of the injury, the morbidity, the potential sites of disruption, the degree of pelvic instability and recommendations for treatment. In fact, the vector of the provocative force is rarely documented. In many instances, scrutiny of the posttraumatic radiographs does not permit a rigorous classification by the mechanism of trauma. For these reasons, Letournel[11] suggests a classification by the site of injury as a combination of two or more of five elementary patterns (Figure 4-25):

**A)** An anterior vertical fracture, which divides the obturator ring vertically or obliquely to separate the superior from the inferior pubic ramus. Less commonly, this anterior fracture divides the body of the pubis with the potential to violate the anterior horn of the acetabular articular surface.

**B)** A transiliac posterior fracture, which usually extends obliquely from the iliac crest to the greater sciatic notch. Alternatively the fracture line may course horizontally from the sciatic notch to the anterior border of the iliac wing. The fracture also may course from the iliac crest to the sciatic notch and progress to the iliac articular surface, where it is associated with a sacroiliac dislocation.

**C)** A transsacral fracture, which extends along the outside or inside of the foramina. The fracture line may propagate

obliquely across the sacrum from superior to inferior.
**D)** A pure separation of the pubic symphysis, which may be accompanied by a separation or overlapping of the opposing rami.
**E)** A pure disruption of the sacroiliac joint.

Recently in an attempt to clarify the precise nature of pelvic ring disruptions, Bucholz[12] undertook an anatomical assessment on multiple trauma victims. Of 150 consecutive victims of multiple trauma examined at autopsy, 47 (31%) were found to have a pelvic injury. Twenty-six of the 32 cadavers that were examined both radiographically and by dissection had a double break in the pelvic ring. An anatomical classification based upon the magnitude of posterior disruption was proposed (Figure 4-26). By radiographic assessment a Group I injury shows an isolated anterior disruption with minimal displacement of a diastasis of the symphysis pubis or ramus fractures. Upon dissection all of the specimens possessed a nondisplaced vertical fracture of the sacrum or minor tearing of the anterior sacroiliac ligament. In the Group II cases, there was radiographic evidence of both an anterior injury to the pelvic ring and a partial disruption of the sacroiliac joint. Upon dissection a complete tear or avulsion of the anterior sacroiliac ligament from the sacrum was visualized but the posterosuperior sacroiliac ligamentous complex was intact. The Group III cadavers possessed a complete disruption of all of the sacroiliac ligaments. A triplane displacement of the hemipelvis was possible with superior migration documented in an anteroposterior radiograph and posterior and external rotational displacement verified by a pelvic inlet view.

An open reduction was attempted in all of the specimens. All of the Group I injuries were virtually nondisplaced. Even with the application of an axial or posterior force to the disrupted hemipelvis there was no displacement. With the application of lateral compression to the iliac crest, two of the five Group II injuries were reduced. In the other three Group II injuries, the interposition of anterior sacroiliac ligament or a sacral avulsion fracture fragment prevented anatomical reduction. Upon excision of the interpositional ligamentous or osseous fragment, anatomical reduction was easily attained. In the 11 Group III injuries, an anatomical reduction could not be achieved and maintained even by the use of manual manipulation, longitudinal traction, and excision of interposed fragments. The anatomic irregularities of the sacroiliac joint inhibited the attempt to reduce the hemipelvis. Even in the few cases where such a reduction was achieved, the intrinsic instability of the sacroiliac articular surfaces precluded maintenance of the

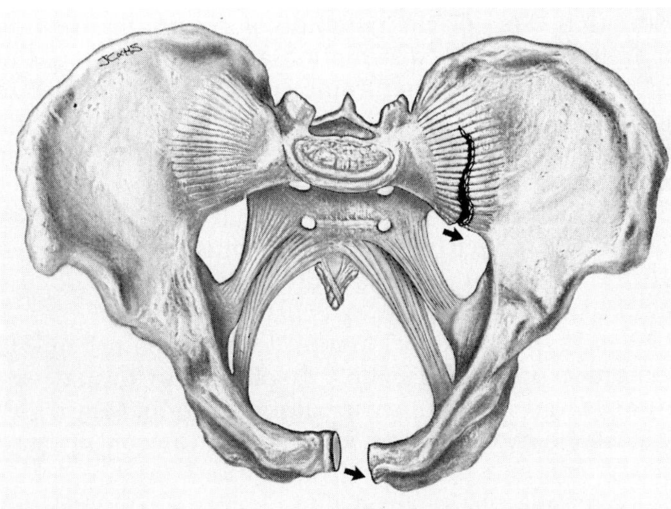

Figure 4-26A.

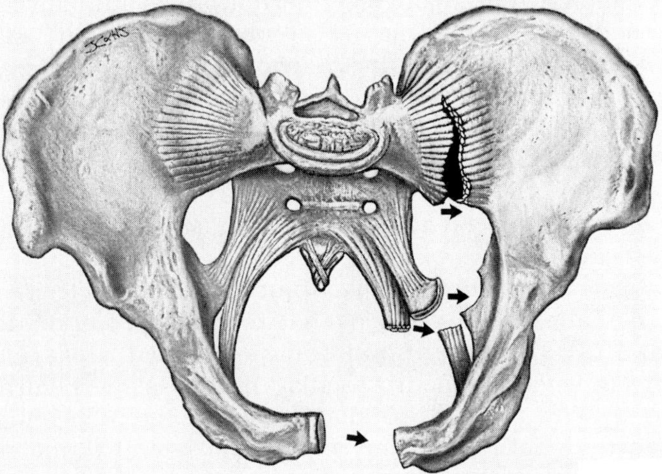

Figure 4-26B.

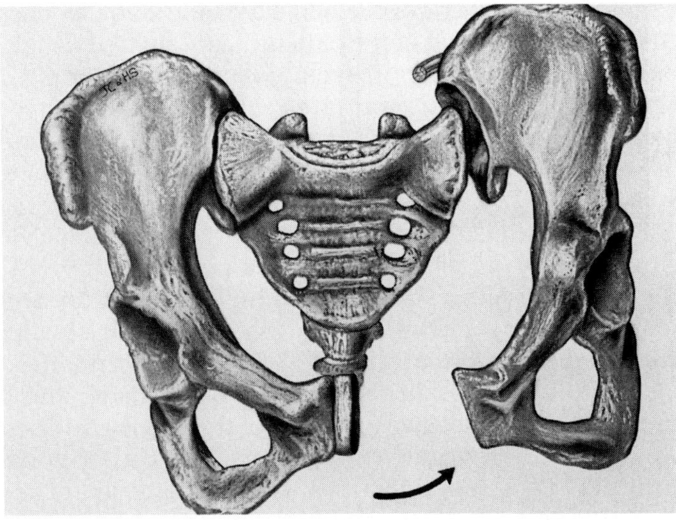

Figure 4-26C.

Figure 4-26. Schematic diagrams to clarify the Bucholz classification scheme for pelvic ring disriptions. A: Group I—minimally displaced ramus fracture and ipsilateral nondisplaced vertical sacral fracture. An alternative injury pattern is a minimally displaced diastasis and a mild tearing of an anterior sacroiliac ligament. B: Group II—an anterior injury such as a diastasis with a complete tear or avulsion injury of the anterior sacroiliac ligament and preservation of the posterosuperior sacroiliac ligamentous complex. By necessity the sacrospinous and sacrotuberous ligaments are torn or avulsed with radiologically evident osseous fragments from the ischial spine. C: Group III—anterior injury and complete posterior disruption.

reduction. This pelvic instability accounts for the loss of an adequate closed reduction achieved by the use of a simple pelvic external frame employed to immobilize a Group III pelvic injury. In the Bucholz study, all of the pelvic reductions were undertaken with the cadaver oriented in a supine position. Both the posterior and external rotational vectors of displacement are much more easily corrected if the closed reduction is performed with the patient in a lateral position, prior to the application of a complex external pelvic frame.

Even if the Letournel anatomically-based scheme is combined with the Bucholz displacement format two other categories of injury merit recognition. Mears and Rubash[13] have described a fourth major category of pelvic injury, complex pelvic ring disruptions (Figure 4-27), which are usefully subdivided into four main subgroups: **A)** bilateral unstable posterior disruptions of the sacroiliac joint or adjacent ilium and sacrum accompanied by an anterior disruption; **B)** a unilateral unstable posterior fracture accompanied by an iliac fracture and an anterior disruption; **C)** a unilateral posterior fracture with an anterior disruption as well as an acetabular fracture; and **D)** various patterns of comminuted injuries with unilateral or bilateral unstable posterior disruptions, bilateral acetabular or iliac fractures, bilateral ramus fractures, and lumbosacral dislocations.

All of the Group IV pelvic injuries are characterized as comminuted disruptions that follow major traumatic insults. The likelihood for associated visceral, appendicular and neurovascular injuries is particularly great. With the multiple disruptions of the pelvic ring either at both sacroiliac joints, the lateral ilium or acetabulum, external fixation cannot be used as the sole method of pelvic stabilization. While it may be used in certain cases to help restore hemodynamic stability, once the general condition of the patient has stabilized usually external fixation requires supplementation or replacement with appropriate techniques of internal fixation. With the multiple sites of pelvic injury, fixation of each unstable site is usually needed to restore adequate stability.

The fifth category of pelvic ring injury is an open pelvic ring fracture. Of all of the types of pelvic disruptions, the Class V fractures possess the highest mortality and morbidity. The complications are associated with a higher energy dissipation at the time of injury, enhanced bleeding in the absence of effective tamponade, and a predilection for massive infection of the pelvis and open wound by Gram negative organisms. The conventional preoperative resuscitative regime and fracture classification is followed by aggressive surgical

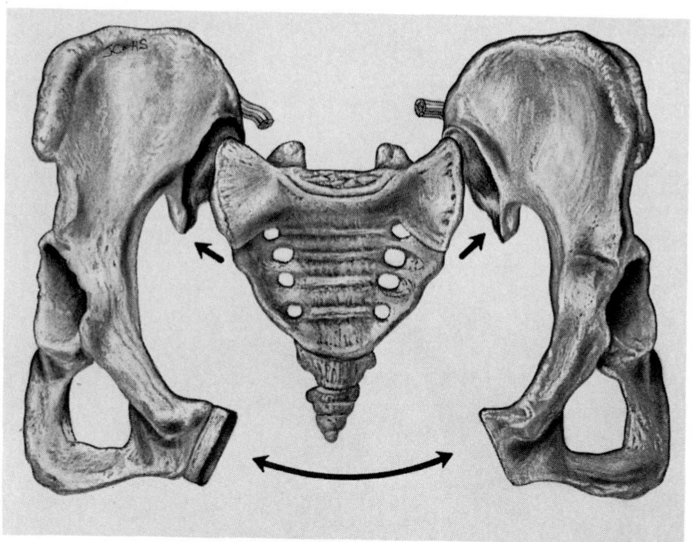

Figure 4-27. Schematic diagram of the representative example of a Group IV pelvic injury with bilateral unstable sacroiliac disruptions.

intervention with external fixation, the creation of a diversion colostomy, and debridement of the perineal wound. Parenteral cephalosporin and aminoglycoside are administered for a 48- to 72-hour period.

Another widely used classification scheme based upon the vector of the provocative force was devised by Pennal and Tile.[2] While in the present state of knowledge it may be somewhat cumbersome, for the past decade it has been widely accepted. When it is correlated with the substantial clinical experience of the Toronto school it, too, provides insight into the magnitude of the traumatic force, the likelihood for associated injuries, the degree of pelvic instability and, thereby, a guideline for the optimal therapeutic methods to restore pelvic stability. For these reasons it is presented in detail.

An anteroposterior compression injury (Figure 4-28) results from a blow that strikes the posterior ilium or the anterior pelvis to disrupt the symphysis and the anterior sacroiliac ligaments of one or both sacroiliac joints. Usually the crucial posterior sacroiliac complex is spared and the injury is defined as a stable disruption. In a very small percentage of anteroposterior injuries, probably less than 5% to 10% of cases, the posterior sacroiliac ligaments are violated to produce an unstable hemipelvis.

A lateral compression injury arises from a direct blow to the lateral ilium (Figure 4-29). An extremely stable impacted fracture of the sacrum or rarely the adjacent sacroiliac joint may ensue. In the presence of an anterolateral or posterolateral force, however, the ipsilateral hemipelvis rotates around the site of the posterior disruption involving the sacroiliac joint or the adjacent sacrum or ilium. This fracture pattern,

Figure 4-28. Anteroposterior compression injuries. A: Computed scan consistent with the minor and moderately severe injuries shown in Figure 4-26A and B. B: Schematic view of more severe bilateral injury with wide diastasis, disruption of the sacrospinous, sacrotuberous and anterior sacroiliac ligaments but preservation of the posterior ligaments. C: Anteroposterior radiograph equivalent of (B). D, E: Anteroposterior radiograph and computed scan to show a wide diastasis with a completely unstable left hemipelvis.

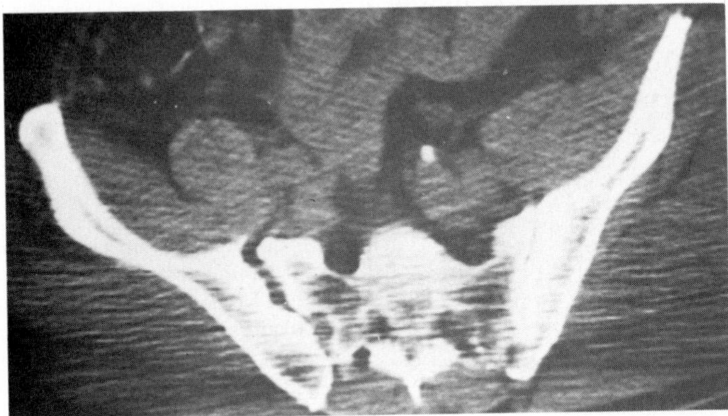

Figure 4-28A.

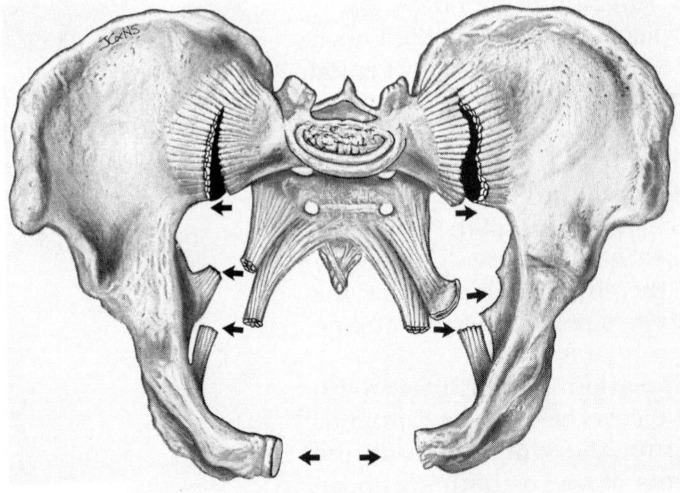

Figure 4-28B.

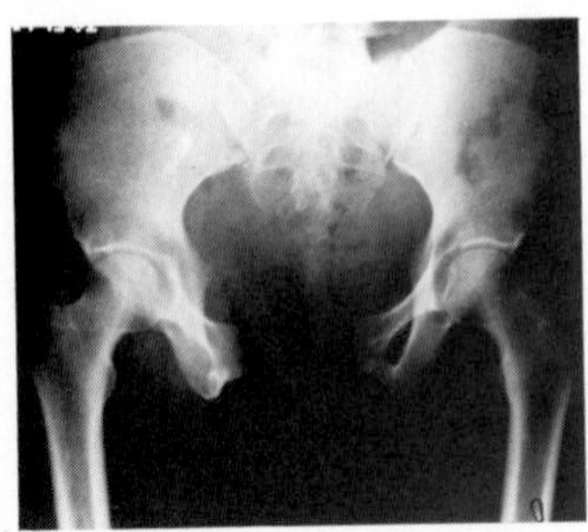

Figure 4-28C.

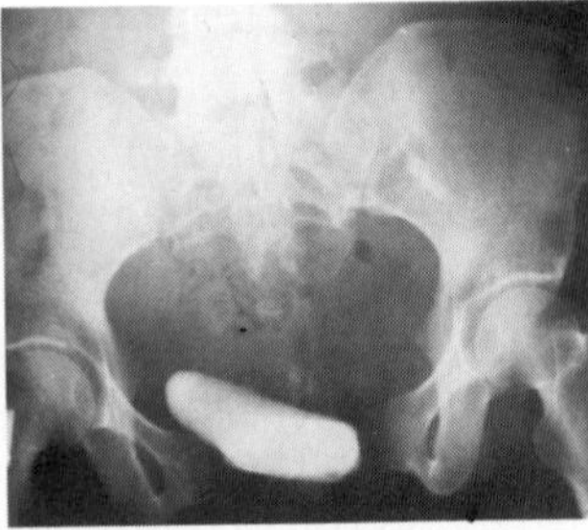

Figure 4-28D.

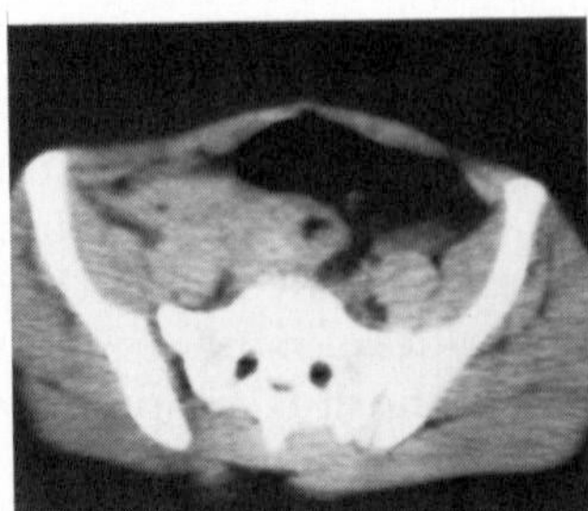

Figure 4-28E.

therefore, includes both stable and unstable injuries. Usually the contralateral rami are fractured, although not infrequently the ipsilateral pubic rami and/or all four rami are disrupted. Both a stable or an unstable lateral compression injury may be complicated by an acetabular fracture. Such a combination of injuries is included in the complex or Group IV category of pelvic disruptions. Previously a fracture of all four rami generally was attributed to a direct blow in the midline immediately superficial to the rami. At present such a "straddle" fracture is recognized as a moderately uncommon type of pelvic injury.

All of the vertical shear injuries are highly unstable and show evidence of complete posterior ligamentous instability of one or both sacroiliac joints (Figure 4-30). Most of these patients are victims of falls from a great height or a high speed motor vehicular accident. Usually the associated anterior disruption is a diastasis of the symphysis pubis. Supplementary radiological findings consistent with an unstable lateral compression or a vertical shear injury are avulsion fractures of the sacrotuberous and sacrospinous ligaments from the ischial spine or the adjacent sacrum. Another example is an avulsion of the transverse process of the fourth or fifth lumbar vertebrae at the sites of the origin of the lumbosacral ligaments. With the marked posterior displacement, especially when it involves the roof of the greater sciatic notch adjacent to the superior gluteal vessels, the likelihood for profuse posttraumatic hemorrhage is considerable.

## Classification of Acetabular Fractures

Historically, acetabular fractures were crudely divided into posterior fracture dislocations of the hip with an acetabular rim fracture and a central fracture of the acetabulum.[14-16] The two injuries were readily distinguished by scrutiny of an anteroposterior pelvic radiograph. This distinction did not permit sufficiently accurate characterization of the central fractures of the acetabulum to determine the degree of anteroposterior displacement of the femoral head the site(s) of principal acetabular disruption and, thereby, the appropriate operative exposure. It was solely of value where nonoperative treatment or skeletal traction was employed to a central fracture group. Later, a more elaborate classification was devised by Rowe and Lowell[17] with six categories of acetabular fracture. This classic work attempted to identify those displaced fractures in which management by resort to a closed reduction with skeletal traction possessed an overwhelming propensity for an incongruous hip destined for early traumatic arthritis. Again, the classification scheme did not accurately

Figure 4-29. Lateral compression injuries.

Figure 4-29A. Stable lateral compression injuries: i and ii) schematic diagram and anteroposterior radiograph with rotation of left hemipelvis and slightly displaced right rami; iii) a computed scan of a stable lateral compression injury with a buckle-type impaction of the left sacral ala; iv) a computed scan with multiple cracks from the right ala into the neural foramen.

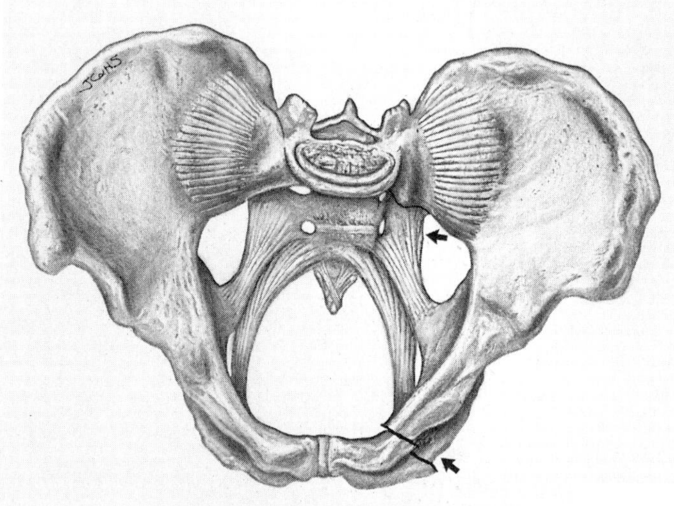

Figure 4-29A i.

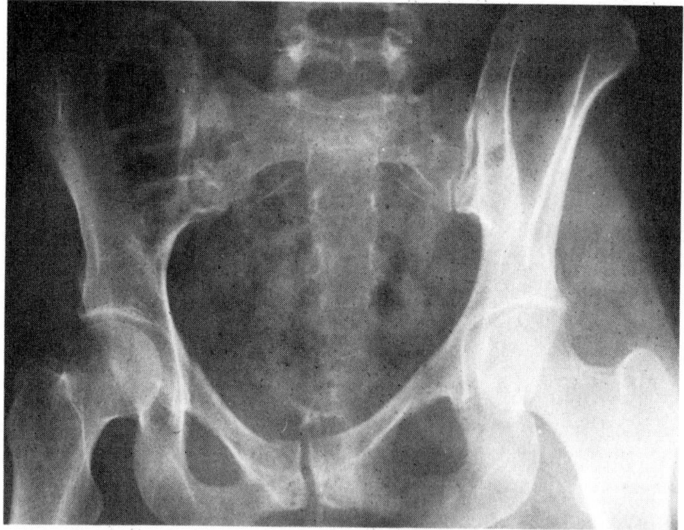

Figure 4-29A ii.

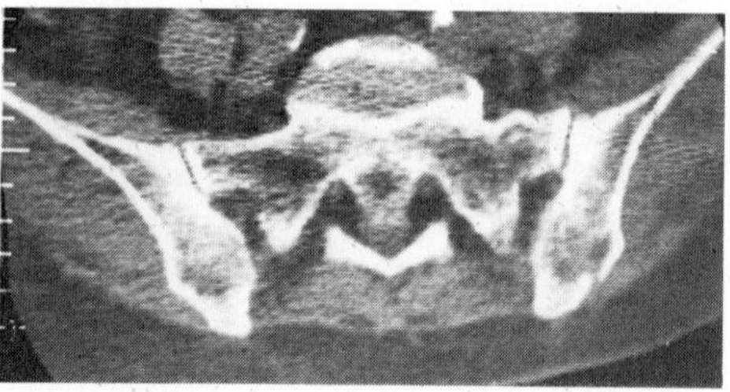

Figure 4-29A iii.

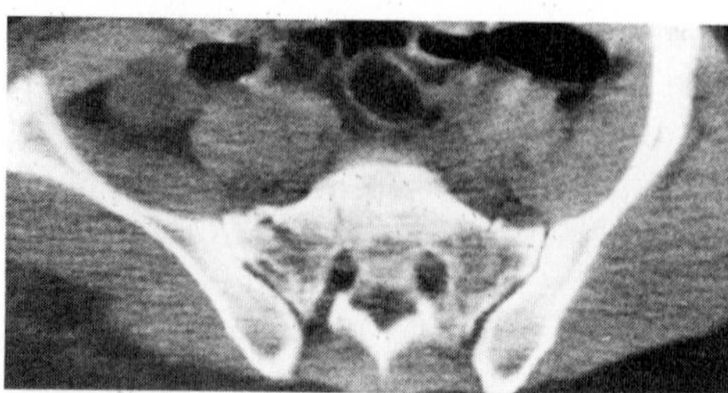

Figure 4-29A iv.

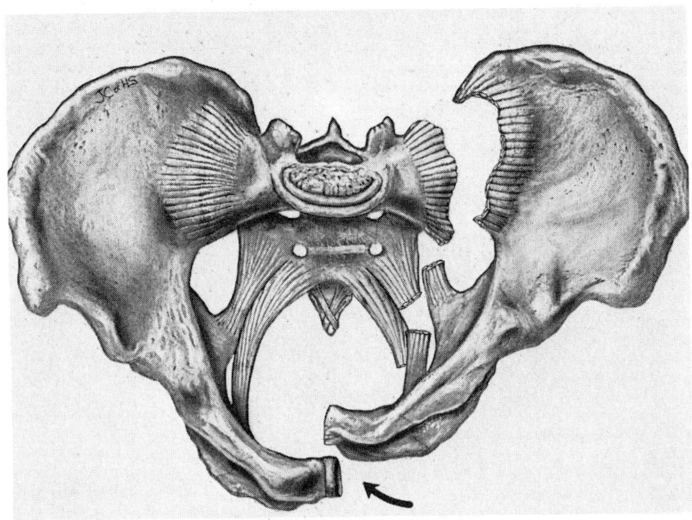

Figure 4-29B. Schematic view of an unstable moderately displaced lateral compression injury with rotational deviation of the left hemipelvis.

characterize the specific regional site(s) of acetabular disruption so that appropriate preoperative planning for an open reduction could be undertaken. In retrospect, the observations of Lowell indicated that most displaced acetabular fractures were unlikely to undergo a concentric realignment under the influence of skeletal traction. As discussed in Chapter 6, this observation has been reaffirmed in a more critical fashion by Matta. If this hypothesis is true, then the principal purpose for a classification scheme is to define the geographic region of the acetabulum that is damaged to permit elucidation of the appropriate technique for exposure, reduction, and stabilization. Such a classification scheme was developed by Letournel in his thesis of 1960,[18] and was published with minor modification by Judet and Letournel in 1965.[19] While at first glance it seems needlessly cumbersome, it permits a precise characterization of acetabular fractures into two large groups. The elementary fractures are distinguished by a disruption of one region or column of the acetabulum or a single disruption as a transverse fracture. A second group of associated fractures includes at least two patterns of the five elementary fractures with five principal variants. Virtually all acetabular fractures can be categorized into one of these ten varieties. Other features of the injury that have been classified include the damage to the weightbearing surface or dome or the medial wall, or quadrilateral surface, and the magnitude of displacement, comminution, and osteoporosis. While these features correlate with prognostication, they do not lend themselves to classification in a way that facilitates the surgical procedure. For the remainder of this discussion, the system of Letournel and Judet[3] will be employed.

Figure 4-29C. Unstable lateral compression injuries: i) schematic diagram; ii) markedly malrotated left rami, anteroposterior radiograph; iii) displaced fractures of all four rami, anteroposterior radiograph.

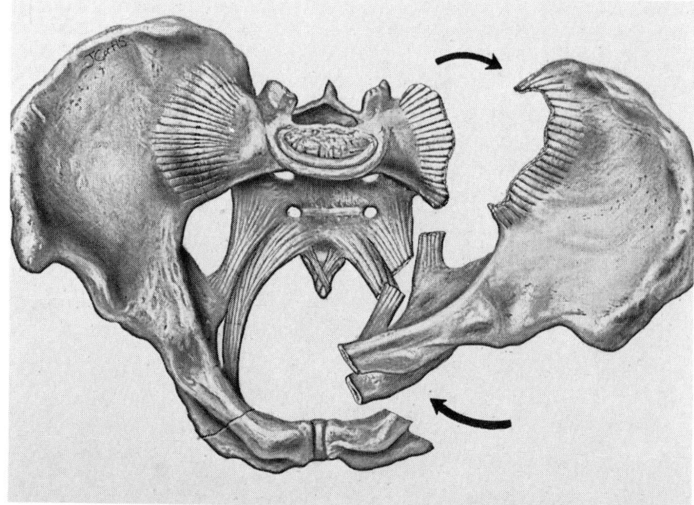

Figure 4-29C i.

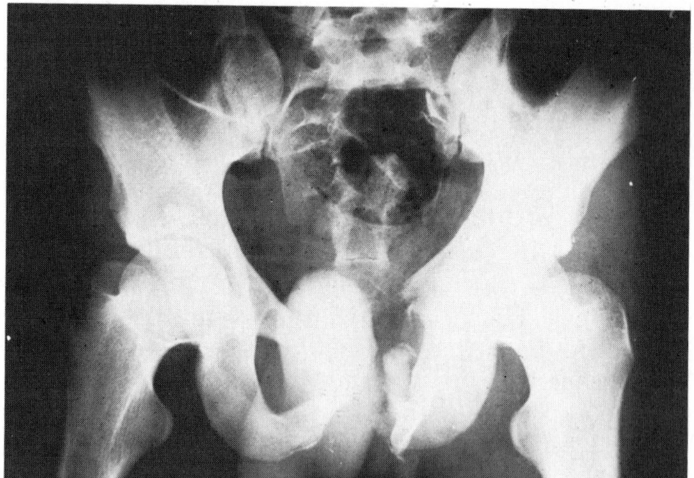

Figure 4-29C ii.

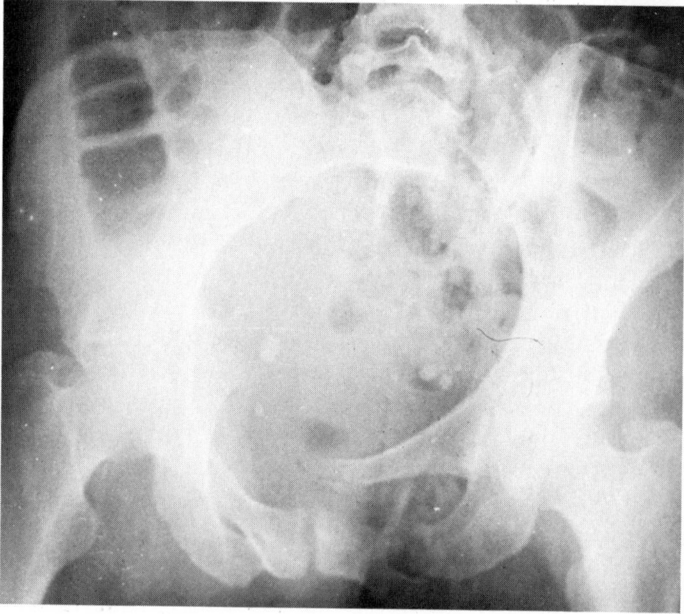

Figure 4-29C iii.

Figure 4-29D. Computed scans of various types of unstable posterior disruptions with lateral compression injuries: i) crack propagating from anterior sacrum, possibly unstable; ii) fracture/dislocation of sacroiliac joint extending into posterior sacrum with considerable likelihood for posterior instability; iii) unstable right-sided sacral fracture; iv) unstable sacral fracture through right neural foramen; v) unstable midline sacral fracture.

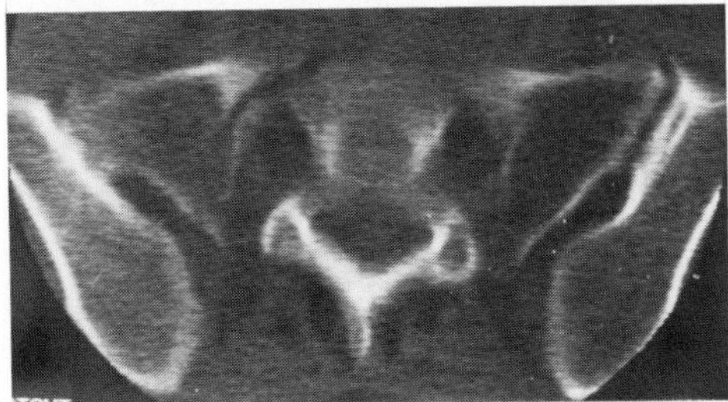

Figure 4-29D i.

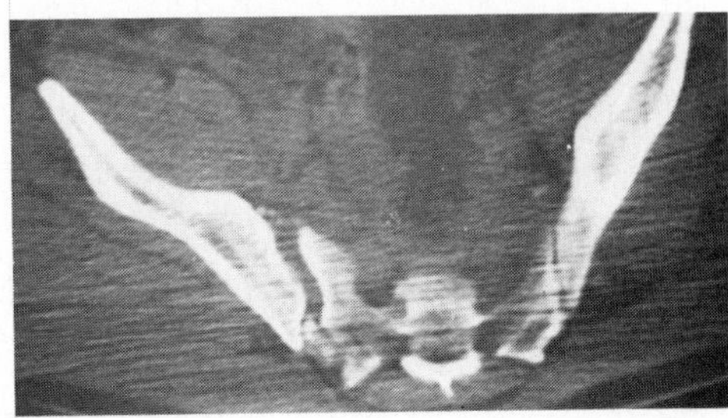

Figure 4-29D ii.

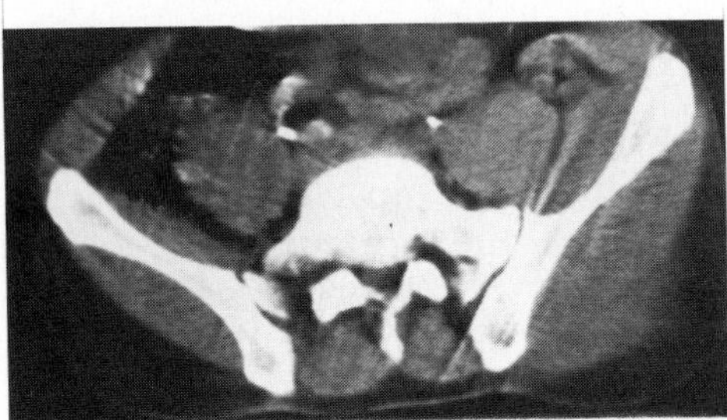

Figure 4-29D iii.

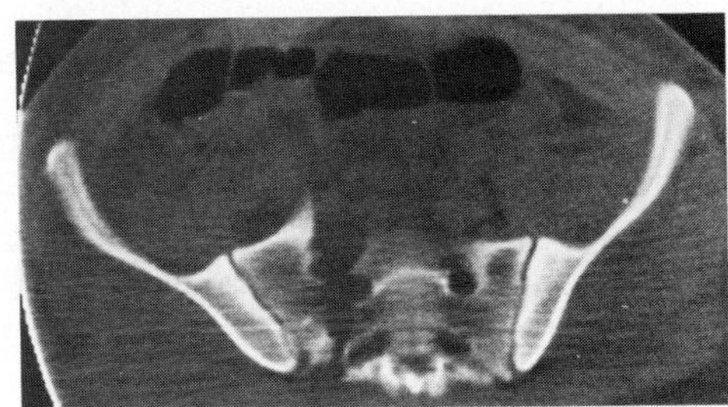

Figure 4-29D iv.

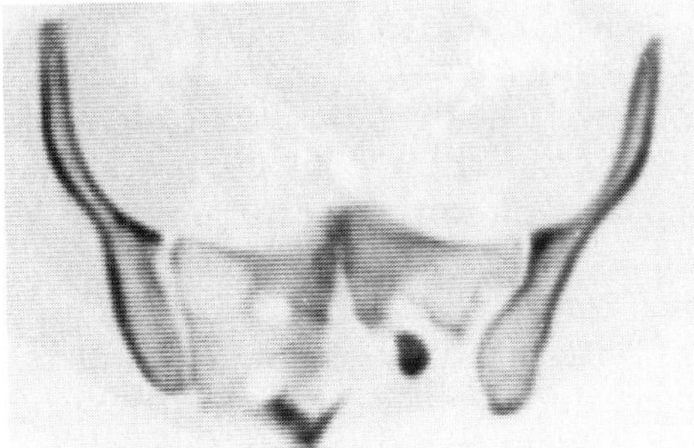

Figure 4-29D v.

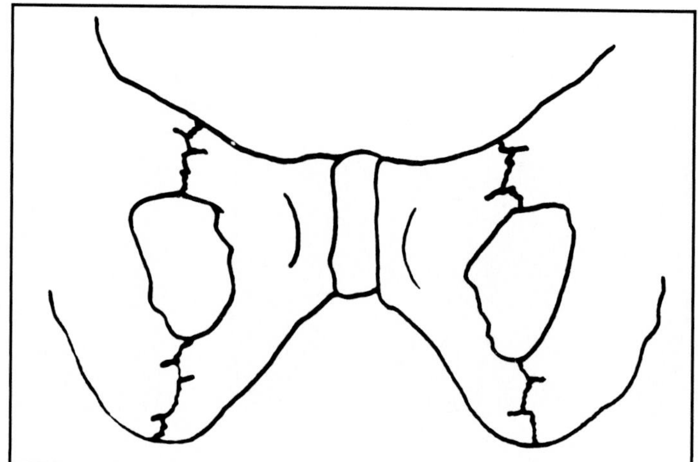

Figure 4-29E. Schematic view of a "straddle fracture." This injury pattern is usually provoked by a lateral compression injury.

## *A. Elementary Fractures*

**1. Posterior Wall Fracture.** This injury involves a separation of a segment of the posterior part of the articular surface to spare the principal part of the posterior column (Figure 4-31). It arises as part of a posterior dislocation of the femoral head with a considerable propensity for a sciatic nerve injury. Posterior wall fractures may be subcategorized by the region of involvement. Mostly they involve the posterior wall inferior to the acetabular roof. A small percentage involve the posterosuperior portion of the posterior wall with the adjacent part of the roof and less frequently the posteroinferior portion including the posterior wall, the horn, and the upper pole of the ischial tuberosity. While the vast majority of these injuries are simple fractures, rarely they are comminuted or they may involve most of the posterior column with transitional forms to complete a posterior column or a transverse fracture. About 16% present with a marginal impaction of the articular surface where the articular cartilage is impacted into the underlying cancellous bone. In a computed scan, the notable features include the position of the femoral head with anatomical reduction or persistent posterior displacement. The size of the wall fragment, including the magnitude of the articular surface, its degree of displacement and site of origin from superior or inferior posterior column are evident. An associated minimally displaced posterior column fracture may be recognized along with a free intraarticular osteochondral fragment, which originates as an avulsion fracture from either end of the ligamentum teres (Figure 4-31E).

**2. Posterior Column Fractures.** In a typical example the entire posterior column is separated as one piece although the acetabular roof is spared (Figure 4-32). In

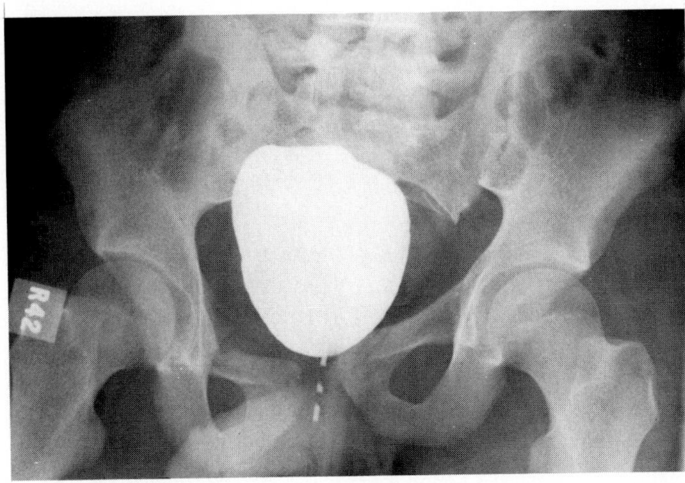


Figure 4-30. Vertical shear injuries of the left hemipelvis, anteroposterior radiograph. A comparable schematic diagram is shown in Figure 4-26C.

the anteroposterior view the head is dislocated centrally to encroach upon the pelvic inlet. The iliopectineal and acetabular-obturator lines are intact and the tear drop is in its proper position. In the obturator oblique view, the integrity of the innominate line and, thereby, the anterior column are confirmed while breaks of the posterior acetabular lip and the ischiopubic ramus are documented. The femoral head is displaced along with the posterior column. In the iliac oblique view, the displaced fragment is clearly delineated, usually to the angle of the greater sciatic notch. The anterior lip of the acetabulum, as well as the roof and the iliac wing, is noted to be intact. In about 25% of the cases of posterior column fractures, the fracture line skirts the pelvic rim so that the tear drop is included within the extended fracture fragment. In a computed scan the size and the magnitude of the posterior displacement of the posterior column fragment are readily evident. The anatomically situated or posteriorly displaced femoral head is documented along with the presence of free osteochondral fragments. Associated minimally displaced posterior wall fragments may be evident.

**3. Anterior Wall Fracture.** This uncommon counterpart of the posterior wall fracture involves a separation of the anterior part of the articular surface along with a large portion of the middle third of the anterior column (Figure 4-33). In the anteroposterior view the anterior inferior iliac spine and the angle of the pubis are spared. Disrupted radiological landmarks include the anterior border of the acetabulum, the innominate line and the superior pubic ramus. Usually the detached segment forms a trapezoid. When visible, generally the tear drop is displaced medially with an oblique orientation. While some portion of the roof is always involved, the relevant

Figure 4-31. Posterior wall fractures.
Figure 4-31A. Schematic view of the typical example to show the outer (i) and inner (ii) pelvic surfaces.

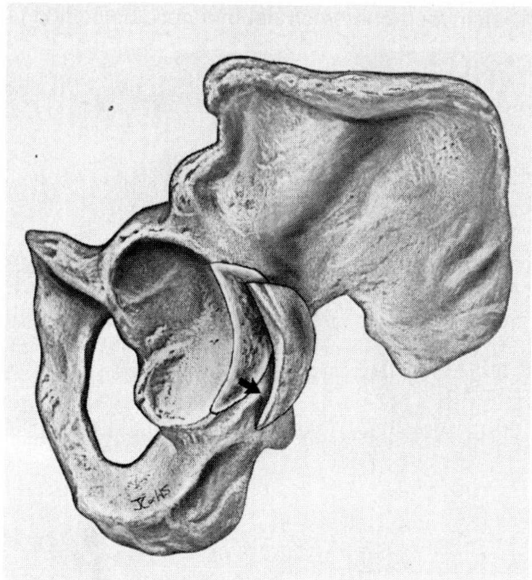

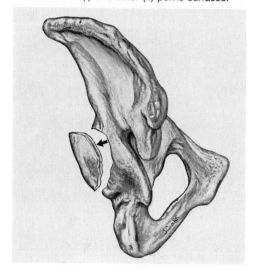

Figure 4-31A i.

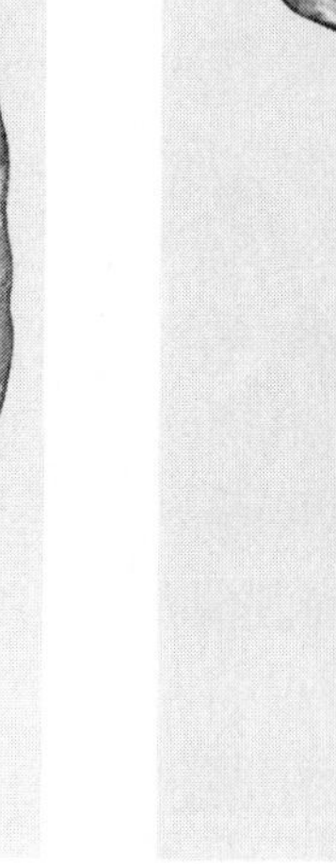

Figure 4-31A ii.

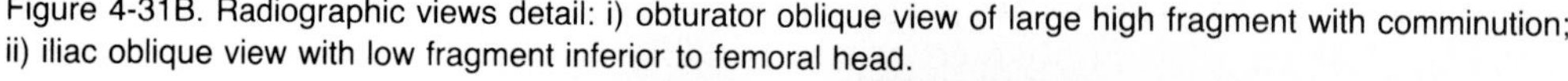
Figure 4-31B. Radiographic views detail: i) obturator oblique view of large high fragment with comminution; ii) iliac oblique view with low fragment inferior to femoral head.

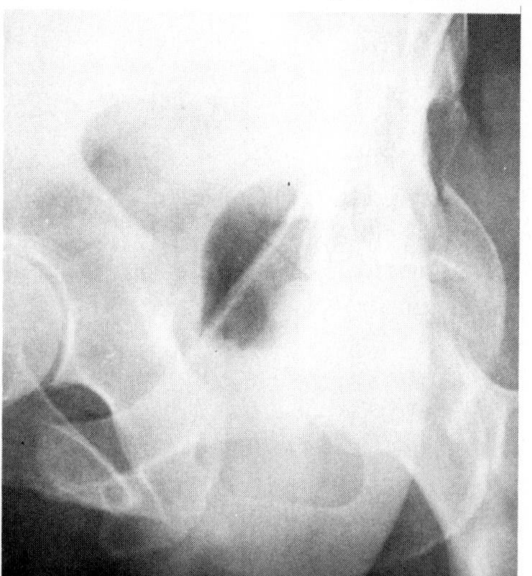

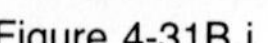
Figure 4-31B i.

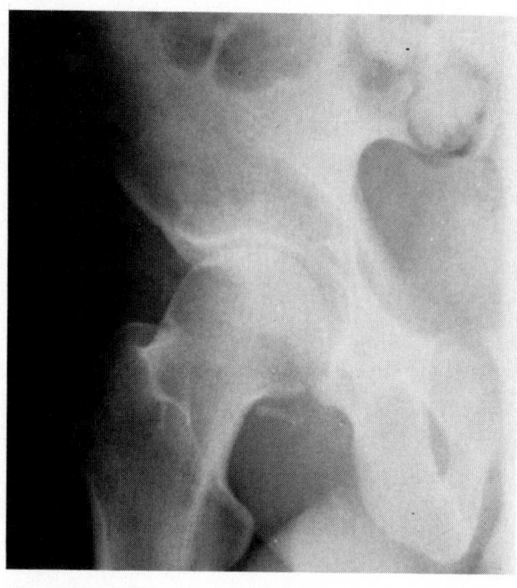

Figure 4-31B ii.

area is of very variable size. The femoral head is dislocated anteriorly with external rotation to overlap the ilioischial line. In the iliac oblique view, the integrity of the posterior border of the innominate bone is confirmed along with the anterior inferior iliac spine and the anterior border of the ilium. The site of rupture of the anterior acetabular wall is confirmed. In the obturator oblique view, the anterior wall fragment is clearly seen with preservation of the posterior border of the acetabulum. The degree

Figure 4-31C. Computed scan: i) high fragment; ii) middle comminuted fragments; iii) low fragment.

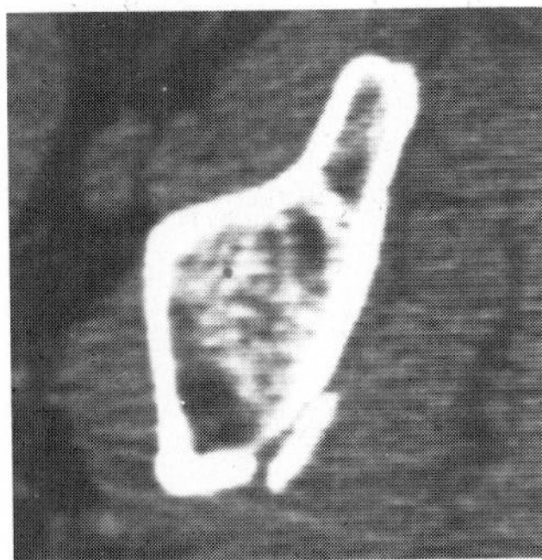

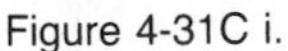

Figure 4-31C i.

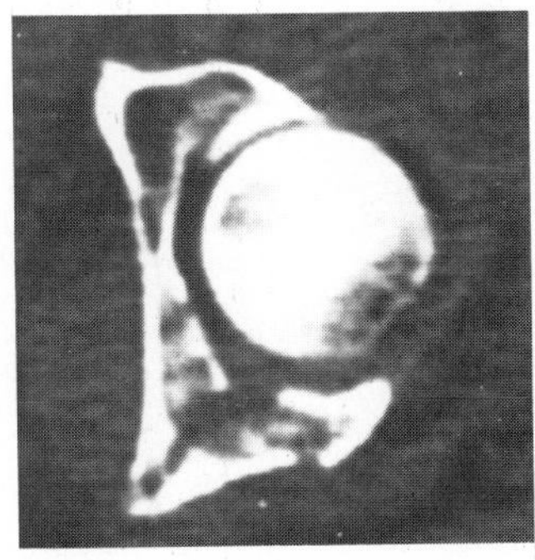

Figure 4-31C ii.

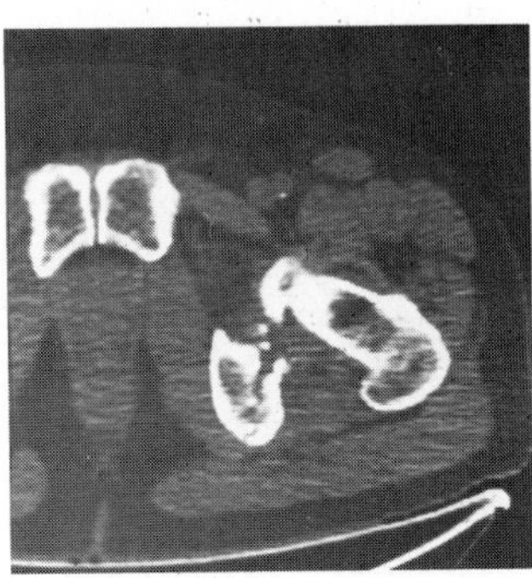

Figure 4-31C iii.

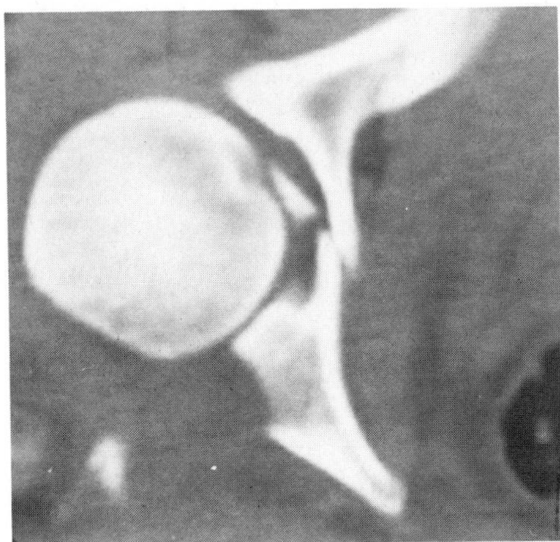

Figure 4-31D. Computed scan of posterior wall/ posterior column fracture with intraarticular avulsion fracture fragment from ligamentum teres.

of medial displacement of a trapezoidal wall fragment and the extent of articular disruption can be assessed. The computed scan provides the most direct evidence of the degree of displacement of the anterior wall fragment and the presence of comminution. Many of these fractures are highly comminuted and minimally displaced so that an open reduction is technically difficult but, fortunately, unnecessary.

**4. Anterior Column Fracture.** Another uncommon pattern of injury creates a fracture line extending from the middle of the ischiopubic ramus to the iliac crest. The fractures can be subcategorized by the level at which the upper end of the fracture line divides the innominate bone (Figure 4-34). The very low group involves an anterior and inferior portion of the acetabulum with minimal acetabular disruption. As the fracture line ascends progressively to a very high group, the degree of weightbearing involvement of the acetabulum increases correspondingly. The striking radiographic feature of all of the anterior column fractures is the

Figure 4-32. Posterior column fractures.

Figure 4-32A. Schematic views: i) outer; ii) inner.

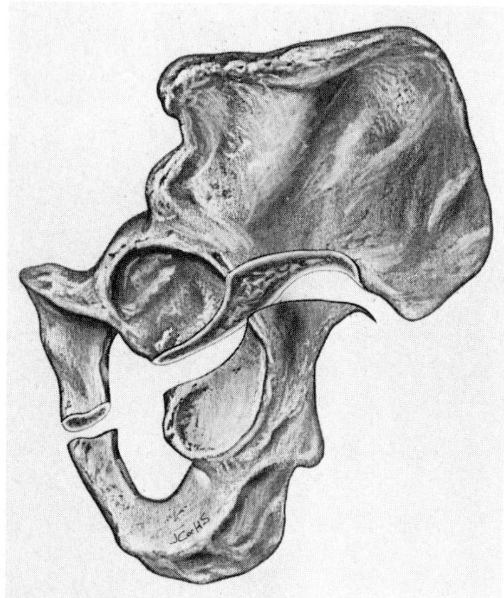

Figure 4-32A i.

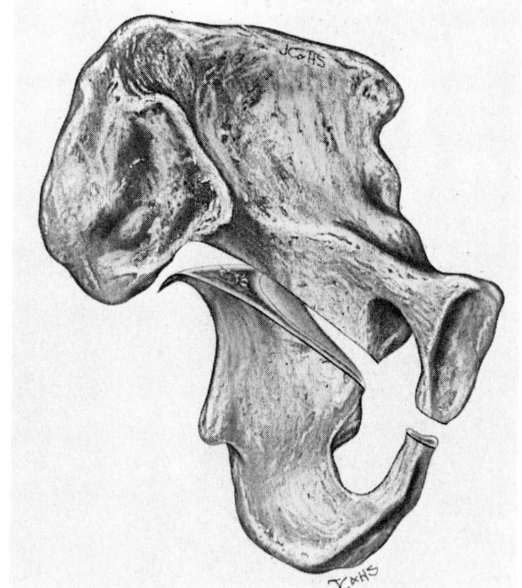

Figure 4-32A ii.

Figure 4-32B. Radiographic views: i) anteroposterior view, fracture is easily overlooked; ii) iliac oblique view with characteristic posterior column displacement.

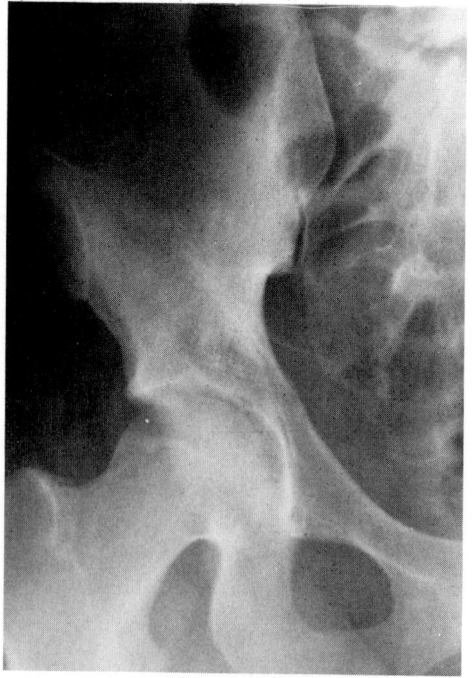

Figure 4-32B i.

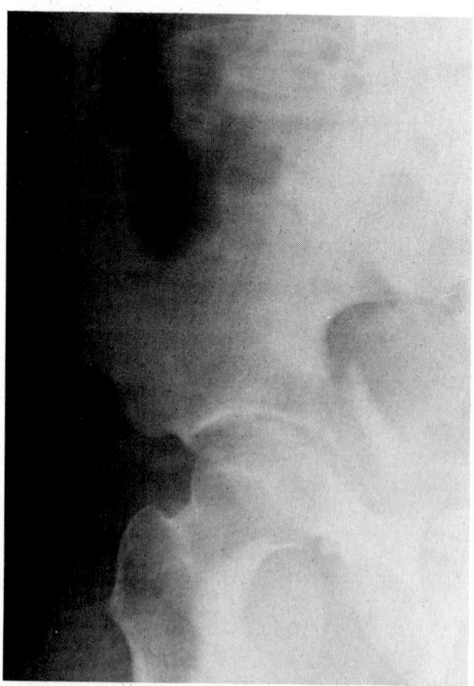

Figure 4-32B ii.

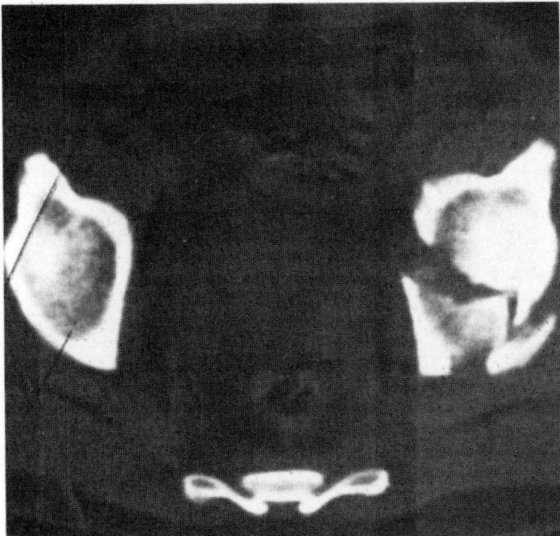

Figure 4-32C. Computed scan of posterior column fracture with a supplementary wall fragment.

preservation of the posterior column with sparing of the ilioischial line, the posterior border of the acetabulum, and the innominate bone. With all of the fracture variants the anteroposterior film reveals a break in the iliopectineal line as well as the inferior pubic ramus. Usually the anterior column is medially displaced and malrotated with a corresponding medial displacement of the femoral head. In the iliac oblique view the size of the anterior column fragment is evident. The very low fracture variants possess fracture fragments involving the anterior and lower quadrant of the acetabulum. With the intermediate group the anterior fracture line exits through the anterior inferior or anterior superior iliac spine while the high group possesses a fracture line exiting through the iliac crest. From this crucial observation, the required extent of surgical visualization of the anterior column is determined. In the obturator oblique view, medial displacement of the anterior column is confirmed with corresponding migration of the femoral head so that the two structures remain congruent. As the fracture variant progresses from low to high the fracture line is observed to change position from the medial acetabulum to the acetabular roof or the adjacent ilium. In a computed scan the size of the displaced articular fragment is readily evident. In many cases the entire dome portion of the acetabulum is involved, whereas in other lower quadrant injuries a negligible part of the articular surface is implicated. In the higher lesions marked comminution of the lateral ilium may be recognized so that an appropriate surgical exposure is planned. In the three-dimensional computed scan, the magnitude of anteromedial displacement is optimally characterized. With the more displaced fracture variants, a surgical approach that visualizes the inner pelvis is preferred to a lateral exposure.

Figure 4-33. Anterior wall fracture.
Figure 4-33A. Schematic views: i) outer; ii) inner.

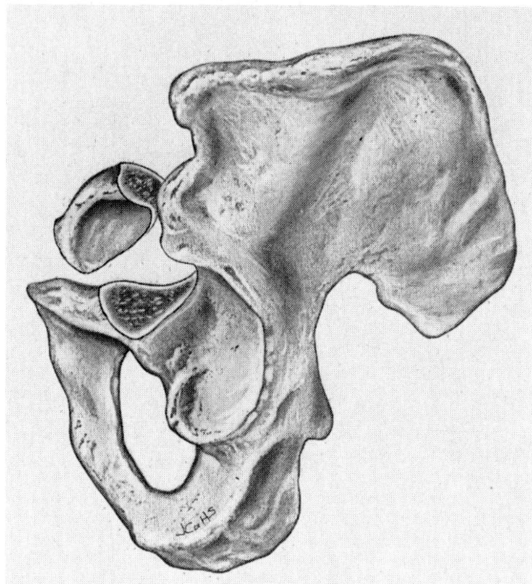

Figure 4-33A i.

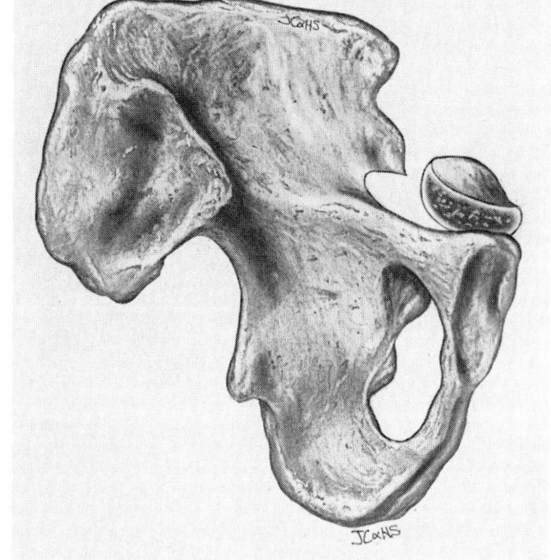

Figure 4-33A ii.

Figure 4-33B. Radiographs: i) obturator oblique; ii) iliac oblique view; iii) tomograph.

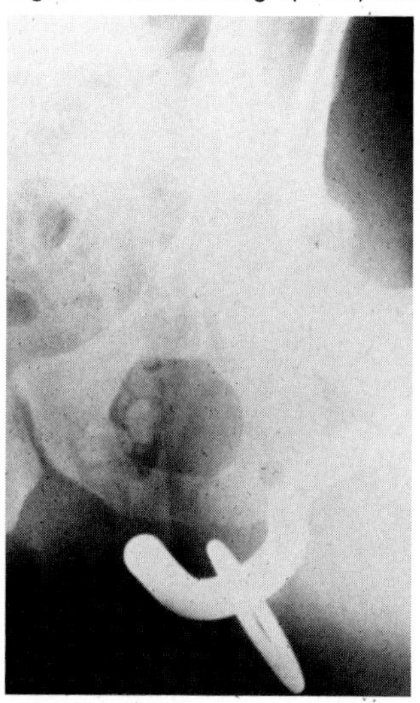

Figure 4-33B i.

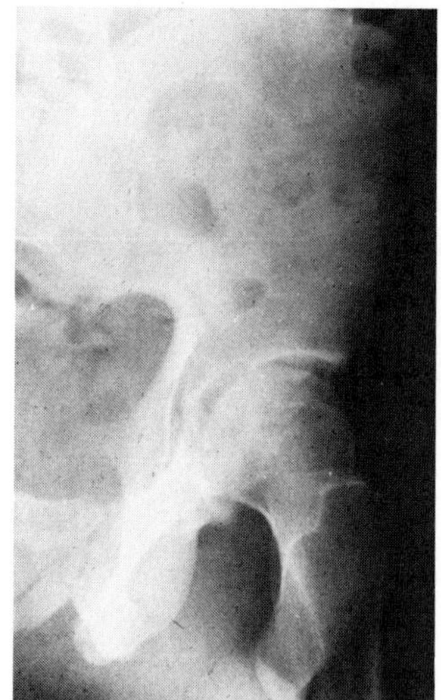

Figure 4-33B ii.

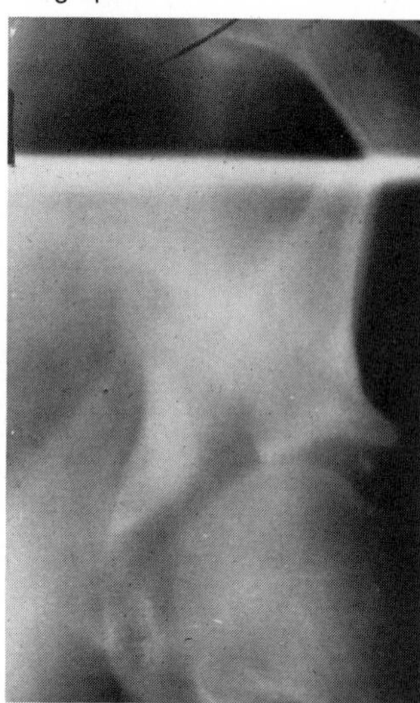

Figure 4-33B iii.

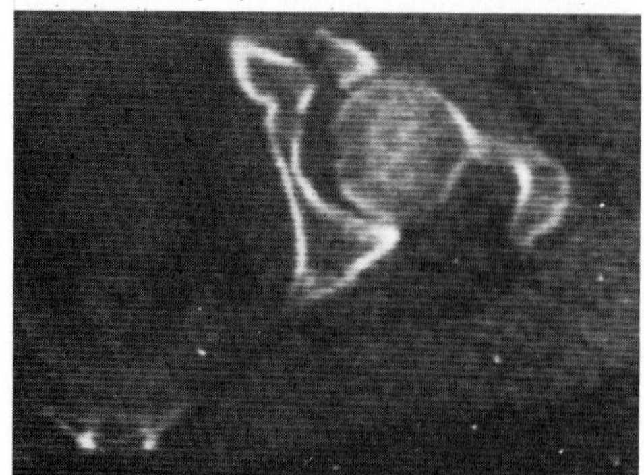

Figure 4-33C. Computed scan.

Figure 4-34. Anterior column fractures.
Figure 4-34A. Schematic views of outer and inner pelvis: i) low pattern, involving a small portion of articular surface; ii) intermediate pattern, with moderate portion of articular surface; iii) intermediate pattern with most of articular surface; iv) high with only about one third of the articular surface displaced; v) high with most of the articular surface displaced.

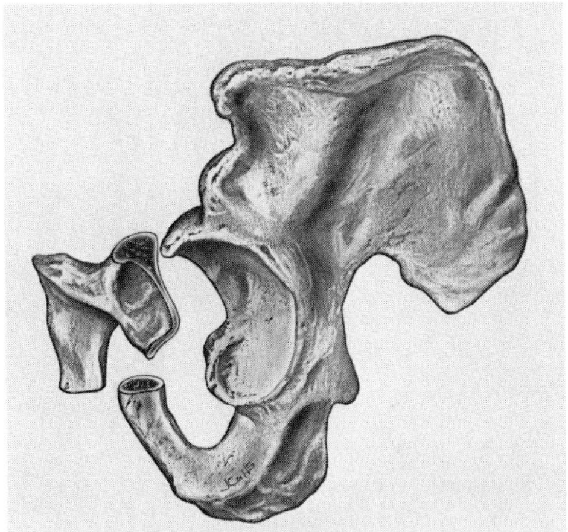

Figure 4-34A i.a. Outer surface.

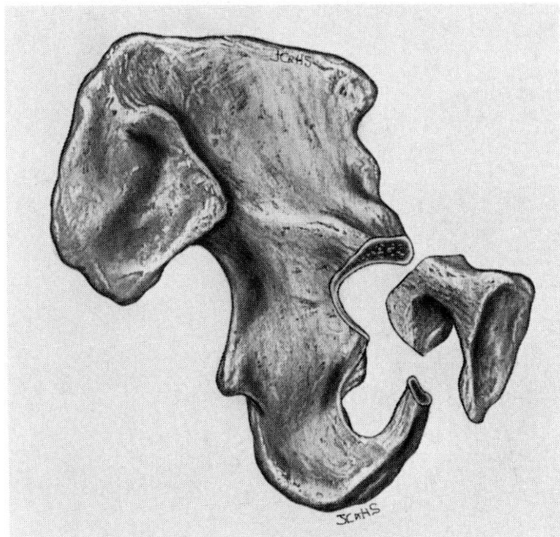

Figure 4-34A i.b. Inner surface.

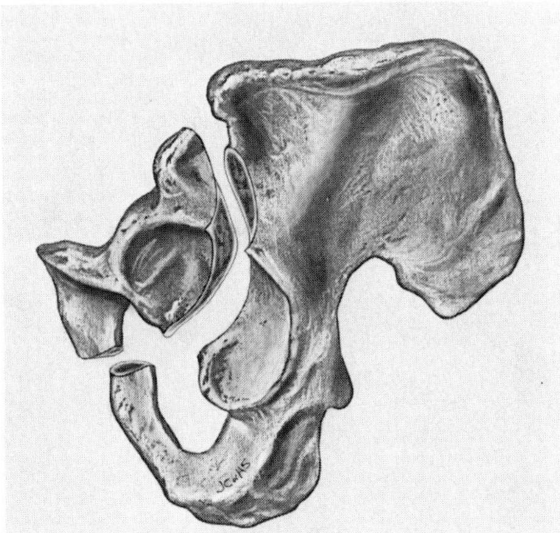

Figure 4-34A ii.a. Outer surface.

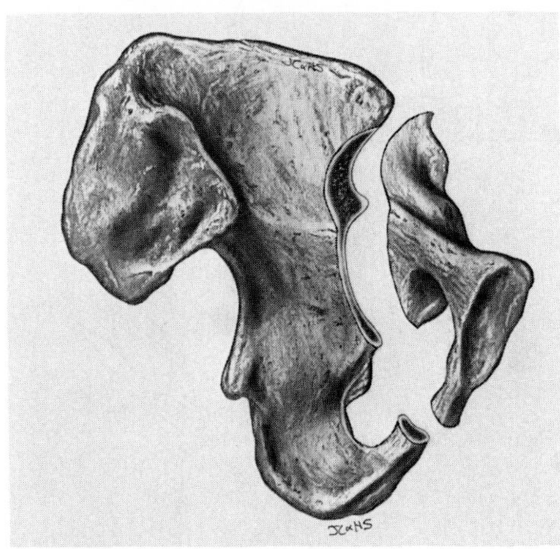

Figure 4-34A ii.b. Inner surface.

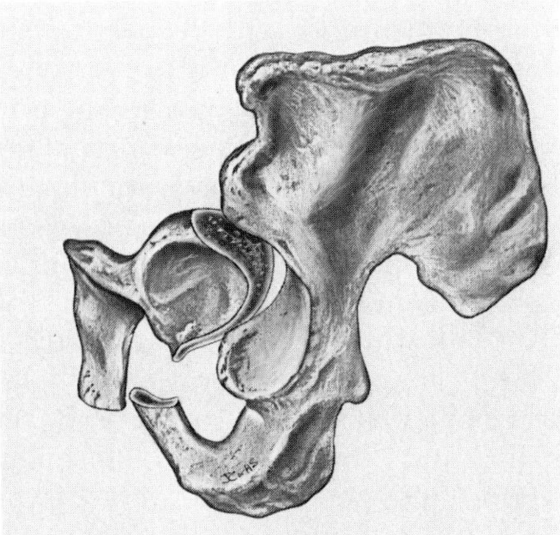

Figure 4-34A iii.a. Outer surface.

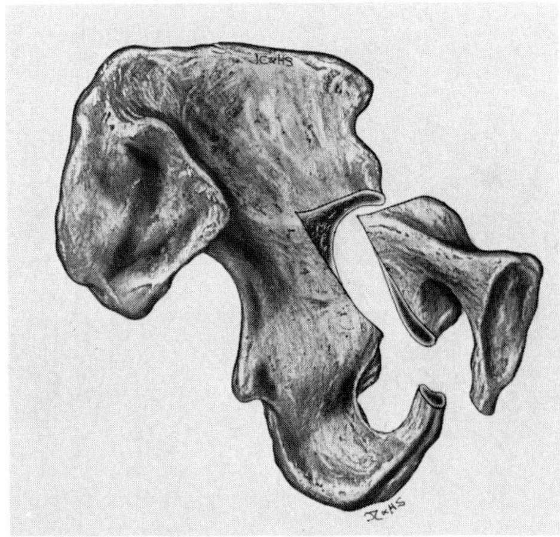

Figure 4-34A iii.b. Inner surface.

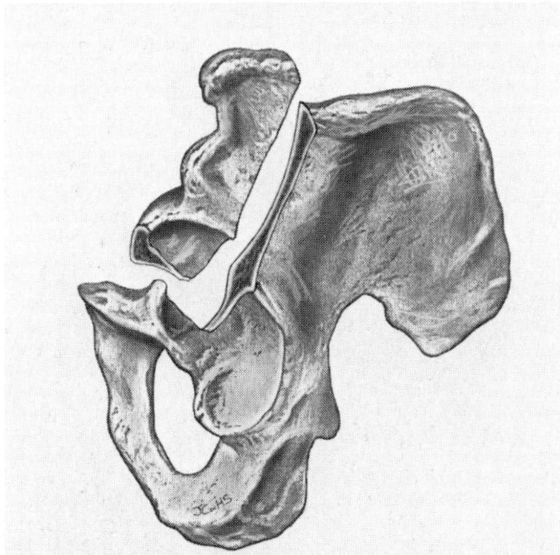

Figure 4-34A iv.a. Outer surface.

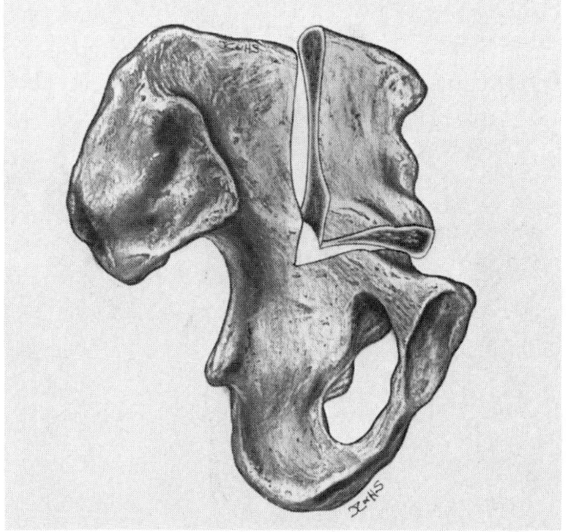

Figure 4-34A iv.b. Inner surface.

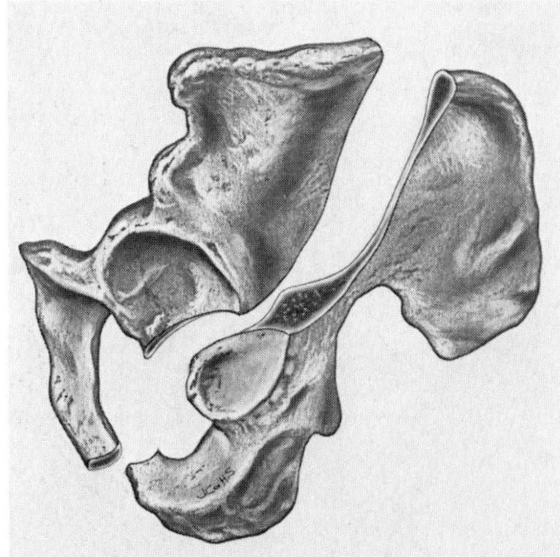

Figure 4-34A v.a. Outer surface.

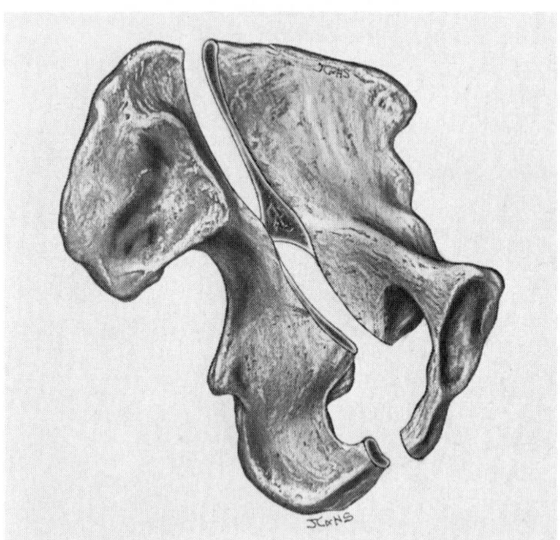

Figure 4-34A v.b. Inner surface.

**5. Pure Transverse Fractures.** The transverse fracture line divides the innominate bone into an upper iliac portion and a lower ischiopubic segment. The upper and lower segments remain intact with respect to one another. The orientation of the fracture varies considerably to create infratectal, juxtatectal and transtectal categories (Figure 4-35). Progression along these categories is associated with an ever-increasing displacement of the roof. The fracture lines possess a varying degree of obliquity from the outer to the inner portion of the pelvis and from anterior to posterior. The ischiopubic segment is displaced medially with a rotational displacement or superior migration.

In the anteroposterior view virtually all of the vertically aligned structures, including the pelvic brim, ilioischial line, and the anterior and posterior borders of the acetabulum, are disrupted although the obturator ring is spared. The obliquity of the fracture and the site of

Figure 4-34B. Radiographs: i, ii) obturator and iliac oblique views of a simple, low anterior column fracture with minimal articular involvement; iii-v) anteroposterior, obturator, and iliac oblique views respectively of comminuted high anterior column disruption.

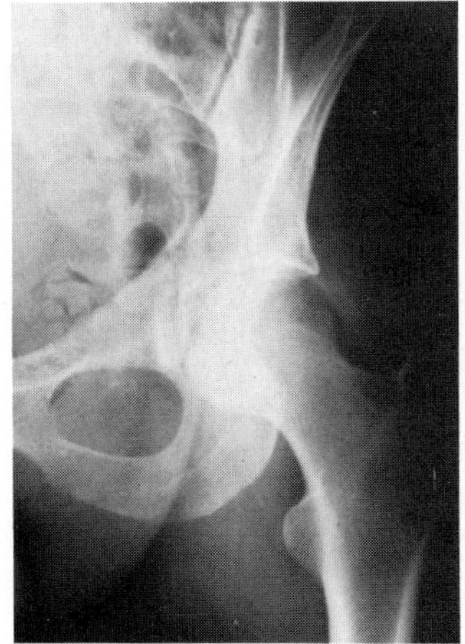

Figure 4-34B i.

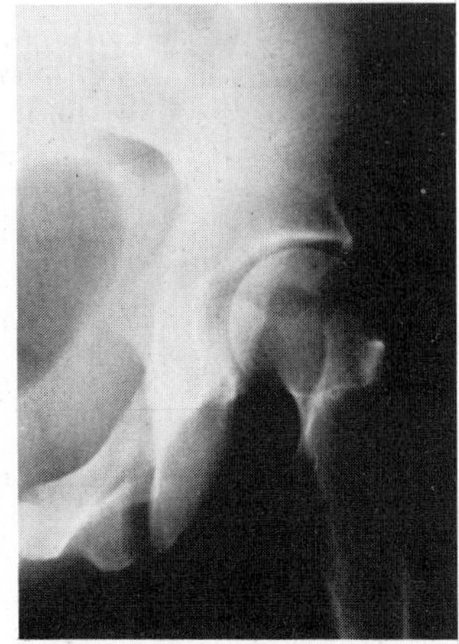

Figure 4-34B ii.

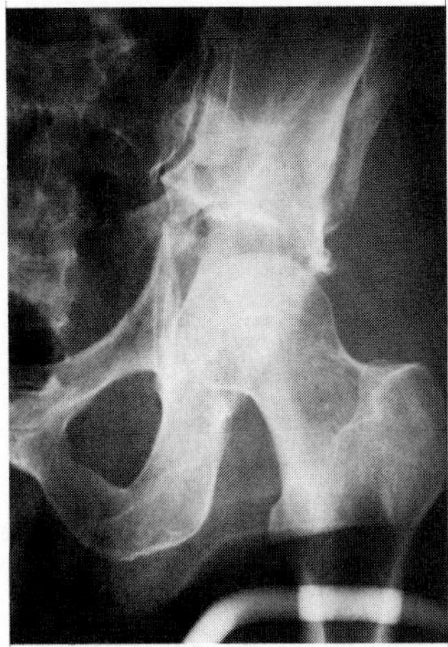

Figure 4-34B iii.

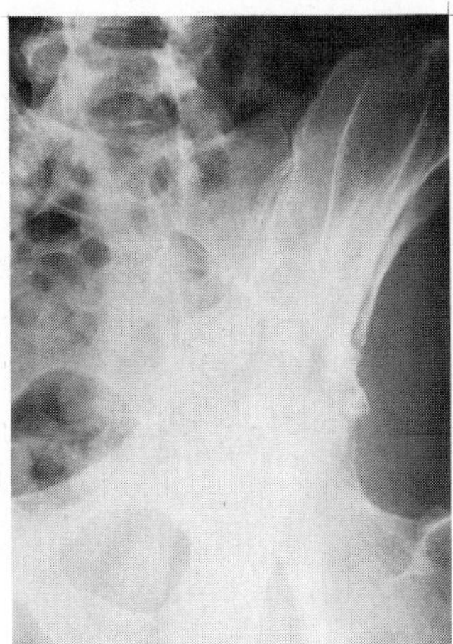

Figure 4-34B iv.

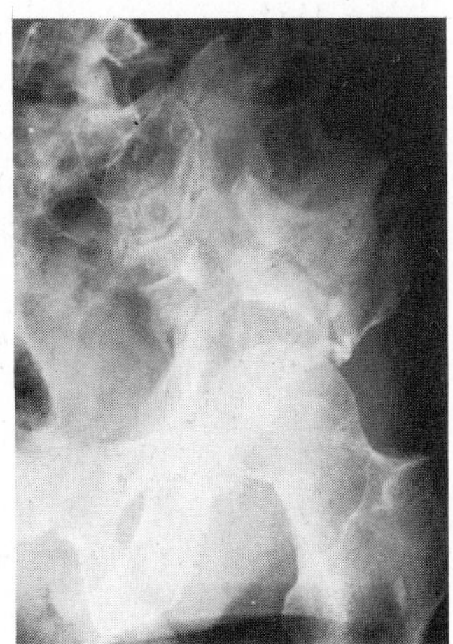

Figure 4-34B v.

Figure 4-34C. Computed scans: i) simple displaced fracture involving half of quadrilateral surface; ii) comminuted with displacement of entire dome surface.

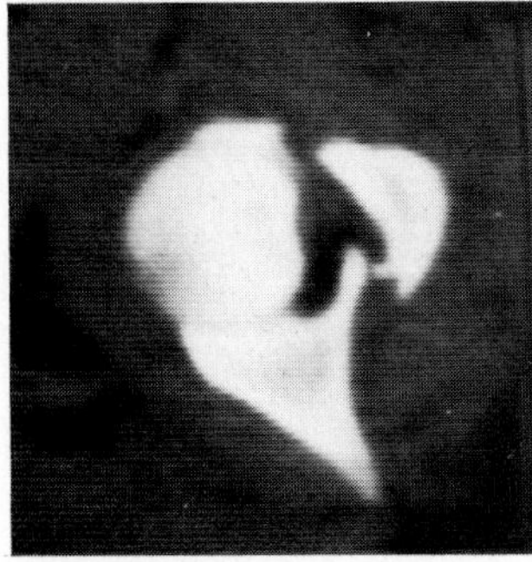

Figure 4-34C i.

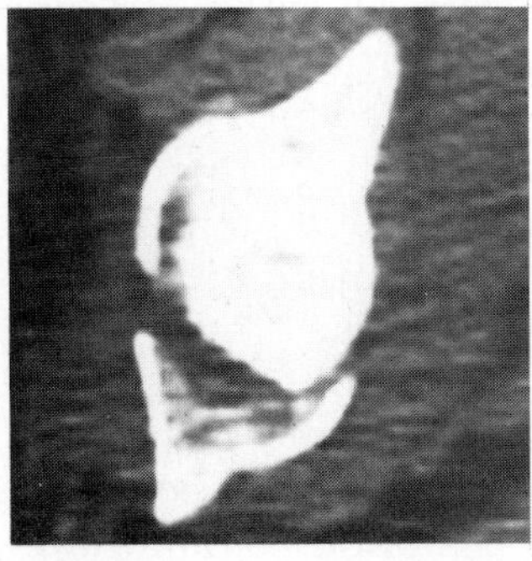

Figure 4-34C ii.

Figure 4-34D. Computed 3-D scan: i) anterosuperior view with femoral head displaced through pelvic wall; ii) superior view with medial displacement; iii) medial view.

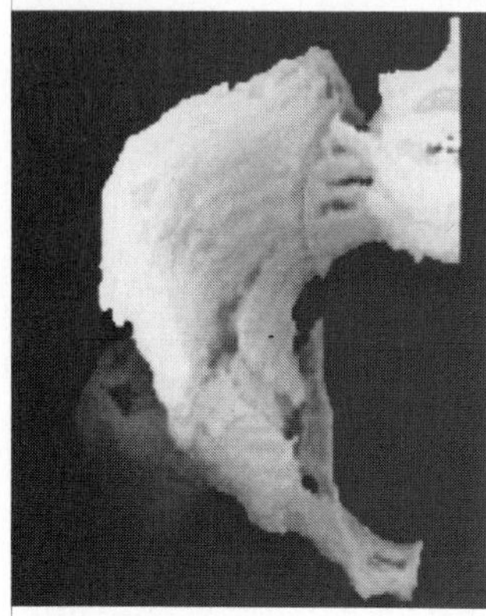

Figure 4-34D i.

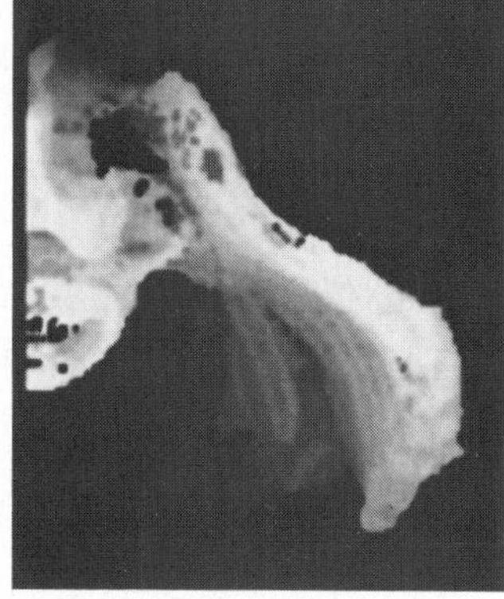

Figure 4-34D ii.

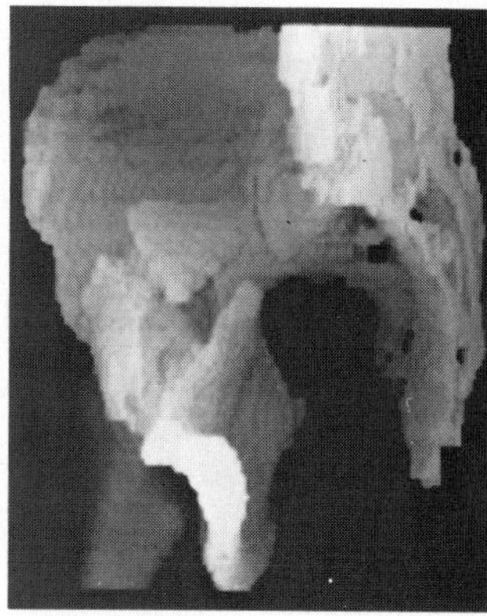

Figure 4-34D iii.

Figure 4-35. Transverse fractures.
Figure 4-35A. Schematic views: i) infratectal; ii) juxtatectal; iii) transtectal; iv) comminuted involving lateral ilium.

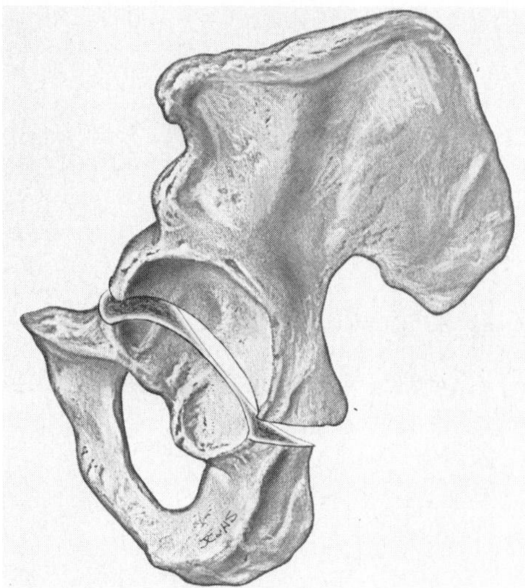

Figure 4-35A i.

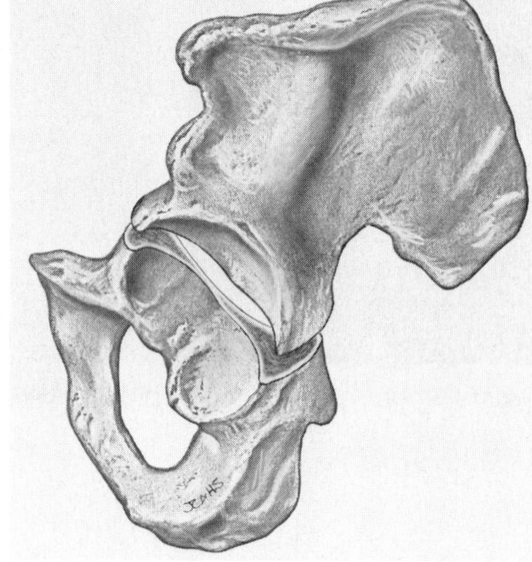

Figure 4-35A ii.

involvement within the cotyloid fossa or roof are evident. Some portion of the roof remains intact, however. In the iliac oblique view, the site of involvement of the fracture on the quadrilateral surface of the ischium is evident along with the point of rupture of the greater sciatic notch. In the obturator oblique view, the preservation of the obturator ring is confirmed. The level of the fracture at the posterior border of the acetabulum as well as the magnitude of central dislocation are documented. In a computed scan, the degree of central or posterior comminution is readily evident. When conventional imaging techniques are employed, the scan

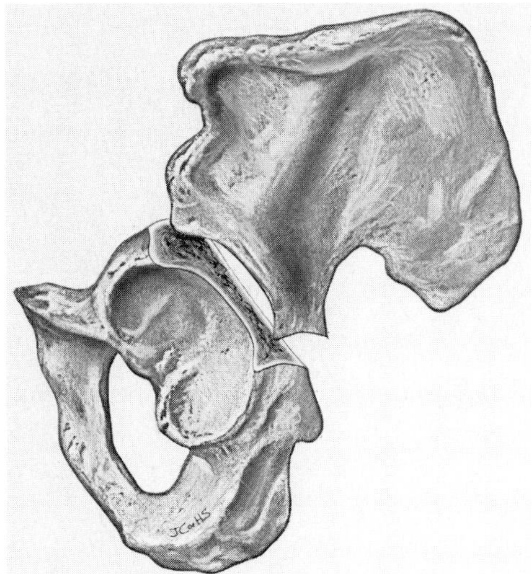

Figure 4-35A iii.

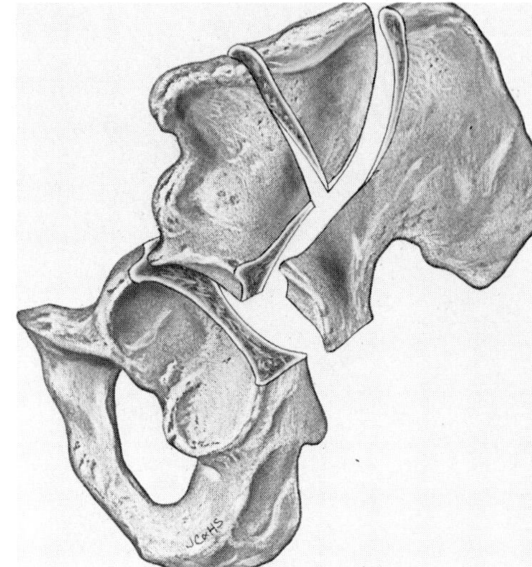

Figure 4-35A iv.

Figure 4-35B. Anteroposterior radiograph (i) and computed scan (ii) of a simple truly transverse transtectal pattern.

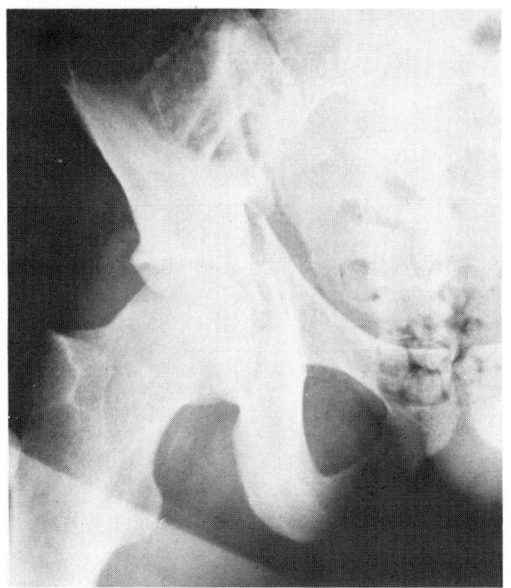

Figure 4-35B i.

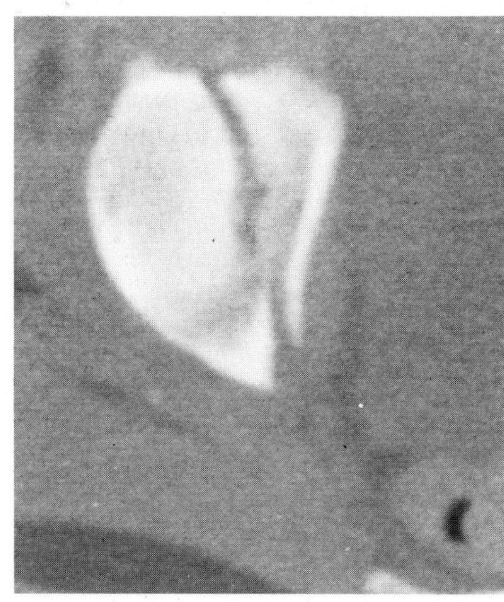

Figure 4-35B ii.

represents an oblique section of the pelvis. The obliquity hampers an identification of the part of the acetabular roof that is injured unless the three dimensional scan is available. A conventional scan also permits the recognition of an undisplaced T-component of a transverse fracture.

## *B. Associated Fractures*

**1. Associated Posterior Column and Posterior Wall Fractures.** This uncommon injury is characterized by

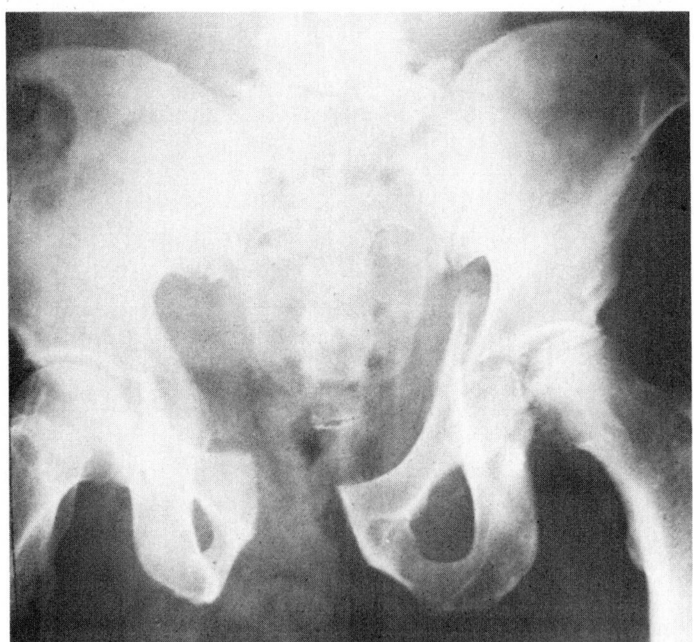

Figure 4-35C. Anteroposterior radiograph of an oblique type of transverse fracture that is juxtatectal anteriorly and transtectal posteriorly.

Figure 4-35D. Outlet (i) and iliac oblique (ii) views of an oblique type transverse fracture that is high or transtectal anteriorly and low or infratectal posteriorly.

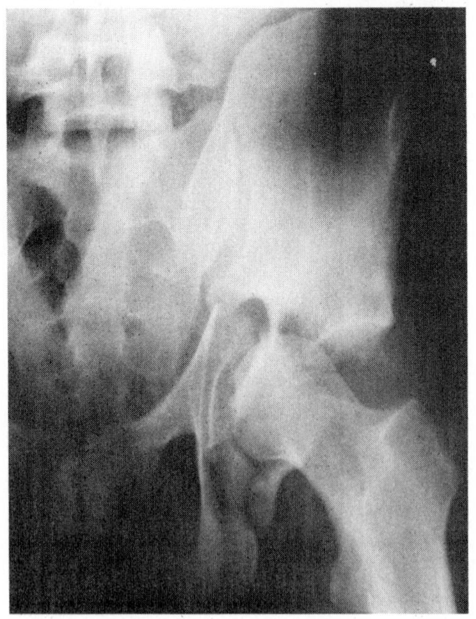

Figure 4-35D i.

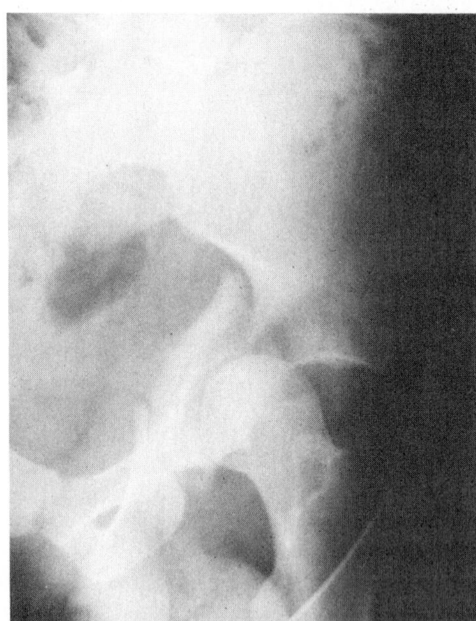

Figure 4-35D ii.

a posterior column fracture usually with minor rotational displacement and a crucial posterior wall fragment that generally is completely displaced often with marked rotation of up to 180° (Figure 4-36). The injury represents

Figure 4-35E. i-iii) Anteroposterior, iliac, and obturator oblique views of transverse fracture with comminution of dome and quadrilateral surface.

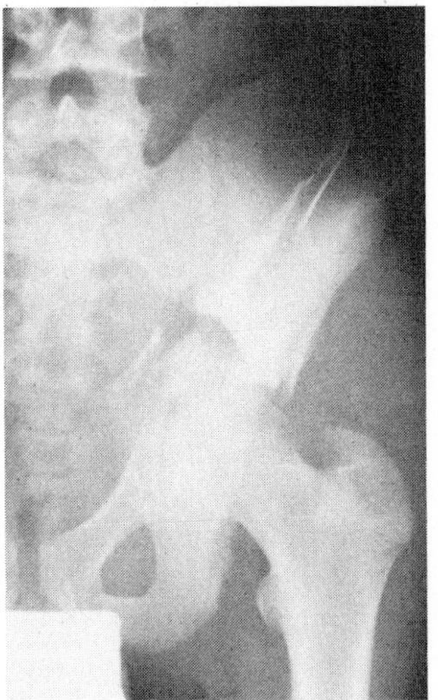

Figure 4-35E i.

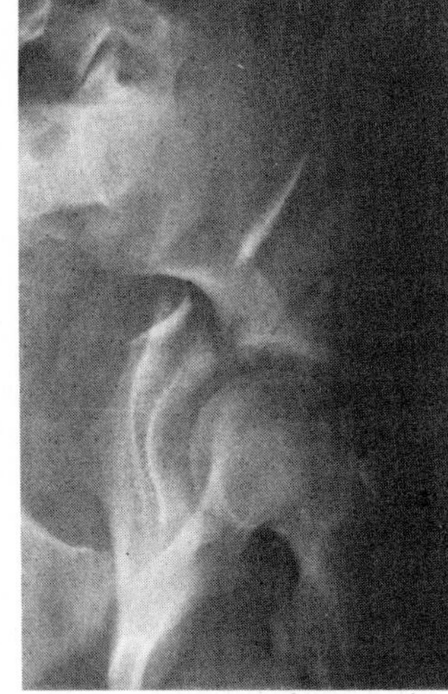

Figure 4-35E ii.

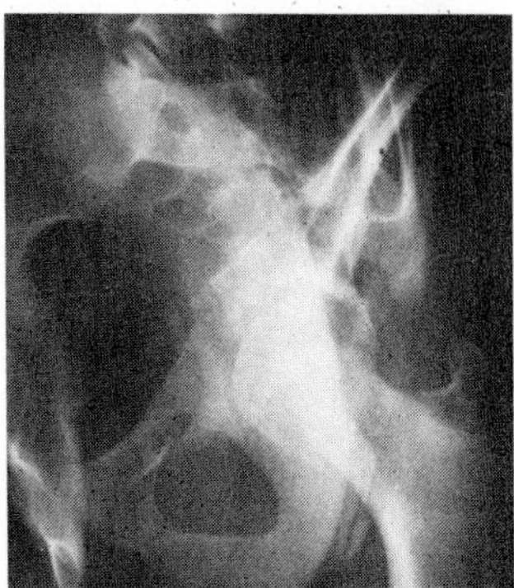

Figure 4-35E iii.

Figure 4-35F. Transverse fracture with iliac comminution in which the fracture progresses from high anteriorly to low posteriorly: i, ii) anteroposterior and obturator oblique radiographs; iii-v) computed scans through ilium, dome, and quadrilateral surface.

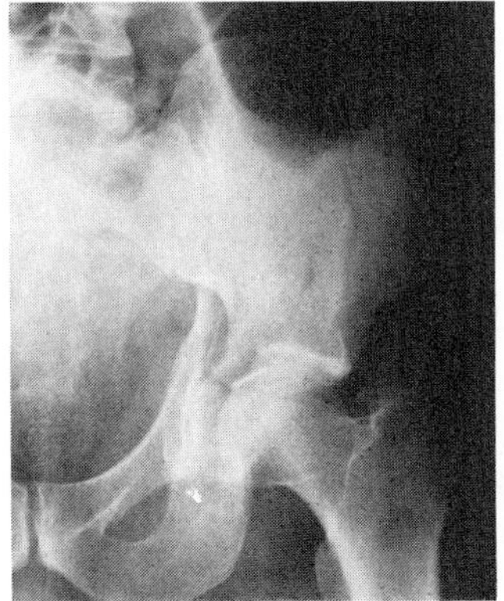

Figure 4-35F i.

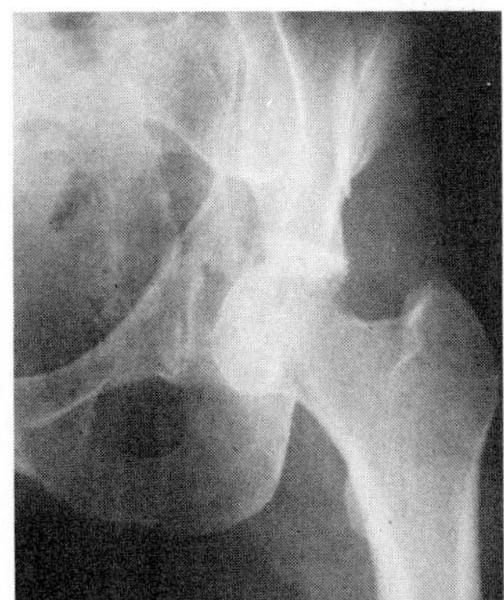

Figure 4-35F ii.

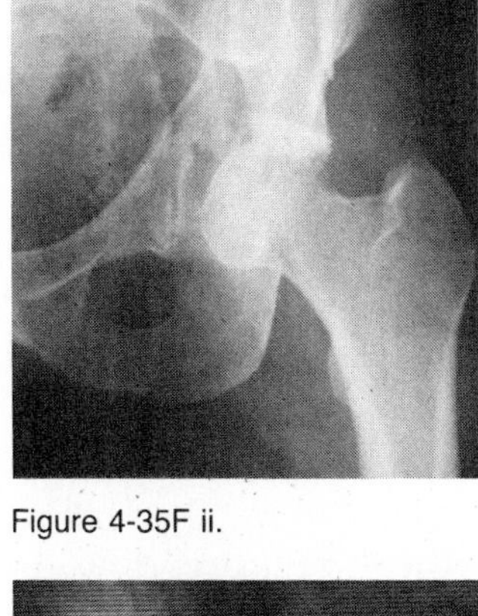

Figure 4-35F iii.

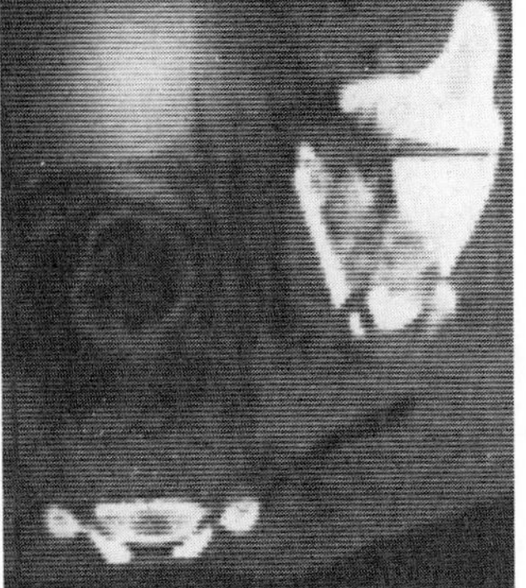

Figure 4-35F iv.

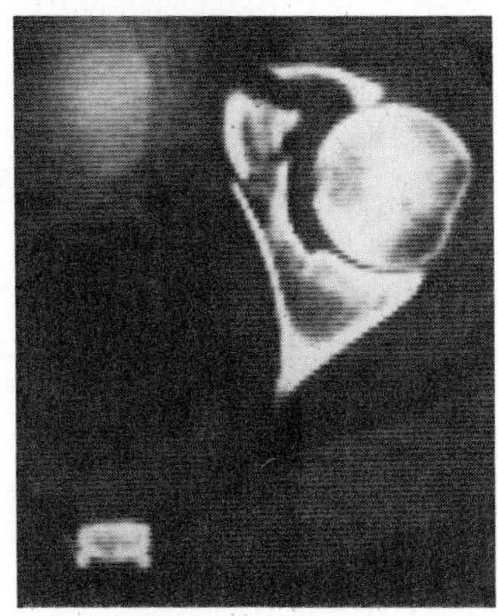

Figure 4-35F v.

Figure 4-36. Associated posterior column/posterior wall fractures.

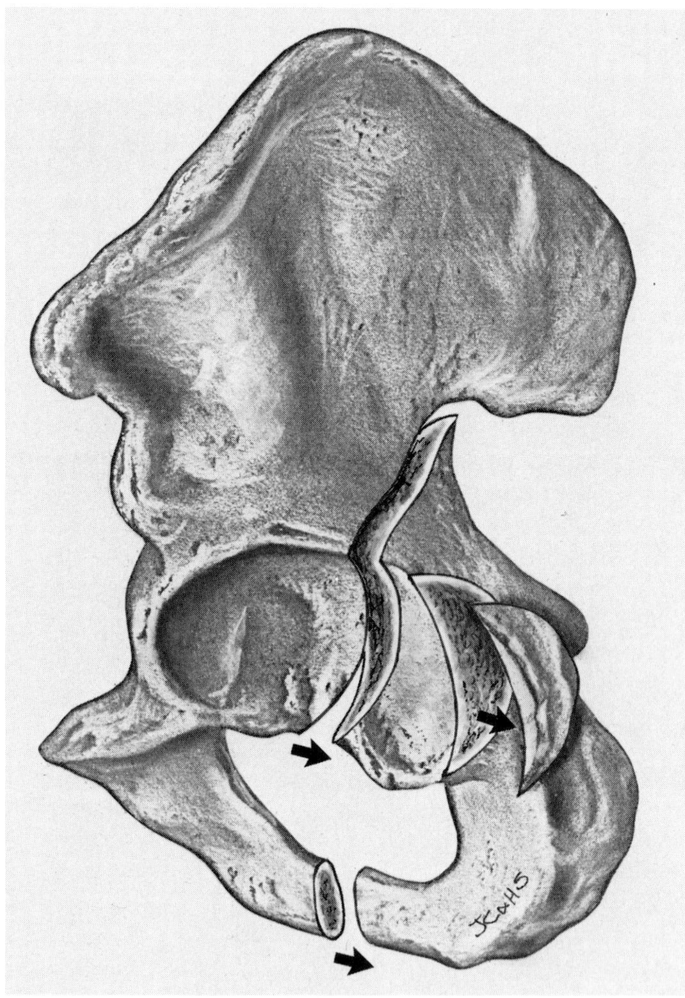

Figure 4-36A. Schematic diagram of posterior column fracture with associated posterior wall fragment.

one pattern of a posterior fracture-dislocation of the hip, which frequently is accompanied by injury to the sciatic nerve. Marginal acetabular impaction may be evident. The posterior column fracture is well seen in the anteroposterior view and especially the iliac obturator view. In contrast the wall fragment is best seen in the obturator oblique view. In the last view, the inlet landmarks of the anterior column referable to the iliopectineal line are documented. A computed scan permits recognition of minimally displaced posterior wall fragments and marked comminution of the posterior rim. A particularly large posterior wall fragment can be identified that precludes the initial stabilization of the posterior column with a plate, prior to the reduction of the wall fragment and its attached capsule. Once the wall fragment is replaced, the hip joint cannot be inspected so that preliminary fixation of the posterior column has to be achieved solely with a lag screw prior to the application of the plate across both the posterior column and wall fragments.

Figure 4-36B. Anteroposterior and iliac oblique view (i, ii) and computed scans (iii, iv) presenting a high wall fragment and impaction of the posterior column.

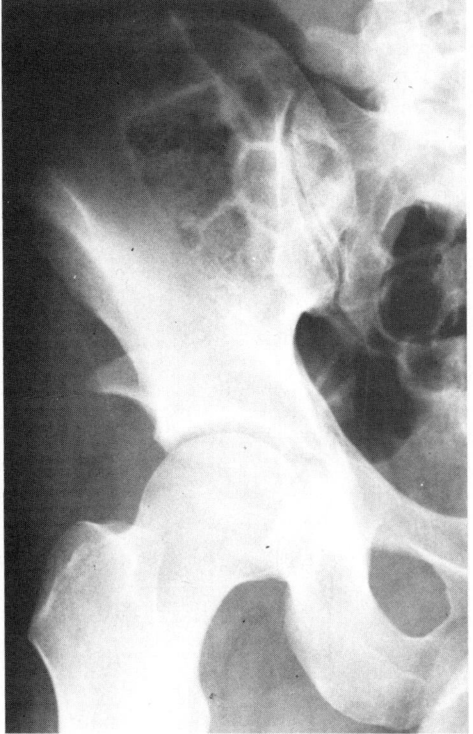

Figure 4-36B i.

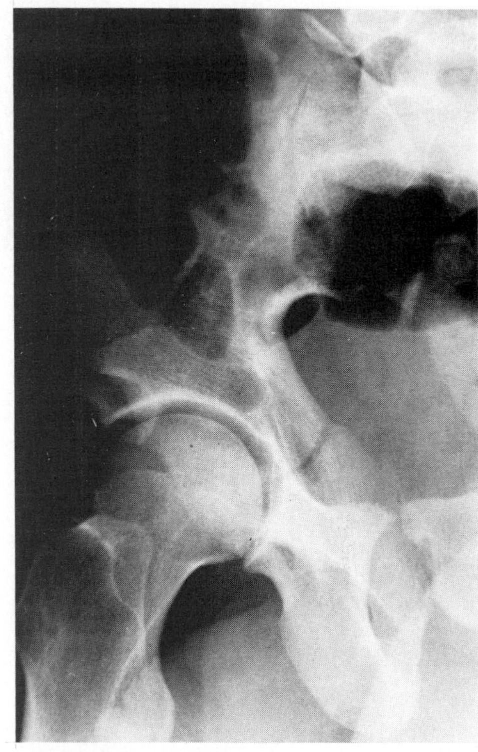

Figure 4-36B ii.

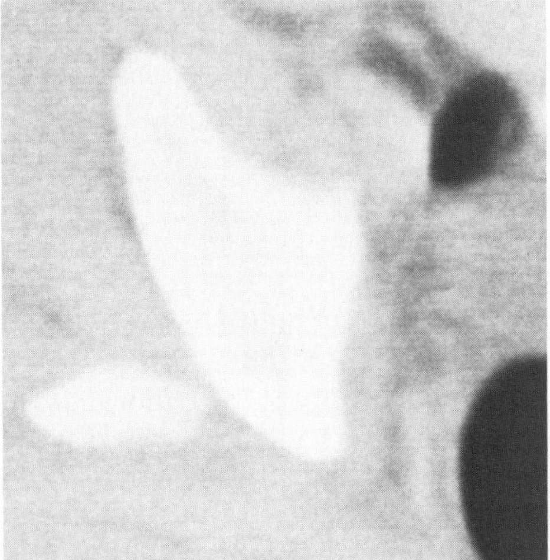

Figure 4-36B iii.

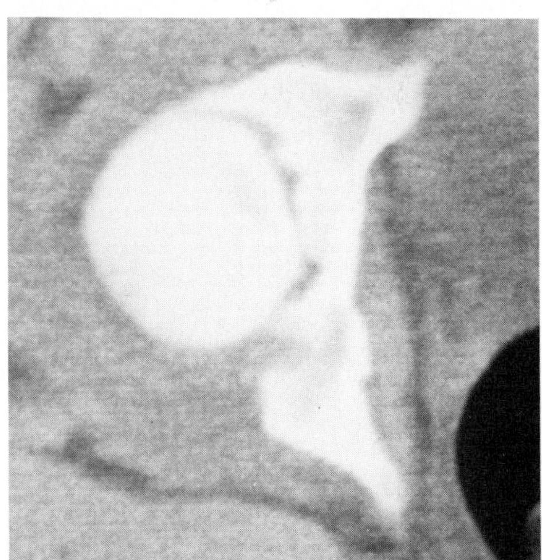

Figure 4-36B iv.

**2. Associated Transverse and Posterior Wall Fracture.** This pattern of injury can be produced either by a central dislocation or a posterior dislocation of the femoral head (Figure 4-37). With the former, the displaced transverse fracture component creates the principal source of

Figure 4-36C. Computed scans (i-iii) with marked comminution of posterior wall and column fracture.

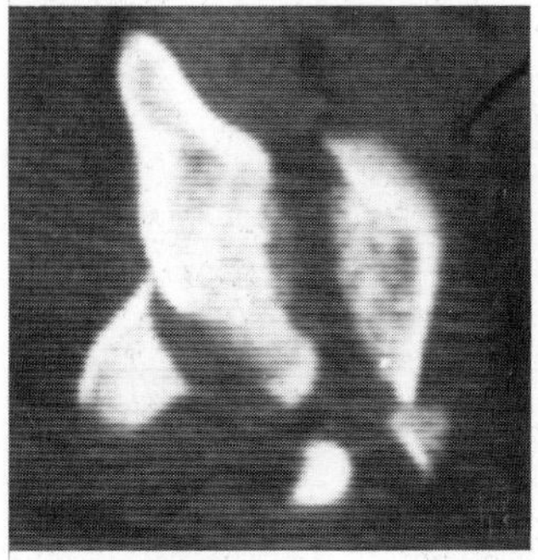

Figure 4-36C i.

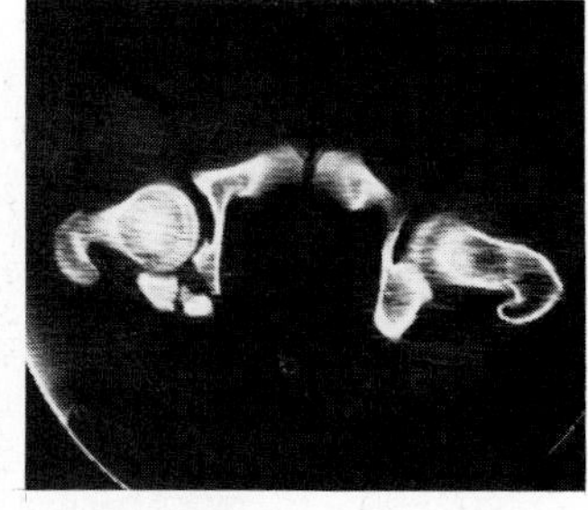

Figure 4-36C ii.

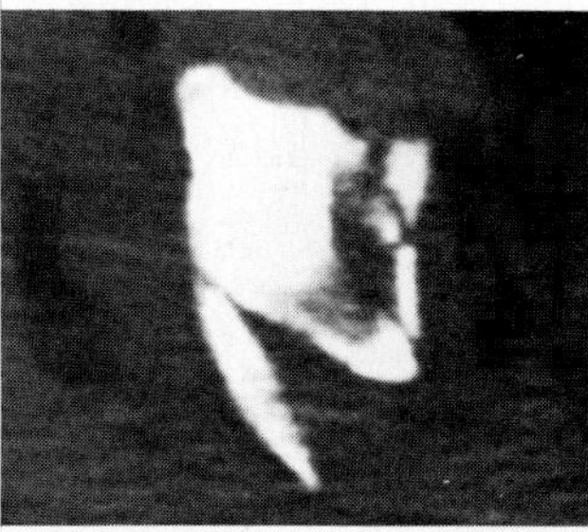

Figure 4-36C iii.

Figure 4-37. Associated transverse and posterior wall fracture.
Figure 4-37A. Schematic views: i) pattern with central dislocation of femoral head; ii) pattern with posterior dislocation of femoral head.

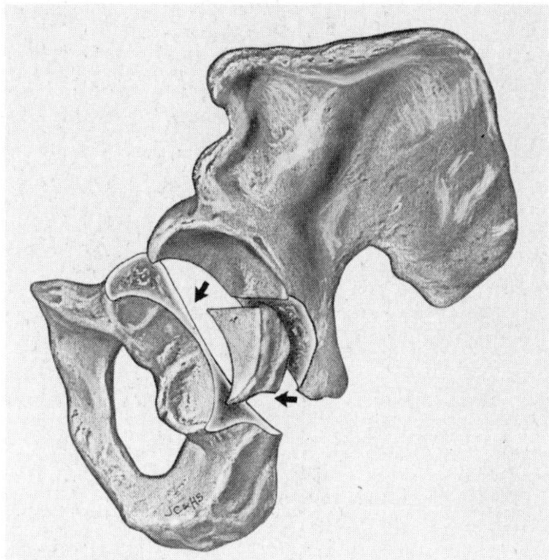

Figure 4-37A i.

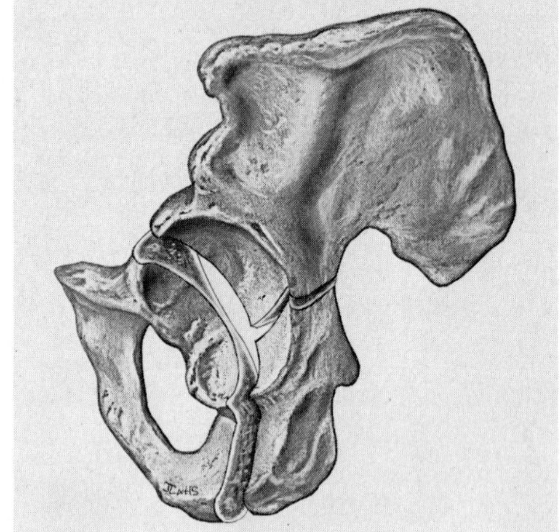

Figure 4-37A ii.

instability of the femoral head while the posterior wall fracture is an accessory lesion. In the latter, the posterior wall fracture dictates the instability of the femoral head. The central fracture-dislocation is best seen in the anteroposterior view. The medially displaced femoral head is no longer congruous with the intact portion of the acetabular roof. A disruption of the iliopectineal and ilioischial lines is confirmed. A displaced posterior wall fracture is best seen in the obturator oblique view, while the inward displacement of the ischiopubic fragment is most prominent in the iliac oblique view. In a computed scan the degree of comminution of the posterior wall is visualized along with the central or posterior displacement of the femoral head. The magnitude of anterior acetabular displacement also can be recorded. If the anterior displacement is minimal, a posterior

Figure 4-37B. Example of pattern with central dislocation of femoral head: i-iii) anteroposterior, obturator, and iliac oblique radiographs; iv) computed scan as transverse pelvic section; v-viii) iliac oblique, lateral, obturator oblique, and superior three-dimensional views.

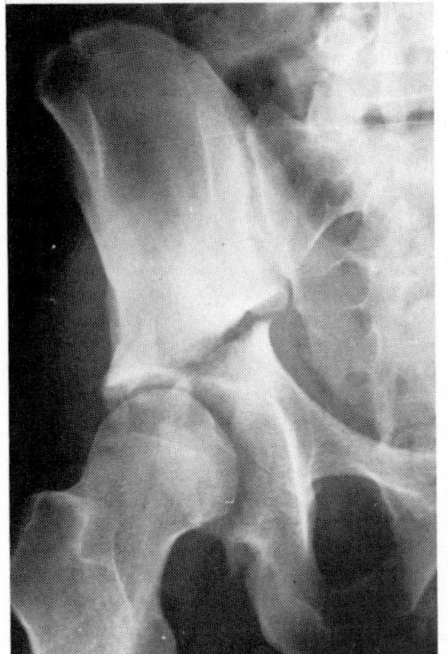

Figure 4-37B i.

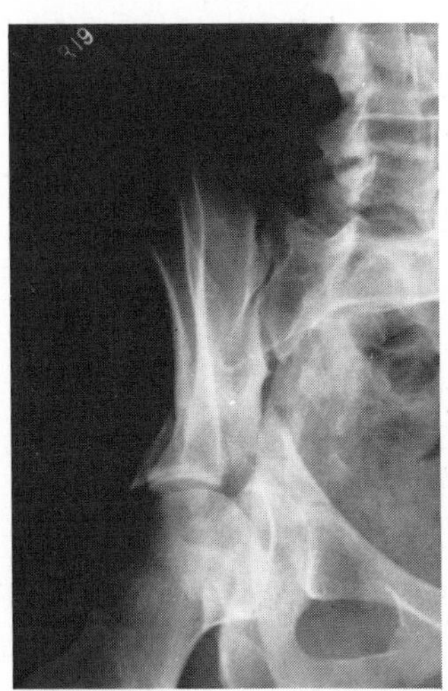

Figure 4-37B ii.

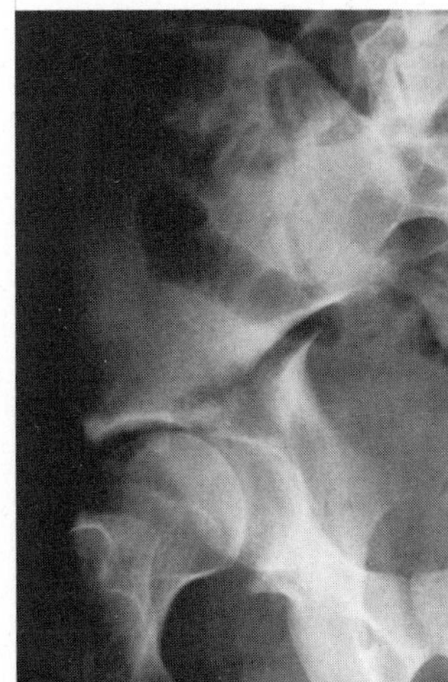

Figure 4-37B iii.

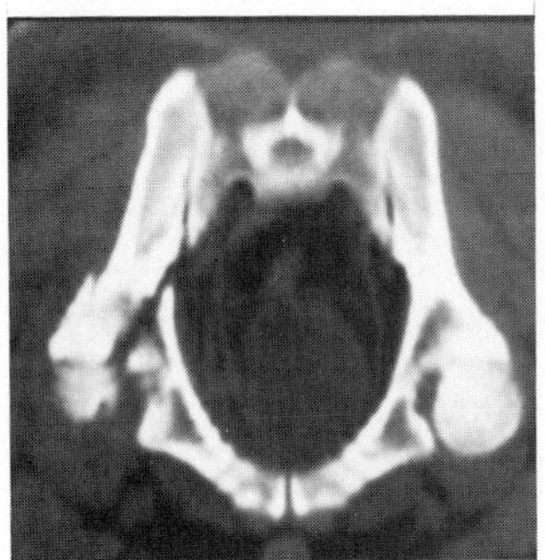

Figure 4-37B iv.

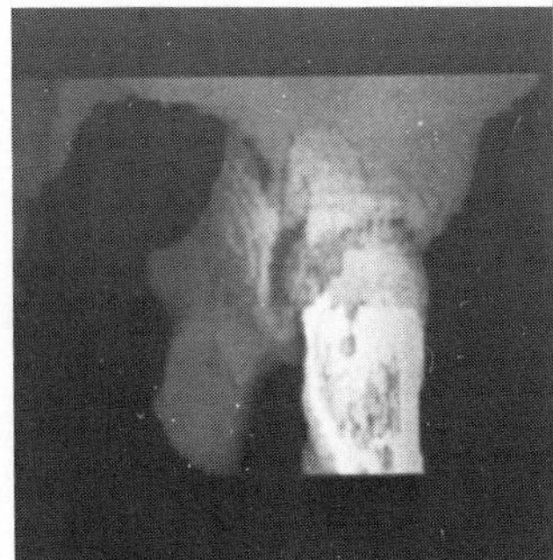

Figure 4-37B v.

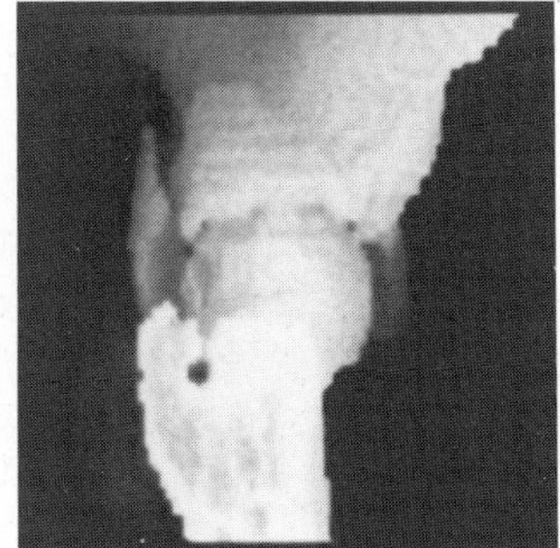

Figure 4-37B vi.

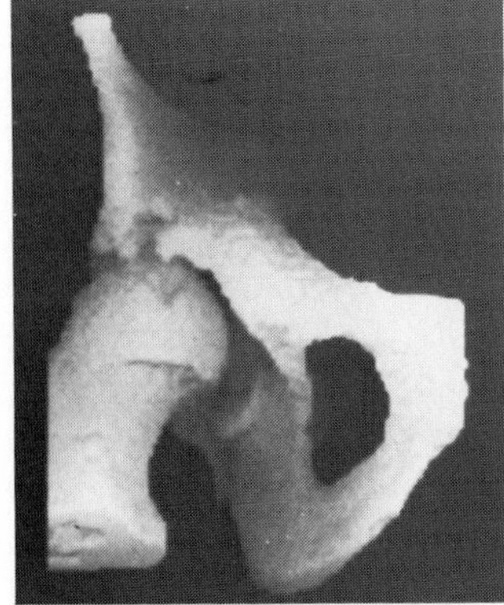

Figure 4-37B vii.

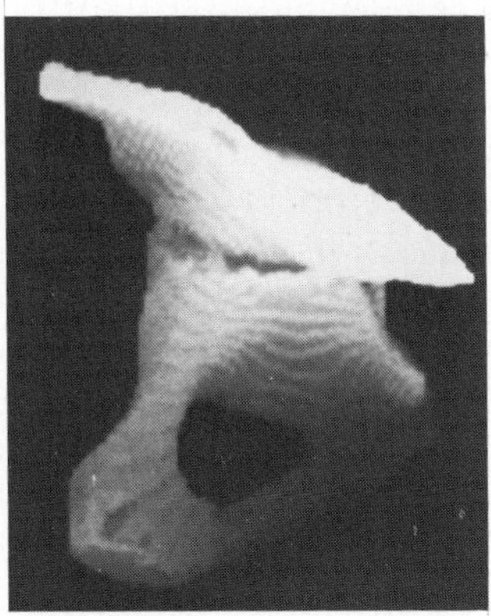

Figure 4-37B viii.

Figure 4-37C. Example of pattern with posterior dislocation of femoral head: i, ii) anteroposterior and obturator oblique radiographs; iii, iv) computed scans through dome and quadrilateral surface.

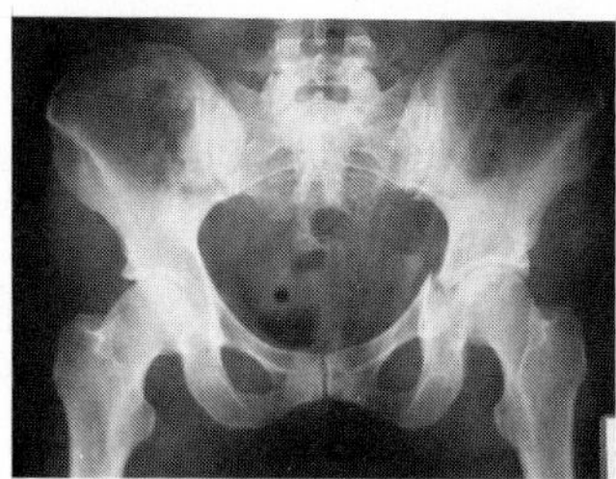

Figure 4-37C i.

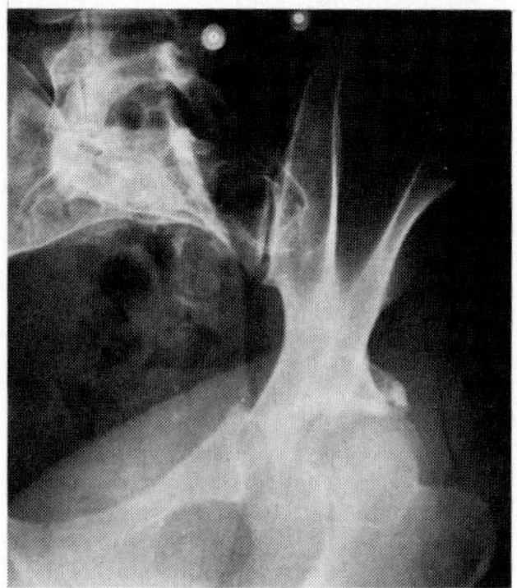

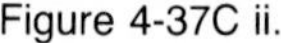

Figure 4-37C ii.

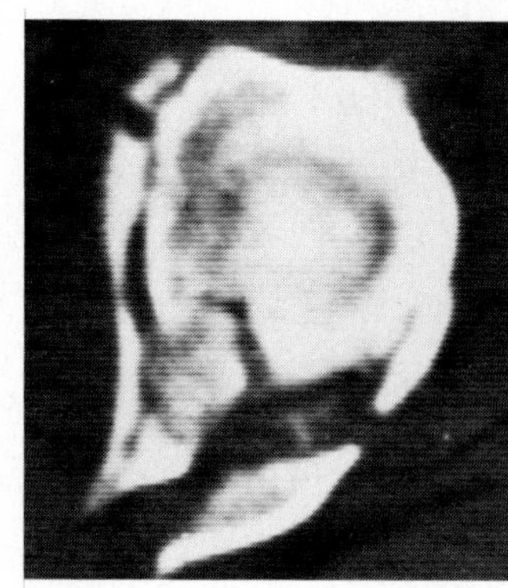

Figure 4-37C iii.

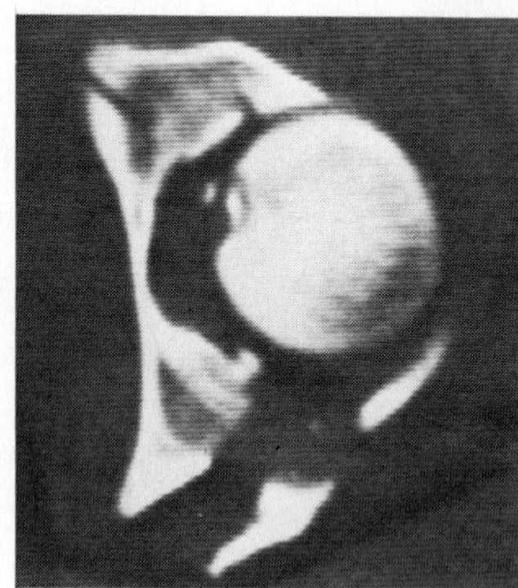

Figure 4-37C iv.

surgical approach may be undertaken instead of a more extensile exposure.

**3. Associated Anterior and Posterior Hemitransverse Fracture.** This injury comprises an anterior wall or column fracture together with a posterior column fracture (Figure 4-38). The posterior column disruption is equivalent to the posterior half of a transverse fracture usually with relatively minor displacement. The femoral head is driven against the anterior fragment usually with marked anterior dislocation of the femoral head and a corresponding displacement of the fracture fragment. A portion of the articular cartilage of the posterior acetabular roof always remains intact with the wing of the ilium to distinguish this injury from a both-column fracture. The pattern of disruption on the inner aspect of the pelvis is wholly different from a "T" fracture, which also spares a portion of the acetabular roof. On the anteroposterior and obturator oblique views, the anteriorly displaced femoral head is confirmed along with the presence of the anterior fracture fragment. The posterior fracture line is seen on the obturator oblique view along with the intact portion of the posterosuperior acetabular roof. The introduction of three dimensional scanning techniques has greatly facilitated the recognition of this fracture pattern. It permits an assessment of posterior column displacement, as well as the displacement and comminution of the anterior

Figure 4-38. Associated anterior and posterior hemitransverse.

Figure 4-38A. Schematic views: i, ii) associated anterior wall and posterior hemitransverse; iii, iv) associated anterior column and posterior hemitransverse.

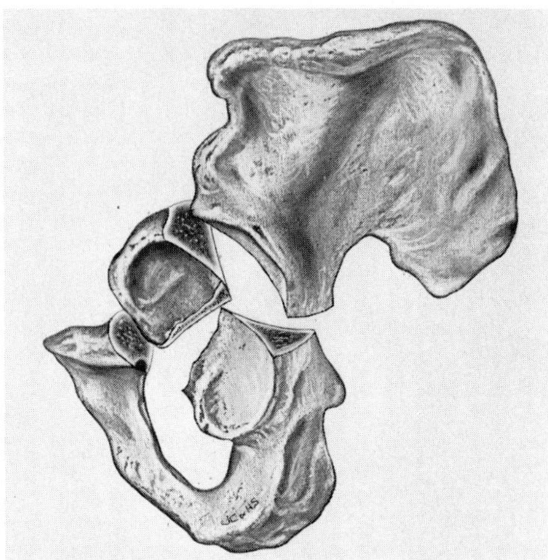

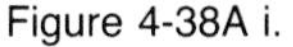

Figure 4-38A i.

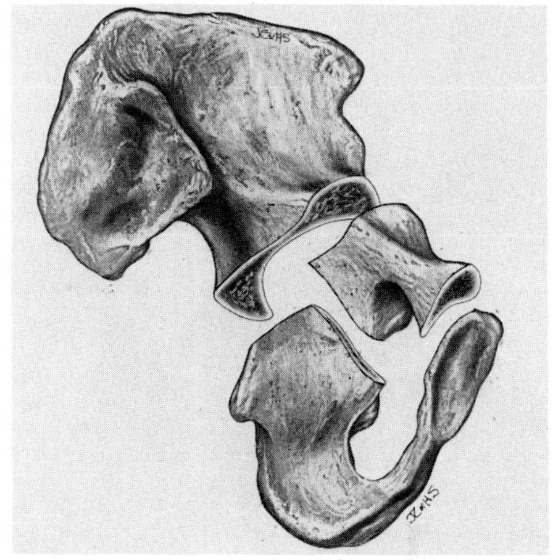

Figure 4-38A ii.

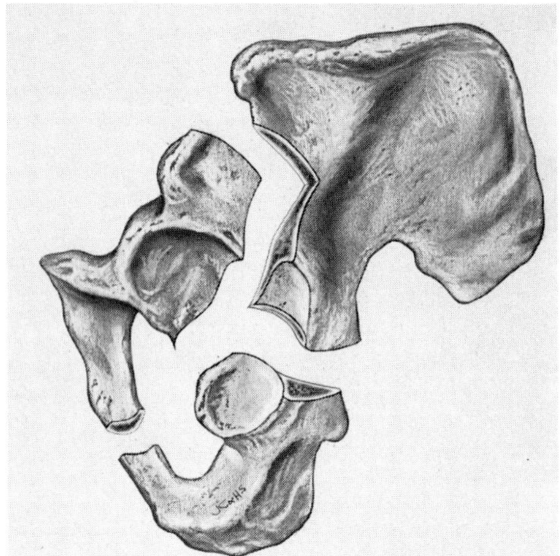

Figure 4-38A iii.

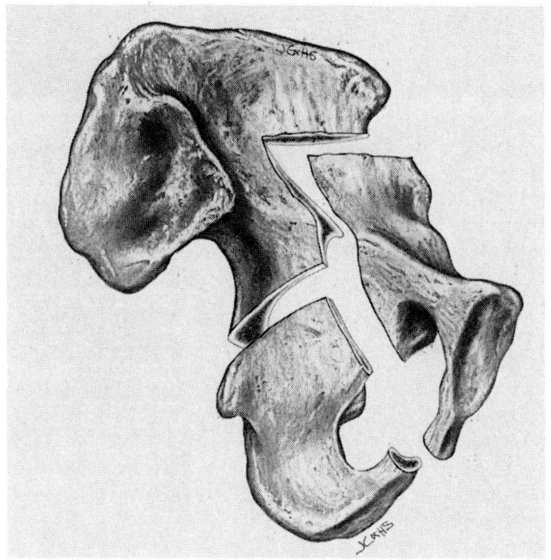

Figure 4-38A iv.

column, including the inner pelvic wall. The optimal surgical approach depends heavily upon these detailed features of the injury.

**4. "T" Fracture.** This uncommon injury possesses a transverse fracture component with a vertical element that divides the ischiopubic component into two portions (Figure 4-39). The transverse constituent can occur at all of the various levels previously described for the simple transverse fracture. The vertical or "stem" fracture constituent can exit anteriorly, inferiorly or posteriorly depending upon the vector of the provocative force. Radiological features are comparable to those described

Figure 4-38B. Associated anterior wall and posterior hemitransverse: i) anteroposterior view; ii) obturator oblique view, highlighting anterior wall fragment and intact portion of posterior roof; iii) iliac oblique view, with displaced posterior column; iv, v) computed scans through the dome and quadrilateral surface with the anterior wall and posterior column fragments and intact acetabular segment; vi-viii) 3-D computed scans confirming anterior wall and posterior column fragments with intact acetabular segment.

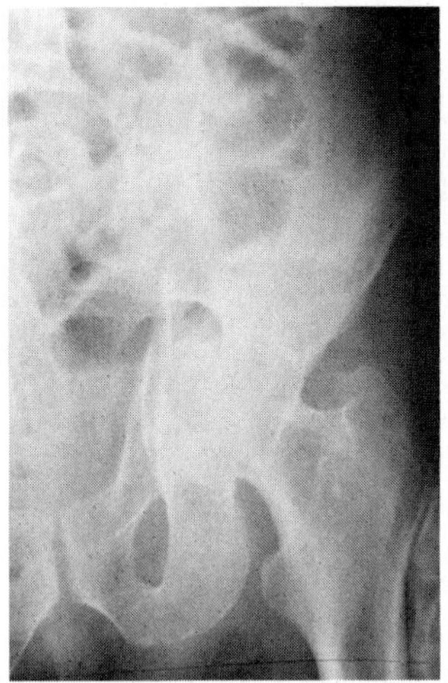

Figure 4-38B i.

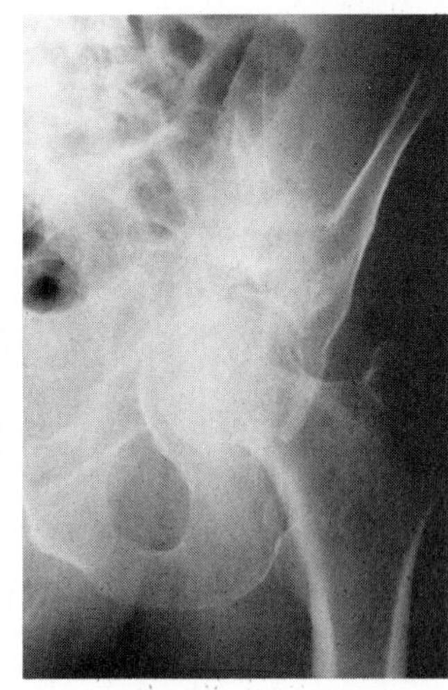

Figure 4-38B ii.

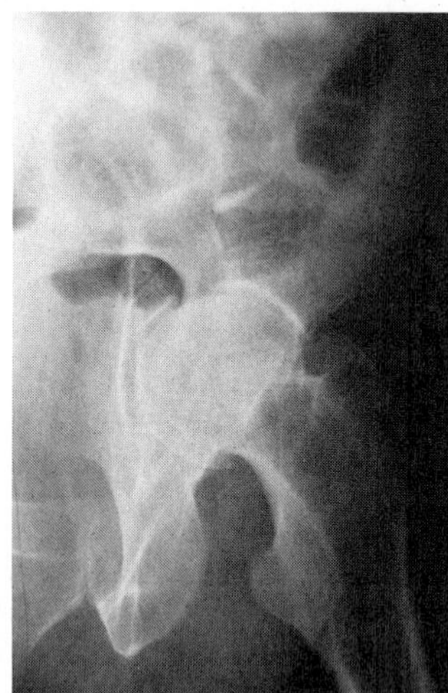

Figure 4-38B iii.

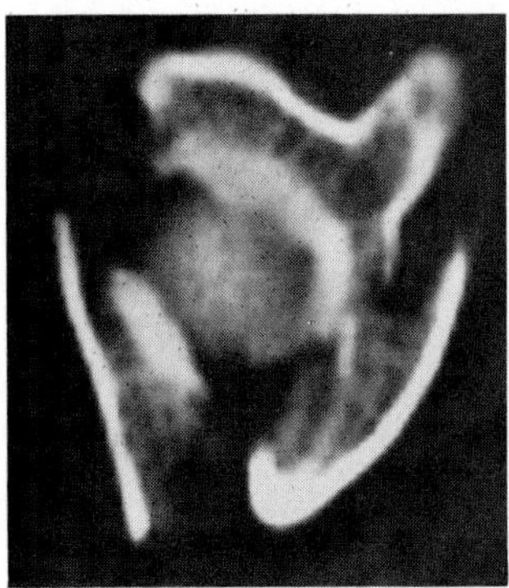

Figure 4-38B iv.

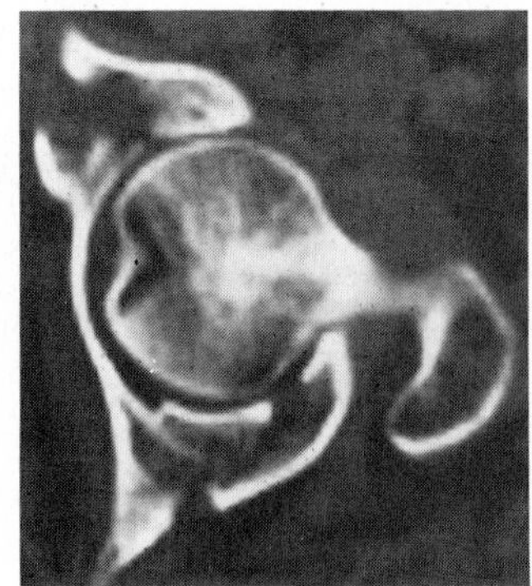

Figure 4-38B v.

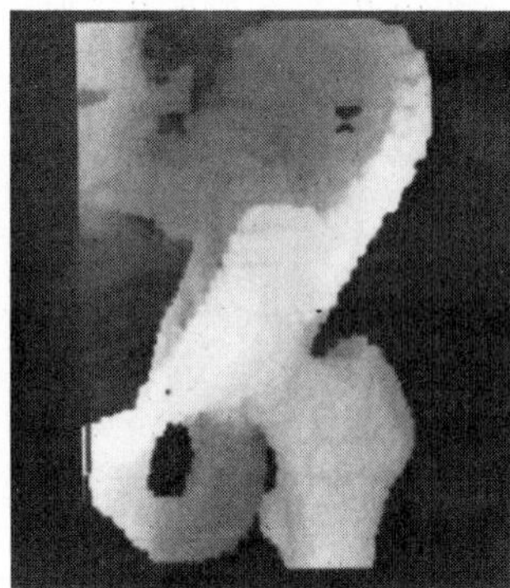

Figure 4-38B vi.

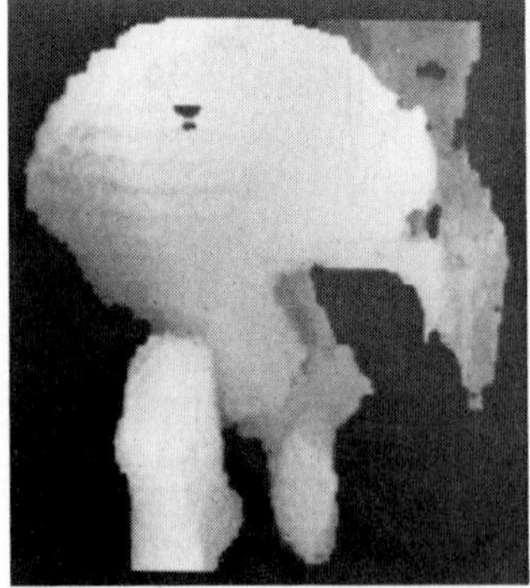

Figure 4-38B vii.

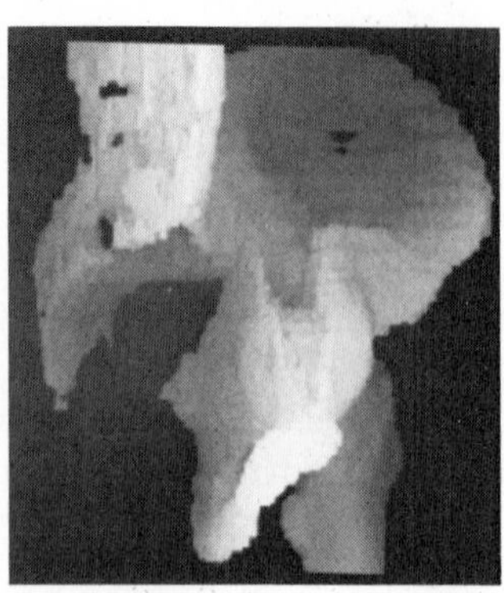

Figure 4-38B viii.

Figure 4-38C. Associated anterior column and posterior hemitransverse: i) anteroposterior view; ii) obturator oblique view with anterior column fragment; iii) iliac oblique view with posterior column fragment including displaced quadrilateral surface; iv) computed scan through quadrilateral surface with displaced anterior and posterior columns.

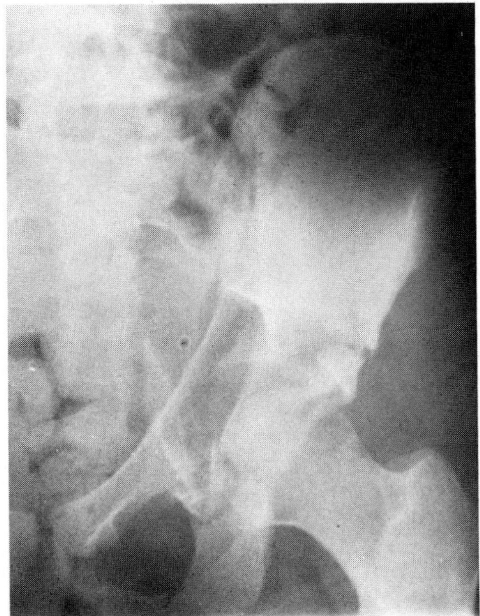

Figure 4-38C i.

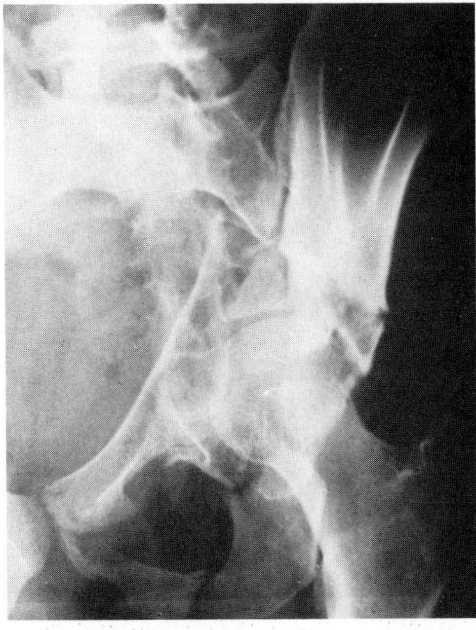

Figure 4-38C ii.

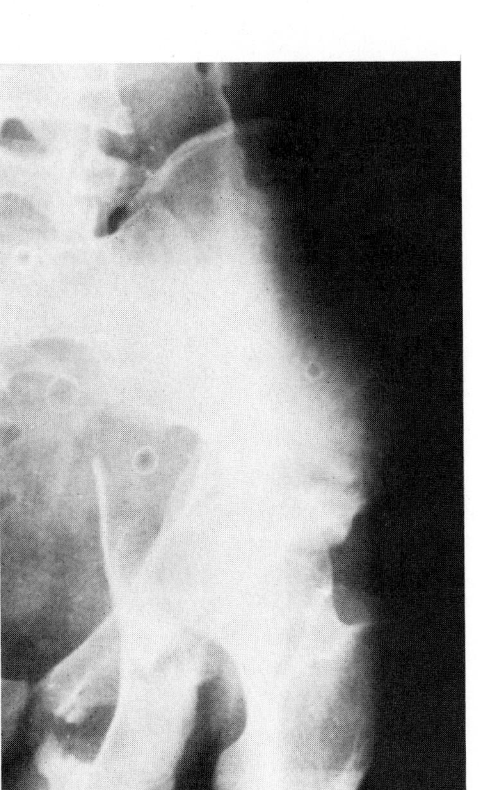

Figure 4-38C iii.

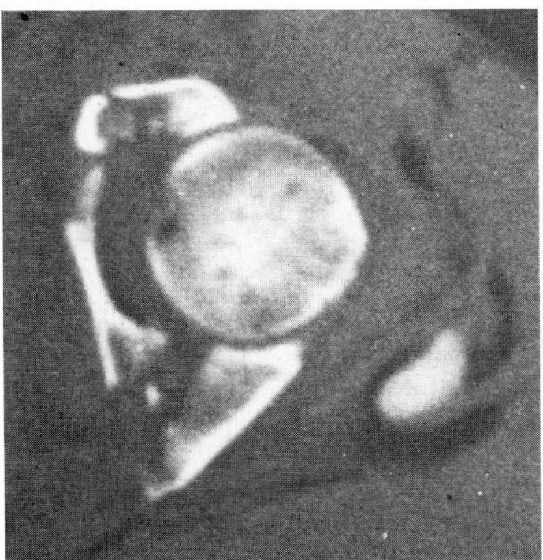

Figure 4-38C iv.

Figure 4-38D. Associated anterior column and posterior hemitransverse: i) anteroposterior view; ii) obturator oblique view; iii) iliac oblique view; iv) anteromedial 3-D scan; v) superior view 3-D scan; vi) inferior view 3-D scan.

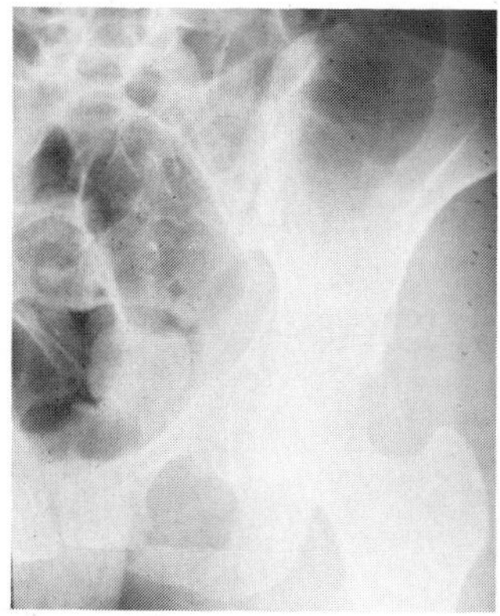

Figure 4-38D i.

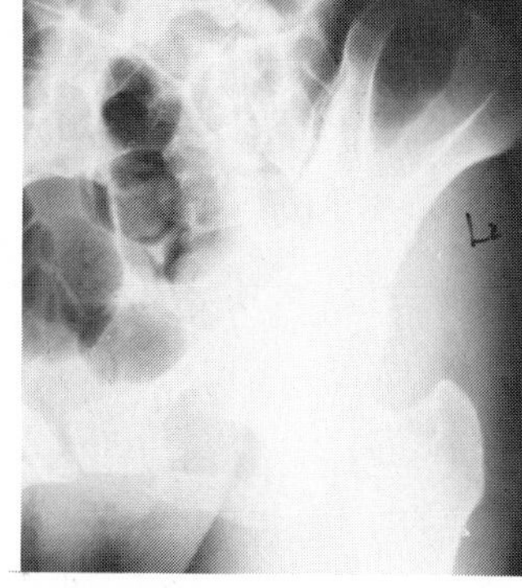

Figure 4-38D ii.

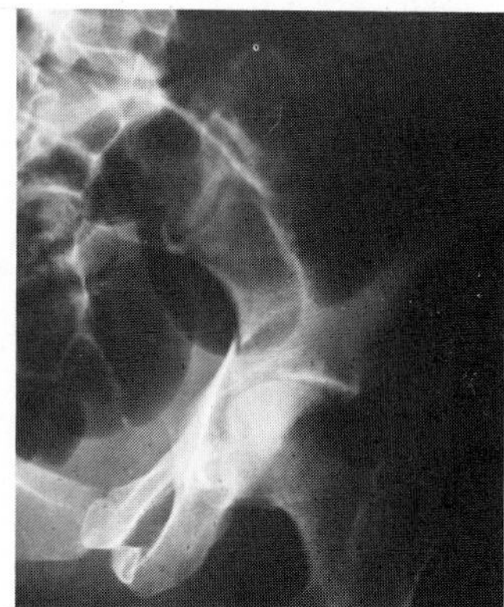

Figure 4-38D iii.

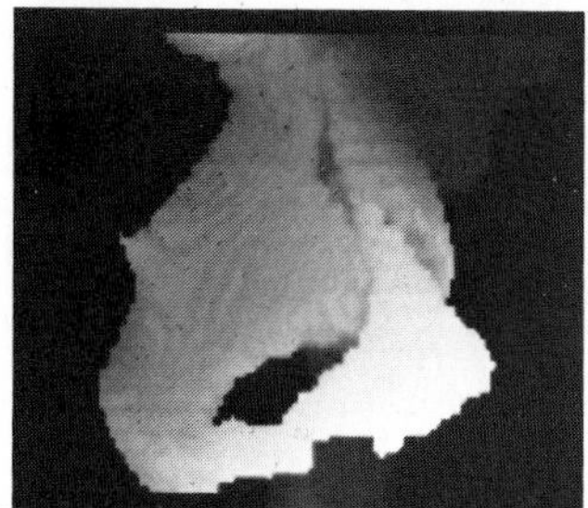

Figure 4-38D iv.

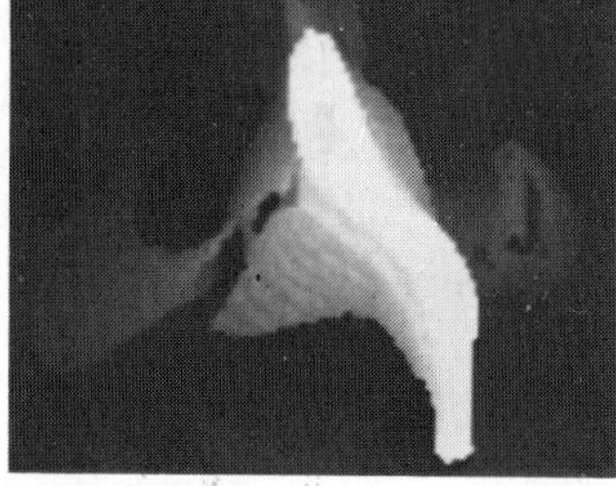

Figure 4-38D v.

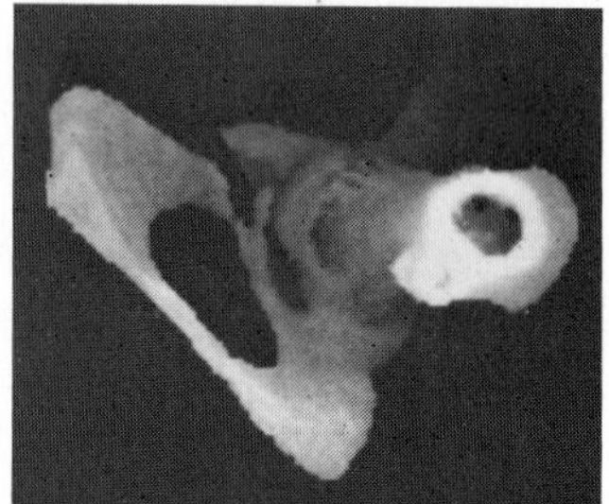

Figure 4-38D vi.

previously for a transverse fracture. In the anteroposterior, obturator oblique, and iliac oblique views, all of the vertically aligned landmarks are disrupted by the displaced transverse element of the fracture. While difficult to recognize, the vertical limb of the "T" fracture is best seen on the obturator oblique view, although it may be evident in the anteroposterior view. The iliac oblique view clearly shows the posterior part of the transverse fracture. Usually the iliac wing is spared, although a stable disruption of the ipsilateral sacroiliac joint is commonly encountered. In a conventional computed scan, the vertical component of the "T" can be recognized. With the obliquity of the pelvis in a supine individual the "T" fracture is readily confused with an isolated posterior or anterior column or a both-column fracture line unless other radiographic features are employed. The three-dimensional scan is particularly valuable to ascertain the vector of displacement of the principal fracture fragments. The conventional scan illustrates the degree of central or iliac comminution so that the degree of technical difficulty anticipated at the time of an open reduction can be estimated.

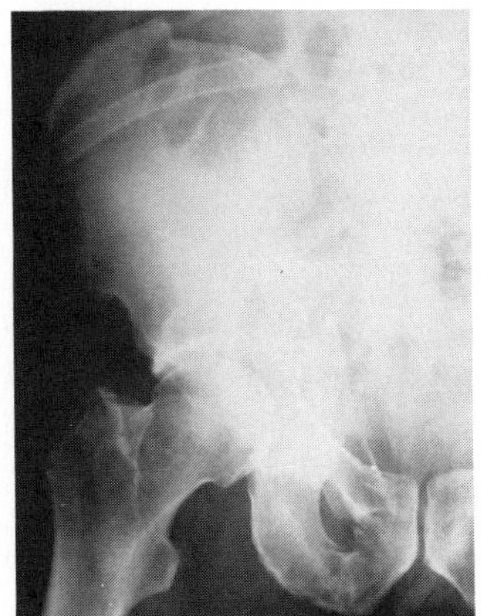

Figure 4-38E i.

Figure 4-38E. Associated anterior wall, anterior column, and posterior hemitransverse: i) anteroposterior view; ii) computed scan through ilium with superior anterior column disruption; iii) computed scan through dome with posterior column displacement; iv) computed scan through quadrilateral region with comminution of anterior wall; v) anteroposterior 3-D scan highlighting posterior column displacement; vi) 3-D obturator oblique-type scan featuring comminution of anterior wall, the intact roof segment, and the displaced posterior column; vii) 3-D posterior scan with posterior column disruption and intact roof segment.

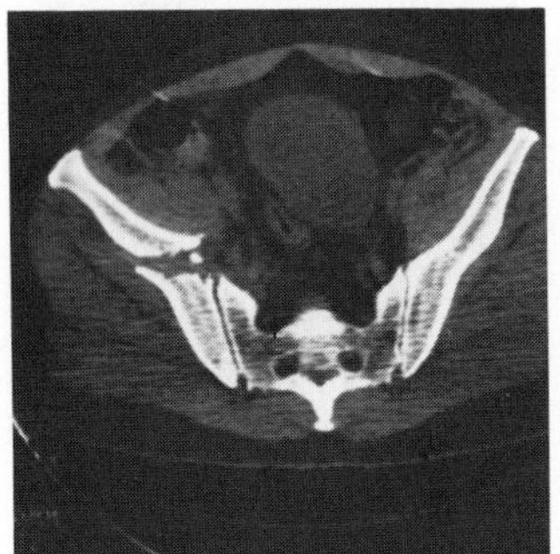

Figure 4-38E ii.

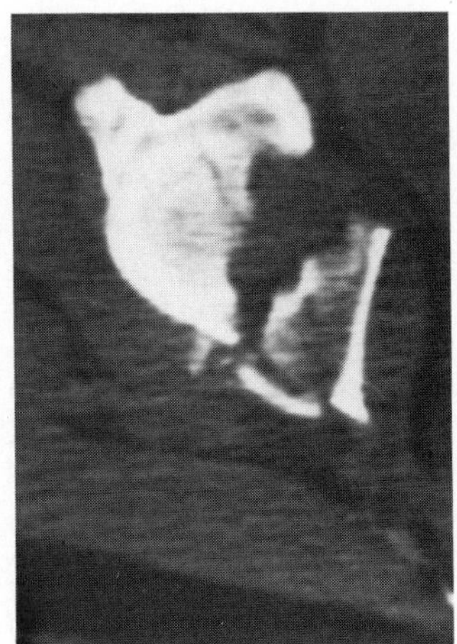

Figure 4-38E iii.

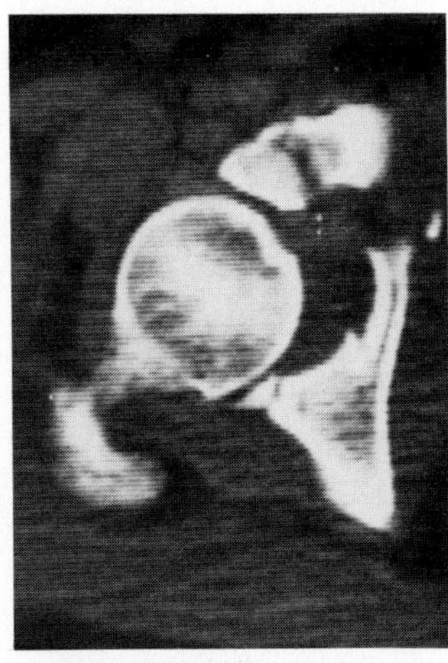

Figure 4-38E iv.

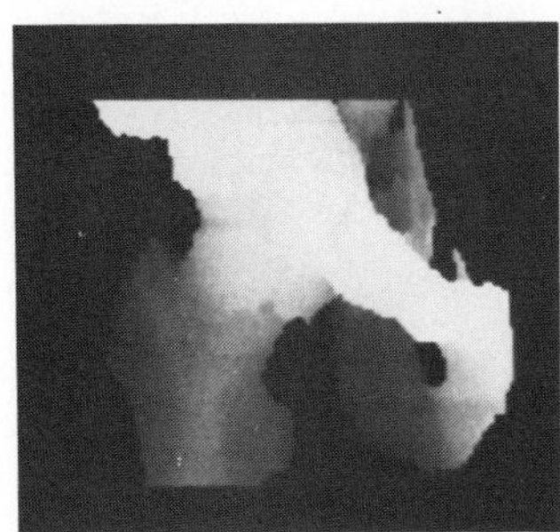

Figure 4-38E v.

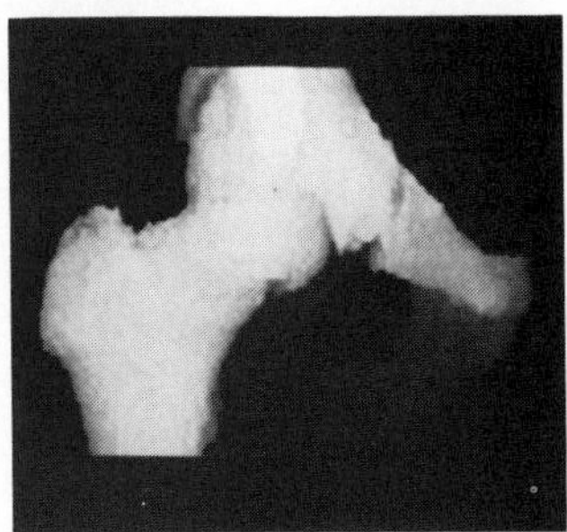

Figure 4-38E vi.

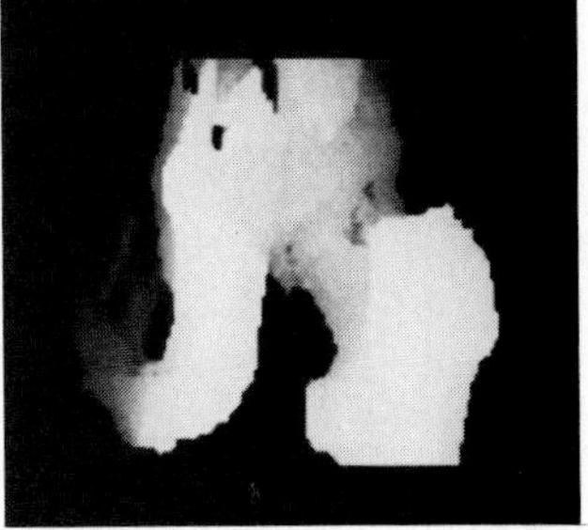

Figure 4-38E vii.

Figure 4-39. "T" fractures.

Figure 4-39A. Schematic diagrams (i, ii) of typical variants.

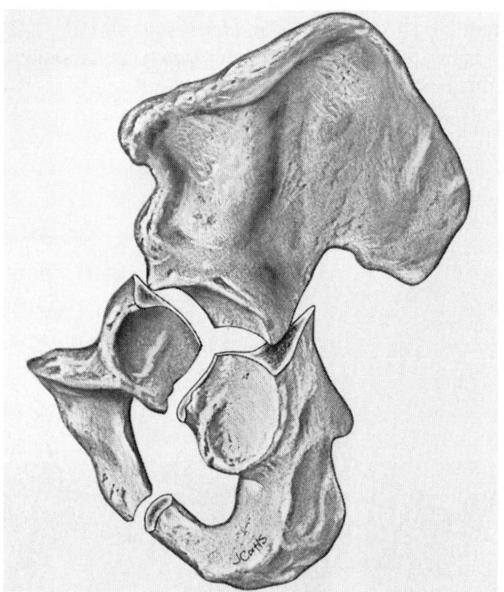

Figure 4-39A i.

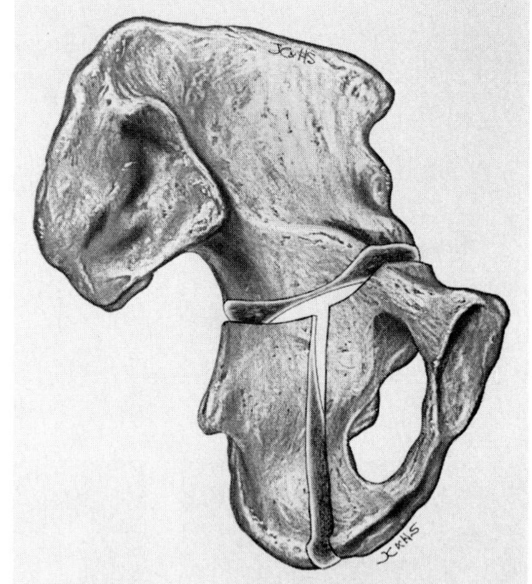

Figure 4-39A ii.

Figure 4-39B. Schematic diagrams (i, ii) of anterior "T" fracture where the stem exits anteriorly across the obturator foramen.

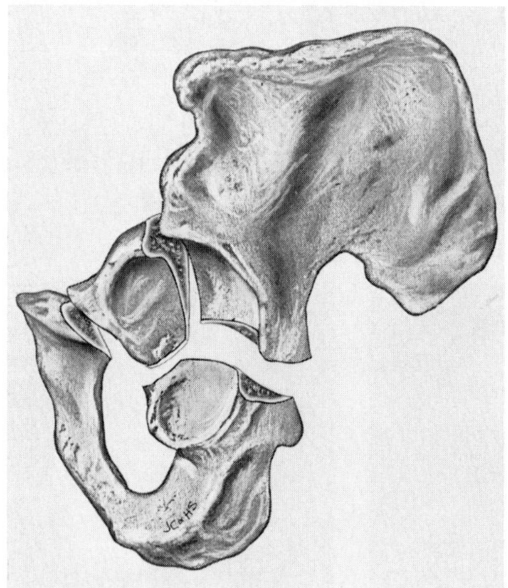

Figure 4-39B i.

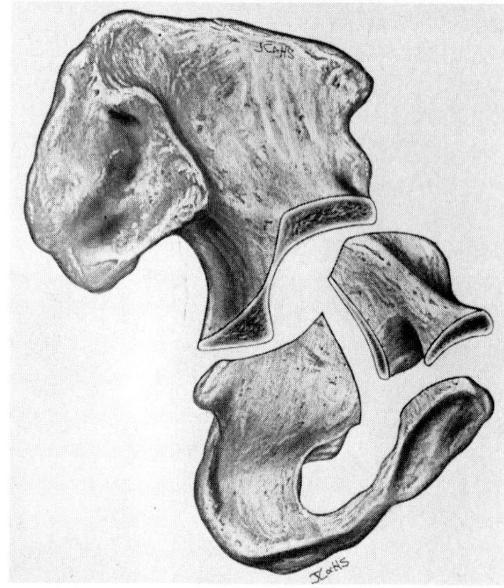

Figure 4-39B ii.

Figure 4-39C. Clinical example of typical "T" fracture: i) Anteroposterior view; ii) obturator oblique view; iii) iliac oblique view.

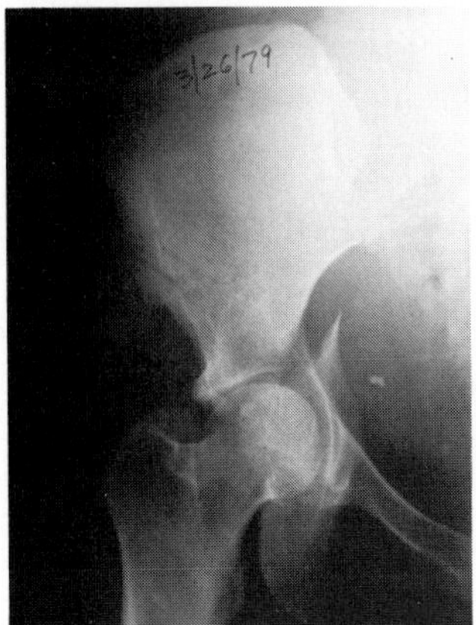


Figure 4-39C i.

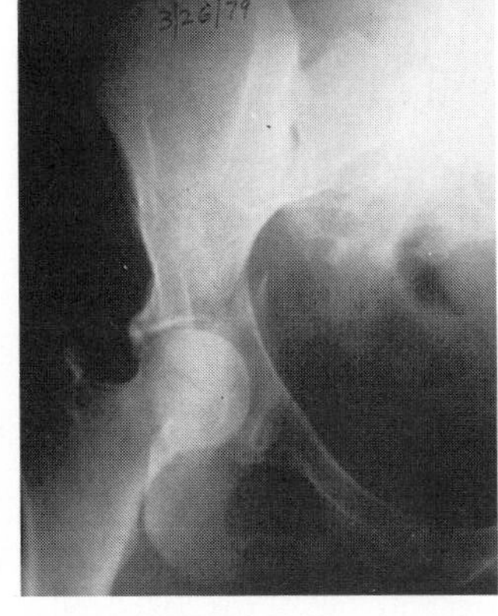


Figure 4-39C ii.

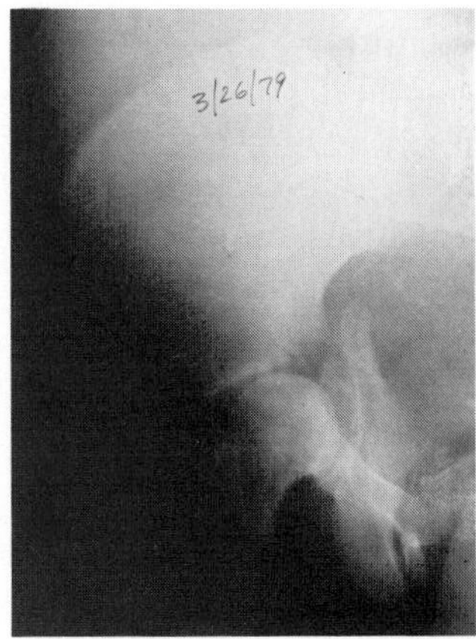


Figure 4-39C iii.

Figure 4-39D. Clinical example of posterior "T" fracture: i) anteroposterior view; ii) pelvic inlet view highlighting central and posterior displacement; iii) computed scan of dome with the three principal acetabular fragments and the femoral head; iv) 3-D computed scan with anteroposterior view featuring transverse fracture element; v) 3-D computed scan with posterior view highlighting posterior column displacement and comminution of posterior wall; vi) 3-D computed scan with medial view confirming stem fracture through posterior column.

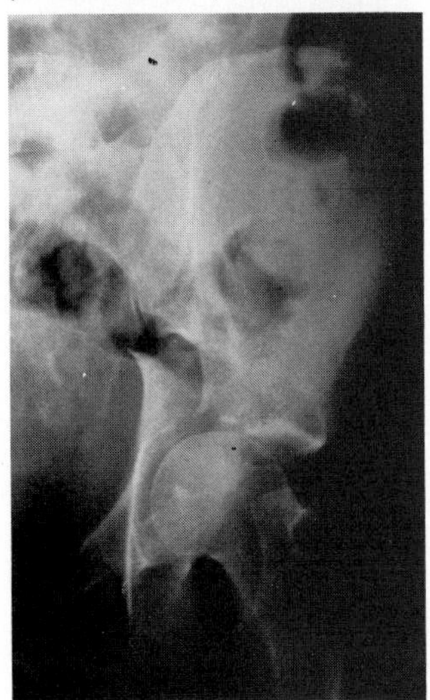

Figure 4-39D i.

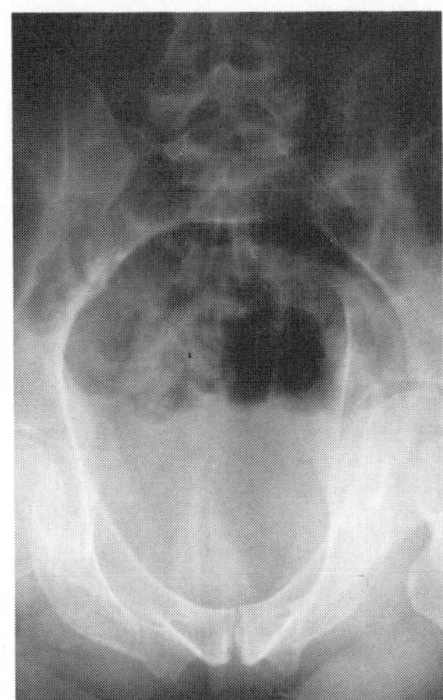

Figure 4-39D ii.

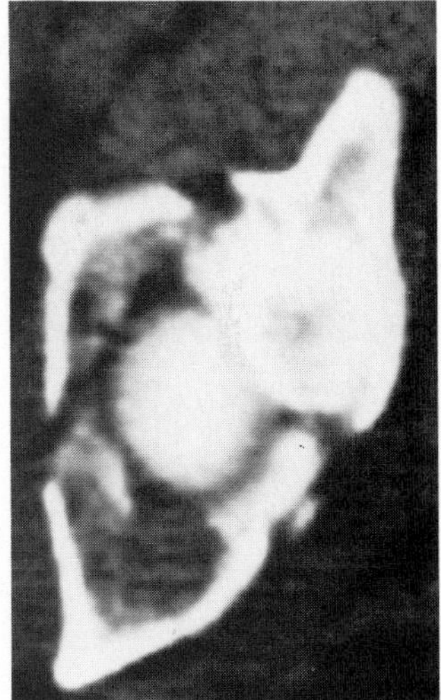

Figure 4-39D iii.

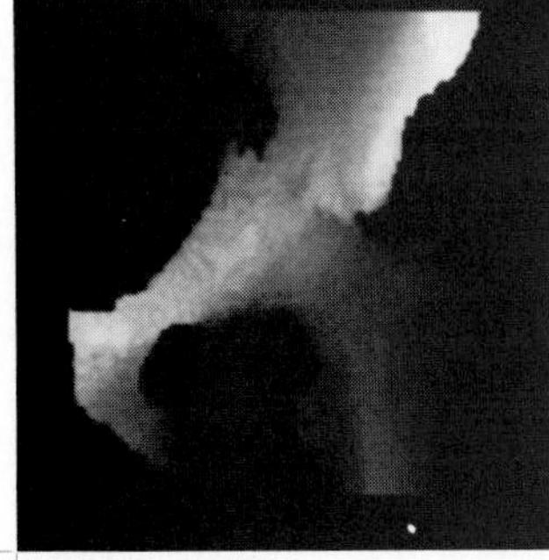

Figure 4-39D iv.

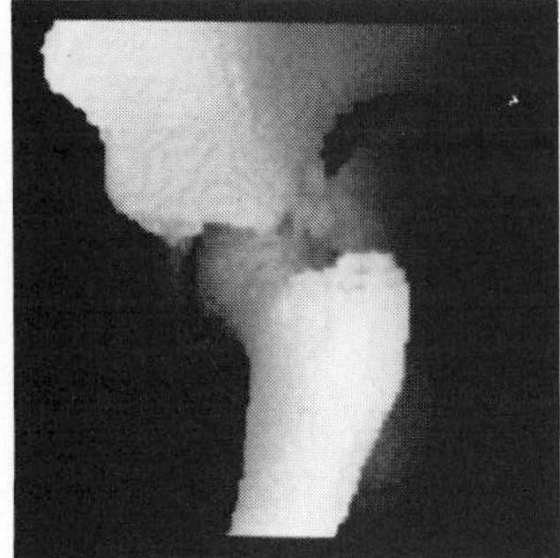

Figure 4-39D v.

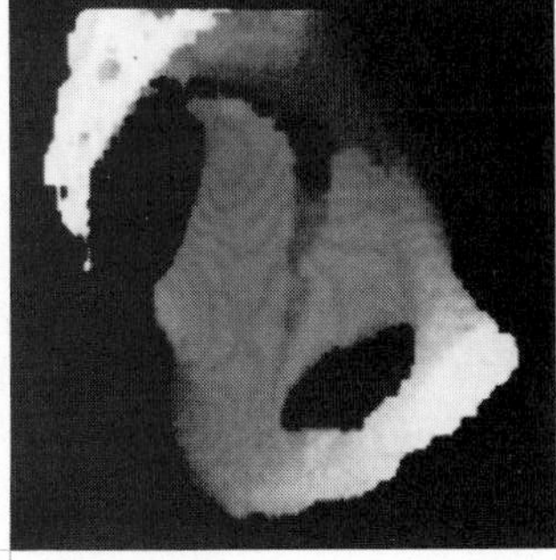

Figure 4-39D vi.

Figure 4-39E. Clinical example of anterior "T" fracture: i) anteroposterior view; ii) obturator oblique view; iii) iliac oblique view.

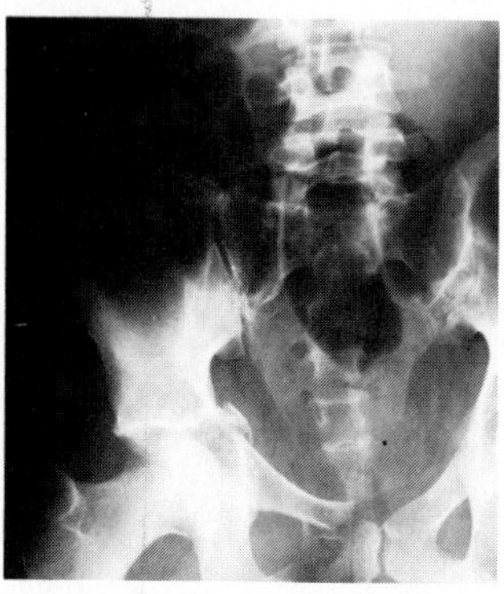

Figure 4-39E i.

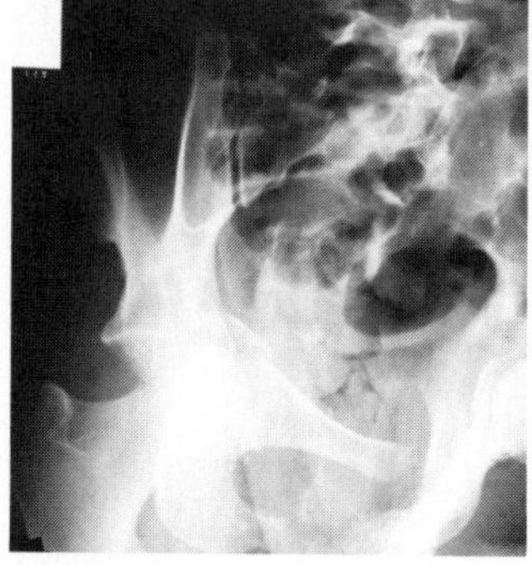

Figure 4-39E ii.

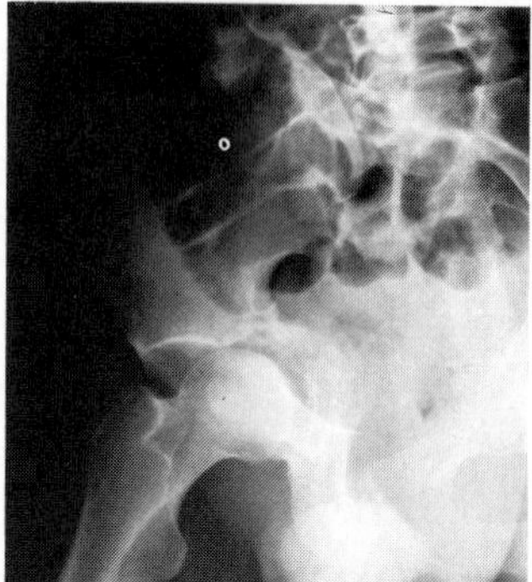

Figure 4-39E iii.

Figure 4-39F. Clinical example of posterior "T" fracture with stable, Grade II ipsilateral sacroiliac disruption: i) anteroposterior view with transverse fracture element; ii) obturator oblique view with posterior stem and sacroiliac disruption; iii) computed scan through sacroiliac joints.

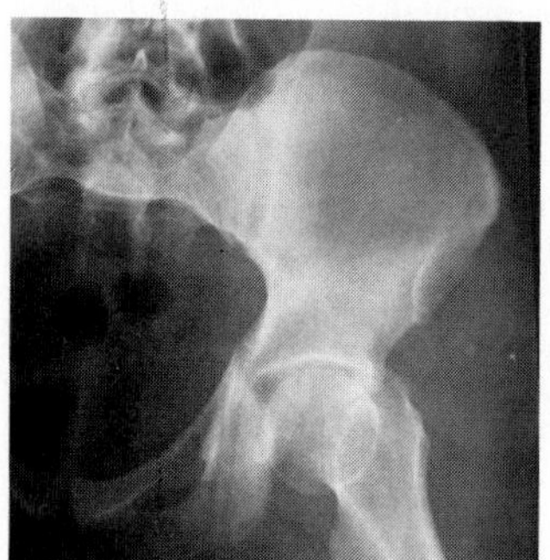

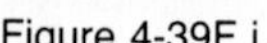

Figure 4-39F i.

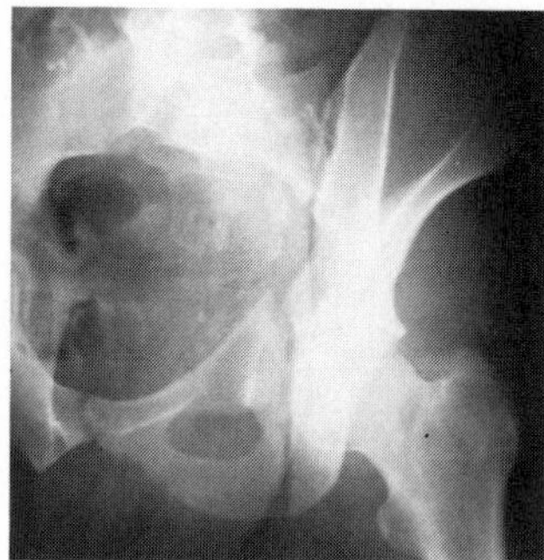

Figure 4-39F ii.

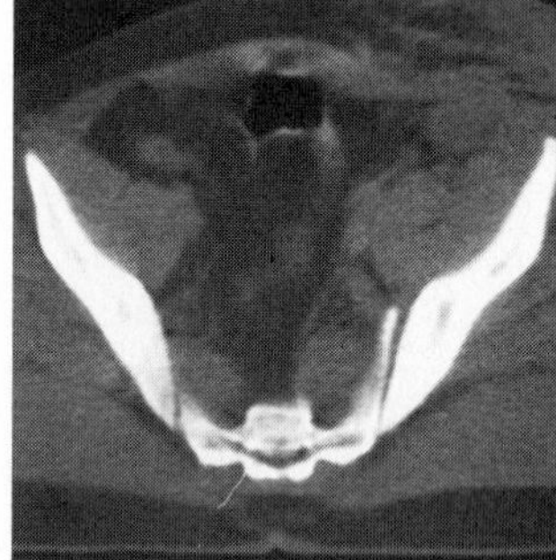

Figure 4-39F iii.

**5. Both-Column Fracture.** This comminuted injury constitutes the most complex type of acetabular fracture and historically was termed a "central acetabular fracture." The anterior and posterior columns along with their respective adjacent segments of articular surface are separated from one another (Figure 4-40). A portion of iliac wing, of variable size, remains attached to the sacrum at the ipsilateral sacroiliac joint. Frequently, these fractures are highly comminuted with the presence of numerous osseous fragments that do not possess an articular surface. The posterior part of the fracture complex including its direction of displacement is similar to a simple posterior column fracture. The principal posterior column fragment is detached superiorly by a fracture that begins anywhere on the posterior border of the innominate bone in the region of the greater sciatic notch and extends inferiorly. Secondary fracture lines may be present in the posterior column. Frequently, the anterior column fracture begins confluent with the fracture of the posterior column and extends across the iliac wing to the iliac crest or to the anterior border of the iliac bone. Anterior comminution can be anticipated along with the disruption of the articular surface into several large irregular osteochondral fragments. Central dislocation of the femoral head is a constant feature. Unlike a "T" fracture, no iliac portion of the acetabular roof remains undisplaced. The discrete iliac fracture fragment generally undergoes a marked rotational deviation and may be displaced secondarily at the sacroiliac joint or at an adjacent fracture site in the posterior ilium or sacrum. In the anteroposterior view the central displacement of the femoral head is evident, frequently with an accompanying portion of the acetabular roof. A large, medially displaced ilioischial fragment and an iliac fracture line extending across the iliac wing to the anterior iliac margin or the iliac crest are identified. In the obturator oblique view the separate anterior column fragment is clearly seen, as well as an anterior wall fracture and secondary comminution. Superior to the centrally displaced acetabular roof a characteristic "spur" of bone can be seen, indicative of a both-column fracture and the corresponding pattern of iliac disruption. The iliac oblique view demonstrates a fracture of the posterior column as well as the iliac fracture line. The anterior iliac fracture fragment with a portion of the articular roof is tilted so that it remains congruent with the femoral head. In the presence of a central dislocation of the femoral head, the iliac wing fracture and the "spur" sign permit a radiological distinction of a both-column fracture from a "T" fracture, an anterior column and posterior hemitransverse fracture, and an associated transverse fracture with comminution of the iliac wing. Unlike a both-column fracture in all of the latter examples, an articular segment of acetabulum remains attached to the iliac wing.

A conventional computed scan characterizes the degree of comminution, especially of an associated iliac portion of the anterior column disruption. The three-dimensional scan is most valuable to determine the vector of displacement of the anterior and posterior columns. The triplane deformities of the columns with the "barroom door" appearance is a classic feature. The columns migrate centrally with a characteristic malrotation provoked by the inward displacement of the femoral head. An accurate recognition of this deformity is crucial in the preoperative period so that the appropriate vector for the open reduction of the columns is achieved at the time of surgery.

Figure 4-40. Associated both-column fractures.

Figure 4-40A. Schematic views (i, ii) of both-column fracture with a high anterior disruption extending to the iliac crest.

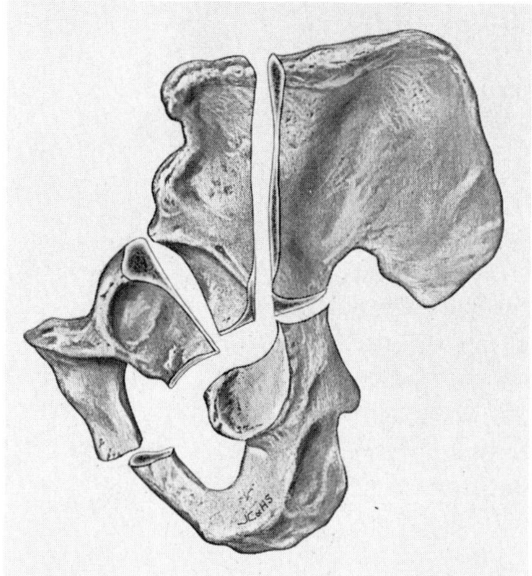

Figure 4-40A i.

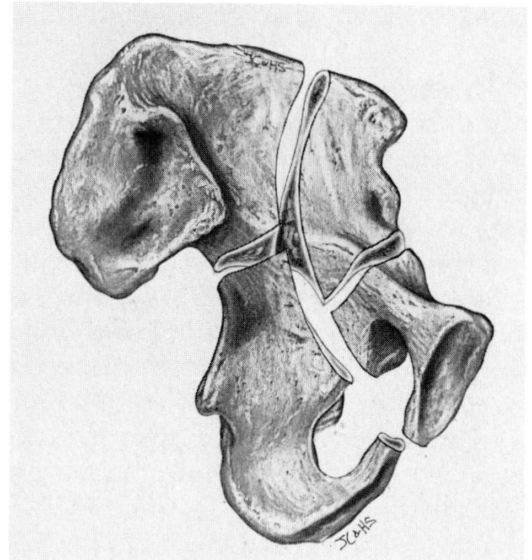

Figure 4-40A ii.

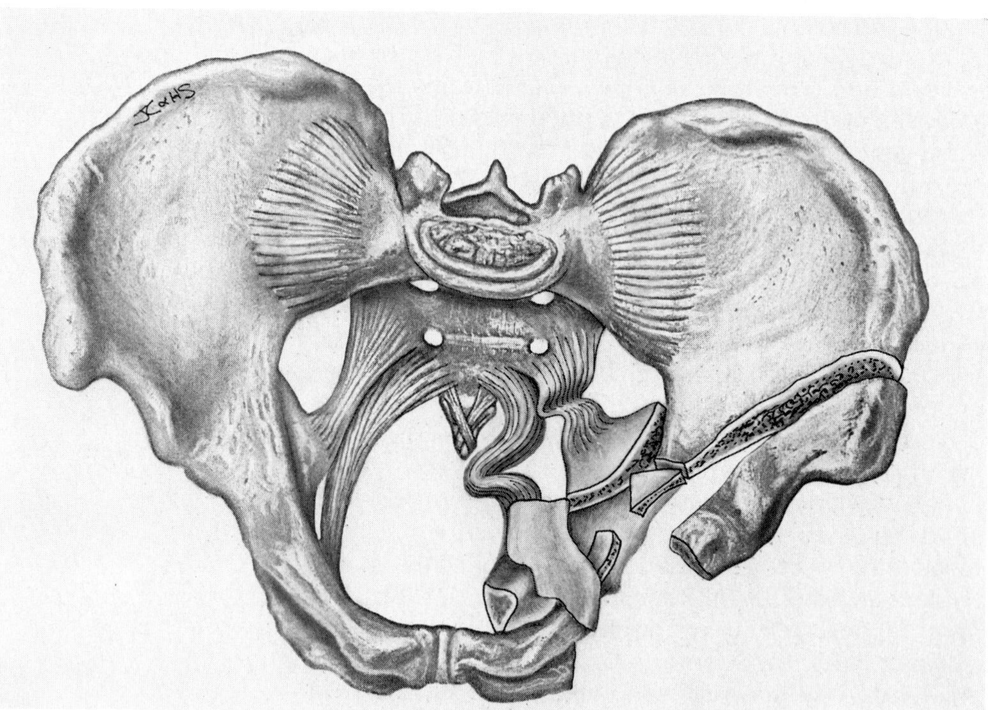

Figure 4-40B. Schematic view of an example with an intermediate anterior disruption extending to the anterior border of the ilium.

Figure 4-40C. Schematic views of one comminuted variant with a segmental anterior column disruption (i, ii), and another with marked iliac comminution (iii, iv).

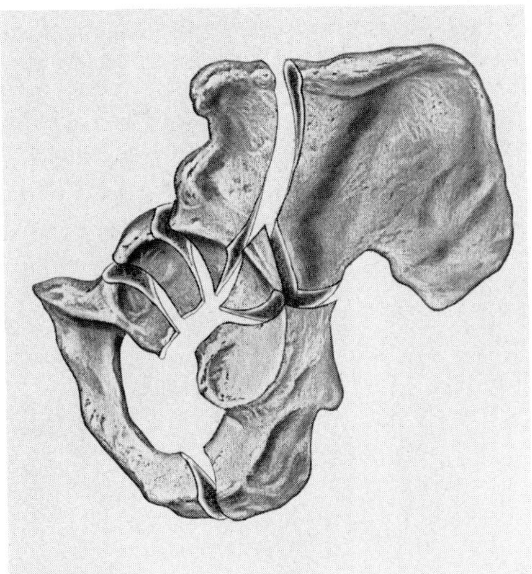

Figure 4-40C i.

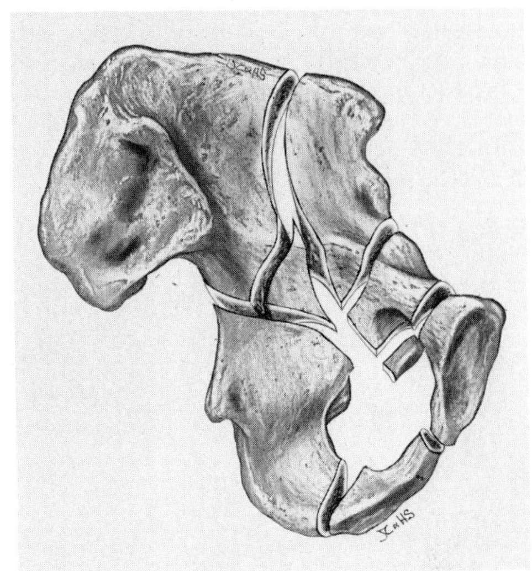

Figure 4-40C ii.

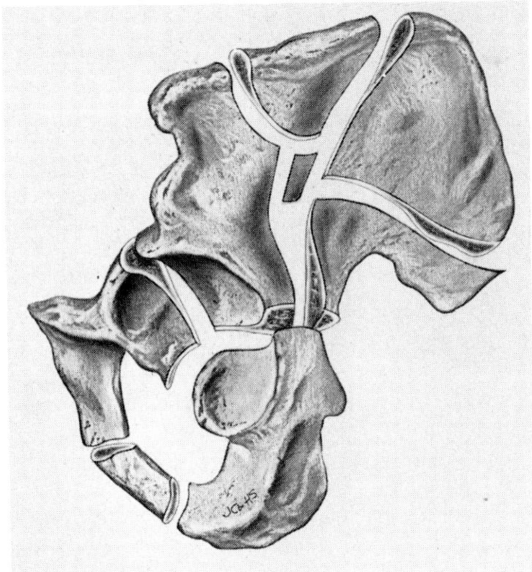

Figure 4-40C iii.

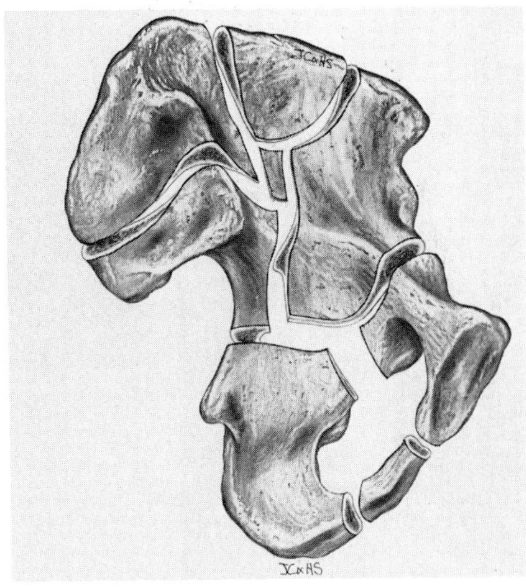

Figure 4-40C iv.

## C. Complex Pelvic Injury

**1. Acetabular and Pelvic Ring Fracture.** A separate category is an acetabular fracture complicated by other disruptions of the pelvic ring, which the authors[13] identify as a complex or Group IV pelvic injury (Figure 4-41). The concomitant fractures in the pelvic ring can occur on either side of the ring and at one or several sites including the contralateral acetabulum. Virtually

Figure 4-40D. Clinical example of a both-column fracture with a high segmental anterior column disruption: i) anteroposterior view; ii) inlet view; iii) obturator oblique view; iv) iliac oblique view; v) computed scan with iliac anterior column disruption; vi) computed scan with dome comminution; vii) computed scan through the quadrilateral region, which is characteristically included in the posterior column fragment; viii) 3-D computed scan: anterior inferior view highlights anterior column fracture; ix) 3-D computed scan; posterolateral view with posterior column disruption and iliac extension of anterior column fracture; x) 3-D computed scan; anterior, medial view with medially displaced quadrilateral surface, as an extension of the posterior column and the anterior wall segment; xi) 3-D computed scan of medial view with segmental anterior column fragments and large posterior column fragment.

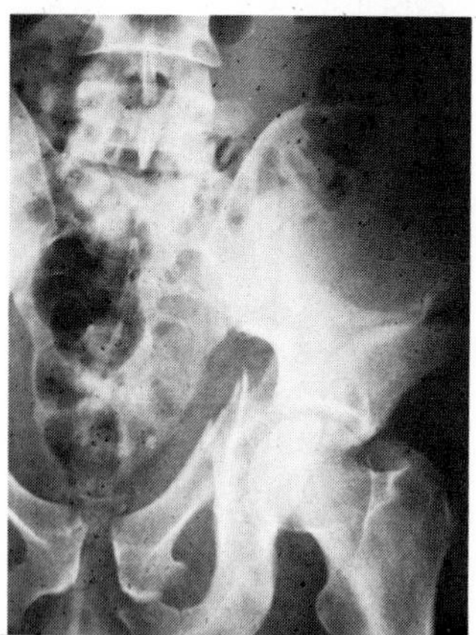

Figure 4-40D i.

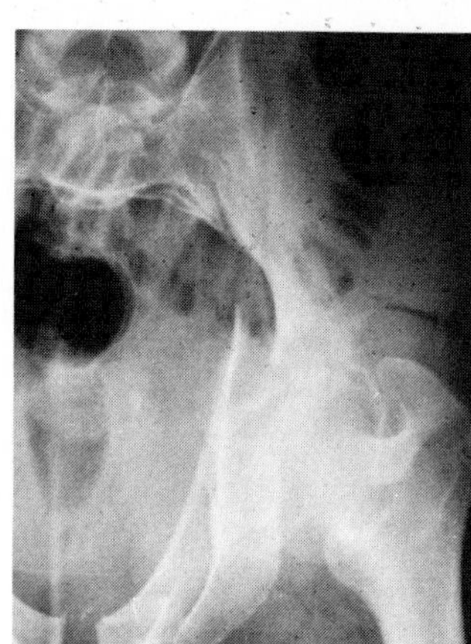

Figure 4-40D ii.

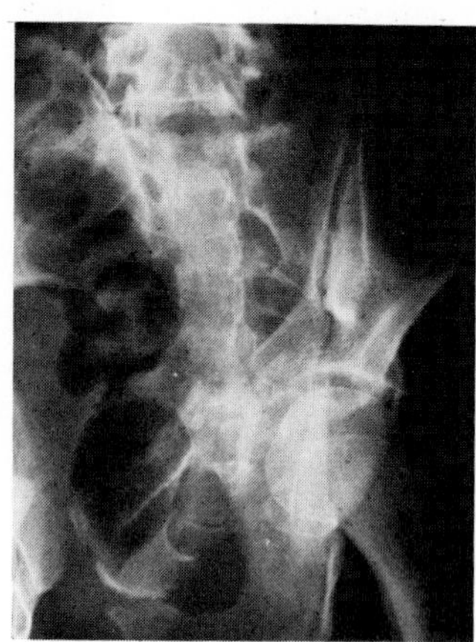

Figure 4-40D iii.

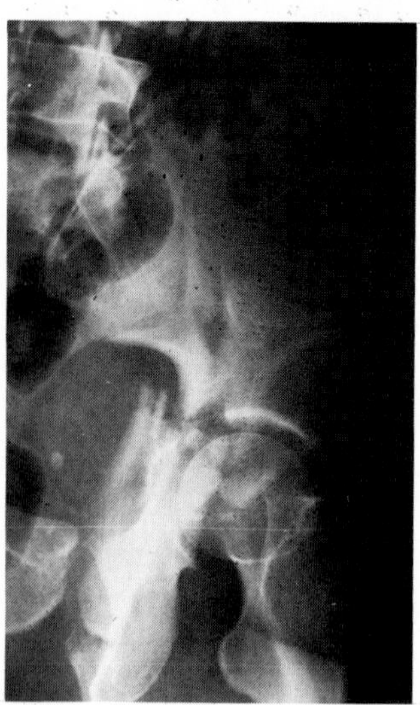

Figure 4-40D iv.

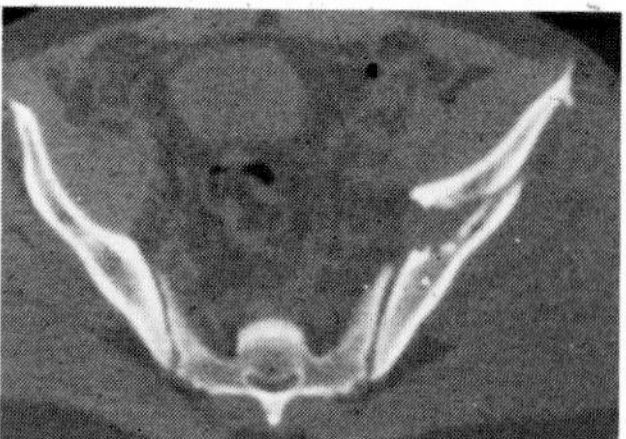

Figure 4-40D v.

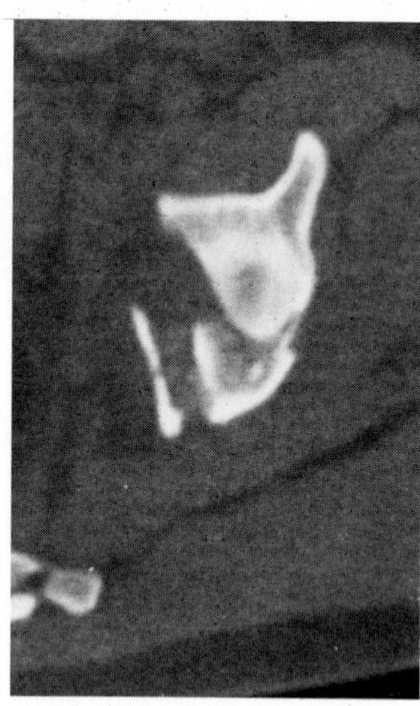

Figure 4-40D vi.

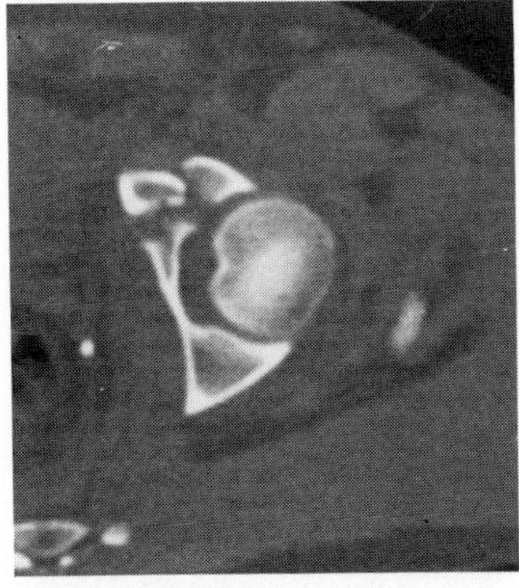
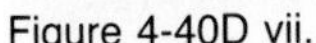

Figure 4-40D vii.

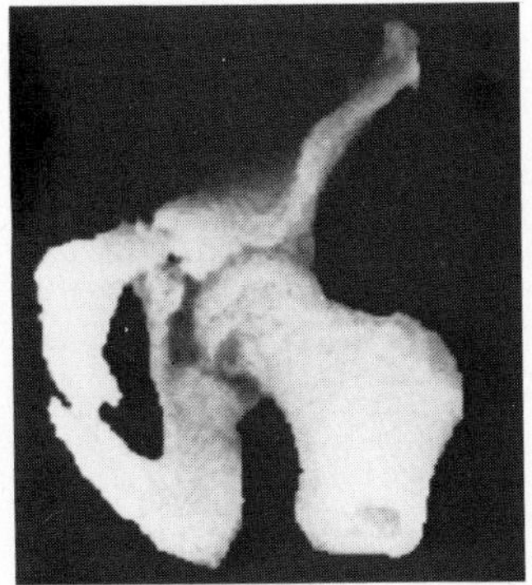

Figure 4-40D viii.

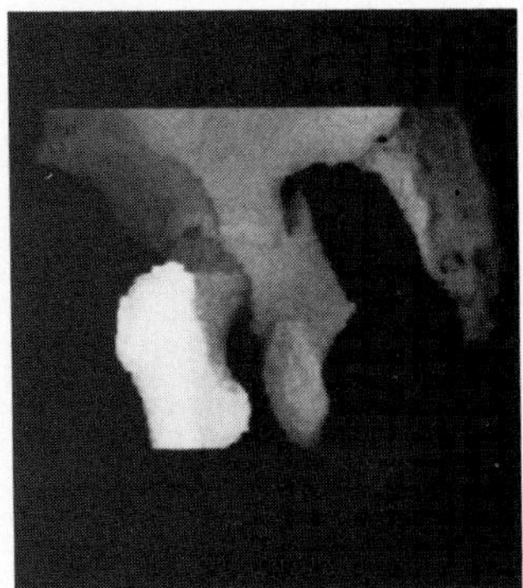

Figure 4-40D ix.

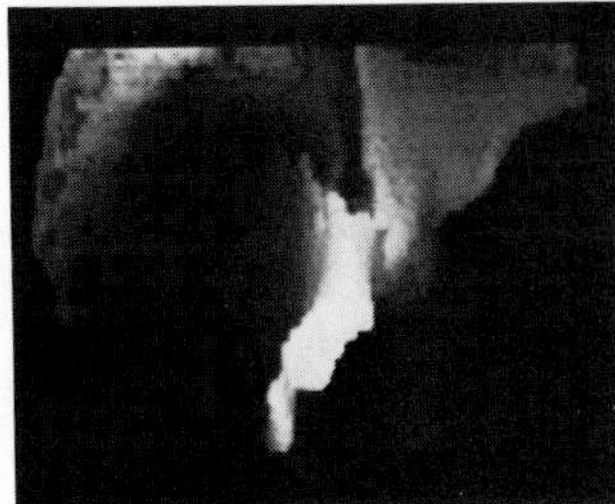

Figure 4-40D x.

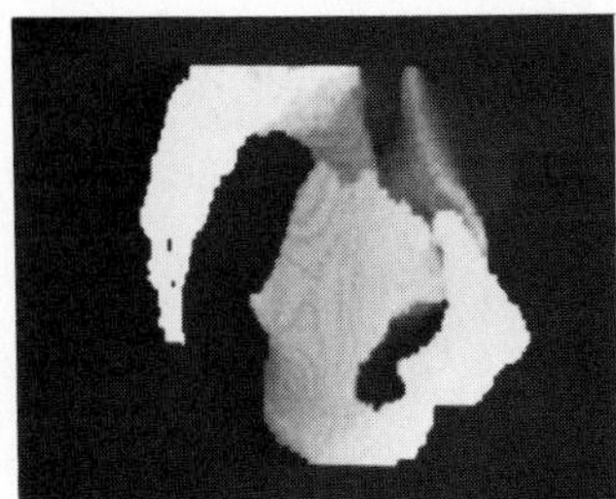

Figure 4-40D xi.

all of the acetabular fractures with supplementary pelvic disruption are variants of a lateral compression injury. Previously, about 10% of all acetabular fractures were characterized as a complex disruption. With the more recent availability of routine computerized axial tomography probably a more accurate percentage is 20% to 25%. The larger incidence is related to stable and minimally displaced ipsilateral or contralateral sacroiliac disruptions and sacral fractures which are invisible in conventional radiographs but readily distinguished in a computed scan.

When an ipsilateral sacroiliac subluxation or dislocation is present, the lateral ilium and adjacent portion of the acetabulum is thereby displaced. The initial anatomic restoration of some portion of the acetabulum or adjacent ilium necessitates an initial reduction of the ipsilateral sacroiliac joint. A computed scan of the posterior pelvis provides crucial information about the sacroiliac joint so that a surgical approach to an associated acetabular fracture can be appropriately planned. Marked three-dimensional displacement of the principal pelvic fragments is a common feature of the Group IV pelvic injuries with acetabular involvement. The application of a three-dimensional scan permits accurate characterization of the deformities to facilitate the operative reduction.

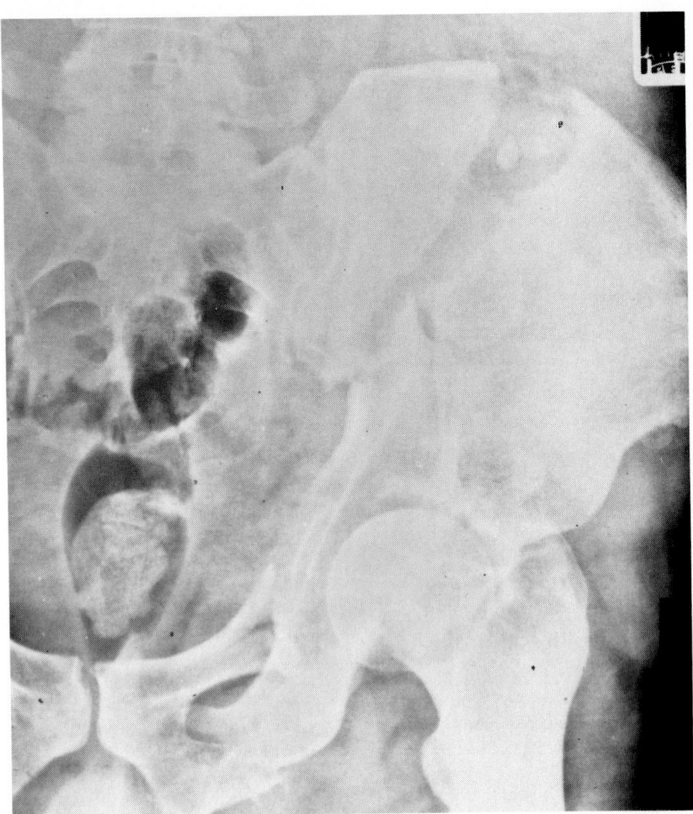

Figure 4-40E. Anteroposterior view of both-column fracture with exceedingly high anterior column involvement vertically across the ilium from the greater sciatic notch.

Figure 4-40F. Clinical example of both-column fracture with intermediate anterior column extension: i) anteroposterior view; ii) obturator oblique view with "spur" sign fragment on lateral iliac surface and anterior column disruption; iii) iliac oblique view with posterior column displacement.

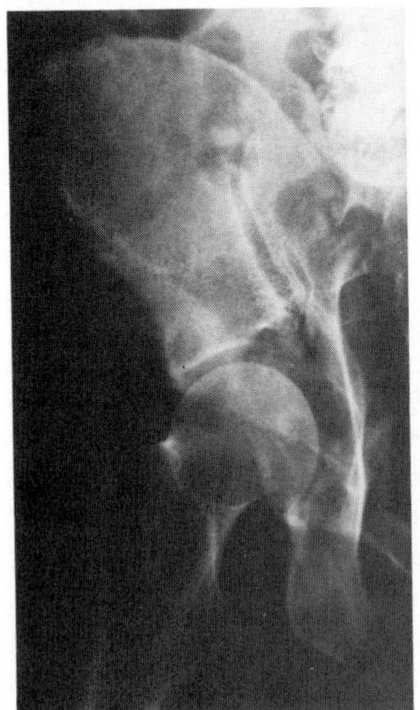

Figure 4-40F i.

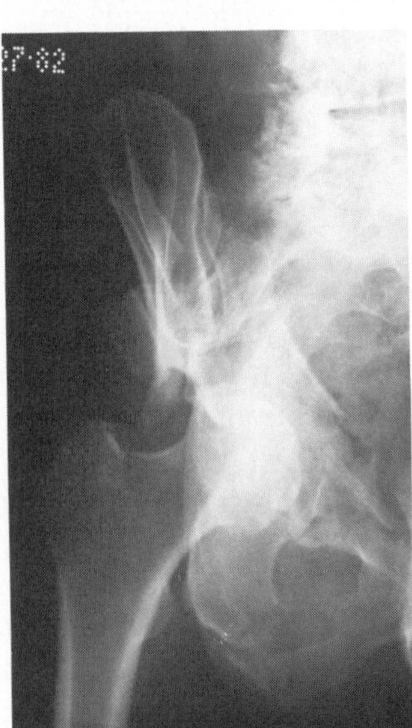

Figure 4-40F ii.

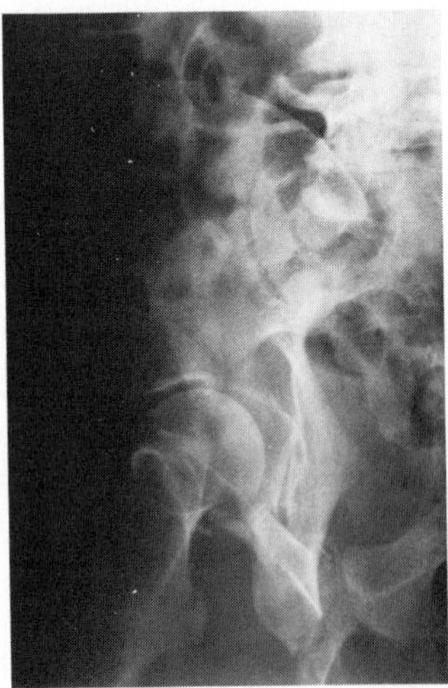

Figure 4-40F iii.

Figure 4-40G. Clinical example of highly comminuted both-column fracture in 250-pound woman, consistent with technically difficult surgical reconstruction: i) anteroposterior view; ii) close-up anteroposterior view illustrating the numerous shards of displaced iliac fragments; iii) obturator oblique view with comminuted anterior wall segment and "spur" sign; iv) iliac oblique view with displaced posterior column; v) computed scan with sacral fracture and anterior column extension across the ilium; vi) computed scan through quadrilateral surface with comminution of anterior and posterior walls.

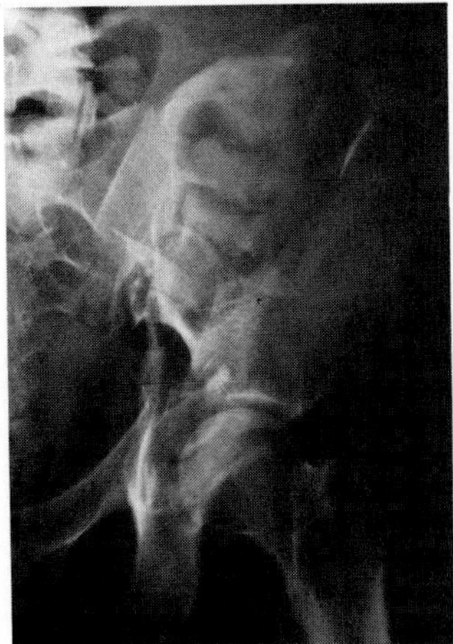

Figure 4-40G i.

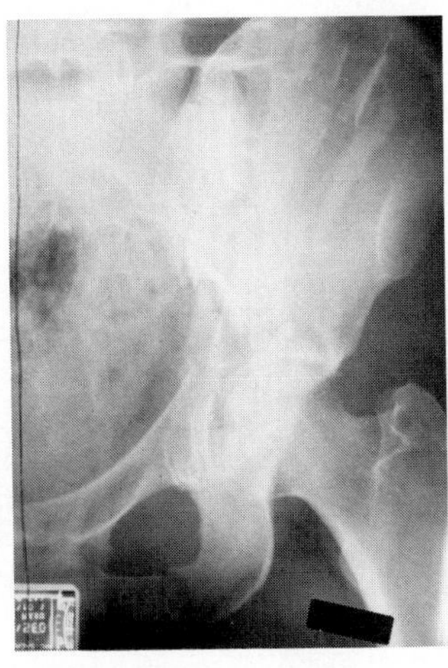

Figure 4-40G ii.

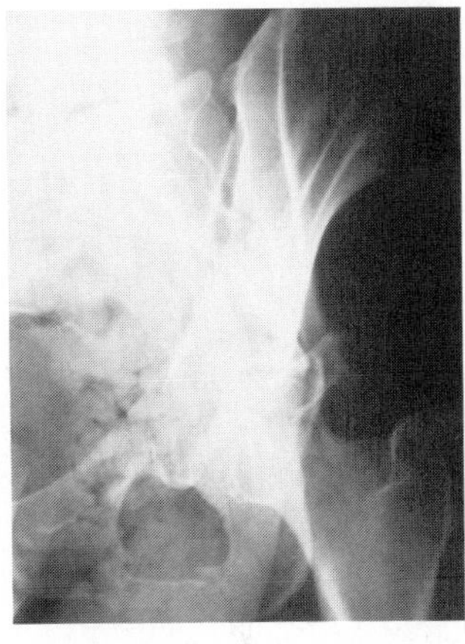

Figure 4-40G iii.

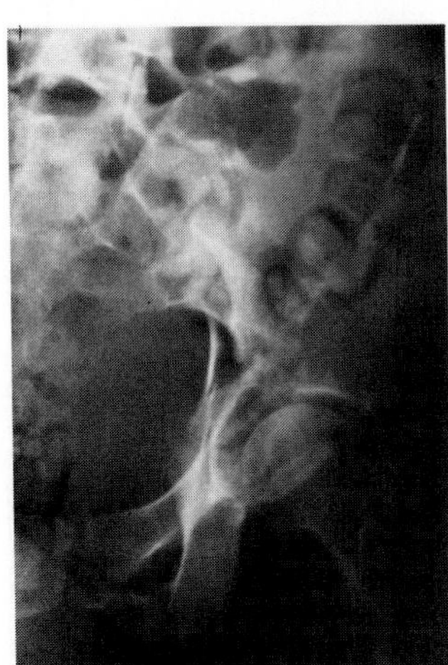

Figure 4-40G iv.

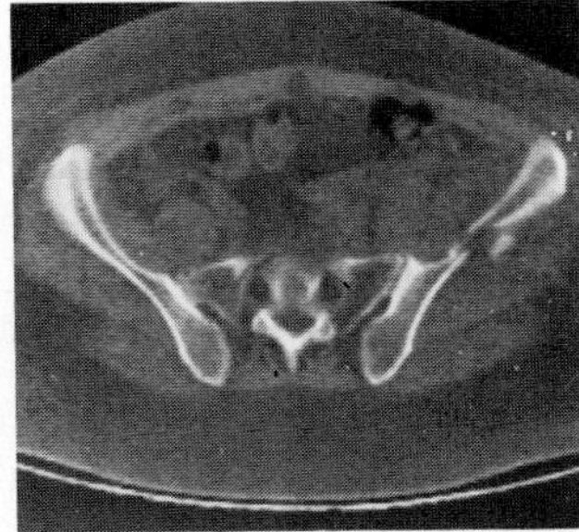

Figure 4-40G v.

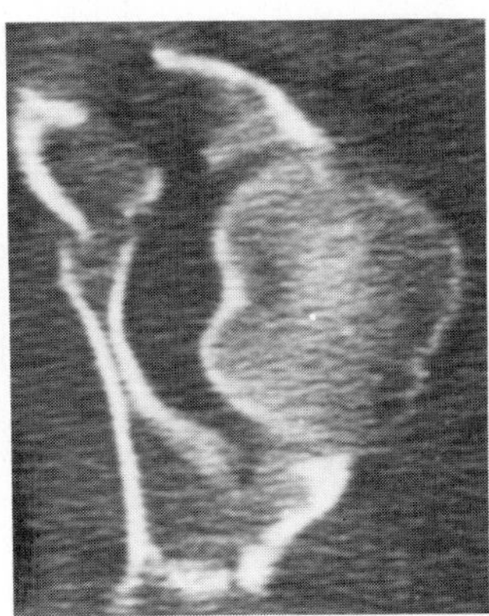

Figure 4-40G vi.

Figure 4-41. Complex pelvic disruptions.

Figure 4-41A. Markedly comminuted "T" fracture with ipsilateral sacroiliac disruption: i) anteroposterior view; ii) computed scan through dome and quadrilateral surface with comminution.

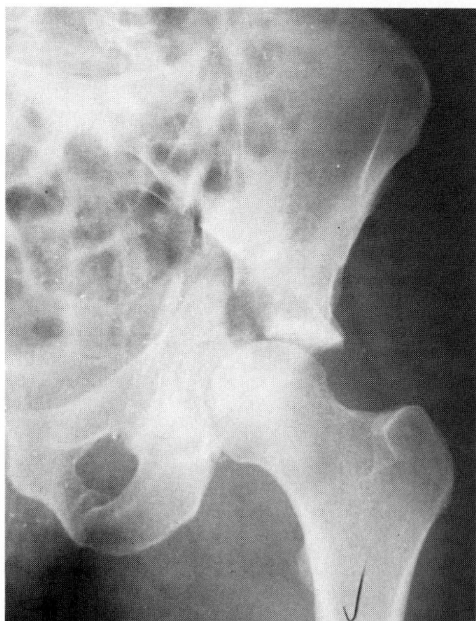

Figure 4-41A i.

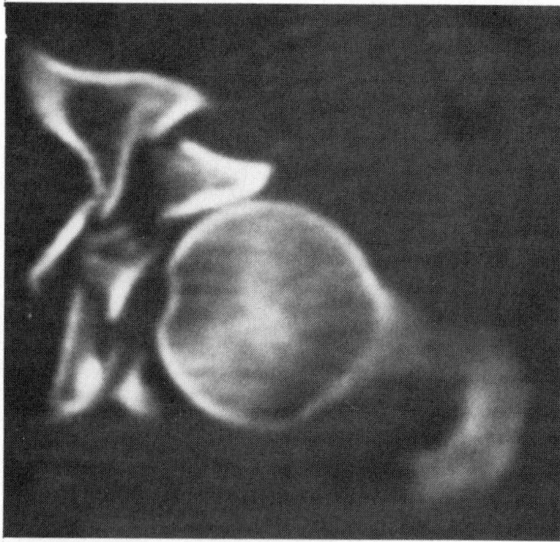

Figure 4-41A ii.

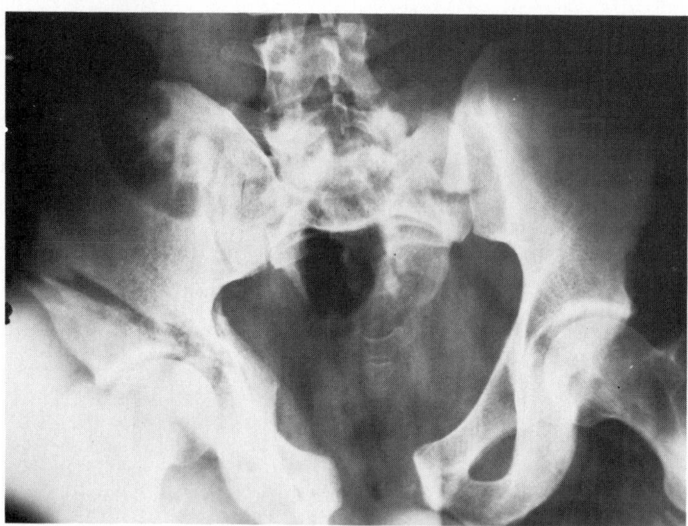

Figure 4-41B. Both-column fracture with diastasis of the symphysis and a contralateral sacroiliac dislocation.

Figure 4-41C. Bilateral transverse acetabular fractures with a unilateral sacroiliac dislocation: i) Anteroposterior view; ii) Inlet view; iii) Computed scan through sacroiliac joints.

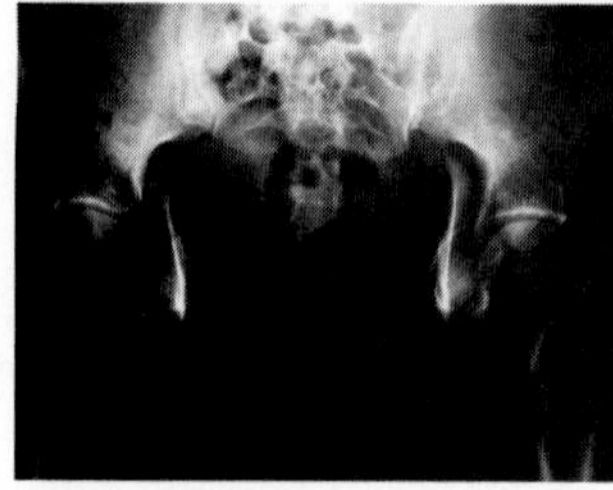

Figure 4-41C i.

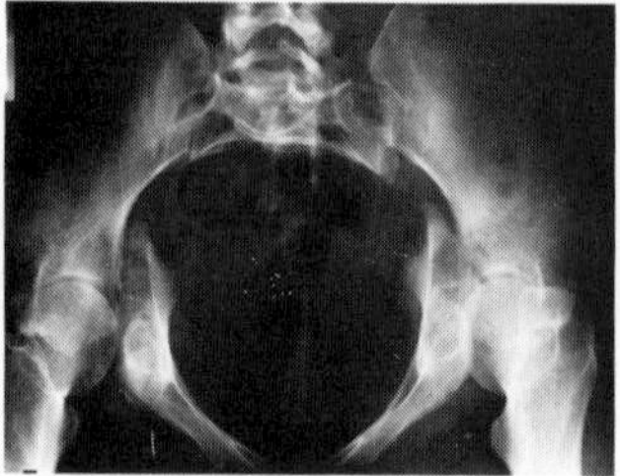

Figure 4-41C ii.

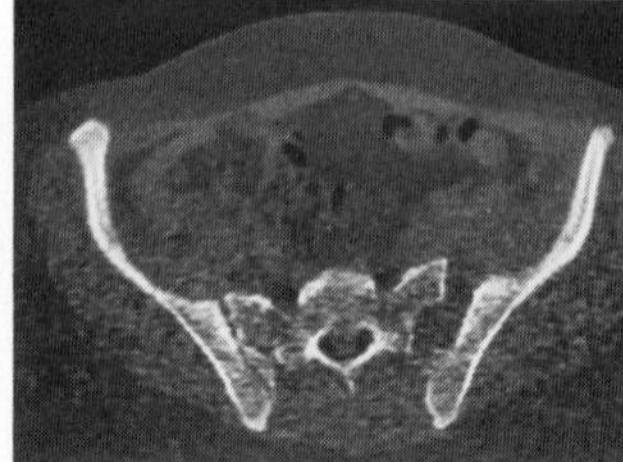

Figure 4-41C iii.

## References

1. Pennal GF, Sutherland GO: Fractures of the Pelvis. Motion picture in AAOS Film Library, 1961.
2. Pennal GF, Tile M, Waddell JP, Gardie H: Pelvic disruption: Assessment and classification. Clin Orthop 151:12, 1980.
3. Letournel E, Judet R: Fractures of the Acetabulum. New York, Springer-Verlag, 1981, p 22.
4. Mears DC: External Skeletal Fixation. Baltimore, Williams and Wilkins, 1983, p 339.
5. Mack LA, Harley JD, Winquist RA: CT of acetabular fractures: Analysis of fracture patterns. Am J Radiol 138:407, 1982.
6. Harley JD, Mack LA, Winquist RA: CT of acetabular fractures: Comparison with conventional radiography. Am J Radiol 138:413, 1982.
7. Burk DL, Mears DC, Herbert DL, Straub WH, Cooperstein LA, Beck EA: Pelvic and acetabular fractures: Examination by angled CT scanning. Radiol 153:548, 1984.
8. Herman GT: Three-dimensional display of computed tomographic scans. Radiol 151:805, 1984.
9. Totty WG, Vannier MV: Complex musculoskeletal anatomy: Analysis using three-dimensional surface reconstruction. Radiol 150:173, 1984.
10. Burk DL, Mears DC, Kennedy WH, Cooperstein LH, Herbert DL: Three-dimensional computed tomography of acetabular fractures. in press, 1985.
11. Letournel E: Fractures of the Acetabulum and Pelvis, lst International Symposium, Paris, May 5-13, 1984.
12. Bucholz RW: The pathological anatomy of Malgaigne fracture-dislocations of the pelvis. J Bone Joint Surg 63A:400, 1981.
13. Mears DC, Rubash HE: External and internal fixation of the pelvic ring, in: AAOS Instructional Course Lectures. St. Louis, Mosby, 1984, 33:144.
14. Thompson VP, Epstein HA: Traumatic dislocation of the hip, A survey of 204 cases covering a period of twenty-one years. J Bone Joint Surg 33A:746, 1951.
15. Knight RA, Smith H: Central fractures of the acetabulum. J Bone Joint Surg 40A:1, 1958.
16. Carnesale PG, Stewart MJ, Barnes SN: Acetabular disruption and central fracture-dislocation of the hip. J Bone Joint Surg 57A:1054, 1975.
17. Rowe CR, Lowell JD: Prognosis of fractures of the acetabulum. J Bone Joint Surg 43A:30, 1961.
18. Letournel E: Les fractures du cotyle, Etude d'une serie de 75 case, Thesis, Paris, 1961.
19. Judet R, Letournel E: Fractures of the acetabulum: Classification and surgical approaches for open reduction. J Bone Joint Surg 46A:1615, 1964.

# CHAPTER 5

# Acute Resuscitation of the Patient with a Pelvic Ring or Acetabular Fracture

## Introduction

The management of the multiple trauma victim involves the rapid initiation of a complex array of diagnostic and therapeutic measures. Prior to the presentation of a patient to a trauma service, a multidisciplinary protocol is needed to define the priorities in diagnosis and management. The general surgical, orthopaedic, urological and neurosurgical members of the trauma team have to identify the optimal sequence for various diagnostic and operative procedures for the prospective pelvic fracture patient who is a multiple trauma victim.[1,2] To characterize the extent and severity of the injuries, a quantitative assessment or Injury Severity Scale has been devised.[3] Such a numerical rating encourages a prompt recognition of those particular patterns of injury that merit rapid aggressive threapeutic intervention, as well as those which almost inevitably culminate in a fatal outcome. The following account highlights a multisystem approach and focuses upon the essentials of management (Figure 5-1). The conventional priorities assigned to the injured systems[4] (i.e. the six Bs) are

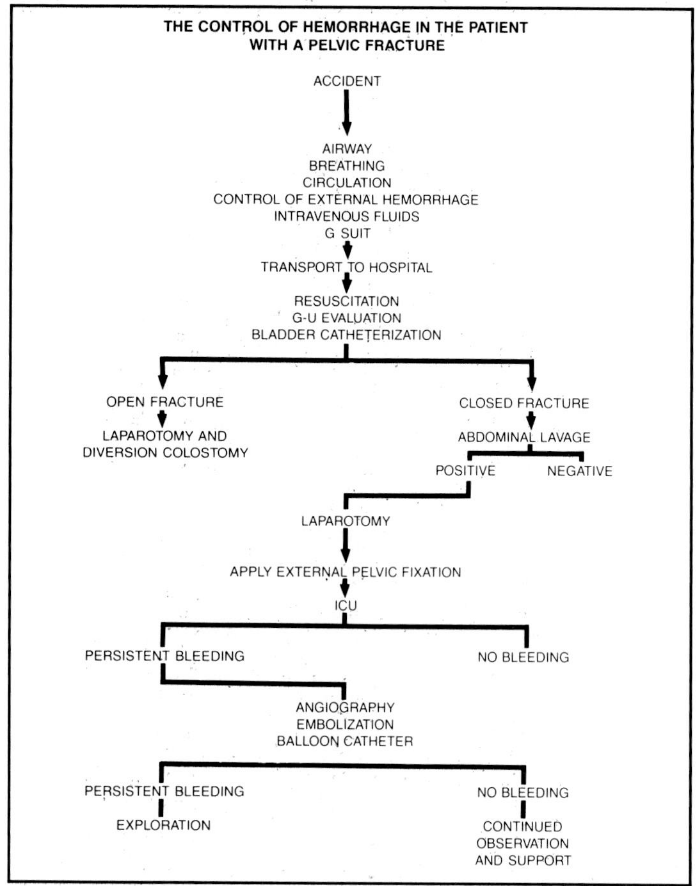


Figure 5-1.

employed: breathing, bleeding, brain injury, bladder, bowel and bone.

## Breathing

Prior to transportation, cardiopulmonary stabilization is the foremost priority. Initial resuscitation includes the provision of a patent upper airway secured by suctioning and positioning, supplementary oxygen, and an oral or endotracheal airway as indicated. In the hospital emergency room, the vast majority of thoracic injuries with compromise of the lower airway are adequately managed by the use of two thoracostomy tubes. In those unusual cases with maxillofacial or laryngeal trauma, an emergency tracheostomy is performed. Rarely, persistent profuse intrathoracic hemorrhage or failure to obtain an effective seal around the chest tubes warrants immediate thoracotomy. Persistent hypoxemia despite the administration of supplementary oxygen and an appropriate attempt to restore an adequate red blood cell mass may provide an indication for the use of mechanical ventilation and positive end expiratory pressure (PEEP). If PEEP is employed, serial measurements of the blood pressure, pulse, central venous pressure, and pulmonary arterial wedge pressure are needed as an estimate of the cardiac output (c.o.) to ensure that a secondary decrease in c.o. does not occur.

## Bleeding

As part of the initial resuscitation of the patient who sustains a pelvic or acetabular fracture, consideration of the potential for massive hemorrhage is of paramount importance.The principal sources of blood loss are: **1)** intrathoracic, **2)** external, **3)** intraperitoneal, **4)** retroperitoneal, and/or **5)** intravascular (coagulopathy). Intrathoracic bleeding is recognized by clinical examination supplemented by a chest x-ray and thoracostomy tubes. Sources of external bleeding are obvious and are managed by the use of pressure dressings and splints or other types of immobilization. Recognition and treatment of the other three sources of bleeding necessitate the institution of special methods. Irrespective of the source of hemorrhage, the initial treatment protocol addresses volume resuscitation. At the scene of the accident the paramedic team applies and inflates a MAST suit (military anti-shock trousers, otherwise known as a pneumatic anti-shock garment or G-suit) to the unstable bleeding patient.[5,6] This maneuver restores one to two units of blood from the lower extremities of the patient into the circulating blood volume. The MAST suit functions: **a)** to increase the cardiac output by augmentation of peripheral vascular resistance and, thereby, supplementation of venous return to the heart; and **b)** partly to discourage hemorrhage by reduction and immobilization of the pelvic fracture. A potential contraindication to the use of the MAST suit, the presence of pulmonary edema, is extremely unlikely to arise in a patient with hemorrhagic shock.

Also prior to transportation, fluid replacement with a suitable asanguinous fluid is begun. The protocol employed at Sunnybrook Hospital in Toronto[2] merits scrutiny as a guideline for fluid replacement once the patient reaches the emergency unit. During the first 30 to 60 minutes three to five liters of asanguinous fluid are given. Initially, one to two liters of Ringer's lactate or normal saline solution are used followed by two to three liters of 5% albumin and Ringer's lactate buffered to a pH of 7.2. The protocol encourages prompt restoration of the circulating blood volume with widely available intravenous solutions. Such fluids also improve the microcirculation by decreasing the viscosity of the blood.[7] In addition, the patency of the renal tubules is maintained through a solute diuresis.[8] Its foremost limitation is a lack of oxygen-carrying capacity. In a seriously volume-depleted patient, type specific or 0 negative blood can be employed within 15 minutes after a blood specimen has been collected. In contrast, at least 45 minutes is needed to obtain a suitable cross-match. Continued hypotension despite the application of an inflated MAST suit indicates either inadequate volume resuscitation or continued hemorrhage or both. Exceedingly large numbers of units of blood may be necessary. As a protocol, the initial cross-match provides from eight to ten units of blood.[2] For the replacement of every five to six liters of blood and fluid, supplementary administration of two to three units of fresh frozen plasma and six to eight units of platelets is undertaken.

During the resuscitative phase of management, the response of the patient to the volume replacement is carefully documented. Massive hemorrhage is defined as a blood volume replacement in 12 hours. A torrential hemorrhage represents a blood volume replacement within 30 to 60 minutes. When the previously described fluid replacement protocol is used, a failure to respond is defined as the inability of the patient to maintain a systolic blood pressure of greater than 100mmHg, a pulse of less than 100, a central venous pressure of greater than 5mmHg and a urine output of greater than 30ml/hr after the replacement of a patient's estimated blood volume by the use of fluid or blood or both within 1 to 1.5 hours.[2] If the patient fails to respond to the volume replacement, a rapid initiation of supplementary diagnostic techniques is needed to identify the source of persistent hemorrhage.

In the Emergency Room, deflation of the MAST suit may be needed to facilitate both the clinical examination and the application of supplementary diagnostic methods. Clearly, abrupt deflation of the MAST suit can provoke a catastrophic fall in the blood pressure and the circulating blood volume. With the potential for life-threatening hemorrhage at the time of deflation of the MAST suit, prolonged application of the garment for a two to three day period of hemodynamic stabilization has been previously recommended.[6] Considerable liabilities associated with prolonged application of the MAST suit include a diminution in the circulation to the lower extremities, possible initiation of a compartment syndrome, limited access to the patient, and initiation of the pulmonary, urological and thromboembolic complications associated with enforced recumbency. With the anticipated multiple traumatic insults in the pelvic fracture victim, the limited access imposed by the presence of the MAST suit is a substantial liability, especially if a laparotomy is required. As a rule, the MAST suit is deflated in small increments so that the blood pressure does not fall by more than 5mmHg. If an attempt to deflate the suit is accompanied by significant hypotension it is abandoned. Upon completion of the initial examination, the patient is transported rapidly to the operating room so that immediately upon removal of the suit, alternative surgical measures to restore hemodynamic stability can be undertaken.

## Resuscitative Urological Management

Catheterization of the urinary bladder to document urinary output provides the optimal determinant of adequate volume resuscitation. In the presence of a major pelvic fracture, urinary catheterization requires special consideration. The incidence of concomitant injury to the bladder or urethra approximates 20%.[9] Features of the physical examination that indicate a possible bladder or urethral injury include bloody drainage from the meatus or a highly mobile or abnormally situated prostate. Microscopic hematuria indicates a supplementary genitourinary injury. A Foley catheter can be placed directly into the bladder of a female patient. In the male, however, a urethrogram is first obtained. Attempts to pass a catheter blindly through a partially disrupted male urethra can result in a stricture, incontinence or impotence. Moreover, a partial urethral tear, which might heal spontaneously, may be converted into a complete disruption, thereby creating a formidable reconstructive problem with a substantial likelihood for surgical complications. While a partial urethral tear is distinctly uncommon in women, the incidence in males is up to 14%.

If the urethrogram indicates a passage of contrast medium into the bladder without extravasation, the catheter is advanced into the bladder. A cystogram is performed to exclude a rupture of the bladder. Finally, an intravenous pyelogram is undertaken to assess the kidneys and ureters. A large pelvic hematoma, frequently documented in such patients, is represented on the cystogram or the intravenous pyelogram as an intact but elevated bladder, often with a tubular configuration. This benign finding merits no specific treatment, although it is indicative of a large blood loss and of the need for supplementary fluid or blood replacement. If a urethral injury is identified, a suprapubic cystostomy is performed. The procedure can be rendered technically difficult to perform by the presence of a large pelvic hematoma.

Frequently, the initial abdominal examination performed upon a patient who presents with a pelvic fracture is highly misleading. If the findings are consistent with profuse intraabdominal hemorrhage or a visceral disruption, an exploratory laparotomy is indicated. Clinical findings such as unexplained hypotension or anemia, or an inconclusive physical examination, provide an indication for peritoneal lavage or preferably a minilaparotomy as described by Gill et al.[10]

## Technique for Peritoneal Lavage

A peritoneal dialysis catheter is inserted by a cutdown technique above the umbilicus with the catheter directed toward the pelvis. Free bloody aspirate withdrawn from the peritoneal cavity constitutes a positive lavage. If, however, there is no return of blood, the abdomen is lavaged with one liter of normal saline and a sample of fluid is aspirated from the peritoneal cavity. The presence of greater than 500 red blood cells per milliliter of lavaged fluid or of bile, bacteria, amylase, or vegetable matter is a positive indication of significant intraabdominal injury. In typical trauma patients, Shires and Polk[6] recorded false positive rates of 2% to 3% and a false negative rate of 2%. The false positive rate is much higher in patients who possess a major pelvic fracture. For example, Hubbard et al[11] observed a false positive rate of 16%. This discrepancy can be explained by several factors. The pelvic hematoma may dissect anteriorly and can be entered inadvertently by the surgeon during the insertion of the peritoneal lavage catheter. Also, red cells can pass into the peritoneal cavity by diapedesis or directly from a tear into the distended pelvic or posterior peritoneum. On the other hand, a negative lavage provides good evidence that there is no significant intraabdominal injury.

The principal advantage of the minilaparatomy is the elimination of the 10% to 15% false-positive results associated with the percutaneous lavage.[2] False-negative minilaparotomies are so uncommon (i.e. less than 1%) that a negative result is indicative of extraperitoneal bleeding. False positive minilaparotomies have been documented in about 18% of pelvic fracture victims in association with retroperitoneal hematomas. With the substantial anticipated mortality of pelvic fracture victims who have an unrecognized abdominal visceral injury, in the presence of a positive minilaparotomy, a formal laparotomy is indicated.[12] If the result of the minilaparotomy is equivocal, with greater than 100,000 cells/mm$^3$, either the lavage is repeated or the catheter is left in situ for serial evaluation during the subsequent 24 hour period.[13]

## Open Pelvic Fracture

In the presence of an open pelvic fracture with a laceration of the rectum, vagina or perineum, communication to the bone with the potential for a deep pelvic infection is a possibly fatal complication.[14-16] In our experience with 12 open pelvic fractures, ten cases presented with lacerations in the perineal region and only two possessed an open sacroiliac joint. Even in the presence of an intact anal sphincter, a divided colostomy is performed to lessen the great likelihood for bacterial contamination of the typically anterior open fracture site. The colostomy is most easily created in the transverse colon remote from the true pelvis and the pelvic hematoma. After the operation, the defunctionalized rectal segment is irrigated to minimize contamination from residual fecal material. A patient who presents with an open fracture does not require peritoneal lavage in the emergency room because the abdomen will be explored at the time of creation of the colostomy. During the laparotomy, if another intraabdominal injury is identified it is repaired immediately.

## Pelvic Stabilization

A new approach to control the intrapelvic bleeding associated with a major pelvic fracture, and one that does not require surgical violation of the retroperitoneum, is the use of a closed reduction of the fracture with external fixation.[1,17] Reduction of the pelvic fracture produces an increase in the interstitial tissue pressure and provides a tamponade of the retroperitoneal bleeding. The reduction of the fracture markedly reduces the volume of the true pelvis and therefore lessens the size of the potential cavity in which extravasated blood may accumulate. In a laboratory study of the volume of the true intrapelvic space (Figure 5-2), Rubash and Mears[17] recorded figures of 1.5L in the anatomic pelvic, 3.0L in the presence of a 3.0cm diastasis of the symphysis pubic, 6.0L with a 6cm diastasis and 0.75L with an overriding of the symphysis of 3.0cm. These findings are not surprising since the volume of a sphere is a cubic function of its radius (i.e. $V = \pi r^3$). A closed reduction of the fracture also diminishes the rate of osseous bleeding with the approximation and immobilization of the cancellous bony fragments. As part of the resuscitative protocol external fixation is strongly recommended for application to the

Figure 5-2. Photographs show a cadaveric pelvic fracture model for measurement of the intrapelvic volume. A balloon was filled with water until it rested upon the brim of the true pelvis. Subsequently, the volume of the water within the balloon was recorded: A: anatomical pelvis—1.5L volume; B: 3.0 cm diastasis of the symphysis—3.0L volume; C: 3.0 cm overriding of the symphysis—0.75L volume.

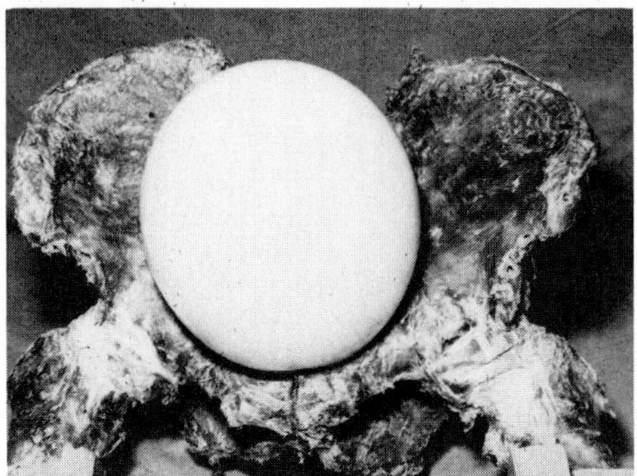

Figure 5-2A.

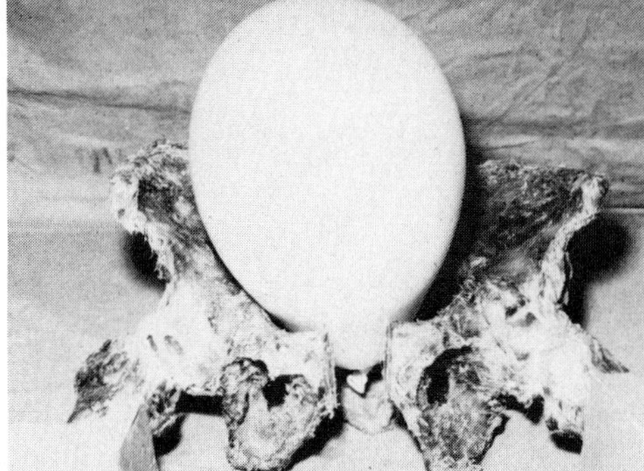

Figure 5-2B.

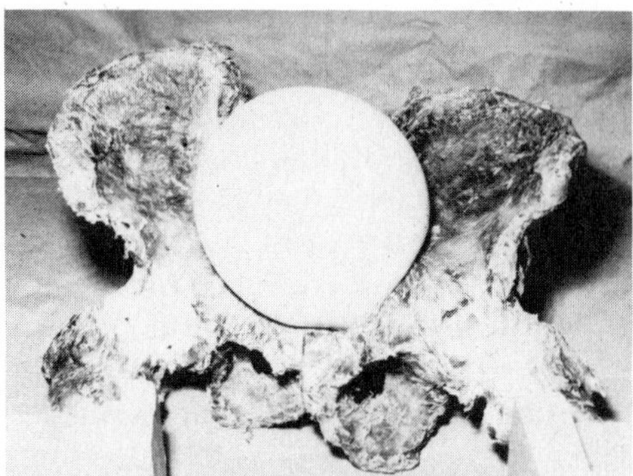

Figure 5-2C.

patient who sustains a pelvic ring fracture complicated by profuse hemorrhage.

As a method to control intrapelvic hemorrhage, the use of internal pelvic fixation also merits consideration.[1,18] While pelvic stability and diminution of intrapelvic volume can be most effectively achieved by the use of internal fixation, direct operative exposure of the fracture can provoke further, potentially catastrophic hemorrhage. If the pelvic fracture is exposed at the time of an emergency resuscitative surgical procedure such as a laparotomy, retroperitoneal exploration or reconstruction of a ruptured urinary bladder, an experienced surgical team knowledgeable in techniques of pelvic reconstruction can usefully consider supplementary internal pelvic fixation as a means to control hemorrhage. Otherwise, for the hemodynamically unstable patient, the acute application of external pelvic fixation generally is preferred. In many of these cases where multiple sites of pelvic instability or acetabular comminution is documented, a secondary reconstruction of the pelvis with open reduction and internal fixation is undertaken once the hemodynamic stability has been restored.

A patient with a negative or a weakly positive laparotomy, or one who fails to respond hemodynamically to a laparotomy and/or external pelvic fixation, remains a surgical emergency. Arterial and venous bleeding secondary to a laceration or avulsion of a major vessel is a well recognized complication of a pelvic fracture.[19] Even with a pelvic external frame in place, selective arteriography or venography permits identification of the source of persistent retroperitoneal hemorrhage and the size of the bleeding vessel.[20,21] Examples of a small-bore bleeding vessel include the superior gluteal artery and a branch of the iliac system in the posterior pelvis. Alternatively, examples of a large-bore vessel include the femoral and iliac arteries. If the provocative source is a small-bore vessel, control of the hemorrhage can be achieved by angiographic embolization of autologous blood clots or gelfoam clots.[2,21] The procedure is available in most institutions and can be performed rapidly. Emboli are thought to flow selectively to the point of bleeding because of the lower peripheral vascular resistance of the traumatized vessel. In contrast to the surgical approach to bleeding in the retroperitoneum, this angiographic embolization does not violate the peritoneal barrier, does not risk disturbance of the tamponade effect, and does not provide a significant risk of infection. Selective angiography and embolization does provide a small potential risk for misdirected emboli. The method is not applicable for the management of venous bleeding.

In conjunction with angiography, bleeding has been controlled by the use of balloon catheter occlusion.[22,23] For this technique, a balloon is inserted under radiographic control into the bleeding vessel and is inflated to occlude the vessel for 24 to 48 hours. Unlike the use of embolization, this method eliminates the potential for misdirected emboli. Also, it is suitable for application in conjunction with venography to control persistent venous hemorrhage.

If angiographic assessment provides the recognition of persistent bleeding from a large bore vessel, direct surgical exploration for repair or ligation is indicated.[19,24,25] In an unusual case where uncontrolled massive hemorrhage from a large-bore vessel is recognized during a laparotomy, control of the abdominal aorta by compression or clamping distal to the renal arteries is undertaken. Angiography performed on the operating table provides a rapid means to identify the large bleeding vessel so that a direct surgical exposure can be undertaken immediately. Certain features of an anteroposterior pelvic radiograph are indicative of potential sites of bleeding.[2,26,27] A disruption of the ilium or sacroiliac joint is suggestive of injury to the iliac vessels. A fracture violating the sciatic notch is likely to be associated with bleeding from a superior gluteal vessel. A fracture of the superior pubic ramus implicates the obturator artery as the source of persistent hemorrhage. Such knowledge can be helpful when emergency or intraoperative arteriography is performed. In those unusual situations where arteriography cannot be performed, and in the presence of persistent "torrential" hemorrhage, direct surgical exposure of the presumed site of the vascular injury can be undertaken.

Another surgical technique described for the control of hemorrhage from intrapelvic organs is ligation of the hypogastric artery.[28,29] When gynecologists employed this method they observed that it was not associated with an ischemic insult of the intrapelvic organs. The extensive collateral intrapelvic circulation, which perfuses the intrapelvic structures, explains why ligation of the hypogastric artery has not provided significant success when it has been employed to control intrapelvic bleeding.

### Coagulopathy

In massively traumatized patients, especially those who require major blood replacement, coagulopathy is a well recognized cause of persistent bleeding. The initial coagulogram is compared with serial studies that are repeated after each blood volume replacement. Such early recognition of the coagulopathy encourages prompt replacement of clotting factors and platelets. Clinical signs of an impending coagulation defect include persistent bleeding from lacerations, intravenous puncture wounds and mucous membranes. Prophylactic administration of two to three units of fresh frozen plasma and six to eight units of platelets following each blood volume replacement of fluid and/or blood minimizes the risk of coagulopathy.[2]

## Radiological Assessment and Surgical Planning

During the early resuscitative phase of management, the immediate value of a full radiological survey of the pelvis is judged against the time required to undertake the studies and the urgency for completion of other diagnostic procedures or for surgical intervention. An anteroposterior pelvic view combined with a pelvic inlet or true obstetric view are crucial to permit the recognition of disruption of the pelvic ring with cephalad or caudad migration as well as anteroposterior displacement of a hemipelvis.[30] The latter deformity is evident in the inlet view. At some stage in management, but with a lesser priority in the acute setting, a pelvic outlet view provides a characterization of the rami and obturator foramina and a more critical assessment of vertical migration of a hemipelvis. Also, at that time the obturator and iliac oblique views or Judet views permit a detailed assessment of the anterior and posterior supportive elements of the acetabulum.[31] Computerized axial tomography of the pelvic ring provides the optimal method for examination of the posterior portion of the pelvic ring, especially the sacrum and the sacroiliac joints.[32,33] The degree of pelvic instability and appropriate surgical methods to restore pelvic stability are determined primarily by a scrutiny of computed scans. In the majority of pelvic fracture patients where hemodynamic instability is not an overriding concern, a full pelvic radiological series and a computed tomographic study can be undertaken safely during the early posttraumatic period. Supplementary urological investigations and appendicular radiography are interspersed with the other investigations. In a typical case, all of the diagnostic studies can be reviewed by the surgical team so that a therapeutic protocol encompassing all of the major organ systems is prepared. When an emergency laparotomy or reconstruction of the bladder is indicated, pelvic stabilization is performed under the same general anesthetic. Provided that hemodynamic stability can be restored and maintained, reconstruction of the long bones and appendicular joints is undertaken. When an unstable spinal injury complicates a pelvic fracture, the relative urgency of the spinal surgery and the pelvic stabilization is assessed and a suitable plan of surgical intervention is designed. If a displaced acetabular fracture complicates a pelvic ring disruption, the degree of hemodynamic stability and the resources and skill of the surgical team to undertake emergency pelvic reconstruction is examined. Prompt effective surgical stabilization of all of the pelvic, spinal, and appendicular disruptions undertaken by highly trained surgical teams provides the optimal likelihood for survival with the least morbidity and the best chance for return to gainful employment. Nevertheless, contraindications to such an approach merit careful appraisal: hemodynamic instability, limitations of the surgical team or its resources, and the presence of heavily contaminated open wounds.

## Summary

The optimal protocol for a patient who sustains a major pelvic fracture starts with appropriate immediate resuscitation and follows sequentially with transportation and careful clinical and radiological assessment. At each stage of management, diagnostic and therapeutic facets of care are interspersed under the direction of a previously organized protocol that accounts for the widely varied patterns of multiple trauma. The management of life-threatening hemorrhage includes early fluid and blood replacement, the use of a MAST suit, diagnostic scrutiny of the sources of bleeding, and frequently rapid surgical intervention. The last step includes the application of a laparotomy combined with pelvic stabilization, usually by resort to external fixation. External fixation provides a means of immediate pelvic reduction and fixation with a minimum potential for supplementary hemorrhage. In the presence of continued postoperative hemorrhage, selective arteriography provides a way to identify the site of bleeding. Control of such bleeding from a small-bore artery can be achieved by the use of embolization of blood clots or gelfoam clots or balloon catheterization. In the presence of persistent hemorrhage from a large-bore bleeding vessel, direct surgical repair or ligation is indicated. The emergency protocol includes diagnostic scrutiny of the urological and other systems so that a master therapeutic plan can be defined. Such a plan outlines the timing and scope for visceral and osseous reconstruction of all of the principal injuries. It is fashioned in such a way to account for complicating problems such as hemodynamic instability. In general, if appropriate resources are available, an attempt is made to stabilize the pelvis and long bones under the initial general anesthetic.

## References

1. Rubash HE, Steed DL, Mears DC: Fractures of the pelvic ring. Surg Rounds 5:8, 16, 1982.
2. McMurtry R, Walton D, Dickinson D, Kellam J, Tile M: Pelvic disruption in the polytraumatized patient: A management protocol. Clin Orthop 151:22, 1980.
3. Baker SP, O'Neill B, Haddon W, Long W: The injury severity score: A method of describing patients with multiple injuries and evaluating emergency care. J Trauma 14:187, 1974.
4. Meyers MH: The multiple-injured patient, in Evarts C McC (ed): Surgery of the Musculoskeletal System. New York, Churchill Livingstone, 1983, p 1:19.
5. Batalden DJ, Wickstrom PH, Ruiz E, Gustilo RP: Value of G suit in patients with severe pelvic fracture. Arch Surg 109:326, 1974.
6. Shires GT, Polk H: The management of pelvic fractures. Arch Surg 109:215, 1974.
7. Shoemaker WC, Monson DD: The effect of whole blood and plasma expanders on volume flow relationships in critically ill patients. Surg Gynecol Obstet 137:453, 1973.

8. Lowery BD, Clowtner CJ, Carey L: Electrolyte solutions in resuscitation in human hemorrhagic shock. Surg Gynecol Obstet 133:273, 1971.
9. Colapinto V, Flint LM: Trauma to the pelvis: Urethral injury. Clin Orthop 151:46, 1980.
10. Gill W, Champion HR, Long W, Jamaris JN, Cowley RA: Abdominal lavage in blunt trauma. Br J Surg 62:121, 1975.
11. Hubbard SG, Bivens BA, et al: Diagnostic errors with peritoneal lavage in patients with pelvic fractures. Arch Surg 114:844, 1979.
12. Hawkins L, Pomerants M, Eiseman B: Laparotomy at the time of pelvic fracture. J Trauma 10:619, 1970.
13. Root HD, Hauser CW, McKinley CR, LaFave JW, Mendiola RP Jr: Diagnostic peritoneal lavage. Surgery 57:633, 1965.
14. Rothenberger DA, Fischer RP, et al: Mortality associated with pelvic fractures. Surgery 8(4):356, 1978.
15. Maull KI, Sachatello CR: Current management of pelvic fractures. South Med J 69:1285, 1976.
16. Perry JF Jr: Pelvic open fractures. Clin Orthop 151:41, 1980.
17. Rubash HE, Mears DC: External and internal fixation of the pelvis, in: AAOS Instructional Course Lectures. St. Louis, Mosby, 1983, 32:329.
18. Mears DC, Rubash HE: Internal fixation of the pelvic ring, in: AAOS Instructional Course Lectures. St. Louis, Mosby, 1984, 33:144.
19. Thompson GA: Operative control of massive hemorrhage in comminuted pelvic fractures. Internat Orthop 3:141, 1979.
20. Sclafani SJ, Becker JA: Traumatic presacral hemorrhage: Angiographic diagnosis and therapy. Am J Radiol 138:123, 1982.
21. Stock JR, Harris WH, Athanasoulis CA: The role of diagnostic and therapeutic angiography in trauma to the pelvis. Clin Orthop 151:31, 1980.
22. Paster SB, VanHowton FX, Adams DF: Percutaneous balloon catheterization. J South Med Assoc 230:573, 1974.
23. Davidson AT Sr: Direct intralumen balloon tamponade. Am J Surg 136:394, 1978.
24. Rothenberger DA, Fischer RP, Perry JF: Major vascular injuries secondary to pelvic fractures: An unsolved clinical problem. Am J Surg 136:660, 1978.
25. Flint LM, Brown H, Richardson JD, Polk HC: Definitive control of bleeding from severe pelvic fractures. Amer Surg 189:709, 1979.
26. Margolies RN, Ring EJ, Athanasoulis C, Baum S, Waltman AC: Arteriography in the management of hemorrhage from pelvic fractures. N Engl J Med 287:317, 1972.
27. Smith K, Ben-Menachem Y, Duke JH, Hill GL: The superior gluteal—an artery at risk in blunt pelvic trauma. J Trauma, 16:273, 1976.
28. Hawser CW, Perry JF: Control of massive hemorrhage from pelvic fractures by hypogastric artery ligation. Surg Gynecol Obstet 121:313, 1965.
29. Severs R, Lynch J, Ballord R, Jernigan S, Johnson J: Hypogastric artery ligation for uncontrollable hemorrhage in acute pelvic trauma. Surgery 55:516, 1964.

30. Pennal GF, Tile M, Waddell JP, Garside H: Pelvic disruption: Assessment and classification. Clin Orthop 151:12, 1980.
31. Letournel E, Judet R: Fractures of the Acetabulum. New York, Springer-Verlag, 1981, p 13.
32. Hansen ST Jr: Computerized axial tomography for pelvic fractures. Am J Radiol 138:592, 1982.
33. Mach LA, Harley JD, Winquist RA: CAT of acetabular fractures: Analysis of fracture patterns and comparison with conventional radiography. Am J Radiol 138:407, 1982.

# Chapter 6

# Planning Definitive Care

## Introduction

Once the acute resuscitative phase of management has been completed and the hemodynamic stability of the patient has been restored, then the definitive plan for management of the pelvic or acetabular fracture can be initiated. The first crucial stage in planning is the completion of a suitable diagnostic protocol to permit the identification of any problem involving multiple organ systems. A standard protocol, prepared by the various surgical subspecialties, includes the preferred sequence and timing for various diagnostic procedures, so that the examinations are undertaken in a timely and orderly way.[1-4] Once this information is available, it is reviewed to ascertain whether the medical center possesses the resources necessary to manage the various traumatic problems. If the local resources are not suitable, then prompt transfer of the hemodynamically stabilized patient to a regional trauma center is strongly advised. If a period of a few days or weeks is lost prior to such a transfer, generally the optimal long-term results of surgery such as acetabular reconstruction are substantially compromised. Such procrastination greatly increases the complexity of the surgical procedure. It provides further opportunity for the onset of various medical complications associated with enforced recumbency,[5-9] such as thromboembolic problems and urinary or pulmonary tract infections, which in turn culminate in a still longer deferral of the reconstructive surgery. Once hemodynamically stable, the patient can be transported readily on a stretcher, with or without traction applied to the lower extremity, by an ambulance or by a suitable aircraft for virtually any distance.

Even though the initial scrutiny of the hemodynamically unstable trauma victim may permit solely an anteroposterior radiograph of the pelvis, ultimately a complete radiological series is needed so that certain relatively obscure but crucial disruptions of the pelvis are not overlooked. Once a high degree of suspicion of a pelvic or acetabular fracture exists, then a complete radiographic study of the pelvis with anteroposterior, inlet, outlet, iliac, and obturator oblique views is obtained. Assessment of the multiple views minimizes the likelihood of failure to recognize a minimally displaced but potentially comminuted and unstable pelvic or acetabular fracture. Once a displaced pelvic ring fracture has been documented by plain radiographs and whenever posterior disruption of the pelvic ring is suspected, computerized axial tomography is undertaken. This method permits the confirmation of an obscure injury such as a sacral fracture, as well as documentation of the degree of posterior instability. After a closed reduction of the pelvic ring with application of external fixation has been undertaken as part of the resuscitative protocol, a computed scan provides confirmation of the adequacy of the closed reduction and the degree of posterior instability, and thereby, the need for supplementary posterior internal fixation. In the presence of a fracture dislocation of the hip or an acetabular fracture, a computed scan provides the best diagnostic tool to identify a free intraarticular osteochondral fragment, an impacted fracture fragment in the acetabular rim, malrotation of a dome fragment, or the presence of marked comminution. In a skeletally immature individual, a computed scan of the pelvis and acetabulum also provides optimal resolution for the detection of an injury to a growth plate or any other unmineralized portion of the bone.

Admittedly, from the time of scrutiny of even an anteroposterior radiograph of the acutely injured and unstable patient, a tentative plan for management of the pelvic injury is formulated. In a patient who apart from the pelvic disruption is generally stable, the definitive plan for management is established as soon as the appropriate diagnostic tests are completed. When multiple systemic disruptions are documented, then the pelvic reconstruction is planned in collaboration with other surgical specialists so that the priorities of management and the optimal timing of each procedure can be defined. Once a regional trauma center prepares a general protocol for the management of typical patterns of multiple trauma, then such a guideline prioritizes the surgical management of spinal, pelvic, and appendicular fractures along with intracranial, intrathoracic and intraabdominal disruptions.

The urgency for pelvic and acetabular reconstruction of the hemodynamically stable patient has been questioned by many surgeons.[2,9,10] Historically, these surgical procedures have been subject to considerable deferral either in favor of other surgical procedures or of convenience for the surgeon. While pelvic reconstruction is rarely a surgical emergency, nevertheless it is optimally performed within a few days after the time of the injury. Usually such a period suffices to complete the resuscitative and diagnostic protocol. A more prolonged deferral subjects the patient to the potentially life-threatening complications associated with enforced recumbency. Once such a complication arises, it leads to a substantial delay until the pelvic reconstruction can be performed. If a delay of more than a week and especially of two to four weeks ensues, the subsequent reconstructive procedure is greatly increased in the degree of technical difficulty, the anticipated volume of blood loss and, in the case of acetabular procedures, the likelihood of ectopic bone formation.[11]

## Provisional Stabilization of the Pelvis and Acetabulum

As part of the acute resuscitation, external fixation can be employed to assist in the control of hemorrhage and to immobilize a grossly reapproximated or an anatomically reduced pelvic ring.[2,10] Longitudinal skeletal traction can be used to facilitate the correction of superior migration of a hemipelvis secondary to a vertical shear injury. For an acetabular fracture, longitudinal skeletal traction can provide "ligamentotaxis" as an indirect source of acetabular reduction. The traction lessens the posttraumatic pain, and it often separates the femoral head from the acetabular fragments to minimize the abrasive damage to the head. When the interval between the acute injury and the acetabular reconstruction is planned for less than a day or two, the application of skeletal traction does not lessen the degree of technical difficulty encountered at the time of surgery. When a more prolonged deferral of the open reduction and internal fixation is anticipated, the application of skeletal traction permits restoration and maintenance of the femoral head and partially of the acetabular fragments, which simplifies the open reduction.

In acetabular fracture-dislocations complicated by a posterior dislocation of the femoral head, the indication for an emergency closed reduction of the femoral head has also been debated.[12-14] In the presence of a traumatic dislocation of the hip with minimal acetabular disruption, the role of a closed reduction to lessen the likelihood of subsequent avascular necrosis of the hip has been well documented.[12] This maneuver also provides dramatic relief of the severe hip pain that accompanies the dislocation. Once the fracture-dislocation is accompanied by a disruption of the posterior-column or in the presence of the typical lateral compression injury with a central displacement of the femoral head, a closed reduction of the femoral head by manipulation under anesthesia is of dubious benefit. Following such a fracture-dislocation of the hip, the incidence of avascular necrosis of the femoral head is low and apparently unimproved by the application of techniques of closed reduction.[11] If a forceful closed reduction is needed, concomitant abrasive damage of the femoral head is likely to occur. In the presence of a comminuted fracture, generally the displaced femoral head is readily reduced but unstable unless skeletal traction is maintained. The traction suffices to reduce the femoral head but not the acetabular fragments.

## Indications for Surgery

Previously, pelvic ring fractures have been treated by a wide variety of methods, including bed rest, a pelvic sling, a hip spica cast, skeletal traction, and more recently by external and internal fixation systems. While the pelvic sling, skeletal traction and hip spica cast have been used to immobilize many types of pelvic fractures, their application necessitated a prolonged period of recumbency with the associated likelihood for pulmonary, thromboembolic, urologic, and soft tissue complications. The use of these methods helped to achieve an accurate reduction of an open-book type of anteroposterior compression injury, but did not facilitate an accurate reduction of most other types of pelvic fractures. The use of a hip spica cast, however, remains the most efficacious method for the treatment of a child with an unstable displaced pelvic ring fracture, given the smaller size of the patient, the shorter immobilization period, and the lower incidence of thromboembolic problems. For the majority of displaced pelvic ring fractures, external fixation provides a simple and effective method of treatment. A striking reduction in the magnitude of posttraumatic bleeding has been documented when an external fixation device is applied during the initial management of the patient.[2] A simple pelvic frame provides relief of fracture pain and adequate immobilization of a stable disruption such as a stable anteroposterior compression injury with preservation of the posterior sacroiliac ligamentous complex. In such an instance the patient can undertake bed to chair transfers immediately after surgery. In the presence of posterior instability, a three-dimensional frame configuration such as the Pittsburgh Triangular Frame affords adequate stability to permit immediate postoperative bed to chair activity.

In the presence of an open pelvic fracture, the use of external fixation is particularly attractive as a means of immobilization consistent with minimal risk of inadvertent surgical contamination of an alternative internal fixation and minimal surgical devascularization of bone. External fixation does possess limitations that render the method ineffective or unsuitable for application to many pelvic fractures, especially those complicated by bilateral posterior instability, iliac comminution, or an acetabular fracture. In many of these cases, provisional external fixation can be supplemented or entirely replaced with internal fixation. During the past decade, as our experience with techniques of external and internal fixation of the pelvis has grown, we have attempted to establish an algorithm[15] that defines a suitable protocol for the stabilization of virtually all of the patterns of various pelvic ring disruptions (Figure 6-1). For many of the simpler fracture patterns, two or more therapeutic protocols are available that provide highly suitable therapeutic options. As the fracture patterns progress to the more complex variants, the variety of suitable methods of stabilization dwindles. For the past five years this protocol has been satisfactorily employed in Pittsburgh with but minor modification. The goals of the method include the provision for sufficient pelvic stability, so that immediate postoperative bed-to-chair transfers can be undertaken without loss of the reduction by a failure of the fixation. Generally, about six to eight weeks after surgery the bed-to-chair limitation is superseded by gait training with a partial weight bearing restriction for another six to eight weeks. This therapeutic objective has been consistent with a rapid discharge of the patient from the hospital to his home and minimization of thromboembolic problems despite the absence of routine anticoagulation. Where a simple unstable pelvic ring disruption is managed with stable internal fixation at both the anterior and posterior sites, then crutch walking with a touchdown or partial weightbearing gait is encouraged from the early postoperative period.

Figure 6-1. Algorithm to define a suitable protocol for the stabilization of various pelvic ring disruptions. A: Simple fractures. B: Complex injuries.

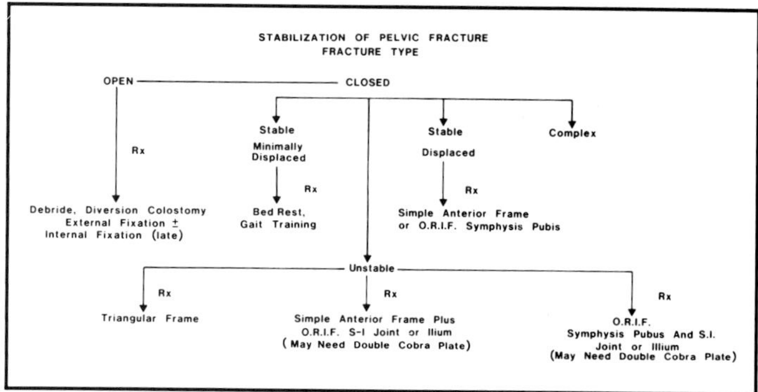


Figure 6-1A.

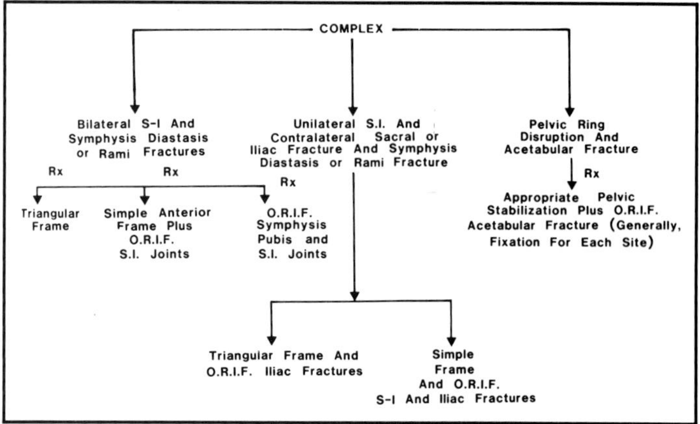


Figure 6-1B.

At the time of presentation of many of the complex pelvic fractures, provisional external fixation by the application of a simple frame facilitates the control of hemorrhage. Once hemodynamic stability has been achieved, replacement or supplementation of the external frame with suitable internal fixation is undertaken.

## Classification and Treatment

The algorithm (Figure 6-1), which defines a suitable protocol for the stabilization of almost every type of pelvic ring disruption, categorizes pelvic fractures into four distinct groups.

The first category comprises stable minimally displaced injuries, usually resulting from low velocity lateral compression insults (Figure 6-2). Following a temporary period of bed rest, a partial weightbearing gait is maintained for a few weeks. For a second large group including most stable anteroposterior and lateral compression injuries, such as a diastasis of the symphysis with preservation of the posterior sacroiliac ligaments and the sacrum, the most suitable treatment is a simple anterior external frame (Figure 6-3). When

Figure 6-2. A stable lateral compression injury suitably managed by conservative treatment. A: Anteroposterior pelvic radiograph. B: Computed scan.

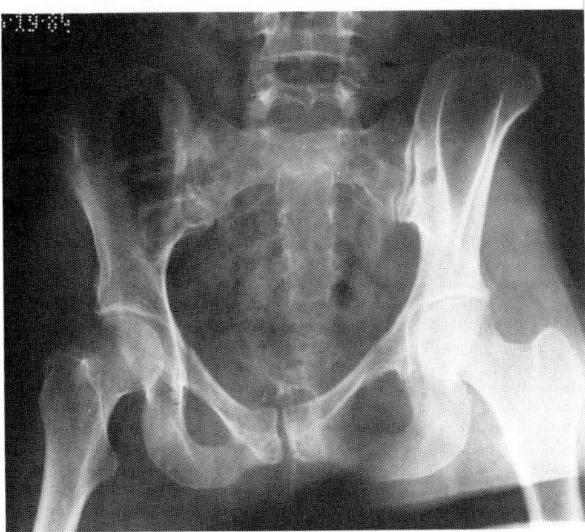

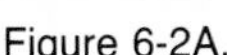
Figure 6-2A.

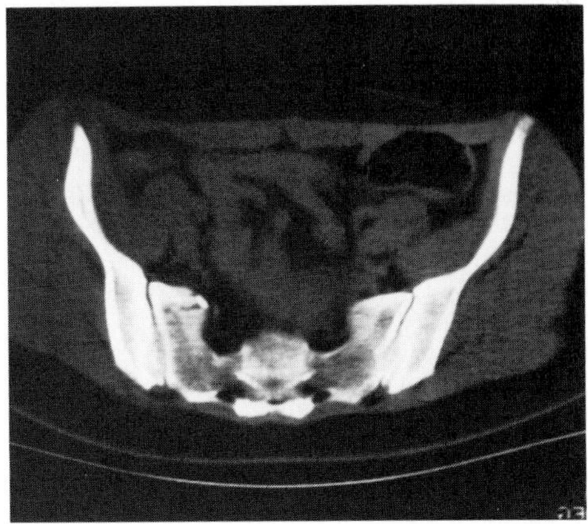
Figure 6-2B.

Figure 6-3. A stable anteroposterior compression injury with a diastasis and mild rotation of the left hemipelvis managed with a simple external pelvic frame. A: Preoperative outlet view. B: Postoperative outlet view.

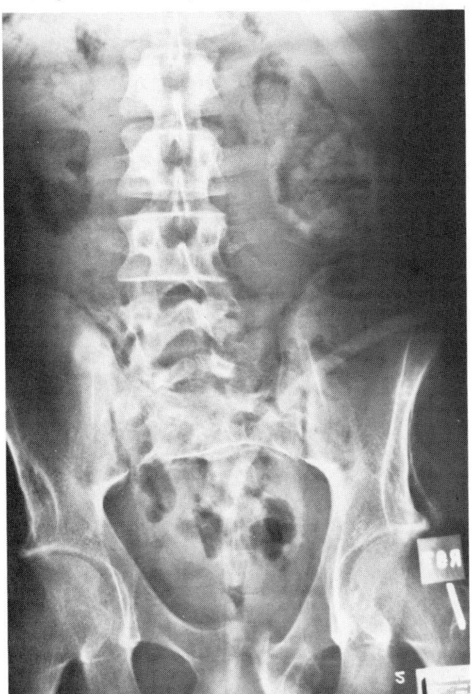
Figure 6-3A.

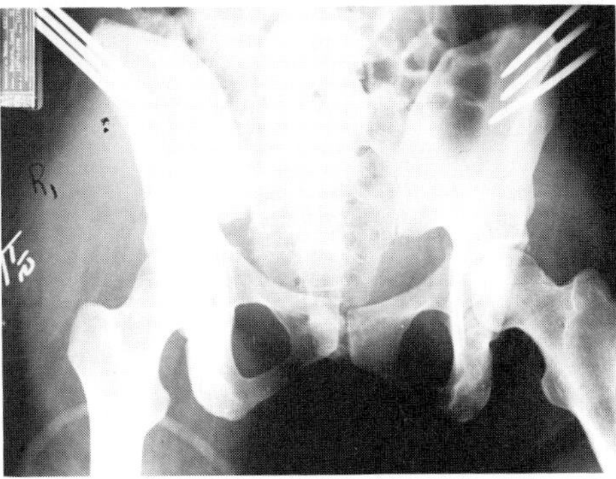
Figure 6-3B.

an emergency laparotomy is undertaken, possibly for the repair of a ruptured bladder, another equally efficacious method of pelvic immobilization for this injury is the application of an open reduction of the symphysis with plate fixation (Figure 6-4). While plate fixation can be applied to immobilize ramus fractures apart from those fractures that approximate the symphysis, the surgical exposure of the rami by resort to an ilioinguinal

Figure 6-4. A stable anteroposterior compression injury with a diastasis managed with internal fixation. A: Preoperative inlet view. B: Postoperative anteroposterior view. C: Postoperative inlet view.

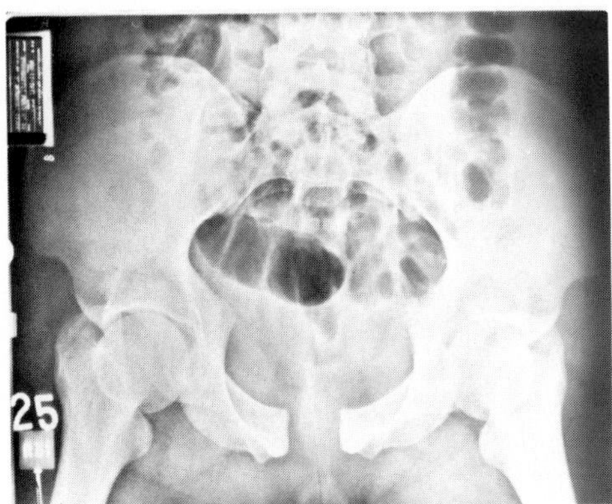

Figure 6-4A.

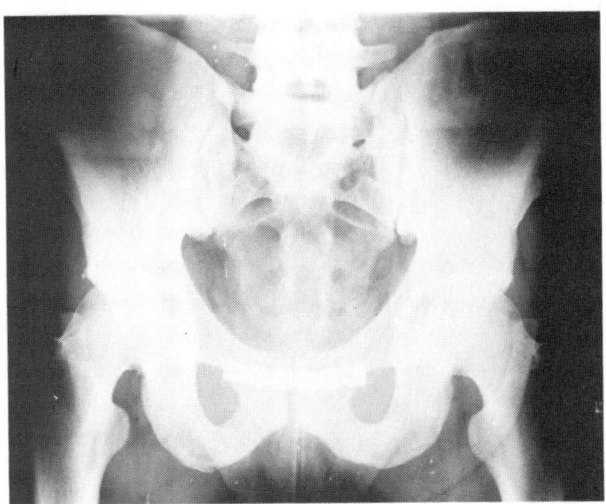

Figure 6-4B.

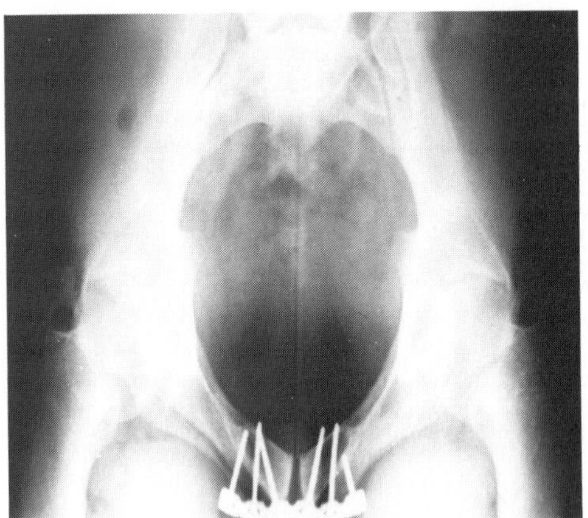

Figure 6-4C.

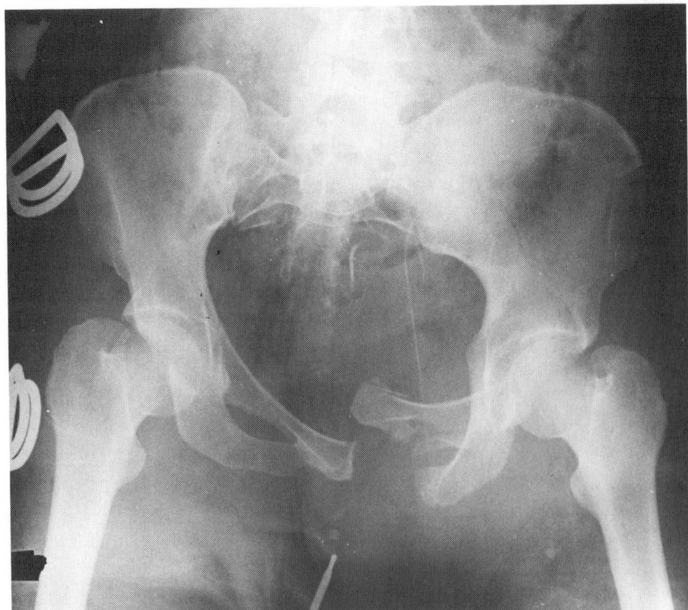

Figure 6-5. An anteroposterior radiograph with markedly displaced rami and a fracture dislocation of the right sacroiliac joint. In this 20-year-old woman, open reduction of the rami as well as the posterior injury is indicated.

approach is difficult and associated with possible injury to the femoral nerve and the external iliac vessels. Generally, when surgical stabilization of an anterior injury with multiple displaced ramus fractures is indicated, the use of external fixation is preferred. One exception is the presentation of markedly displaced rami in a young woman (Figure 6-5), where an accurate open reduction is needed to prevent dyspareunia and to reconstruct the birth canal.

A second category of displaced pelvic disruptions presents with an unstable posterior injury, either of a sacroiliac joint or of a posterior ilium, frequently adjacent to the sacroiliac joint (Figure 6-6). Virtually all of the vertical shear injuries with a unilateral posterior disruption, many lateral compression injuries, and a few anteroposterior compression injuries reside within this category. The simplest therapeutic solution is a closed reduction with the application of a Pittsburgh Triangular Frame. For a vertical shear fracture accompanied by superior migration of a hemipelvis, a closed reduction is achieved by resort to longitudinal traction applied on a fracture table. After external fixation has been applied, a pelvic inlet radiograph and, usually, a computed scan of the pelvis are assessed to determine the accuracy of the reduction. In many instances a satisfactory reduction is documented, so that no further surgical intervention is needed. If the closed reduction is unsatisfactory, open reduction and internal fixation of the posterior disruption is indicated. Two other appropriate methods of treatment are the application of a simple external frame combined with an open reduction and internal fixation of the sacroiliac joint or the ilium (Figure 6-7), or internal fixation of both the symphysis and the posterior disruption (Figure 6-8). A somewhat similar problem is an unstable sacral fracture, although in this case, previously no satisfactory technique of internal fixation has been available. The simplest solution is the application of a Pittsburgh Triangular Frame. Alternatively, the recently developed Double Cobra plate (Howmedica, Inc., Rutherford, New Jersey) provides highly effective posterior stabilization for those unstable displaced sacral fractures that necessitate an open reduction. The accompanying anterior disruption can be immobilized by the use of a simple external frame or with internal fixation.

The third major category of pelvic fractures is a so-called complex ring disruption, with four main subgroups: **a)** bilateral unstable posterior disruptions with an anterior disruption; **b)** a unilateral unstable posterior fracture accompanied by an iliac fracture and an anterior disruption; **c)** a unilateral posterior fracture, an anterior disruption, and an acetabular fracture with

Figure 6-6. An unstable lateral compression injury with a diastasis, dislocation of the right sacroiliac joint, and left ramus fractures in a woman of 24 years is managed with a Pittsburgh Triangular Frame. A: Preoperative anteroposterior radiograph. B: Pelvic inlet view after external fixation. C: An anteroposterior radiograph taken three months after injury when fully active.

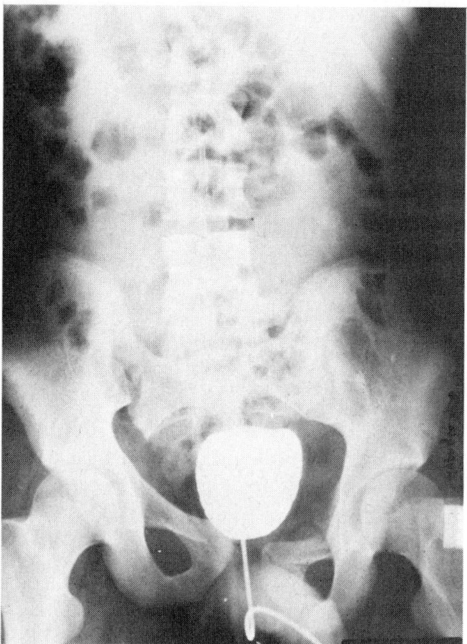

Figure 6-6B.

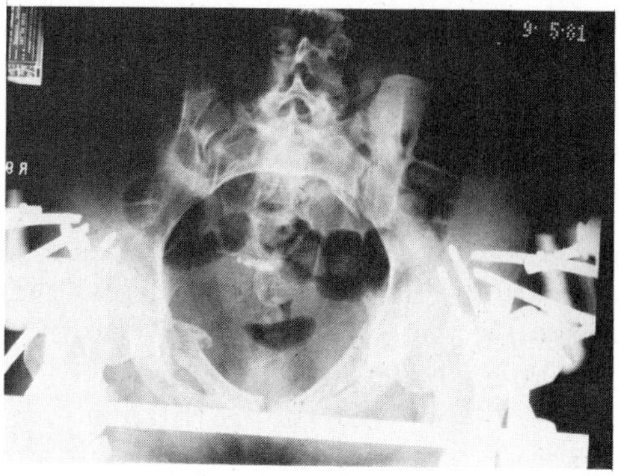

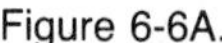

Figure 6-6A.

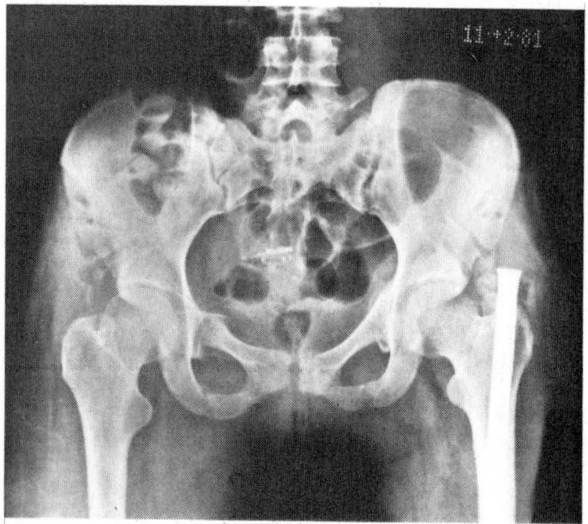

Figure 6-6C.

or without an iliac fracture; and **d)** various patterns of comminuted injuries with unilateral or bilateral unstable posterior disruptions, bilateral acetabular and/or iliac fractures, and bilateral ramus fractures with or without a diastasis of the symphysis. These groups are reviewed in sequence.

Most pelvic fractures with bilateral unstable sacroiliac dislocations and a diastasis of the symphysis are sustained as a vertical shear injury. Where the sacroiliac dislocations possess modest displacement, one technique of immobilization is a closed pelvic reduction with the

Figure 6-7. A female pedestrian of 15 years who was struck by a car sustained an unstable lateral compression injury of the left hemipelvis. A: Initial anteroposterior view. B: Initial inlet view. C: Initial computed scan with unstable left sacroiliac joint. D: Anteroposterior view after the application of a simple external pelvic frame and lag screw fixation of the left sacroiliac joint. E: Anteroposterior view four months later.

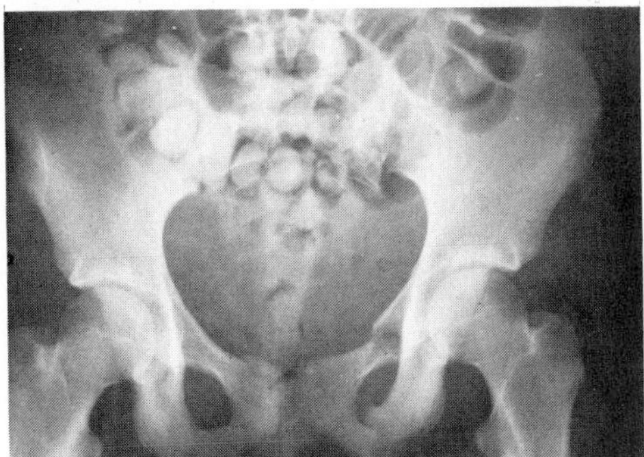

Figure 6-7A.

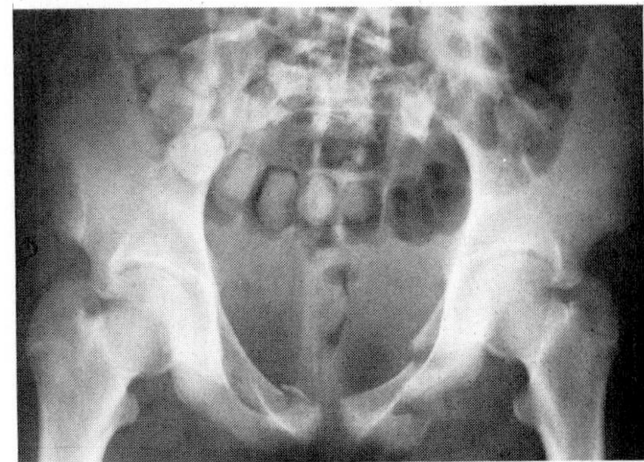

Figure 6-7B.

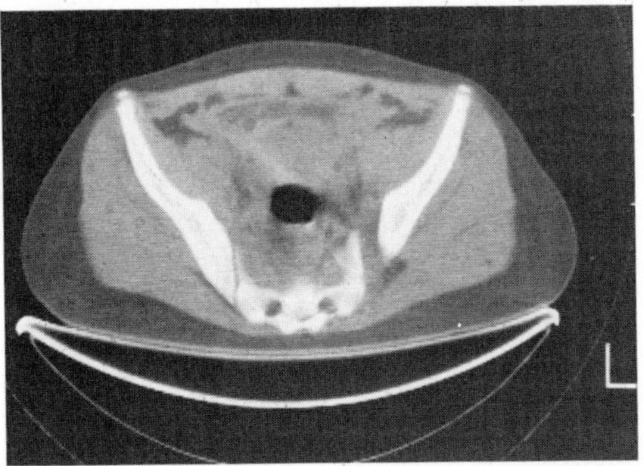

Figure 6-7C.

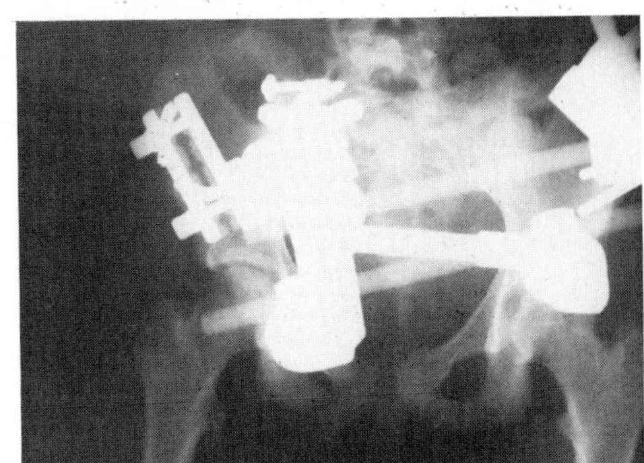

Figure 6-7D.

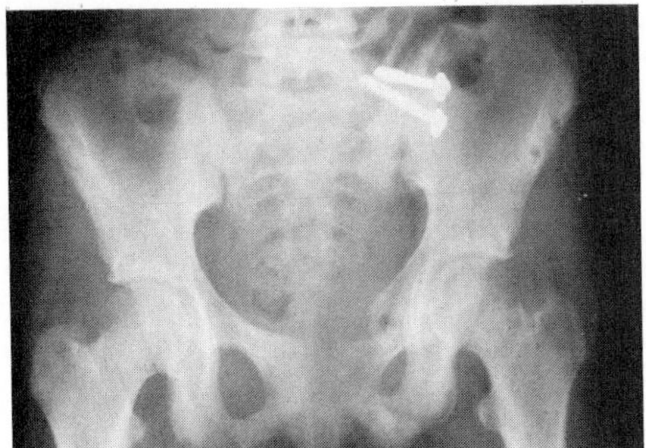

Figure 6-7E.

application of a triangular frame followed by open reduction and internal fixation of one or both persistently displaced sacroiliac joints as documented by a pelvic inlet radiograph or preferably a computed scan (Figure 6-9). Admittedly, a simple external frame is sufficient for anterior stabilization, provided that open reduction and internal fixation of the sacroiliac joints is undertaken

Figure 6-8. A motorcyclist of 26 years who presented with an unstable right sacroiliac joint and diastasis along with a right femoral shaft fracture and a lumbar fracture/dislocation. Open reduction and internal fixation of the sacroiliac joint and symphysis was undertaken along with internal fixation of the femur and the lumbar spine. A: Preoperative pelvic inlet view. B: Preoperative computed scan of the pelvis. C: Postoperative anteroposterior radiograph.

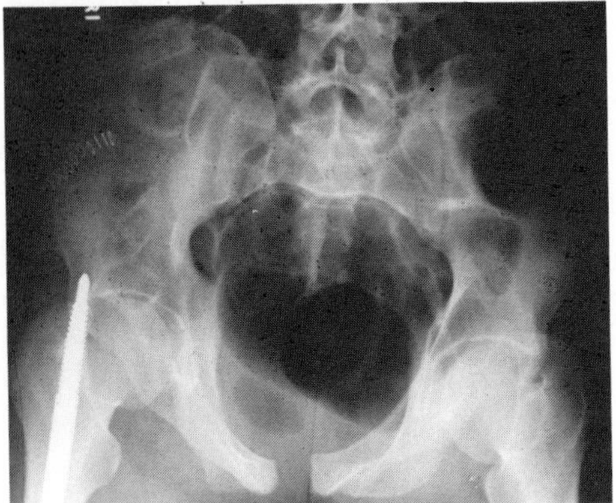

Figure 6-8A.

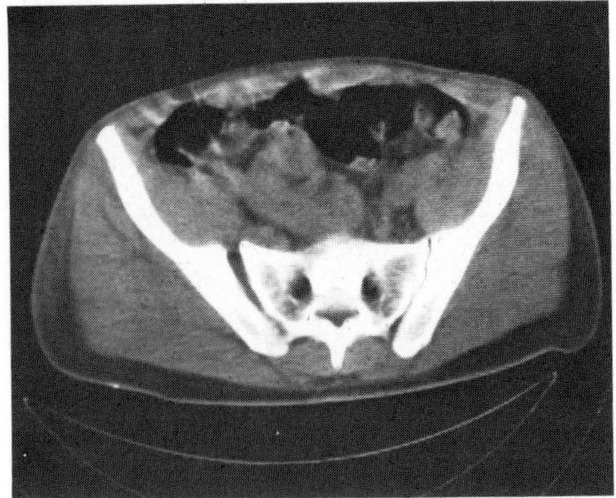

Figure 6-8B.

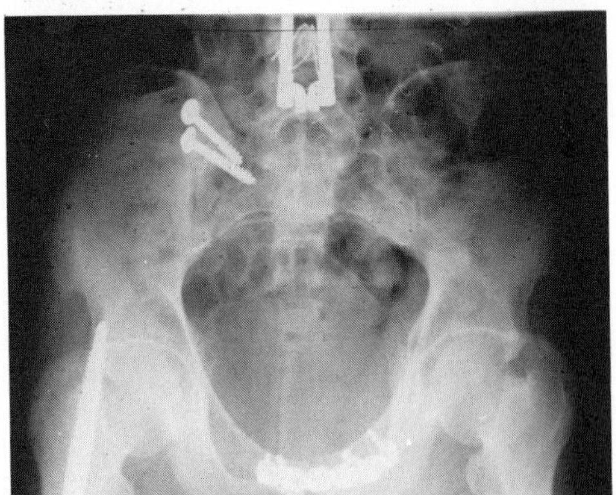

Figure 6-8C.

with resort to a lag screw technique or by the use of the Double Cobra plate. When the patient presents initially with hemodynamic stability, open reduction and internal fixation of the symphysis, as an alternative to the application of an external frame, along with internal fixation of the sacroiliac joints, is preferred.

In the presence of an unstable sacroiliac joint or a lateral or posterior iliac fracture, with multiple ramus fractures or a diastasis, either of these patterns of lateral compression injury is suitably immobilized by a combination of external and internal fixation or by the use of internal fixation of the multiple fracture sites. With the former solution a simple external frame is employed to immobilize the anterior disruption while an open reduction and internal fixation is undertaken to stabilize the sacroiliac disruption and the iliac fracture. Alternatively, a triangular frame is employed to secure

Figure 6-9. A motorcyclist of 26 years struck a telephone pole to sustain bilateral sacroiliac injuries and multiple ramus fractures. A: Preoperative anteroposterior radiograph. B: An inlet view after external fixation with a triangular frame. C: A computed scan after external fixation confirms the accurate reduction of the left sacroiliac joint and the presence of an unstable right sacroiliac disruption. D: An inlet view taken after supplementary open reduction and internal fixation of the right sacroiliac joint.

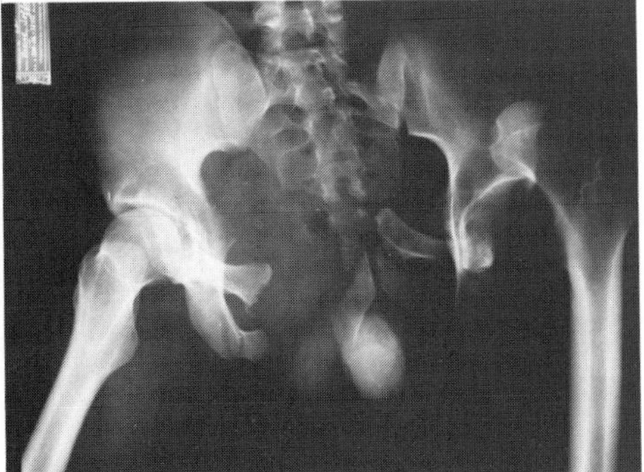

Figure 6-9A.

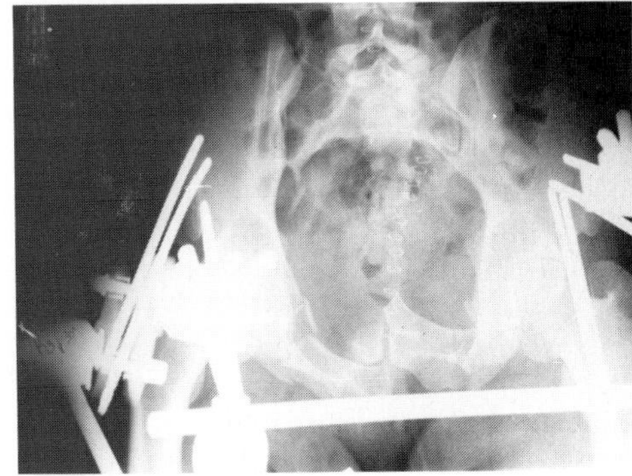

Figure 6-9B.

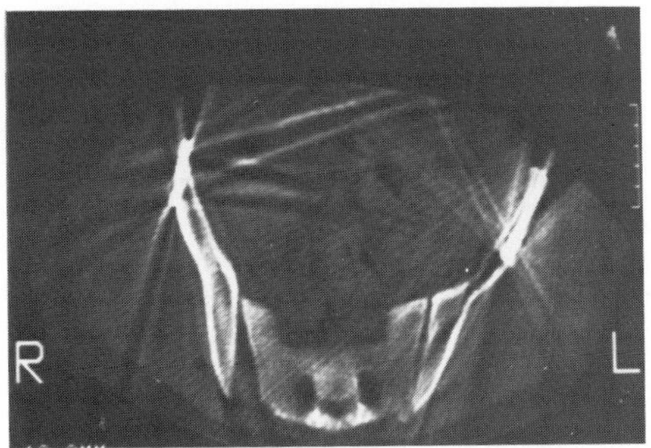


Figure 6-9C.

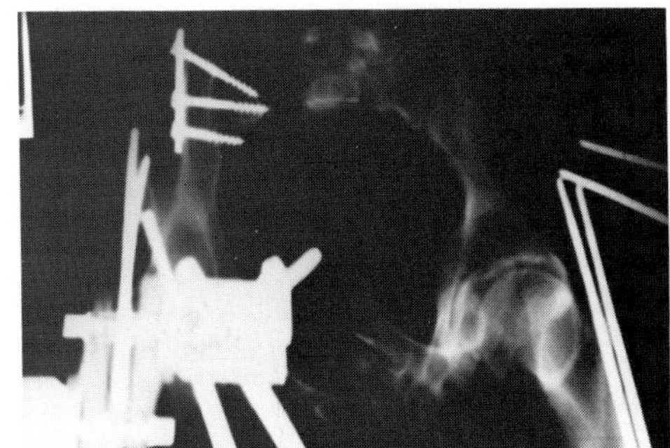

Figure 6-9D.

the anterior disruption and the sacroiliac joint or the iliac fracture, provided that an acceptable closed reduction is documented. In this case, supplementary internal fixation of the third and most displaced disruption not stabilized by external fixation is applied (Figure 6-10). The other and more stable form of fixation, particularly applicable to markedly displaced fractures, is the use of internal fixation at all of the disrupted sites. Generally, whenever multiple ramus fractures are encountered apart from the few markedly displaced instances, especially in young women, external fixation is preferred for the anterior immobilization to avoid the extensive bilateral ilioinguinal dissection necessary to apply the appropriate alternative form of internal fixation.

An unstable sacroiliac disruption with multiple ramus fractures or a diastasis and an acetabular fracture, with or without propagation into the ilium, is another pattern of a lateral compression injury. While the details of acetabular fixation will be reviewed shortly, as a general principle open reduction and internal fixation of the

Figure 6-10. In a mining accident, this 27-year-old man sustained a diastasis, an unstable left sacroiliac disruption, and a right-sided sacral fracture, confirmed by a computed scan. A: Preoperative anteroposterior view. B: Postoperative inlet view with a triangular pelvic frame. C: Anteroposterior view taken one year later when a full functional recovery was documented.

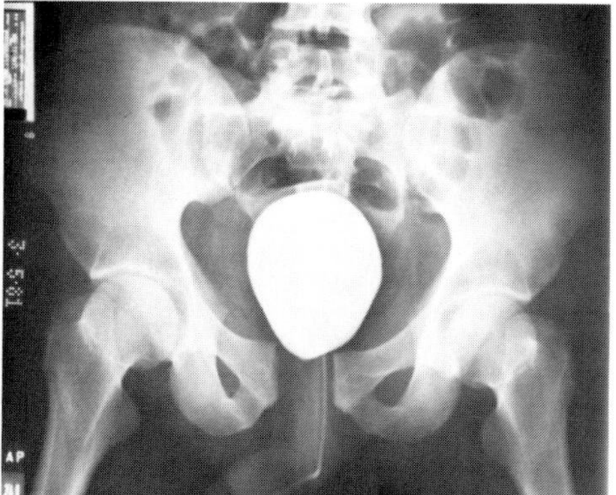

Figure 6-10A.

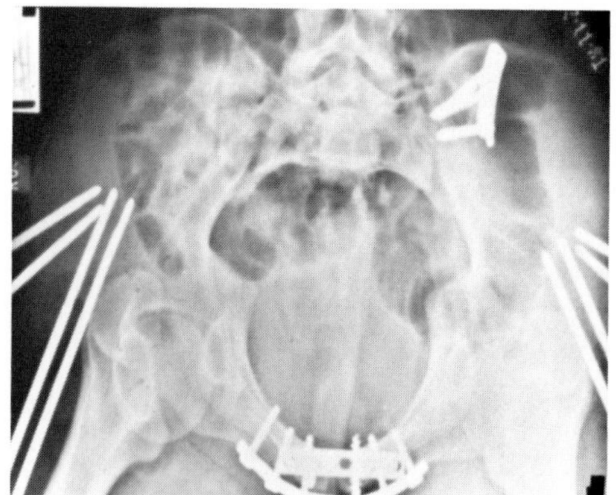

Figure 6-10B.

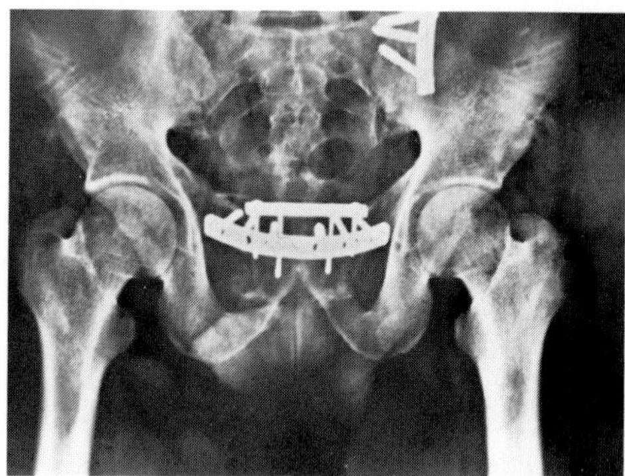

Figure 6-10C.

acetabulum is undertaken through a suitable extensile exposure (Figure 6-11). In the presence of an ipsilateral sacroiliac fracture, such an exposure permits lag screw fixation of that disruption along with acetabular reconstruction, while the rami are immobilized with a simple external frame. In the presence of a contralateral sacroiliac disruption or an unstable sacral fracture (Figure 6-12), both that injury and the ramus fractures are effectively immobilized by the application of a triangular frame. In such examples where a simple anterior frame is applied during the resuscitative period, the contralateral sacroiliac disruption is managed with an open reduction and internal fixation.

Following a violent traumatic insult, several patterns of injury are seen, which include unilateral or bilateral acetabular fractures, bilateral sacroiliac disruptions or other equivalent posterior injuries, and bilateral ramus fractures with or without a diastasis of the symphysis. In most of these cases virtually all of the principal ligamentous supports for the pelvic ring are severely

Figure 6-11. In a vehicular accident this farmer of 35 years sustained a right transverse with a posterior wall acetabular fracture with a diastasis, left ramus fractures, and a stable left sacroiliac disruption. A: Initial anteroposterior radiograph. B: Initial computed scan through the acetabular roof. C: Postoperative outlet view after acetabular reconstruction and the application of a simple external frame. D: Anteroposterior view upon removal of the external frame seven weeks later. The man resumed heavy farming chores about six months after his injury.

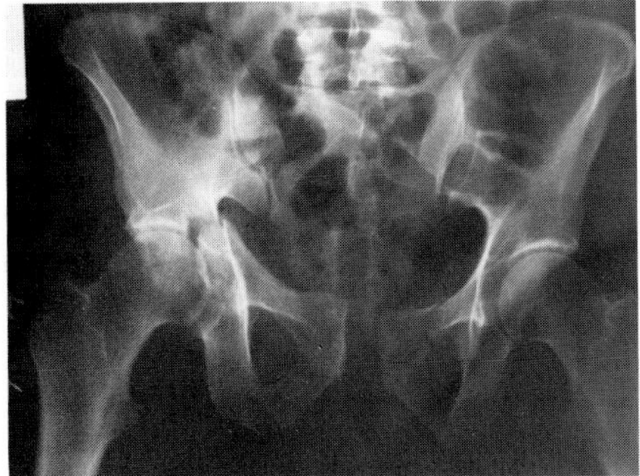

Figure 6-11A.

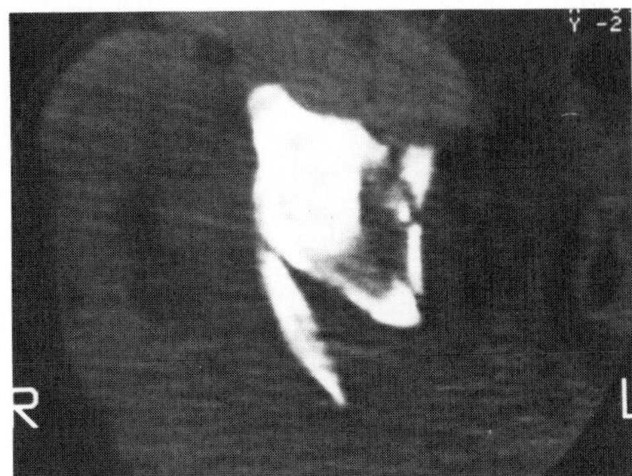


Figure 6-11B.

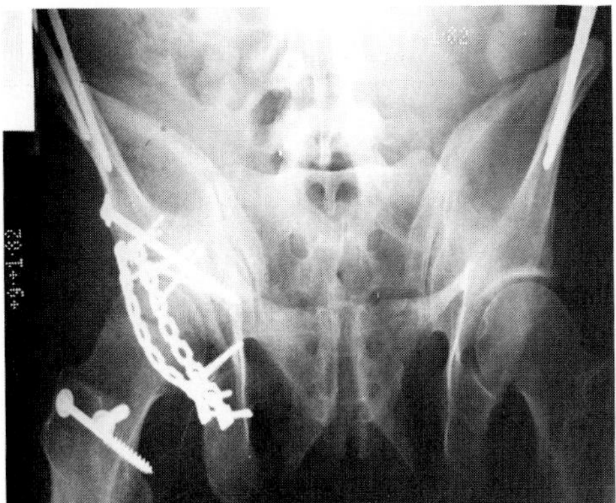

Figure 6-11C.

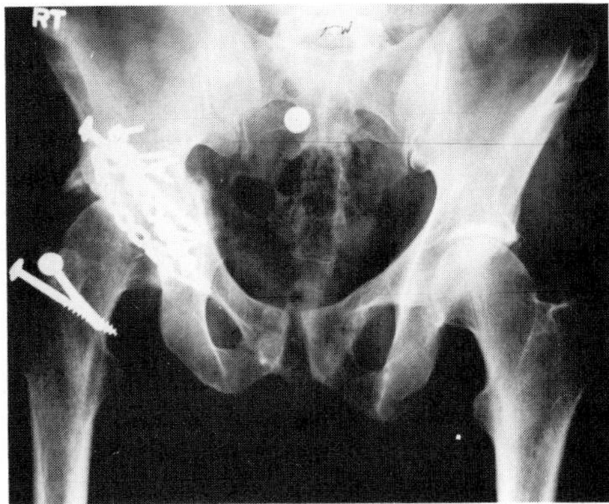


Figure 6-11D.

compromised. As a working rule each site of pelvic disruption is stabilized with the use of an appropriate method of internal or external fixation. With the anticipated degree of displacement and the need for the optimal fixation, even though external fixation is employed for provisional stability, internal fixation is preferred for the definitive reconstruction (Figure 6-13).

The surgical planning involves a careful consideration of the preferred sequence of the reductions, as well as the optimal surgical exposures. In the presence of an acetabular fracture accompanied by marked displacement of a posterior column disruption and an ipsilateral sacroiliac disruption, as well as a diastasis and a contralateral acetabular fracture, adequate exposure of the former acetabulum and sacroiliac joint is achieved by the application of a Kocher-Langenbeck or possibly a triradiate approach (Figure 6-14). In

Figure 6-12. This 62-year-old dean of a medical school fell off a horse that landed on him, provoking a right transverse acetabular fracture with a diastasis and left ramus fractures and an unstable sacral fracture. A: Initial anteroposterior view. B: Initial computed scan with sacral fracture. C: Postoperative inlet view after acetabular reconstruction and the application of a triangular frame. D: Anteroposterior view upon removal of the external frame about eight weeks later. One year after his injury he resumed horseback riding and mountain climbing.

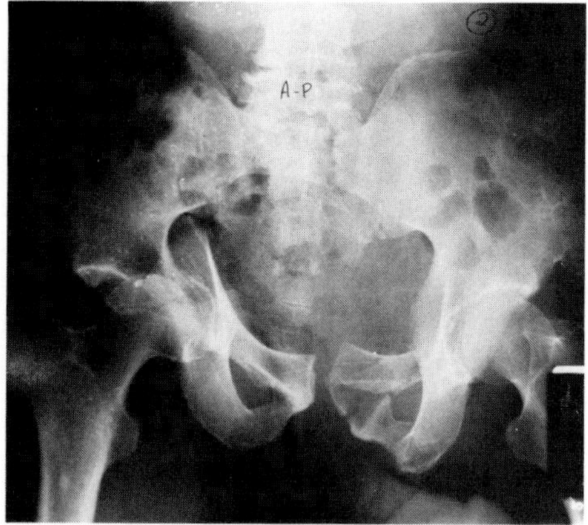


Figure 6-12A.

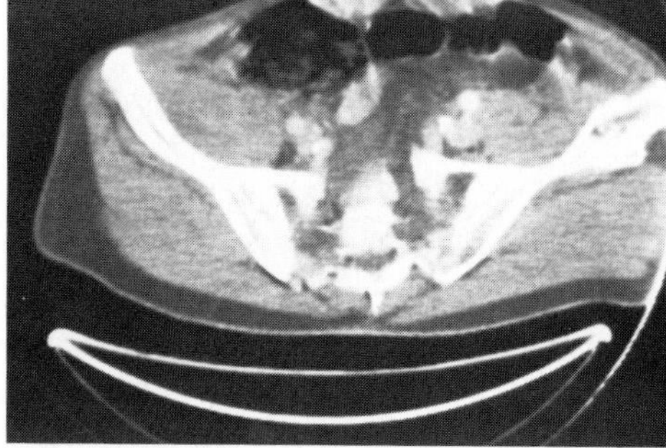

Figure 6-12B.

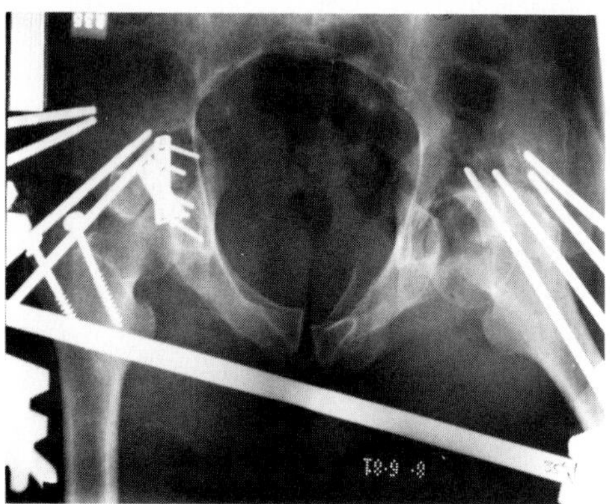

Figure 6-12C.

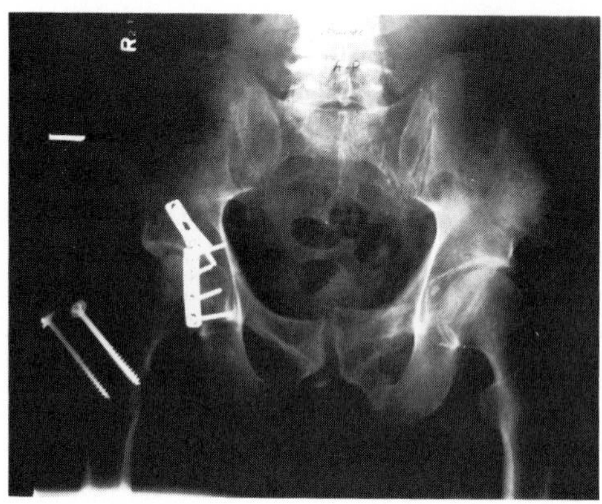

Figure 6-12D.

contrast, if the former acetabular fracture possesses marked anterior displacement with minimal posterior displacement, preservation of the ipsilateral sacroiliac joint, and involvement of the ipsilateral rami or bilateral rami, then a unilateral or bilateral ilioinguinal approach permits adequate exposure to reconstruct both the acetabulum and the superior pubic ramus.

In the presence of bilateral unstable sacroiliac joints with bilateral acetabular disruptions, one option is the application of an appropriate incision such as a Kocher-Langenbeck, a triradiate, or an extended iliofemoral exposure that is suitable for the reconstruction of the acetabulum and the ipsilateral sacroiliac joint, with a comparable procedure on the other hemipelvis. Another option is the use of a transverse posterior incision to

Figure 6-13. A male pedestrian of 26 years who jumped in front of a car traveling at high speed sustained bilateral unstable sacroiliac dislocations, bilateral transverse acetabular fractures, and a diastasis. A simple external frame was applied as part of the acute resuscitation and splenectomy. One week later open reduction of all five pelvic disruptions was undertaken. A: Anteroposterior view after insertion of the external fixation pins. B: Anteroposterior view after assembly of the pelvic frame. C: Inlet view after conversion to internal fixation.

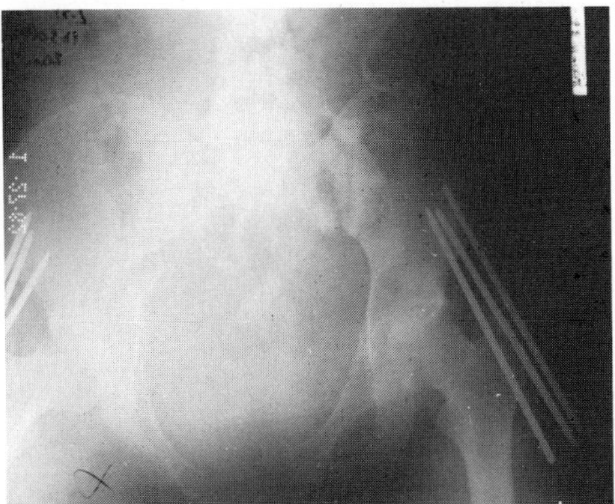

Figure 6-13A.

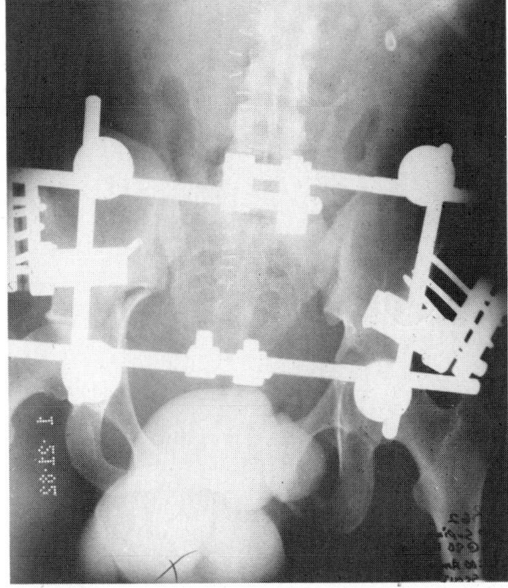

Figure 6-13B.

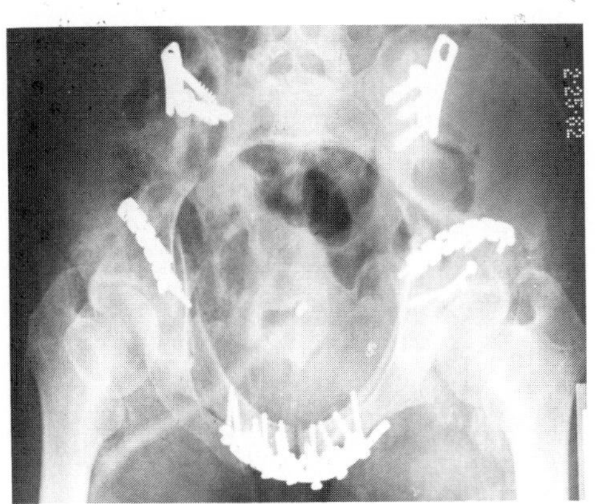

Figure 6-13C.

expose and immobilize both sacroiliac joints, possibly by resort to a Double Cobra plate (Figure 6-15). For the acetabular reconstructions, depending upon the particular patterns of injury, either an extensile lateral exposure or an ilioinguinal approach is selected to maximize the lateral or anterior visualization, respectively.

A fourth major category of pelvic fracture is an open injury. In common with other Grade III open fractures, these injuries are managed by an immediate, thorough debridement, intravenous antibiotics, the application of external pelvic fixation, and a complete diversion

Figure 6-14. A woman of 45 years who was involved in a vehicular accident sustained bilateral transverse acetabular fractures and an unstable left sacroiliac dislocation. At the time of presentation, five weeks afterwards, triradiate approaches were used to undertake the reconstructive procedures. A: Initial anteroposterior view. B: Initial inlet view. C: Initial computed scan with left sacroiliac disruption. D: Postoperative anteroposterior view.

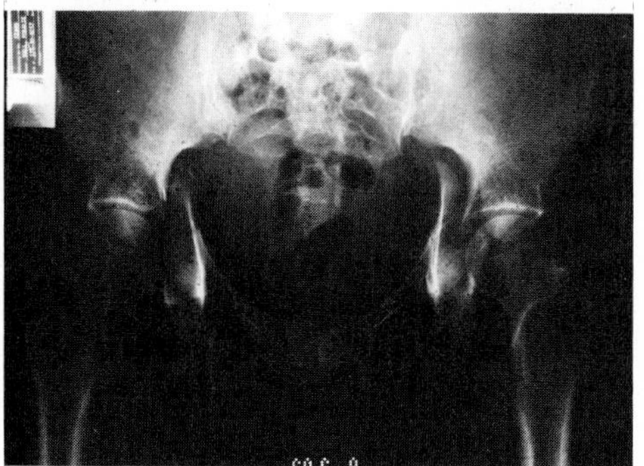

Figure 6-14A.

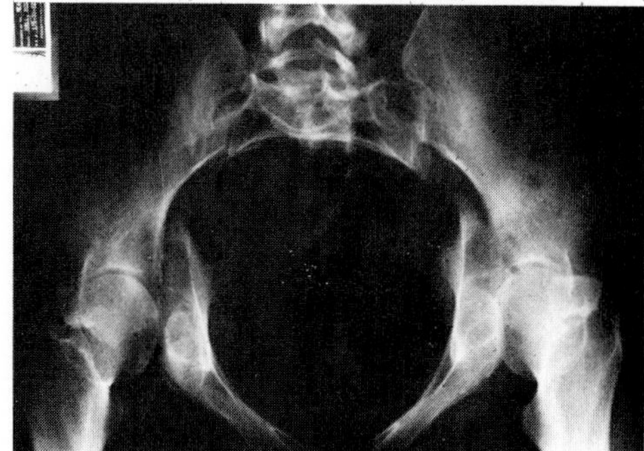

Figure 6-14B.

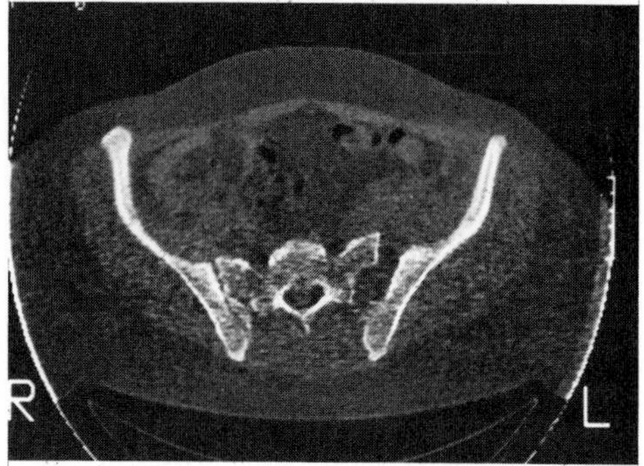


Figure 6-14C.

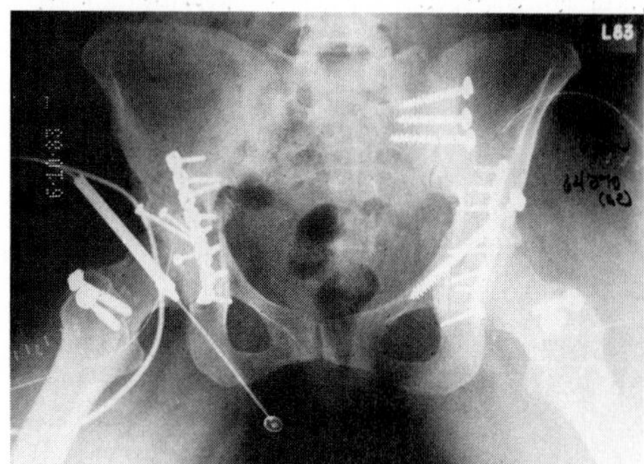


Figure 6-14D.

colostomy. Even in the presence of an intact colon and anal sphincter, the colostomy is mandatory so that the risk of feculent contamination of the open wounds is minimized. The risk of fecal contamination is particularly great when the open wound extends from the groin to or beyond the anal sphincter. An open wound superficial to a ramus or one that violates the scrotum also possesses a substantial risk of secondary infection. In contrast most open fracture dislocations of the sacroiliac joint possess a much smaller risk of fecal contamination, so that a diversion colostomy is rarely necessary. In those open pelvic fractures accompanied by marked instability, delayed supplementary internal fixation is necessary, especially of an unstable posterior disruption. Even in the presence of a Grade I or II open sacroiliac joint, generally such a markedly unstable injury necessitates the use of delayed posterior internal fixation.

Although for the control of hemorrhage and pain the role of external fixation as part of the emergency resuscitation is well established, the optimal time to

Figure 6-15. An intoxicated college student of 21 years was involved in a vehicular accident and sustained a comminuted left transverse acetabular fracture, a diastasis with a low anterior column fracture of the right acetabulum, and an unstable sacral fracture. A: Preoperative anteroposterior radiograph. B: Preoperative computed scan with sacral fracture. C: Postoperative inlet view after left acetabular reconstruction through a triradiate approach, internal fixation of the right acetabulum and diastasis through an ilioinguinal approach, and sacral reconstruction with a Double Cobra plate applied through a transverse incision.

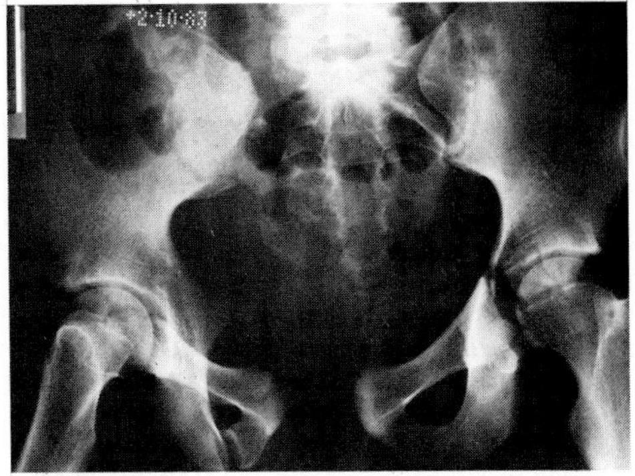

Figure 6-15A.

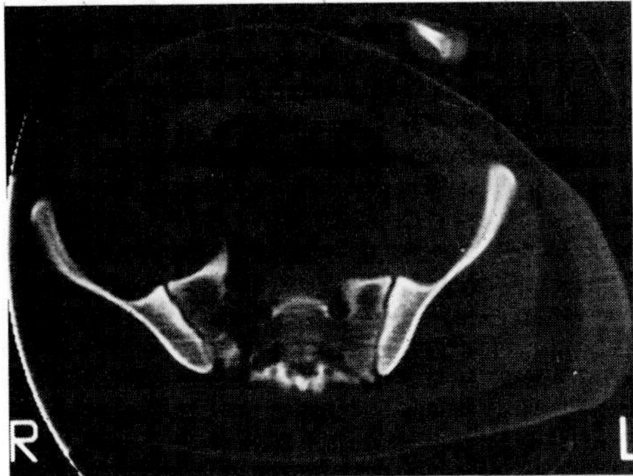


Figure 6-15B.

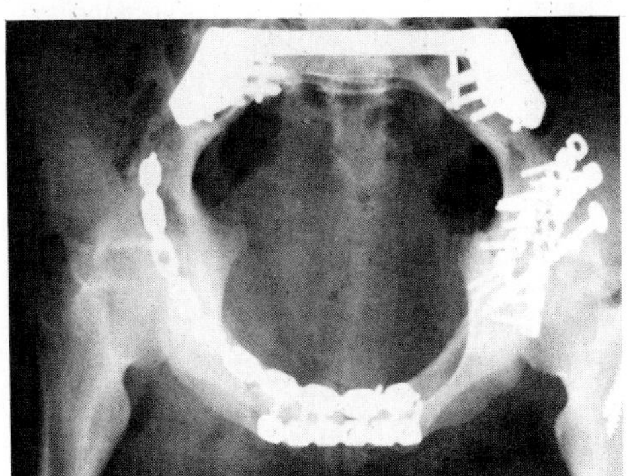

Figure 6-15C.

apply supplementary pelvic internal fixation to a closed disruption remains controversial. Whenever the general condition of the patient—including the hemodynamic status—is questionable, open reduction (with its potential for considerable blood loss) is deferred for 24 to 48 hours after the time of the initial injury. Further delay is likely to culminate in the complications of prolonged recumbency, especially those of pulmonary, thromboembolic and urological origin. When the general condition of the patient is satisfactory, and provided that the surgical team possesses the appropriate resources, early surgical intervention provides the optimal biomechanical environment to achieve rapid recovery with the least likelihood for the complications of enforced recumbency.

# Indications for Nonoperative and Operative Treatment of Acetabular Fractures

Contributed by Joel M. Matta, MD.

## Introduction

The most common late problem following a fracture of the acetabulum is posttraumatic arthritis. Displacement of an acetabular fracture leads to incongruity between the femoral head and the articular fragments of the acetabulum. The incongruity gives rise to markedly altered load transmission of the articular cartilage within the acetabulum, so that the cartilage is subject to a mechanical breakdown or at least the histological and biochemical changes of osteoarthritis. Both the precise physiological loads imposed upon the intact articular cartilage of the acetabulum and the degree to which the cartilage can tolerate enhanced loads prior to the initiation of degenerative change are unknown. Undoubtedly, the articular cartilage tolerates some degree of superficial incongruity and alteration of load bearing, which partly accounts for the successful results documented following nonoperative treatment. The ability of articular cartilage to adapt to incongruity also contributes to the successful results of surgical management in which a less than perfect articular reduction is achieved. In many surgical cases, the clinical result is satisfactory despite 2mm to 3mm of articular displacement following the open reduction.[18,19]

As a rule, an anatomic open reduction and internal fixation of a displaced interarticular fracture of the lower extremity produces the greatest likelihood for a favorable outcome. Despite this generally accepted principle, however, the indications for an open reduction of an acetabular fracture remain controversial. One explanation is the widespread difficulty within the orthopaedic community to accurately characterize radiographically an acetabular fracture pattern and the magnitude of displacement. Another factor is the technical difficulty associated with operative exposure, reduction, and stabilization of the acetabular fracture. In the orthopaedic literature there are markedly conflicting reports on the quality and reproducibility of the results documented following the application of closed and open methods of treatment of an acetabular fracture.[18-26]

A closed reduction by means of manipulation or traction tends to improve the articular reduction, although it rarely produces an anatomic reduction.[18,19] In the presence of a both-column fracture, a closed reduction facilitates a correction of deformity of the pelvic ring. A closed reduction, therefore, is performed with

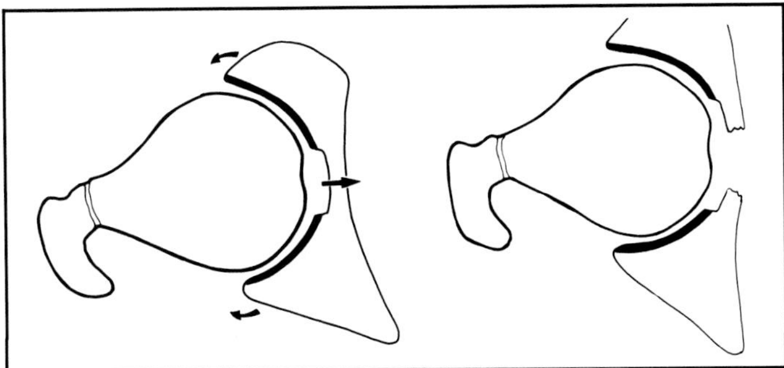

Figure 6-16. Rotational displacement of a complete both-column fracture that can lead to secondary congruence.

the premise that the clinical result will be satisfactory despite the persistent displacement of the articular surface. A major limitation of a closed reduction of a fracture is the inability to control the rotational displacement of the two acetabular columns. With a "T" shaped or a complete both-column fracture, the anterior and posterior columns rotate around the femoral head in opposite directions. The rotational displacement of the two columns is comparable to the opening of swinging doors hinged along the anterior and posterior rims of the acetabulum (Figure 6-16). The maximum displacement is observed medially and the minimum displacement is noted along the acetabular rim. Since a closed reduction achieved by resort to skeletal traction employs "ligamentotaxis" across the intact capsule of the hip to its origin along the acetabular rim, this maneuver does not permit a correction of the principal deformity in the central acetabular region. With a closed reduction, the malrotation of the two columns invariably remains uncorrected. Closed treatment is logically performed with the assumption that the clinical result will be satisfactory despite the residual articular displacement. If a rotational correction is necessary to ultimately achieve a successful clinical outcome, especially with a markedly displaced fracture, then an open reduction is essential.

Some authors[26,27] advocate a closed reduction of the femoral head to its anatomical position with maintenance of that position by skeletal traction despite the failure of this technique to provide a comparable reduction of the displaced acetabular fragments. Recent clinical documentation[18] of those cases where skeletal traction affords an anatomical reduction of the femoral head but not of the acetabulum confirms the inevitable return of the femoral head to its displaced position regardless of the duration of traction. The femoral head cannot be maintained indefinitely in a stable anatomically reduced position unless the displaced acetabular fragments are anatomically reduced and stabilized by surgical intervention.

The decision to perform an open reduction rests upon the findings observed in the initial anteroposterior and 45° oblique radiographs and the computed scan. While a trial closed reduction is rarely indicated, one exception—a posterior dislocation—is managed as a surgical emergency by a closed reduction with a subsequent radiographic assessment to determine if an open reduction is indicated.

## Indications for Nonoperative Treatment

### *Nondisplaced and Minimally Displaced Fractures*

Adequate assessment of any acetabular fracture necessitates a scrutiny of anteroposterior and 45° oblique views of the pelvis. An apparently undisplaced fracture visualized solely by an anteroposterior view actually may have considerable displacement evident in one of the oblique views. In most cases, a supplementary computed scan is examined particularly for determination of the degree of displacement of the posterior wall and for visualization of incarcerated osteochondral fragments. The exact magnitude of a minimal displacement of a fracture fragment that does not merit an open reduction remains unclear. A crucial factor is the site and size of the displaced fragment. A linear displacement even of a small magnitude of 1mm to 2mm in the crucial weightbearing dome of the acetabulum is least well tolerated by the joint.[26] Small and substantially displaced acetabular rim fragments around the inferior aspects of the joint and displaced away from the femoral head are well tolerated. Loss of concentricity of the acetabulum with respect to the femoral head associated with a both-column or a "T" fracture is tolerated to an intermediate degree. Displacement of a major fracture fragment by 2mm to 3mm appears to be consistent with satisfactory remodeling of the incongruent joint.[18,19] Once a displacement of a major fracture fragment greater than 5mm is documented in any radiographic view, an open reduction is indicated.

### *Displaced Fractures of Questionable Significance*

While at first glance the presence of a small avulsion fracture from the posterior rim detected by the scrutiny of anteroposterior and 45° oblique pelvic radiographs appears to be a clinical problem suitably managed by nonoperative treatment, a computed scan also is needed to exclude the possibility of an incarcerated osteochondral fragment, extensive minimally displaced comminution

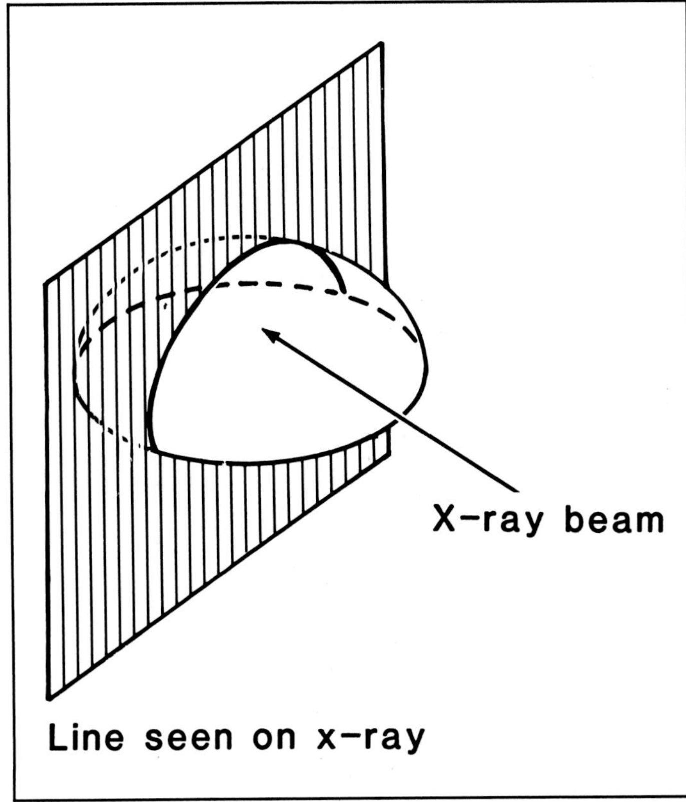


Figure 6-17. Schematic of an anteroposterior view of a transverse fracture and the medial roof arc.

of the adjacent posterior column, and marginal impaction of the adjacent articular surface. Displacement of the superior portion of the acetabulum, defined by Rowe and Lowell[25] as the so-called "weightbearing dome," is prognostically more important than involvement of the more inferior area. Until recently no accurate quantitative method was available to define the magnitude of involvement and displacement of the weightbearing dome. Now a radiographic technique has been devised by the author that permits an anatomical correlation with the specific site of disruption. The method employs three measurements termed the medial, anterior, and posterior roof arcs. The measurements are recorded by examination of the anteroposterior and 45° oblique views of the pelvis. To measure the medial roof arc, a vertical line is drawn through the roof of the acetabulum to the geometric center of the acetabulum. A second line is drawn from the point where the fracture line intersects the acetabulum. The angle subtended by the two lines represents the medial roof arc. Similarly, the anterior and posterior roof arcs are measured by the respective 45° oblique radiographic views (Figures 6-17 through 6-21). With the limitations in the accuracy for proper placement of the patient on a radiographic table, the

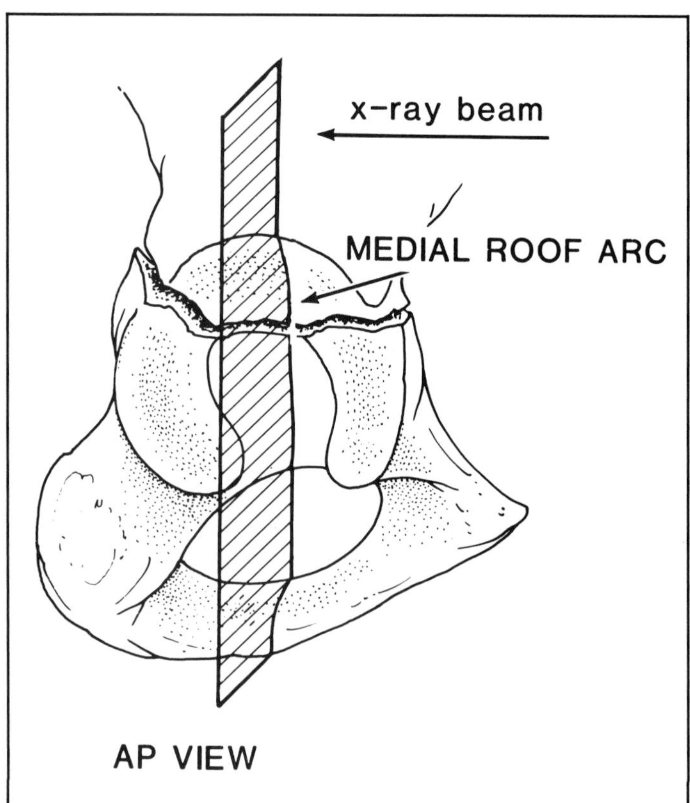


Figure 6-18. Schematic of the obturator oblique view of an anterior column fracture and the anterior roof arc.

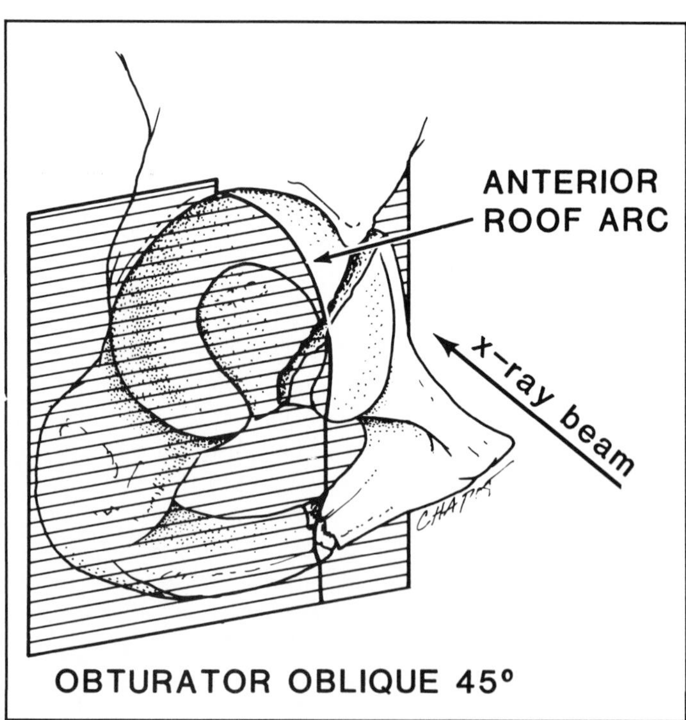


Figure 6-19. Schematic of the iliac oblique view of a posterior column fracture and the posterior roof arc. The posterior roof arc borders the posterior edge of the cotyloid fossa and therefore may not be interrupted despite displacement of a large posterior wall fragment.

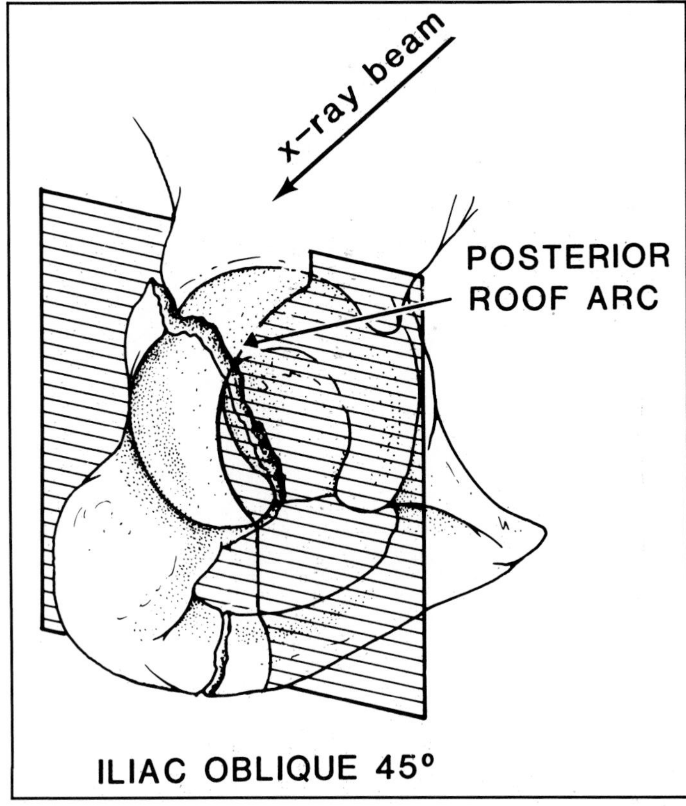


Figure 6-20. The AP and oblique views of a "T" fracture, showing displacement of the femoral head and inadequate roof arc measurements. Operation is indicated.

measurements are quantified to the nearest 5°. Another potential limitation of the method is the two-dimensional radiographic representation of a hemispherical joint that actually consists of a three-dimensional dome (Figure 6-22). Such a quantitative assessment of the disrupted acetabular dome is most useful in the assessment of a posterior or anterior column fracture, a transverse or "T" fracture, and an associated anterior column or wall with a posterior hemitransverse fracture.

Roof arc measurements have limited usefulness for the evaluation of a both-column fracture and a posterior wall fracture. In the former case, with the inevitable separation of the acetabular roof from the iliac wing, the three-dimensional displacement of the acetabular roof cannot be accurately or meaningfully determined. With a typical posterior wall fracture, the displaced segment is positioned posterior to the arc of the acetabulum represented by the posterior roof arc (Figure 6-19). The accuracy of the measurement is thereby greatly reduced. Based upon the measurement of roof arcs, the following types of acetabular fracture patterns are suitable for nonoperative treatment:

- When the patient is not immobilized by traction, the femoral head remains congruous with the roof of the acetabulum.

Figure 6-21. The anteroposterior and oblique views of a "T" fracture, showing congruence of the femoral head out of traction and adequate roof arc measurements. Closed treatment is indicated.

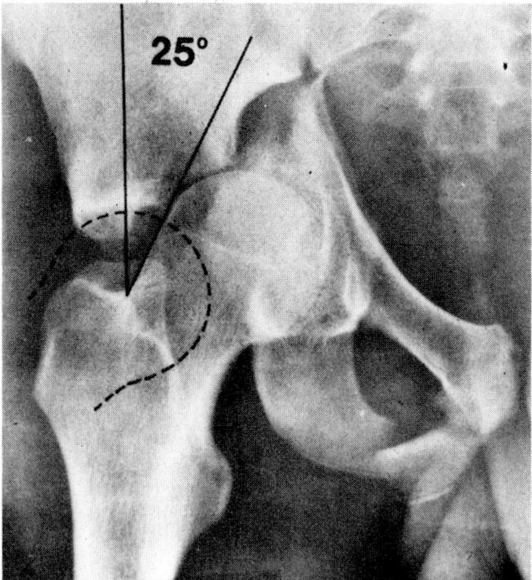


Figure 6-21A.

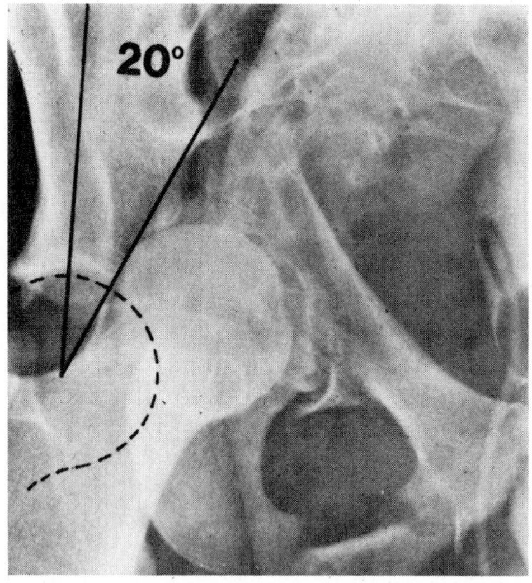


Figure 6-21B.

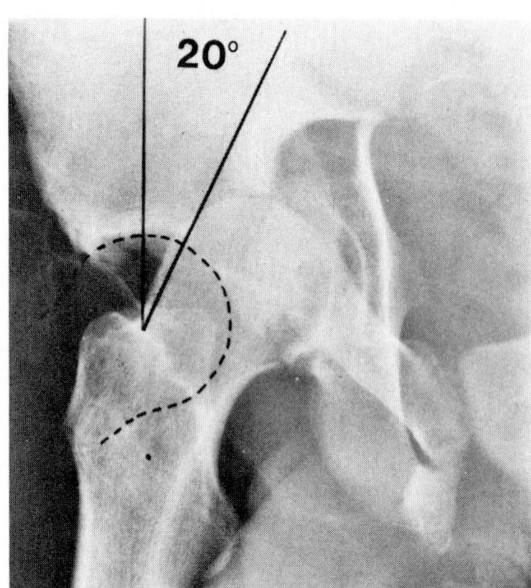


Figure 6-21C.

- The anterior roof arc is greater than 30°.
- The medial roof arc is greater than 40°.
- The posterior roof arc is greater than 50°.
- The posterior wall is assessed separately by resort to conventional pelvic radiographs and a computed scan, as this region is not subject to useful measurements of the roof arcs.

The above values for roof arc measurements constitute the minimum acceptable values consistent with a favorable outcome following nonoperative management. If the roof arc measurements are less than these minimum values, the femoral head is unstable and is unlikely to remain in an anatomically reduced position beneath the acetabular roof.

Figure 6-22. Schematic of a single radiographic view of a hemispherical joint. An arc transversing the hemisphere is represented at the points where the x-ray beam strikes the subchondral bone tangentially.

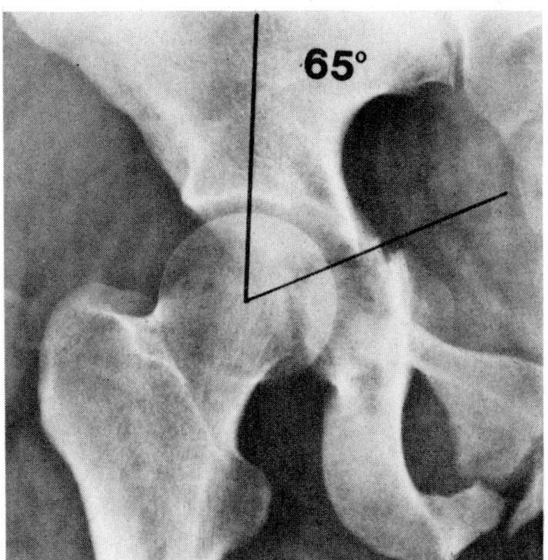


Figure 6-22A.

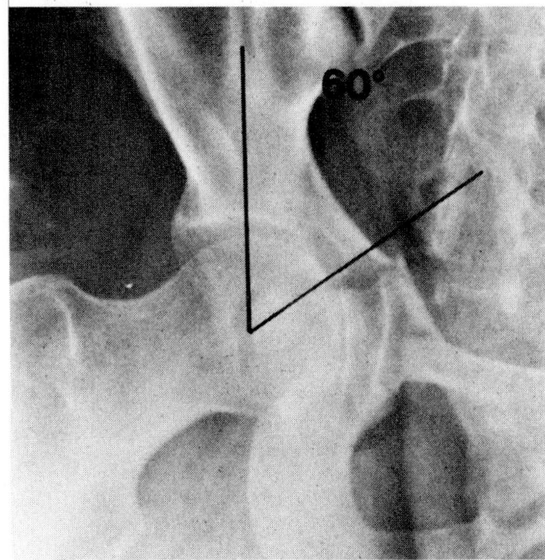


Figure 6-22B.

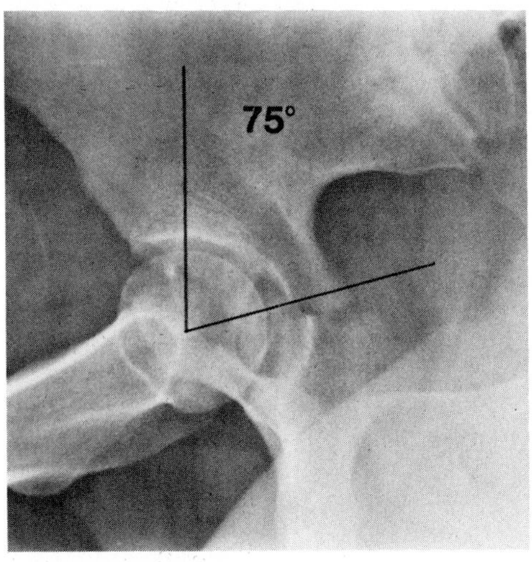


Figure 6-22C.

## *Apparent or Secondary Congruence Associated with a Displaced Both-Column Fracture*

A both-column fracture is a unique situation with the separation of the articular fragments of the entire acetabulum from the intact portion of the ilium that remains attached to the sacrum. Frequently, the articular fragments are displaced along with the femoral head in a superior and medial direction. The displaced fragments, however, retain their congruity with the femoral head.[22] The corresponding roof arc measurements indicate unacceptable displacement of prognostically important portions of the acetabulum. The displacement of the columns, however, is primarily rotational with the creation of gaps between the adjacent acetabular fragments so that the congruity of the acetabulum with the femoral head is preserved (Figure 6-16). This situation is optimally confirmed by the assessment of anteroposterior and 45° oblique pelvic radiographs (Figures 6-23 and 6-24). A computed scan permits the measurement of the degree of separation between the various fracture fragments. If a displacement of more than 10mm is documented, an open reduction is preferred. Secondary congruence does not lead to reproducibly satisfactory results as reliably as an anatomic reduction. Closed treatment of a displaced both-column fracture is preferred for a middle-aged or an older individual, especially in a case with marked osteoporosis, or a case with a late presentation where extraordinary technical difficulties are engendered by the delay in surgical reconstruction. For an adolescent or a young adult with a comparable displaced both-column fracture, generally surgical reconstruction is preferred.

### *Medical Contraindications*

The presence and gravity of various medical disorders and the age of the patient require careful consideration, as well as the likelihood for a satisfactory result following the use of nonoperative methods.

### *Local Infections, Associated Wounds and Associated Soft Tissue Lesions*

Local soft tissue injuries, as well as associated visceral injuries frequently complicate the management of an acetabular fracture. At the site of the blunt trauma that provokes an acetabular fracture, particularly around the greater trochanter, subcutaneous necrosis of fat with an accompanying hematoma and ecchymosis increases the risk of a deep infection following a surgical reconstruction. At the time of acetabular reconstruction, if this so-called Morel-LaValee lesion is encountered, evacuation of the hematoma and excision of the necrotic tissue is undertaken. Subsequently, after rigorous irrigation of the wound with antibiotic solution is completed, exposure of the acetabulum is resumed.

An associated visceral injury—particularly a ruptured bladder or a penetrating injury to the bowel—increases considerably the risk of a postoperative wound infection following an acetabular reconstruction. A visceral injury provides an indication for the application of drainage tubes that course from the pelvis through the skin and provides a conduit for contamination of the pelvis and the adjunct fracture site. In such a case acetabular reconstruction is deferred until the tubes have been removed and the intrapelvic drainage has ceased.

Figure 6-23. Anteroposterior and oblique views of a complete both-column fracture in a 52-year-old woman, demonstrating apparent congruence on all three views.

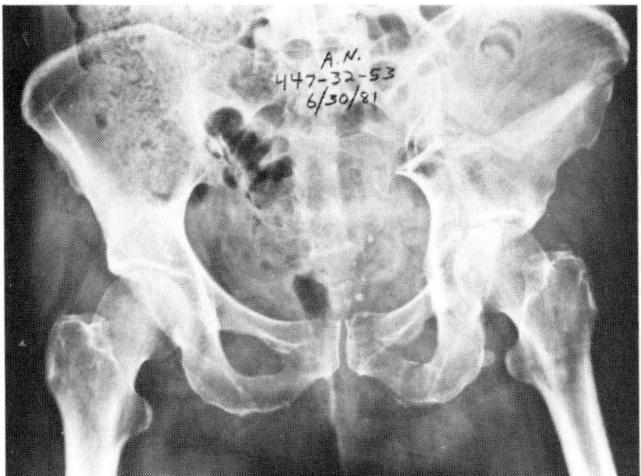


Figure 6-23A.

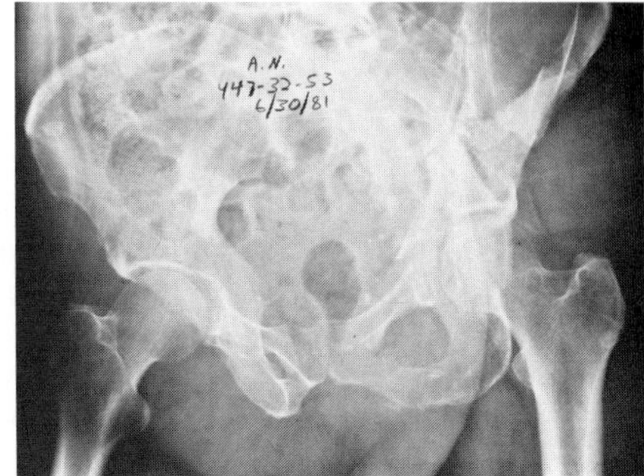


Figure 6-23B.

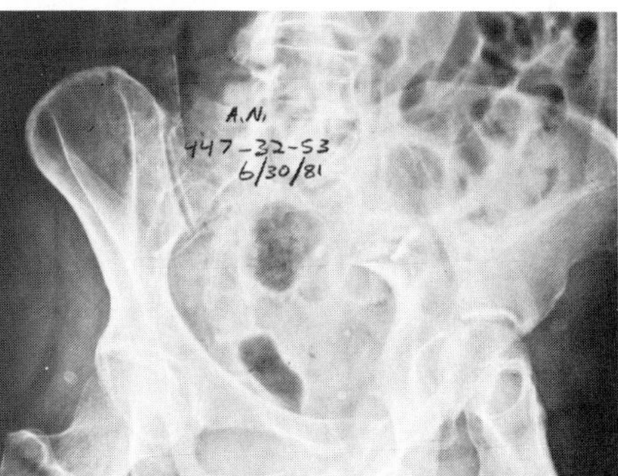


Figure 6-23C.

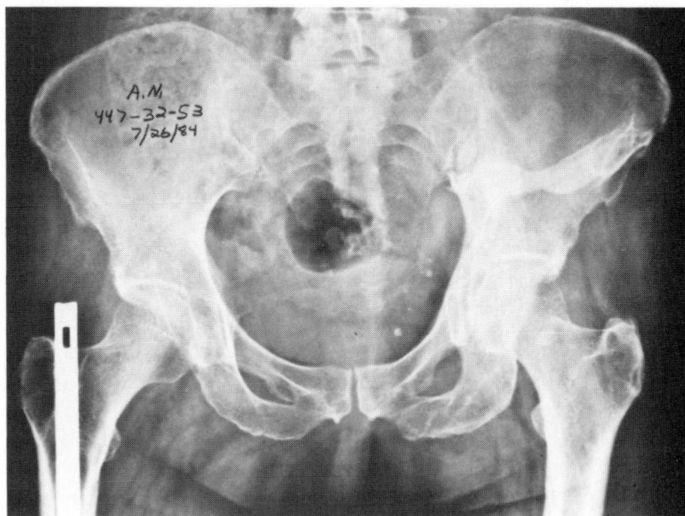


Figure 6-24. Three years later, a good clinical and radiographic result is documented.

## Indications for Operation

The principal indication is the failure to meet the criteria needed for the application of closed treatment.

Following a closed reduction of a posterior dislocation, the presence of an incarcerated osteochondral fragment in the hip joint is an indication for surgical removal of the fracture fragment. An exception is the observation of a minute bony fragment within the cotyloid fossa of the acetabulum in a computed scan taken after a closed reduction of a simple posterior dislocation of the hip. The fragment represents an avulsion injury of the ligamentum teres from either the acetabulum or the femoral head. The osseous fragment can be ignored provided that it is not incarcerated between the cartilaginous surfaces of the femoral head and the acetabulum, and the distance between the femoral head and the tear-drop is not increased. Rarely, a large avulsion fragment attached to the ligamentum teres settles on the femoral head, where it can become adherent. A computed scan taken after the closed reduction confirms the presence of the problem and the need for removal of the fragment.

When mobilization of the patient or ipsilateral lower extremity is deemed to be particiularly important, the indication for an open reduction of an accompanying acetabular fracture is increased. Two examples are an ipsilateral fracture of the femoral shaft and a major ligamentous injury of the ipsilateral knee. Generally when the acetabular fracture is complicated by a major contralateral injury to the lower extremity, the indications for surgical reconstruction of the acetabulum as well as of the other major injury are greatly extended.

In the presence of substantial displacement of an acetabular fracture, an open reduction is necessary to prevent a nonunion and to provide adequate bone stock for a later reconstructive procedure such as a total hip joint replacement.

## Indications in the Elderly

Certain elderly patients possess particularly osteoporotic bone that renders an attempted internal fixation difficult. Impaction of the articular surface is more common in osteoporotic bone and further complicates the reduction and fixation. Generally, an elderly osteoporotic patient with a comminuted displaced acetabular fracture is managed with skeletal traction rather than an extensive acetabular reconstruction. Even though a solid osseous union of the acetabulum is accompanied by an acceptable malalignment and a predilection for traumatic arthritis, ultimately, a total hip joint replacement is likely to provide a highly functional outcome with the least morbidity. In a generally fit elderly patient with an acetabular fracture that is amenable to a limited surgical approach and an accurate stable reduction, and thereby a favorable long term prognosis, prompt open intervention is strongly recommended. In many instances when an open reduction of a displaced fracture is not performed, inadequate bone stock is available for a later reconstructive procedure. For example, in the elderly patient a posterior fracture dislocation of the femoral head with a large displaced posterior wall fragment merits surgical reconstruction. Unless the procedure is undertaken the displaced ununited wall fragment encourages a late subluxation of the femoral head and greatly complicates any attempt to securely anchor an acetabular component at the time of the almost inevitable total hip joint replacement.

The previous criteria were employed prospectively to determine the indications for nonoperative and operative management in 105 displaced fractures of the acetabulum. All of the fractures were displaced by more than 5mm and possessed involvement of at least one entire column.[19] The roof arc technique was used to quantitate the involvement of the acetabular dome in this prospective series and in a retrospective series of an additional 64 fractures.[18] For the prospective series, 17 cases were determined to be suitable for nonoperative treatment while 88 cases were considered to be appropriate for open intervention. Roof arc measurements indicating an adequate acetabular dome were present in only 5% of the fractures. The presence of apparent congruence of a displaced both-column fracture was the principal indication for nonoperative treatment, rather than the preservation of an "intact weightbearing dome."

### Summary

The decision between operative and nonoperative treatment is based primarily upon the configuration and the displacement of the acetabular fracture recorded upon scrutiny of the preliminary pelvic radiographs and a computed scan. An initial period of skeletal traction is unlikely to provide an accurate closed reduction of a displaced acetabular fracture. Although the majority of displaced acetabular fractures require open reduction, careful radiographic analysis permits an identification of the minority that are likely to do well with nonoperative management.

Contribution concludes.

## Accompanying Sciatic Nerve Injury

When a sciatic nerve palsy complicates an acetabular fracture, an additional indication for surgical intervention merits consideration. In such a case, typically in the presence of a displaced posterior wall and/or posterior column fracture, an open reduction of the hip and acetabulum is accompanied by a local sciatic nerve exploration. Impingement of bone fragments upon the nerve is corrected while a bone fragment that impales the nerve is removed. In the presence of epineural or intraneural hemorrhage at the site of the contusion, an epineurotomy is undertaken with preservation of the perineurium.

## Timing for Acetabular Reconstruction

With the likelihood for multiple concomitant injuries and the associated need for extensive diagnostic procedures prior to acetabular reconstruction, generally it is impractical to undertake an open intervention on an emergency basis. Unlike a posterior dislocation of the hip with the increased predilection for avascular necrosis of the unreduced femoral head, an unstable posterior fracture-dislocation with a large posterior wall fragment does not pose a comparable surgical emergency, even though the femoral head cannot be maintained in a reduced position by resort to closed methods. If a closed reduction of a posterior fracture dislocation, however, is followed by the onset of a sciatic nerve palsy, prompt surgical exploration of the sciatic nerve with reconstruction of the acetabulum is indicated.

During the past four years with 35 suitable cases, we have undertaken immediate open reduction and internal fixation of the acetabulum following the completion of the appropriate diagnostic studies. The techniques have been performed with less difficulty than comparable procedures performed a few days later. Once a week after the time of the injury has passed, the technical difficulties associated with an open reduction mount precipitously, making operation extremely difficult within three to six weeks. Also, the likelihood for ectopic bone formation appears to increase substantially when a posttraumatic delay of 10 to 14 days ensues. Our current recommendation, therefore, is for surgical reconstruction as soon as the general condition of the patient is stable, the appropriate radiological and computed scanning protocol is completed, and an experienced operative team is available.

## Complex Pelvic Ring and Acetabular Disruptions

Most complex injuries with disruption of the pelvic ring and acetabulum are markedly unstable and wholly unsuitable for closed methods of treatment. After completion of the radiological series and the computed scan an appropriate and extensive surgical reconstruction is carefully planned and undertaken.

The first step to plan the acetabular approach is critical analysis of suitable radiographs and the computed scan. Unless the extent and specific site of the injury is documented by drawing the fracture lines on the radiographs and a model pelvis, inadequate or inappropriate surgical exposure is likely to follow. While the details of surgical approaches are described in the following chapter, a few general principles are provided here.

A posterior wall or a posterior column fracture is suitably exposed by resort to a Kocher-Langenbeck approach. For those unusual posterior disruptions that propagate into the lateral ilium the exposure is greatly augmented by osteotomy of the greater trochanter and displacement of the glutei.

For a simple transverse fracture with minimal anterior displacement, a posterior approach with a trochanteric osteotomy or a straight lateral longitudinal transtrochanteric approach is suitable. With later presentation, supplementary comminution, or marked displacement, an extensile incision such as a triradiate or extended iliofemoral approach is recommended, so that the entire lateral ilium and adjacent acetabulum are visualized.

Anterior column fractures are divided into lower and higher variants, where the latter are associated with considerable involvement of the lateral ilium. The former are best visualized by a localized anterior incision, such as an ilioinguinal or an iliofemoral approach. For the higher fracture variants where stabilization can be provided by immobilization of the lateral ilium, either a limited version of an extended iliofemoral approach or the anterior limb of the triradiate approach with or without a greater trochanteric osteotomy is suitable. Most of the associated fractures—especially a both-column injury, as well as an associated hemitransverse or a comminuted "T" fracture—merit an extensile approach through a triradiate or an extended iliofemoral incision. Previously, combined anterior and posterior approaches have been used to expose these injuries. With the recent introduction of several extensile incisions generally the use of combined incisions is an outmoded technique. If the two approaches are used sequentially, the initial stage of immobilization of one portion of the fracture greatly impedes the attempt to accurately reduce the other portion of the fracture. If the two approaches are used simultaneously, they do not provide as good a visualization or as rapid an exposure as the use of a single extensile incision.

Currently, the relative roles of intraoperative skeletal traction and the use of onboard reduction aids remain controversial. Judet and Letournel[11] advocate the use of intraoperative traction to anatomically reduce the femoral head and, thereby, to facilitate the acetabular reduction. With their highly sophisticated Judet fracture table and the presence of a suitably trained assistant who can manipulate the table throughout the surgical procedure, the French surgeons have adequately confirmed the merits of their approach. Nevertheless, a wide variety of specialized reduction tools is now available (see Chapter 8) that largely obviates the need for the special fracture table. The authors prefer the use of the latter technique, which appears to be consistent with a much lower incidence of iatrogenically induced sciatic nerve palsy. Subtle adjustments of the position of the femoral head and manipulation of the acetabular fragments are readily achieved by the use of the reduction tools. During the planning of the surgical exposure a dilemma arises about the preference for visualization of the articular surface of the acetabulum versus an exposure of the inner aspect of the pelvis opposite the site of the articular disruption. During the previous decade Letournel[11] employed an ilioinguinal incision, which provides excellent exposure of the inner aspect of the pelvis but poor visualization of the acetabulum. This approach is associated with a low incidence of postoperative ectopic bone formation. Nevertheless, as superior extensile exposures of the acetabular articular surface have evolved, especially the triradiate and extended iliofemoral approaches, ever increasing interest has arisen in visualization of the acetabular articular surface. The principal liability of the lateral extensile exposures is their predilection for postoperative ectopic bone formation.[11,27] Nevertheless, with their greatly enhanced visualization of the site of principal interest, the disrupted articular surface, the newer surgical approaches seem to provide a greater likelihood for accurate reassembly of displaced acetabular fragments. The ilioinguinal approach remains the optimal technique to visualize an extensive comminuted fracture of the entire anterior column with minimal displacement of the posterior column.

To inspect the articular surface of the acetabulum, an extensive capsulotomy around the acetabular rim is required. The insertion of the capsule around the base of the femoral neck is carefully preserved so that the risk of avascular necrosis of the femoral head is minimized. In the presence of a posterior wall fragment, displacement of the fragment permits visualization of the acetabulum. Greater than 50% detachment of the capsule around the acetabular rim is needed to inspect any significant portion of the acetabulum. Routinely in the absence of a posterior wall fragment, 60% to 70% of the periacetabular capsular origin is incised. In the presence of a small wall fragment, the adjacent capsular origin is incised until adequate visualization of the hip joint is achieved. The femoral head can be subluxed in several directions to inspect virtually the entire acetabulum. Nevertheless, the complete acetabular surface cannot be visualized simultaneously unless the femoral head is dislocated. Such a dislocation is possible only when the ligamentum teres has been traumatically or iatrogenically divided. Surgical division of the ligamentum teres is only recommended in an unusual situation where extensive acetabular comminution and displacement greatly complicates the attempt to achieve a congruent reduction. During the exposure of the posterior column as well as during manipulation of the posterior column fragments and of the femoral head, great care is taken to protect the sciatic nerve. Throughout the entire operation the knee is maintained in a position of at least 60° of flexion. The insertion of retractors into the greater sciatic notch is minimized in view of the likelihood for contusion of the nerve. Where drill bits or Steinmann pins are inserted into the posterior column, the proximity of the sciatic nerve is borne in mind to minimize the risk of impalement by a protruding pin. In a somewhat similar way during the exposure of the roof of the greater sciatic notch, or during manipulation of a posterior column fracture fragment that violates the roof of the notch, great care is taken to protect the superior gluteal neurovascular structures. When the fracture is openly reduced more than two to three weeks after injury, frequently fracture callus surrounding the gluteal structures requires meticulous removal prior to the open reduction.

## Summary

Prior to definitive management of a pelvic or acetabular fracture, the preoperative planning phase involves the procurement of appropriate diagnostic studies, determination of the need for nonoperative, limited or extensive surgical management, and rigorous definition of any surgical procedure. The injury is accurately defined and, when necessary, surgical reconstruction is meticulously planned, including the operative approach, the technique of reduction, and fixation. When multiple fractures of the pelvis and acetabulum are present and especially when other major injuries to the lower extremities are encountered, the optimal sequence of the surgical procedures is defined.

## References

1. McMurtry R, Walton D, Dickinson D, Kellam J, Tile M: Pelvic disruption in the polytraumatized patient: A management protocol. Clin Orthop 151:22, 1980.
2. Rubash H, Steed D, Mears D: Fractures of the pelvic ring. Surg Rounds 5:16, 1982.
3. Burns CM: Surgery in the resuscitation of critically injured patients. Canadian J Surg 27:461, 1984.
4. Trunkey DD: Shock trauma. Canadian J Surg 27:479, 1984.
5. Border JR: in Worth M (ed): Trauma and Sepsis in Principles and Practice of Trauma Care. Baltimore, Williams and Wilkins, 1982, pp 330-387.
6. Riska E, von Bondsdorff H, Hackkinen S, Jaroma H, Kiviluoto O, Paavilainen T: Prevention of fat embolism by early internal fixation of fractures in patients with multiple injuries. Injury 8:110, 1976.
7. Riska E, Myllynen P: Fat embolism in patients with multiple injuries. J Trauma 22:891, 1982.
8. Meek R, Vivoda E, Crichton A: Comparison of mortality of patients with multiple injuries according to method of fracture treatment. J Bone Joint Surg 63B:456, 1981.
9. Border JR: Advances in the care of the patient with blunt multiple trauma. Bull Am Col Surg 69:7, 1984.
10. Tile M: Fractures of the Pelvis and Acetabulum. Baltimore, Williams and Wilkins, 1984, p 97.
11. Letournel E, Judet R: Fractures of the Acetabulum. New York, Springer-Verlag, 1981, p 337.
12. Brav EA: Traumatic dislocation of the hip. J Bone Joint Surg 44A:1115, 1962.
13. Epstein HC: Posterior fracture-dislocations of the hip: Long-term follow-up. J Bone Joint Surg 56A:1103, 1974.
14. DeLee JC: Fractures and dislocations of the hip, in Rockwood CA, Green DP (eds): Fractures in Adults. Philadelphia, Lippincott, 1984, p 1287.
15. Mears DC: Pelvic fractures, in Edlich RF, Spyker DA (eds): Current Emergency Therapy. Norwalk, Conn, Appleton-Century-Crofts, 1984, p 124.
16. Rubash HE, Mears DC: External fixation of the pelvis, in: AAOS Instructional Course Lectures. St. Louis, Mosby, 32:329, 1983.
17. Mears DC, Rubash HE: External and internal fixation of the pelvic ring, in: AAOS Instructional Course Lectures. St. Louis, Mosby, 33:144, 1984.
18. Matta J, Anderson J, Epstein H, Henricks P: Fractures of the acetabulum: A retrospective analysis. Orthop Trans 6(3), 1982.
19. Matta J, Mehne D, Roffi R: Fractures of the acetabulum: Early results of prospective study. Orthop Trans 7(3):487-488, 1983.
20. Epstein HC: Traumatic Dislocations of the Hip. Baltimore, Williams and Wilkins, 1980.

21. Letournel E: The results of acetabular fractures treated surgically: 21 years' experience, in The Hip: Proceedings of the Seventh Open Scientific Meeting of the Hip Society. St. Louis, Mosby, 1979, p 42.
22. Letournel E: Fractures of the Acetabulum. New York, Springer-Verlag, 1981.
23. Lipscomb PR: Closed management of fractures of the acetabulum, in The Hip: Proceedings of the Seventh Open Scientific Meeting of the Hip Society. St. Louis, Mosby, 1979, p 3.
24. Mears DC, Rubash HE: The use of the extensile approach to the acetabulum. Contemp Orthop 6(2):21-31, 1983.
25. Rowe CR, Lowell JD: Prognosis of fractures of the acetabulum. J Bone Joint Surg 43A:30-59, 1961.
26. Tipton WW, D'Ambrosia RD, Garrett PR: Nonoperative management of central fracture-dislocations of the hip. J Bone Joint Surg 57A:888, 1975.
27. Mears DC, Rubash HE, Sawaguchi T: Fractures of the acetabulum, in: The Hip. vol 13. St. Louis, Mosby, in press, 1985.

# CHAPTER 7

# Approaches to the Pelvic Ring and Acetabulum

## Introduction

Previously, with the limited indications for surgical reconstruction of the pelvis and acetabulum, the appropriate exposures for this anatomical region have been an enigma to most orthopaedic surgeons. While collaboration with a general or urological surgeon remains a viable alternative, the conventional exposures employed by an abdominal surgeon or a urologist are not designed to visualize the bony pelvis. During the past decade, several standard approaches have been modified to varying degrees so that virtually all aspects of the pelvis can be visualized for the application of newly developed techniques of fixation. The standard approaches to the pelvic ring and the acetabulum are reviewed sequentially. In the presence of a complex pelvic disruption, two or more of the approaches may be needed to expose compromised portions of the pelvis.

## Approaches to the Pelvis

### Symphysis

The approach preferred by the authors is a Pfannenstiel curvilinear transverse approach, although a lower midline vertical incision can be used. For either approach the patient is placed in a supine position and a Foley catheter is inserted for intraoperative identification of the urethra and the base of the bladder. About 2cm superior to the superior pubic ramus, a curvilinear transverse incision is made (Figure 7-1). The intercrural fibers formed by the aponeurosis of the external oblique are incised parallel to the inguinal ligament. The spermatic cords are identified and loosely surrounded with vascular tapes to facilitate their intraoperative recognition. In many instances traumatic disruption of the soft tissues superficial to the symphysis permits a minimally invasive pathway to the bone with negligible devascularization. For example, one or both heads of the rectus abdominus may be avulsed from the proximal rami. Otherwise the aponeurotic insertion of one or both heads of the rectus abdominus is incised near its insertion. Subperiosteal elevation is undertaken on the superior, anterior and deep surfaces of the proximal rami. This elevation is continued in a lateral direction for 4cm to 5cm along either superior pubic ramus until sufficient exposure is achieved. With gentle dissection by the use of scissors or a blunt instrument, both obturator foramina are identified for the subsequent insertion of a tenaculum bone-holding forceps. By manual palpation the urethra with the Foley catheter is identified inferior to the symphysis or the minimally displaced ramus. An anatomical reduction of the symphysis is undertaken by approximation of the opposing rami. If the rami possess a rotational error a second bone holding forceps is applied from the superior surface of one to the inferior surface of the other superior pubic ramus. Stabilization is achieved by the use of an anteriorly or superiorly positioned 3.5mm Reconstruction Plate.

In the presence of unilateral or bilateral ramus fractures this exposure can be extended in the form of a unilateral or bilateral ilioinguinal approach to permit adequate visualization of the entire anterior portion of the pelvic ring. This method is described under the ilioinguinal acetabular approach.

To close the symphysis exposure, the rectus abdominus is repaired with large interrupted sutures. This step is simplified by flexion of the middle of the operating table and, thereby, the patient. Then the aponeurotic portion of the external oblique is carefully repaired to prevent an inguinal hernia. Subsequently, the cutaneous layers and skin are closed in a routine fashion.

## Posterior Exposure of the Sacroiliac Joint

To approach a sacroiliac joint or the adjacent posterior ilium or sacrum, a longitudinal incision is made adjacent

Figure 7-1. Pfannenstiel approach.

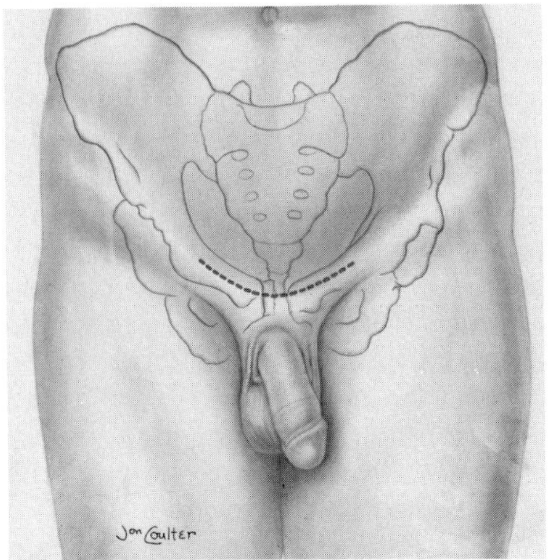


Figure 7-1A. Cutaneous incision.

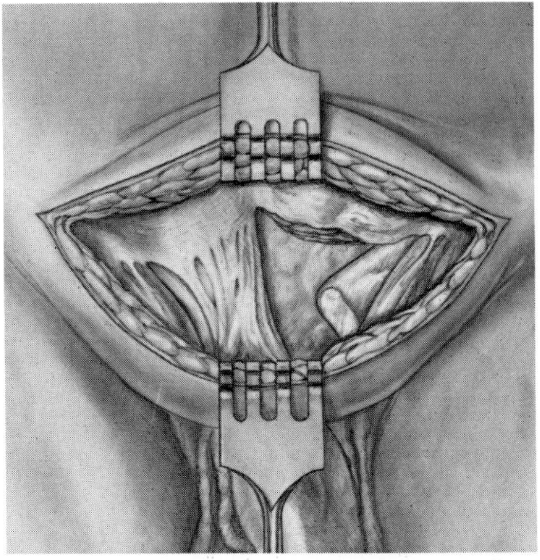

Figure 7-1B. The two parallel insertions of the rectus abdominus immediately superior to the pubic tubercles. The left one has been released.

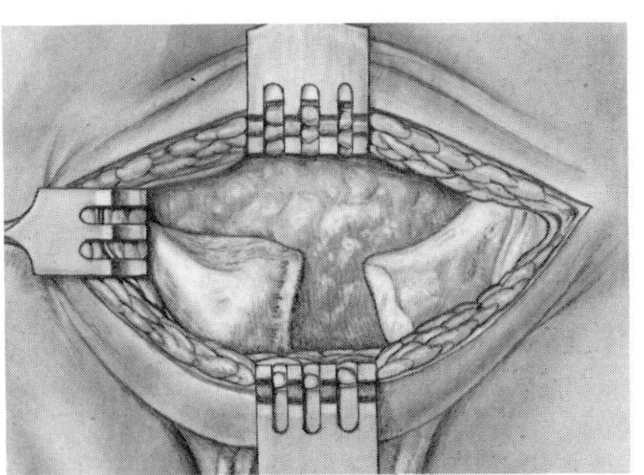

Figure 7-1C. Visualization of the disrupted symphysis.

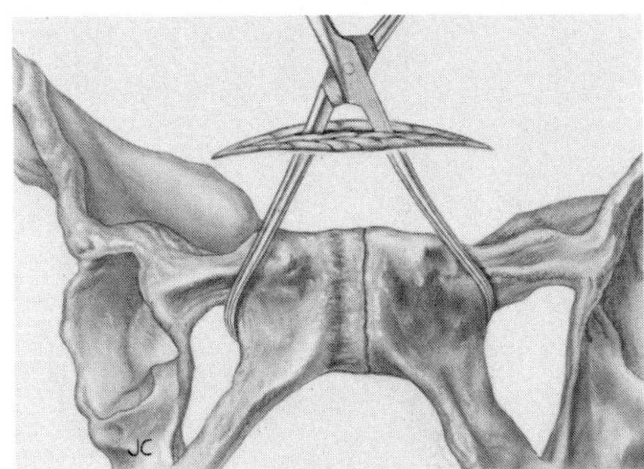


Figure 7-1D. Open reduction with tenaculum forceps inserted into the obturator foramina.

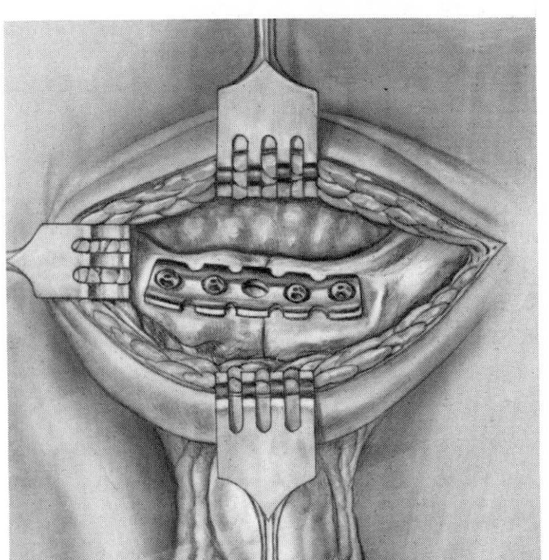

Figure 7-1E. Application of a 3.5mm Reconstruction Plate across the anterior (or superior) surface of the reduced symphysis.

to the posterior superior spine of the ilium (Figure 7-2). It is positioned more medial or lateral to facilitate the exposure of the ilium or sacrum respectively. The incision extends to the diagonal origin of the gluteus maximus. Superiorly the gluteus maximus originates on the posterior superior spine while inferiorly the origin is encountered medially on the midline of the sacrum. By sharp dissection the superior half of the origin is incised. Subperiosteal elevation in a lateral direction is undertaken by the use of an elevator to expose the superficial surface of the posterior ilium. Medial to the iliac crest, the sacroiliac joint is readily approached especially when it is compromised by an unstable disruption. The sacrum is visualized by elevation of the erector spinae and multifidus muscles. The optimal reduction of the sacroiliac joint is achieved by extension of the incision sufficiently inferiorly so that the inferior surface of the sacroiliac joint can be palpated. In the presence of a malunion, the reduction is facilitated by incision of the sacral insertion of the sacrospinous and sacrotuberous ligaments. Subsequently, closure of the wound is initiated by a gentle reposition of the erector spinae muscles and reattachment of the superior origin of the gluteus maximus.

## Exposure of Both Sacroiliac Joints or the Sacrum

Certain pelvic ring disruptions are accompanied by marked instability in the posterior portion of the pelvis, which is the crucial site for transmission of weightbearing forces from the spine to the hips and lower extremities. Bilateral unstable sacroiliac disruptions or comminuted vertical fractures of the sacrum are the two principal examples. As part of an attempt to develop improved techniques of stabilization for these challenging problems an extensile posterior incision has been developed suitable for the application of the Double Cobra plate or for an appropriately contoured 4.5mm reconstruction plate.

### *Technique*

After induction of general anesthesia the patient is turned to a complete prone position on a standard operating table. A straight or curvilinear transverse incision is made across the midportion of the sacrum about 1cm inferior to the posterior superior spines of the ilium (Figure 7-3). For the routine exposure of a bilateral sacroiliac disruption or a displaced sacral fracture, a straight transverse incision is made. If exploration of one or both sciatic nerves from the sacral foramina to the greater sciatic notch is indicated, then the ends of the incision are curved distally to facilitate

Figure 7-2. Unilateral sacroiliac approach.

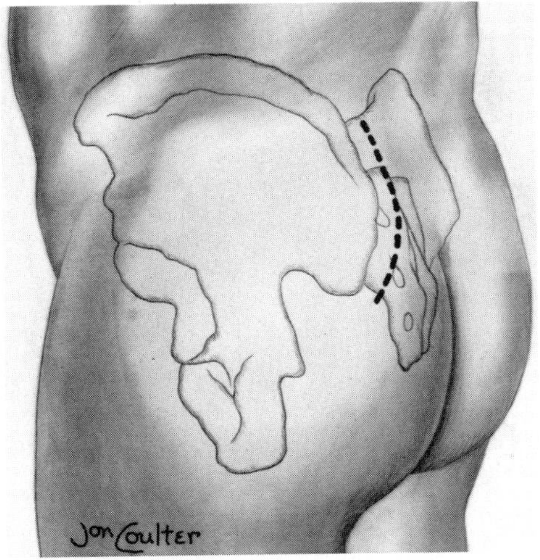

Figure 7-2A. Cutaneous incision.

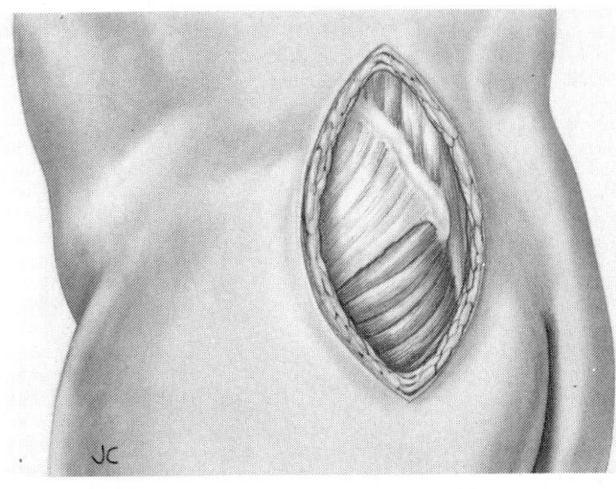

Figure 7-2B. Origin of the gluteus maximus to the posterior superior spine with medially situated paraspinous muscles.

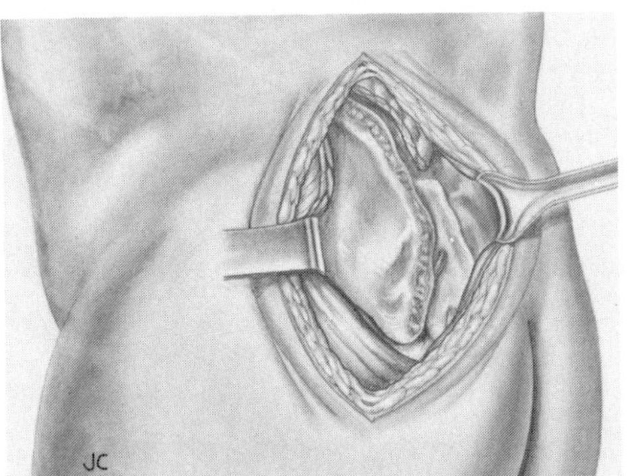

Figure 7-2C. Lateral reflection of the superior origin of gluteus maximus and medial reflection of the paraspinous muscles.

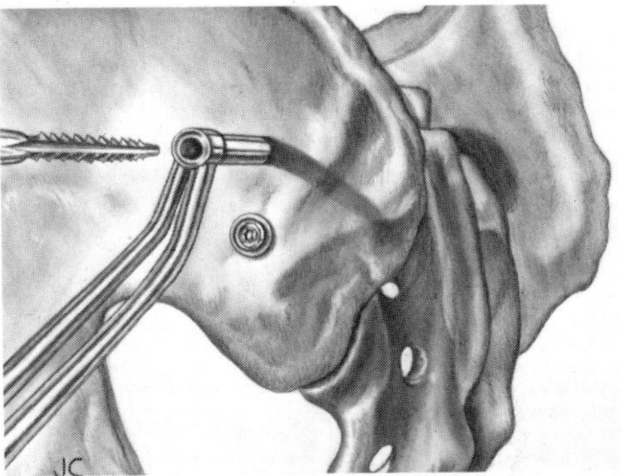

Figure 7-2D. Lag screw fixation from the posterolateral ilium to the sacral ala. Incidentally, the origin of the sciatic nerve at the greater sciatic foramen can be inspected.

such an exposure. If one or both iliac crests are to be visualized for concomitant stabilization of an iliac fracture, then the appropriate side of the incision is curved proximally. The incision is sharply extended through the deep fascia. The superior portions of the origins of gluteus maximus from the posterior superior spines are visualized. The portions of the posterior spines that extend posterior to the sacrum are osteotomized both to provide a distal and lateral reflection of the superior origin of gluteus maximus and to provide a flat surface for application of the plate. Subperiosteal elevation is undertaken on the adjacent parts of the iliac wings. The paraspinous muscles are elevated from the sacrum to either side of the posterior spinous processes. The tips of the posterior spinous processes are osteotomized from the sacrum. A subperiosteal "tunnel"

Figure 7-3. Bilateral sacroiliac or sacral approach.

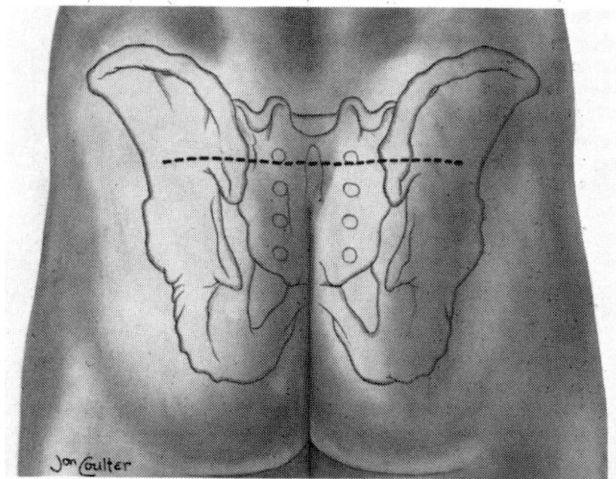

Figure 7-3A. Cutaneous incision.

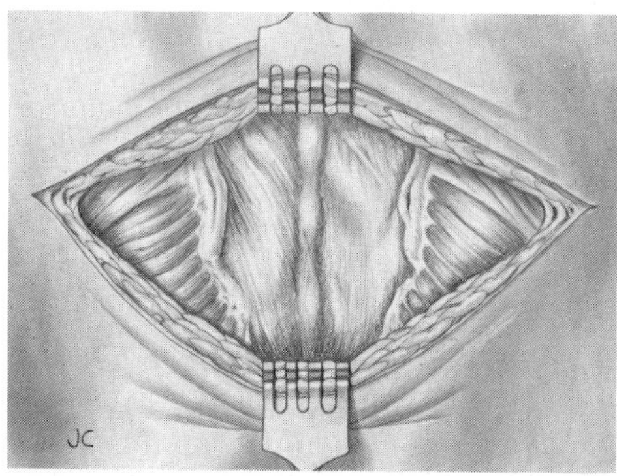

Figure 7-3B. Exposed posterior iliac crests, gluteus maximus, and paraspinous muscles.

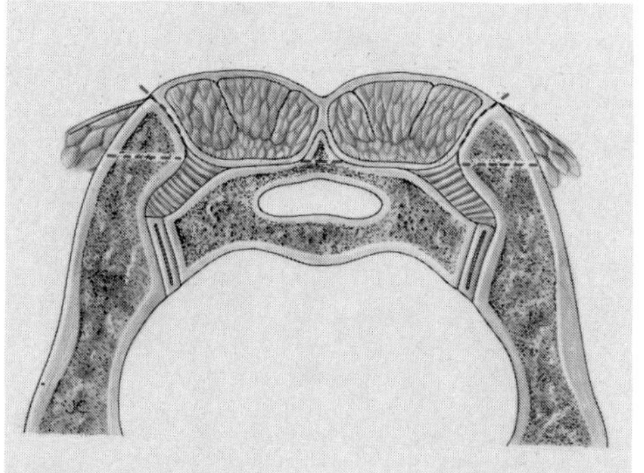

Figure 7-3C. Bilateral dissection between medial border of posterior superior spine and the paraspinous muscles.

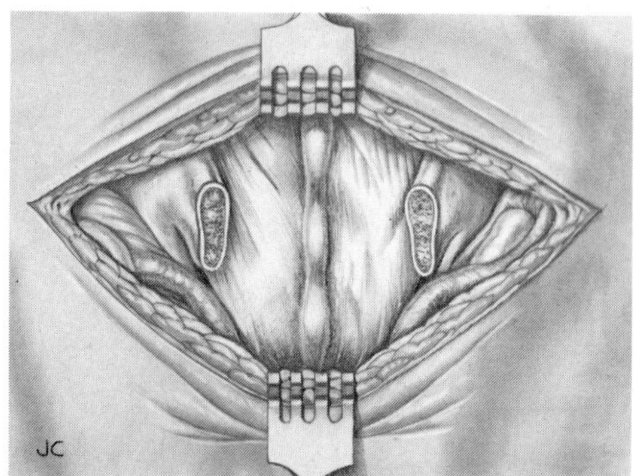

Figure 7-3D. Sites for osteotomies of the posterior superior spines also seen in Figure 7-3G.

is thereby prepared across the back of the sacrum.

The sacral fracture or the sacroiliac joints are reduced by the use of tenaculum bone-holding forceps applied to 3.2mm unicortical drill holes. After measurement of the width of the posterior pelvis adjacent to the edge of the osteotomy sites of the posterior superior spines, a Double Cobra plate of appropriate size is selected. Alternatively, in small individuals weighing less than 120lbs, a 4.5mm Reconstruction Plate of appropriate length is contoured. The plate is inserted in the tunnel deep to the paraspinous muscles and inverted into its final position. Two lengthy, 6.5mm long-threaded, cancellous screws are inserted into the posterior surfaces of the osteotomized posterior superior spines. As the plate approximates the back of the pelvis, it drives the ilia towards the interposed sacrum. Next, the three screw holes in the broadest parts of the plates are filled with 6.5mm cancellous screws of 45mm to 50mm in length. These lag screws are inserted through the ilium into the sacral ala. Finally, two or three 4.5mm cortical screws

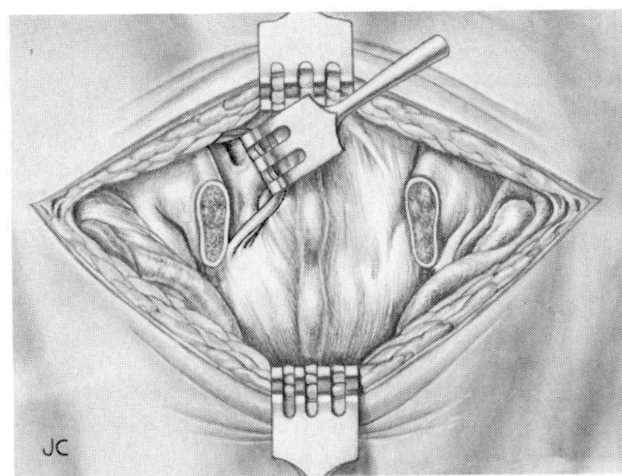


Figure 7-3E. Lateral reflection of the superior portions of the gluteus maximus muscles and preparation of subperiosteal tunnel beneath paraspinous muscles including osteotomy of sacral spinous processes.

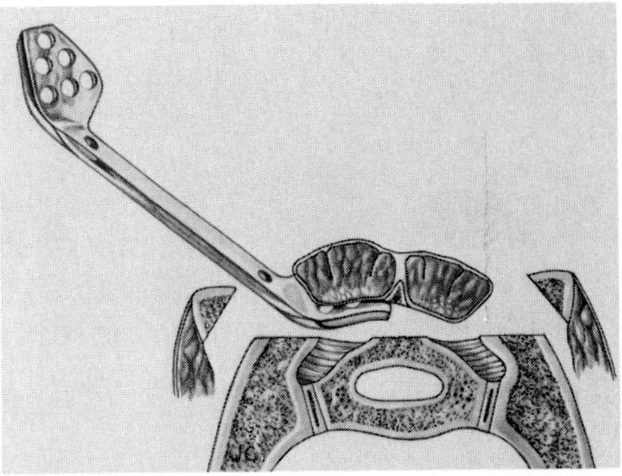

Figure 7-3F. Following the open reduction, insertion of the Double Cobra plate into the tunnel deep to the paraspinous muscles.

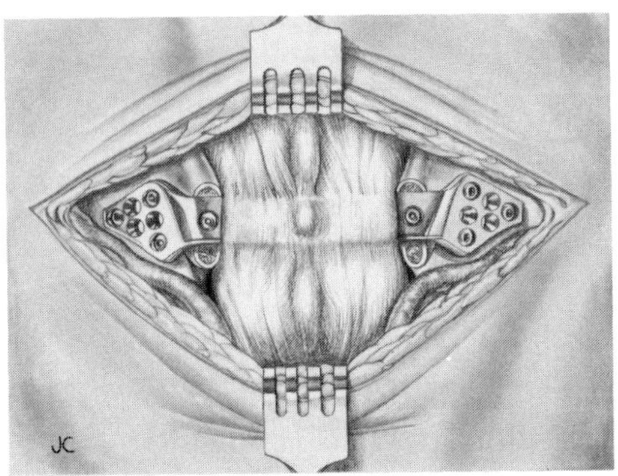


Figure 7-3G. Schematic view of the plate on the posterior pelvis in its final position.

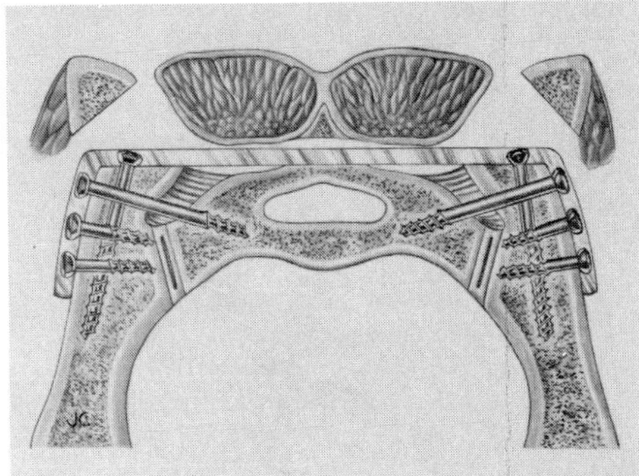

Figure 7-3H. Cross-section of screws in Double Cobra plate.

are inserted in both ends of the plates. These screws anchor the ilia to augment the rotational stability.

Prior to the closure of the wound, the corticocancellous bone fragments attached to the reflected portions of the gluteus maximus are morsalized to provide autologous bone graft for the posterior fracture site(s).

## Extensile Exposure of the Iliac Crest

The patient is placed in a full lateral position on his nontraumatized side. The lower extremity is freely draped and prepared along with the thigh so that during the surgery the extremity can be manipulated to facilitate the reduction of the fracture. A curved incision is made, which follows the iliac crest (Figure 7-4). The incision is prepared about 2cm above or below the most prominent portion of the crest. Frequently a lengthy incision is needed to adequately visualize the comminuted fracture. A typical incision extends from the anterior superior spine around the posterior superior spine to the posterior inferior spine. The region of exposure is selected by the site and extent of the fracture. The gluteal aponeurosis is incised from the iliac crest. The gluteal muscles are elevated from the outer aspect of the wing where the fracture extends into the greater sciatic notch. Subperiosteal elevation continues to the level of the notch for insertion of a blunt tipped Hohmann retractor.

In unusual cases where the ipsilateral sacroiliac joint or the superior pubic ramus adjacent to the anterior superior spine requires visualization, the insertion of the abdominal muscles to the iliac crest is incised for subperiosteal elevation of these muscles and the iliacus from the internal iliac fossa. Soft tissue elevation is continued to the lateral centimeter of sacrum. Hohmann retractors are positioned in the sacrum to maintain visualization of the sacroiliac joint. The soft tissues can be elevated to the iliopectineal line and the lateral 2cm of superior pubic ramus.

## Approaches to the Acetabulum

Once an acetabular fracture has been rigorously characterized as to the region and extent of the osseous disruption, an adequate visualization of the fracture zone is carefully planned. The fracture lines are drawn on a pelvic model although the recently developed three-dimensional computerized imaging scan provides a superior alternative to clarify fully the extent of surgical exposure that is needed. For many years, regional exposures have been available that permit adequate exposure of the posterior, anterior, or lateral aspects of the acetabulum. Gradually, subtle modifications of these incisions have been devised.

For the more complex fracture patterns that violate anterior and posterior portions of the acetabulum or extend to adjacent regions of the hemipelvis, inadequate visualization has been a frequent and formidable problem associated with the use of the conventional surgical incisions. One solution was the application of anterior and posterior incisions undertaken either simultaneously or at separate times. Nearly insurmountable technical difficulties were associated with this method. Once the anterior portion of a fracture had been exposed, reduced, and stabilized, manipulation and fixation of the posterior portion through a second incision was immeasurably complicated by the first stage of the operation. Attempts were made to devise truly extensile exposures that would permit adequate visualization of even the most complex acetabular fractures. One example is the long lateral longitudinal transtrochanteric approach,[1] which permitted satisfactory visualization of a transverse

Figure 7-4. Approach to iliac crest and lateral ilium.

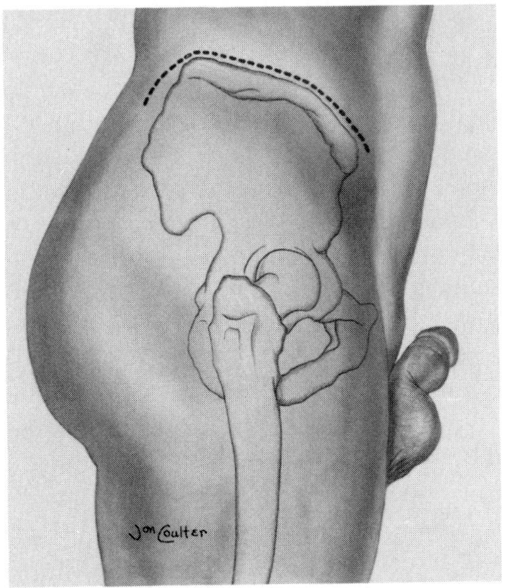


Figure 7-4A. Cutaneous incision.

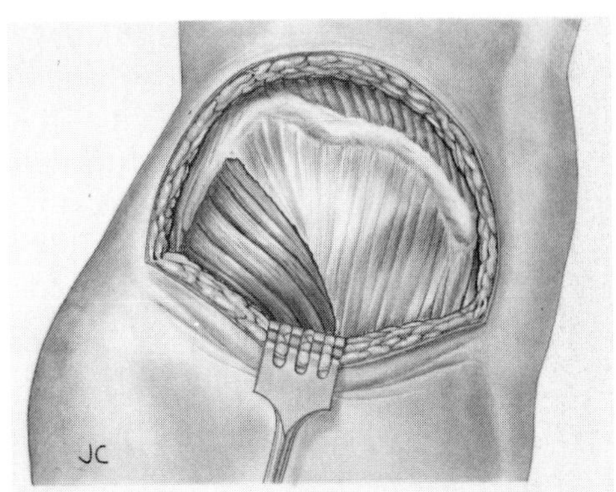


Figure 7-4B. Origins of tensor and glutei and insertions of external oblique to the iliac crest.

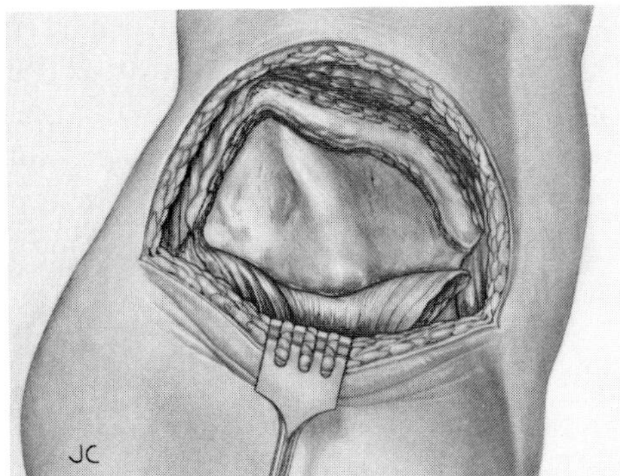


Figure 7-4C. Reflection of tensor and glutei from the iliac crest and adjacent lateral ilium.

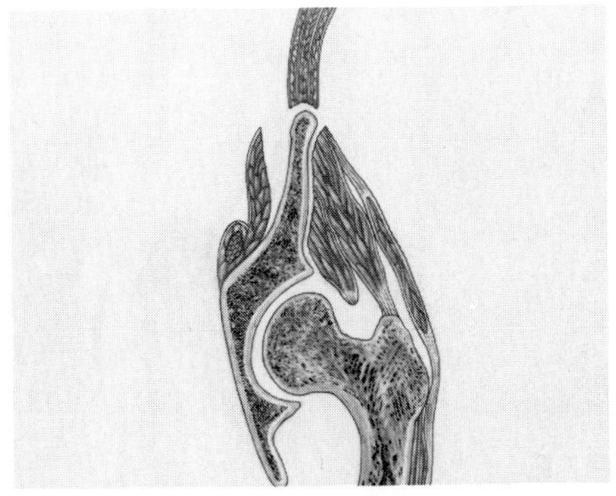

Figure 7-4D. Cross-section of ilium to show reflection of superficial and deep muscles from the ilium.

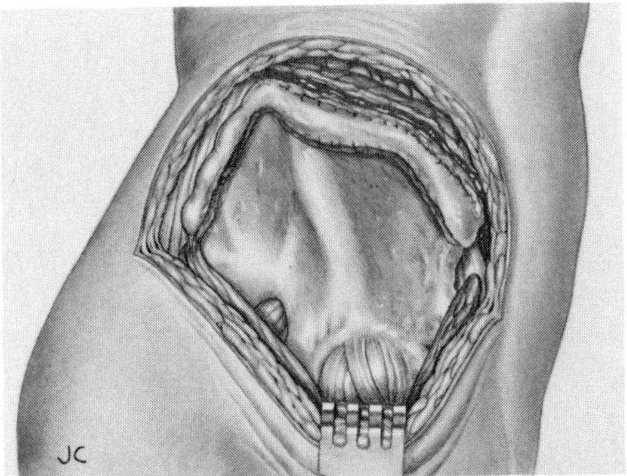


Figure 7-4E. Lateral reflection to expose the greater sciatic notch and capsule of the hip joint.

acetabular disruption. It did not permit reconstruction of the anterior column including the superior ramus or the medial wall of the acetabulum. Another example, the Senegas[2] or modified Ollier approach, shared similar assets and comparable liabilities.

Letournel[3] was encouraged to design an extended iliofemoral approach, which provides excellent exposure of the lateral ilium, acetabulum, and anterior and posterior columns. It was the first truly extensile exposure to eliminate the need for two exposures for the most complex forms of acetabular disruption. With its surgical division of the origins and insertions of the gluteus medius and minimus along the iliac crest and the greater trochanter respectively, it disrupted the blood supply of these vital hip adductors apart from the superior gluteal vessels. If these vessels were damaged as part of the initial traumatic insult or at the time of surgery, unless a satisfactory microvascular reanastomosis could be achieved, the hip abductors would undergo catastrophic ischemic necrosis. In an attempt to eliminate this potential problem and to provide an even more extensive exposure, a triradiate incision[4] with an osteotomy of the greater trochanter was developed that permits visualization of the lateral ilium, the posterior column, and the anterior column within 2cm of the midline. The greater trochanter can be reattached with lag screws to permit an early functional restoration of abductor function. In this section, examples of the exposures for virtually all types of acetabular fractures are presented.

## Anterior Exposure with the Ilioinguinal Approach

Contributed by Joel M. Matta, MD.

The ilioinguinal approach was developed by Letournel[3] as an anterior approach to the pelvis and acetabulum. It provides exposure to almost the entire inner aspect of the innominate bone from the anterior sacroiliac joint to the symphysis pubis. Also included in the exposure is the quadrilateral surface of the innominate bone and the superior and inferior pubic rami. The inner aspect of the ischium is one area not accessible through this approach. A limited exposure to the external aspect of the innominate bone is also possible, primarily to the iliac wing. A reduction of the acetabulum through this approach is done primarily without visualizing the articular aspect of the acetabulum, but rather by restoring the internal contour of the innominate bone. The approach is relatively atraumatic in that the iliacus is the only muscle stripped from the innominate bone. Since the entire hip abductor musculature is left intact, a rapid postoperative recovery is encouraged. The surgical scar is also quite cosmetic. Surgeons who are not familiar with this approach should be cautious in undertaking it for the first time, as the approach proceeds through anatomical areas that are usually unfamiliar to most orthopaedic surgeons. Once the bone is exposed, the reduction can be deceptive and proper placement of the fixation requires a thorough preoperative understanding of the fracture pattern, as well as a knowledge of the normal anatomy of the associated neurovascular structures and the hip joint itself. Prior to undertaking the ilioinguinal approach a surgeon is advised to practice on a cadaver, and to assist a surgeon who is familiar with the exposure.

Indications for the ilioinguinal approach include a fracture of the anterior wall or the anterior column, an associated anterior and posterior hemitransverse fracture, a both-column fracture, and a few types of transverse fracture.

To perform the approach, the patient is positioned supine, preferably on a fracture table with skeletal traction applied by the use of a distal femoral pin. A contraindication for the use of the fracture table is the presence of contralateral superior and inferior pubic ramus fractures that will allow deformity of the lower part of the pelvic ring due to pressure on the symphysis pubis from the perineal post. As the operation proceeds, supplementary lateral traction to the femur can be applied by resort to a traction screw, which is inserted into the trochanter and anchored to a lateral traction attachment on the fracture table. Prior to the operation, the perineal area is completely shaved. A Foley catheter is inserted into the bladder, and adhesive vinyl drapes are applied to the entire iliac crest and the trochanteric area appropriate for the possible insertion of a lateral traction screw.

The incision extends laterally from the midline of the abdomen, three centimeters above the symphysis pubis, across the lower abdomen to the anterior superior iliac spine. It continues posteriorly along the iliac crest to a point about two-thirds of the way along the iliac crest (Figure 7-5). The incision continues beyond the most lateral convexity of the iliac crest to permit an adequate mobilization of the iliopsoas and of the abdominal muscles from their origins on the iliac crest for visualization of the internal iliac fossa. The incision progresses by sharp dissection to the iliac crest without injury to the abdominal muscles that tend to overhang the midportion of the crest. The insertions of the abdominal muscles and the origin of the iliacus are sharply elevated from the crest. By a subperiosteal dissection the iliacus is elevated from the internal iliac fossa as far medially and distally as the anterior aspect of the sacroiliac joint and the pelvic brim. Fracture lines that progress from the anterior column to the ilium are immediately apparent. The internal iliac fossa is temporarily packed with surgical sponges. The incision over the lower abdomen progresses through the superficial fascia to the aponeurosis of the external oblique and the external fascia of the rectus abdominis muscle. The aponeurosis of the external oblique and subsequently the external fascia of the rectus abdominis are sharply incised in the line of the cutaneous incision at least 1cm proximal to the external inguinal ring. To open the inguinal canal, the aponeurosis of the external oblique is elevated distally in continuity with the external fascia of the rectus abdominus. Upon grasping the edge of the incised aponeurosis with surgical clamps the inguinal ligament is visualized. A sponge is used to clean the areolar tissue from the inguinal ligament.

Upon visualization of the spermatic cord or round ligament, a finger is passed posterior to the spermatic cord or round ligament to elevate it and the adjacent ilioinguinal nerve. To provide a method of retraction, a Penrose drain is placed around the spermatic cord or round ligament and the ilioinguinal nerve (Figure 7-5D) progressing from lateral to medial. At this stage, the common origin of the internal oblique and transversalis and the transversalis fascia are detached from the inguinal ligament. The inguinal ligament is sharply incised with a scalpel so that about 1mm of the ligament remains with the aforementioned structures. During this step great care is exercised to avoid injury to the structures that lie directly beneath the inguinal ligament. Upon detachment of the common origin of the internal oblique and transversalis from the inguinal ligament, the psoas sheath is entered. Immediately beneath the inguinal ligament, the lateral cutaneous nerve is situated in a variable position that may be adjacent to or up to 3cm medial to the anterior superior iliac spine. The more medial aspect of the transversalis fascia overlies the external aspect of the external iliac vessels. Upon detachment of the transversalis fascia medial to the external iliac vessels, to open the retropubic space of Retzius, the vessels are subjected to injury unless great care is exercised. Further exposure of the retropubic space is achieved by division of the conjoined tendon of the external oblique and transversalis and the tendon of the rectus abdominus at their insertions on the pubis. The external aspect of the structures that pass under the inguinal ligament are thereby exposed. The femoral nerve is found within the psoas sheath on the medial aspect of the iliopsoas (Figure 7-5E).

The structures passing under the inguinal ligament

lie within one of two compartments or lacunae. The laterally situated lacuna musculorum contains the iliopsoas, the femoral nerve, and the lateral cutaneous nerve of the thigh; the medial lacuna vasorum contains the external iliac vessels and lymphatics. The psoas sheath, or iliopectineal fascia, separates the two lacunae (Figure 7-5F). The psoas sheath is divided and elevated from the pelvic brim for mobilization of the various structures beneath the inguinal ligament and, thereby, exposure of the true pelvis and the quadrilateral surface. To expose the lateral surface of the psoas sheath, the iliopsoas and femoral nerves are retracted laterally. The lymphatics and vessels medial to the psoas sheath are carefully elevated from this fascial septum by blunt dissection with the use of a blunt tipped scissors or a hemostat. The pulse of the external iliac artery is identified adjacent to the pectineal eminence of the innominate bone, medial to the psoas sheath. Upon lateral retraction of the iliopsoas and the femoral nerve, and medial retraction of the iliac vessels and lymphatics, the psoas sheath or iliopectineal fascia is sharply incised by the use of scissors to the pectineal eminence (Figure 7-5 G, H). Subsequently with the same exposure the scissors are used to elevate the psoas sheath sharply from the pelvic brim. In some individuals this maneuver can be undertaken by the use of finger dissection, whereas in other individuals the presence of a tough fascia continuous with the insertion of the tendon of psoas minor on the pectineal eminence necessitates the use of sharp dissection.

A second Penrose drain is placed around the iliopsoas, femoral nerve, and lateral cutaneous nerve of the thigh for subsequent retraction of these structures. The insertion of a finger beneath the iliac vessels, from lateral to medial, and anterior to the superior pubic ramus, permits the application of a Penrose drain around the external iliac vessels and the adjacent lymphatics. The lymphatics and areolar tissue surrounding the vessels are left intact to avoid postoperative impairment of the lymphatic drainage.

Prior to retraction of the external iliac vessels, a search is made medial and posterior to the vessels for the obturator artery and nerve, and for the presence of an anomalous origin of the obturator artery. Occasionally, the obturator artery originates from the inferior epigastric artery rather than the internal iliac artery. This anomalous origin is referred to as the corona mortise. If this anomalous obturator artery is present, it is clamped, ligated, and divided to avoid a subsequent avulsive type of traction injury.

By medial retraction of the iliopsoas, the internal iliac fossa and adjacent pelvic brim can be exposed (Figure

Figure 7-5. Ilioinguinal approach.

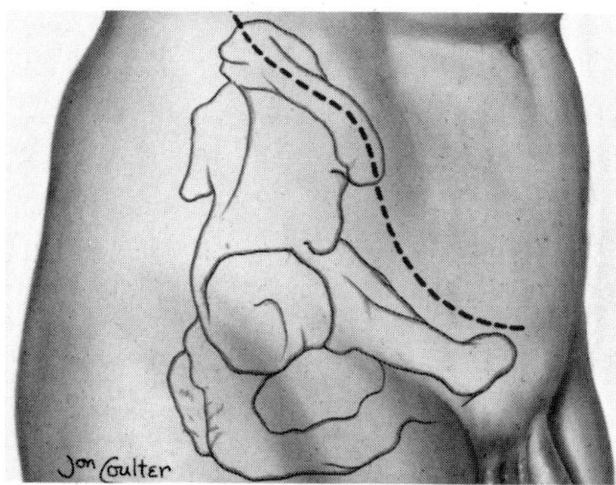


Figure 7-5A. Cutaneous incision.

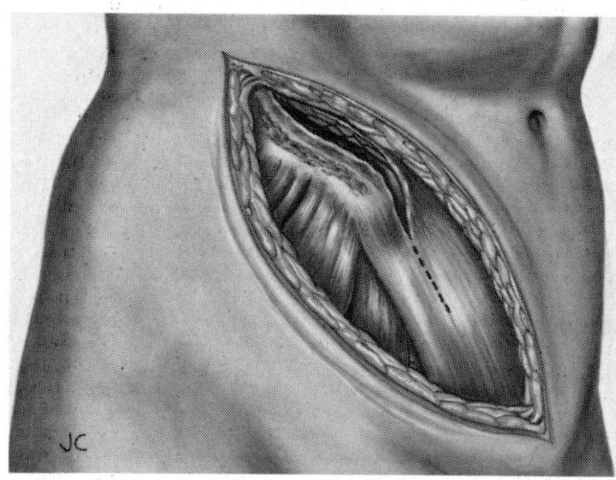


Figure 7-5B. Exposure of the iliac crest with the adjacent aponeurosis of the external oblique medially and hip musculature anteriorly and laterally.

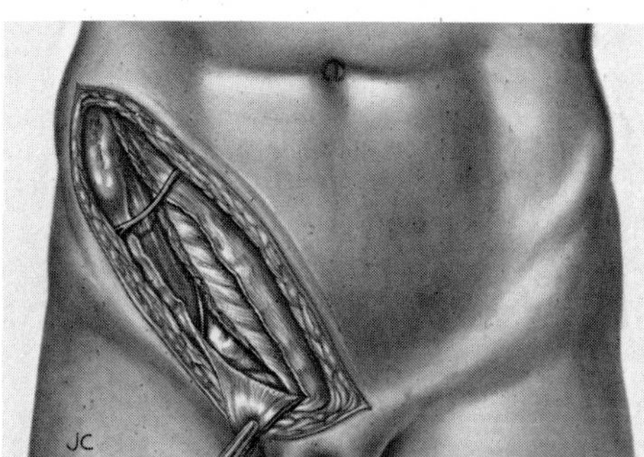


Figure 7-5C. Reflection of iliacus from the iliac crest and incision of the aponeurosis of the external oblique provides exposure of the lateral femoral cutaneous nerve of the thigh.

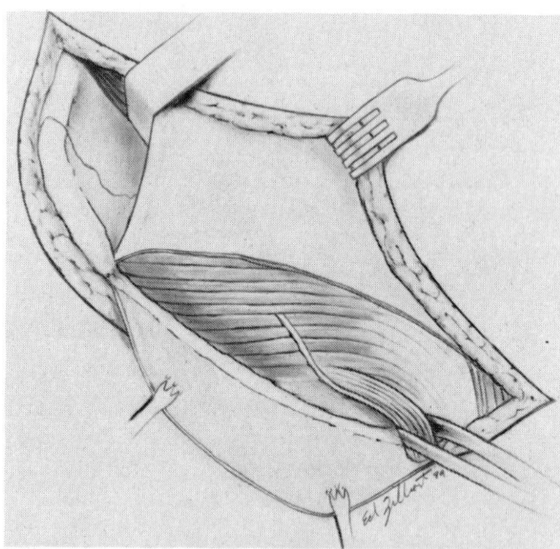

Figure 7-5D. The iliacus has been stripped from the internal iliac fossa, and the aponeurosis of the external oblique has been incised and reflected distally, unroofing the inguinal canal.

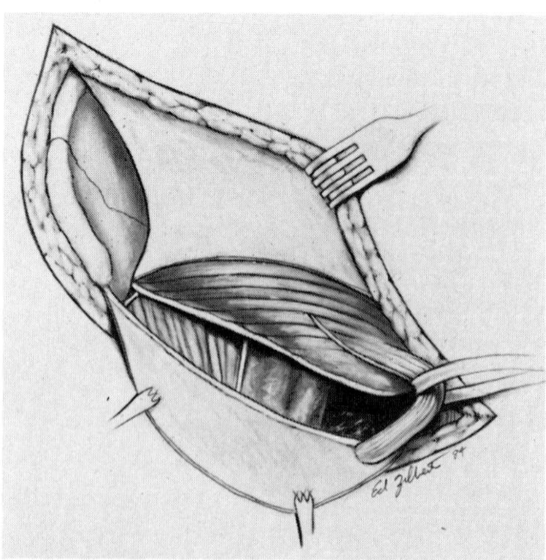

Figure 7-5E. The common origin of the external oblique and transversalis muscles and transversalis fascia have been released from the inguinal ligament.

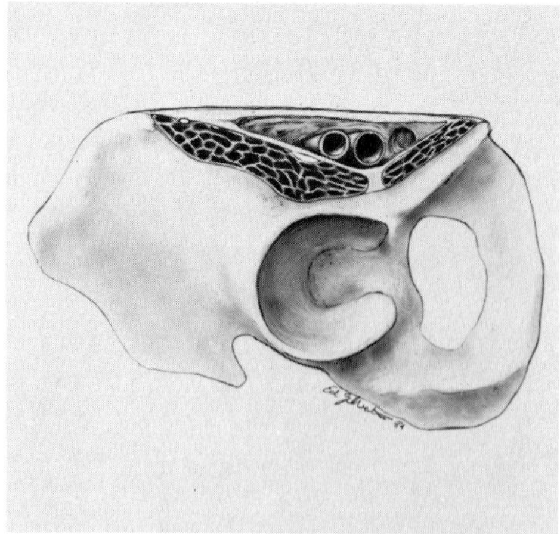

Figure 7-5F. Cross-sections of lacuna musculorum and lacuna vasorum. The iliopectineal fascia separates the two lacunae.

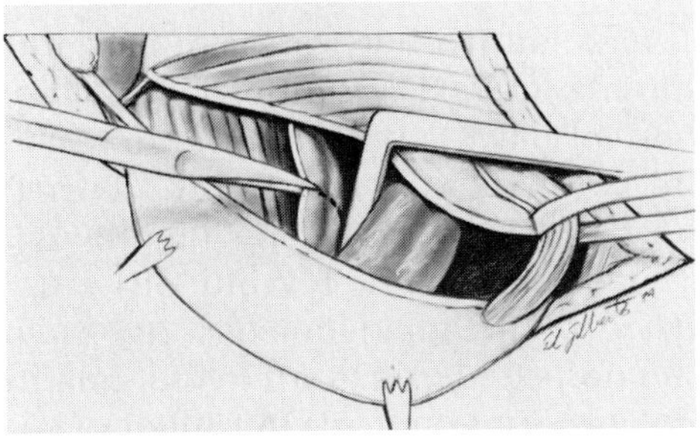

Figure 7-5G. Incision of the iliopectineal fascia toward the pectineal eminence.

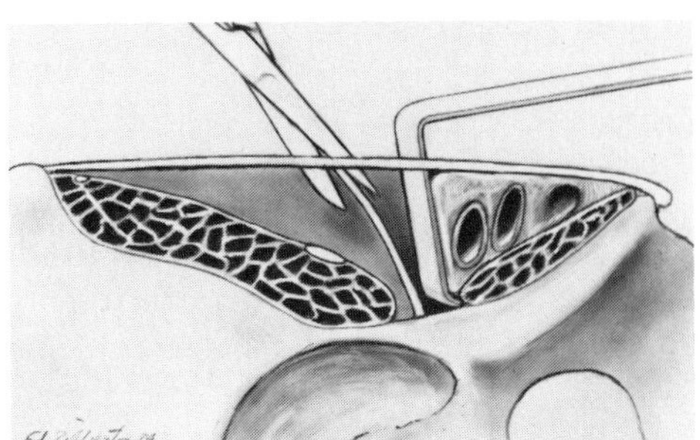

Figure 7-5H. Cross-section of incision of the iliopectineal fascia.

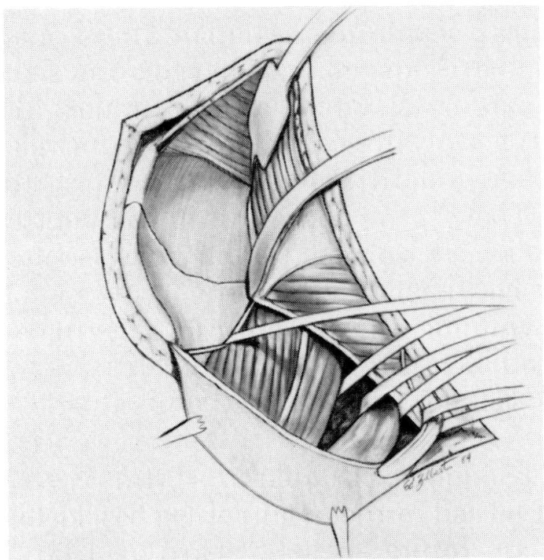

Figure 7-5I. Retraction of the iliopsoas medially to expose the internal iliac fossa.

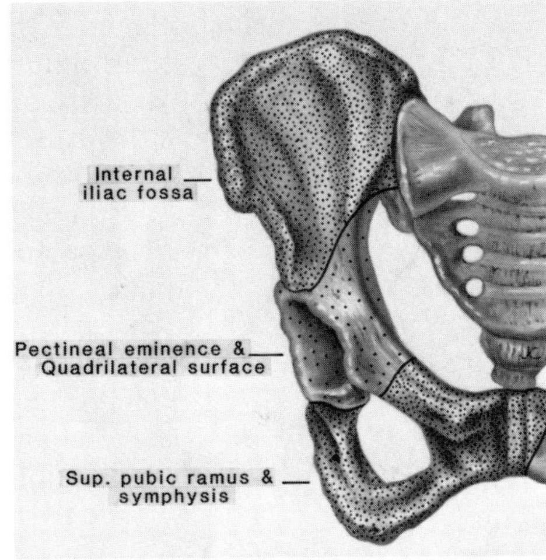


Figure 7-5J. Schematic view of the three regions exposed during various stages of the procedure.

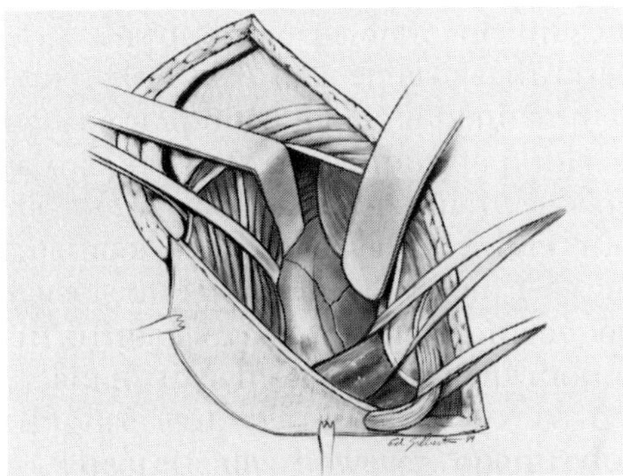

Figure 7-5K. Retraction of the iliopsoas and femoral nerve laterally and external iliac vessels medially to expose the pelvic brim, pectineal eminence and sacroiliac joint.

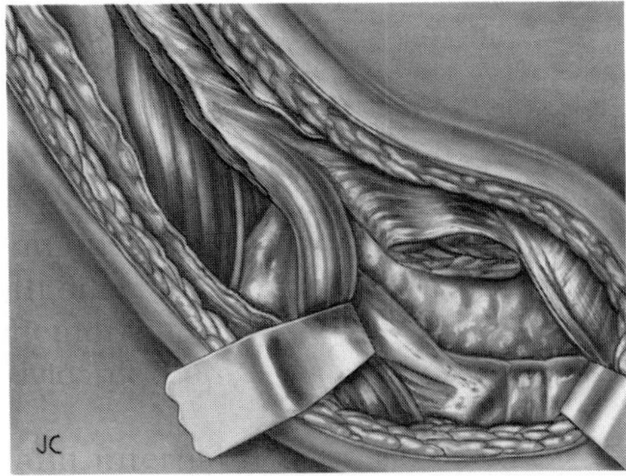

Figure 7-5L. Lateral retraction of the external iliac vessels to expose the medial aspect of the superior pubic ramus and the symphysis pubis.

7-5 I, J). By subperiosteal elevation along the pelvic brim, the fracture lines are visualized with lateral and posterior progression to the quadrilateral surface as necessary. Excessively proximal elevation along the quadrilateral surface inadvertently can provoke an injury to branches of the internal iliac or gluteal vessels or to the main branch of the internal iliac vein. To augment the exposure of the superior pubic ramus, the external iliac vessels are retracted in a lateral direction by manipulation of the Penrose drain. Subperiosteum dissection along the superior aspect of the superior pubic ramus including a release of the origin of the pectineus muscle completes the exposure.

Reduction and fixation of the acetabular fracture is now performed through the various apertures that are available between the several muscular and neurovascular structures that cross the operative field. Medial retraction of the iliopsoas provides access to the entire internal iliac fossa and distally along the anterior column as far as the most superior aspect of the pectineal eminence. The exposure is augmented by the insertion of the tip of a broad Hohmann retractor into the anterior aspect of the sacroiliac joint, with a second similar retractor applied over the pelvic brim.

Lateral retraction of the iliopsoas and femoral nerve combined with medial retraction of the external iliac vessels (Figure 7-5 K) provides access to the entire pelvic brim distally to the origin of the superior pubic ramus, the anterior wall of the acetabulum, the quadrilateral surface, and the superior lateral aspect of the obturator foramen adjacent to the obturator nerve and artery. Medially, retraction is facilitated by the insertion of a malleable ribbon retractor with its tip on the quadrilateral surface near the sciatic notch. During the retraction, the pulse of the external iliac artery is checked periodically. If the pulse is stopped the force of the retraction is lessened. The iliopsoas along with the femoral nerve may be retracted relatively firmly, as a traction injury of the femoral nerve secondary to retraction is rarely seen. Lateral retraction of the iliopsoas and femoral nerve combined with medial retraction of the external iliac vessels provides excellent access to the internal aspect of the innominate bone that cannot be rivaled by the use of any other approach. In most complete column fractures, almost the entire quadrilateral surface remains contiguous with the posterior column. Reduction of the quadrilateral surface with respect to the anterior column thereby provides a reduction of the posterior column. The fracture line between the posterior column and the adjacent ilium may be palpated with a finger where it enters the greater sciatic notch.

Lateral retraction of the iliac vessels with medial

retraction of the spermatic cord provides access to the superior pubic ramus and the superior aspect of the obturator foramen with the obturator vessels and nerve. Lateral retraction of the spermatic cord provides access to the medial aspect of the superior pubic ramus and the symphysis pubis (Figure 7-5 L).

Limited access to the external aspect of the iliac wing is obtained by detachment of the inguinal ligament and sartorius from the anterior superior iliac spine, and elevation of the tensor fascia lata and gluteal muscles from the external aspect of the iliac wing. This maneuver facilitates a reduction of some anterior column fractures and the insertion of a screw from the lateral aspect of the ilium distally along the anterior column into the superior pubic ramus. A substantial muscular attachment to each principal osseous fragment is carefully preserved to avoid devitalization of the bone.

At the completion of the operation, a suction drainage tube is placed in the retropubic space and the internal iliac fossa beyond the pelvic brim to the quadrilateral surface. Heavy sutures are employed to secure the abdominal fascia to the fascia lata along the iliac crest. During this repair vigorous traction is applied to avoid the tendency of the abdominal fascia to retract proximally and posteriorly. The tendon of the rectus abdominis is reattached to the periosteum of the pubis. The transversalis fascia and the common origin of the internal oblique and transversalis are reattached to the inguinal ligament. The narrow strip of inguinal ligament that was harvested with these structures aids in a solid repair. The psoas sheath or iliopectineal fascia that formerly separated the iliopsoas from the iliac vessels is not repaired. Upon closure of the external fascia of the rectus abdominis as well as the aponeurosis of the external oblique, the subcutaneous layer and the skin are repaired in a conventional manner.

Forty-eight hours afterwards the suction drains are removed and active motion exercises of the hip are initiated. Within two to five days, a partial weightbearing gait is encouraged.

Contribution concludes.

## Bilateral Ilioinguinal Anterior Approach

For extensile exposure of the entire anterior half of the pelvic ring including both superior pubic rami, the symphysis, the iliac fossae and the anterior aspect of the sacroiliac joints, a bilateral ilioinguinal incision is employed. With minor modification the contralateral extension of the incision is performed as a mirror image of the ipsilateral portion (Figure 7-6). The cutaneous incision courses from the anterior superior spine across

Figure 7-6. The bilateral ilioinguinal approach.

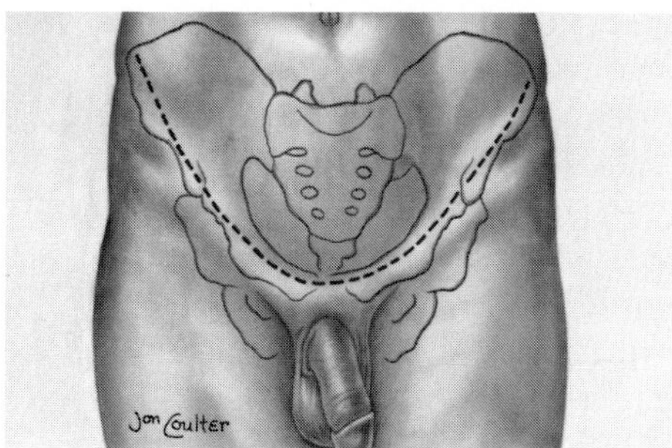

Figure 7-6A. Cutaneous incision.

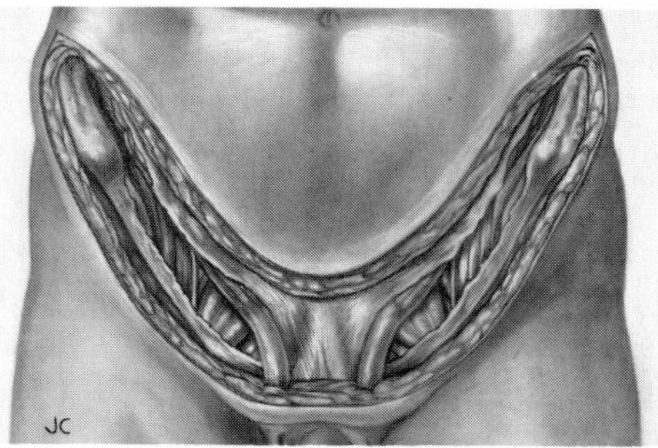

Figure 7-6B. Reflection of the skin deep to the anterior iliac crests with incision of the aponeurosis of both external oblique muscles permits visualization of the iliacus, psoas muscle with the overlying femoral nerve, the external iliac vessels, and the rectus abdominus.

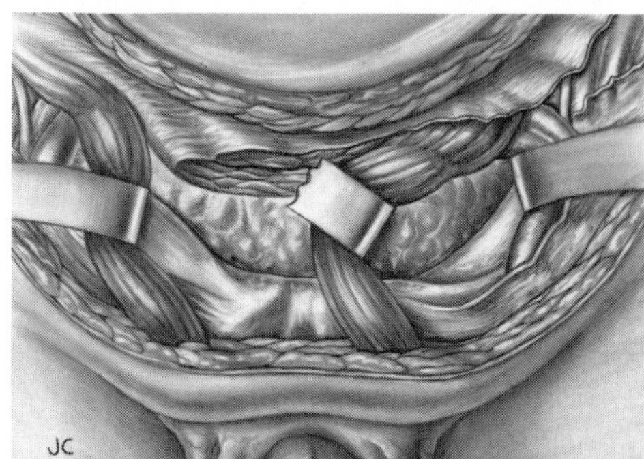

Figure 7-6C. Upon release of the insertions of rectus abdominus and lateral retraction of the external iliac vessels, the symphysis pubis with the adjacent superior pubic rami are visualized.

the superior border of the symphysis to the opposite anterior superior spine. Depending upon the need for exposure of the posterior part of the iliac fossa, the sacroiliac joint and the quadrilateral surface one or both ends of the cutaneous incision are continued posteriorly along the lateral iliac crests. Upon exposure of the iliac crests the aponeurosis of both external oblique muscles is incised. In the midline the insertions of the rectus abdominus muscles on the superior pubic rami are visualized. One or both heads are incised to complete the medial visualization of the symphysis and the adjacent superior pubic rami. The more peripheral parts of the incision are developed as previously described under the unilateral ilioinguinal approach.

## Modified Smith-Petersen or Iliofemoral Anterior Approach

Another suitable exposure for an anterior column fracture is a modified Smith-Petersen approach, in which the muscles on the inner wall of the ilium are elevated. Letournel[3] has further improved this approach and

Figure 7-7. The modified Smith-Petersen or iliofemoral approach.

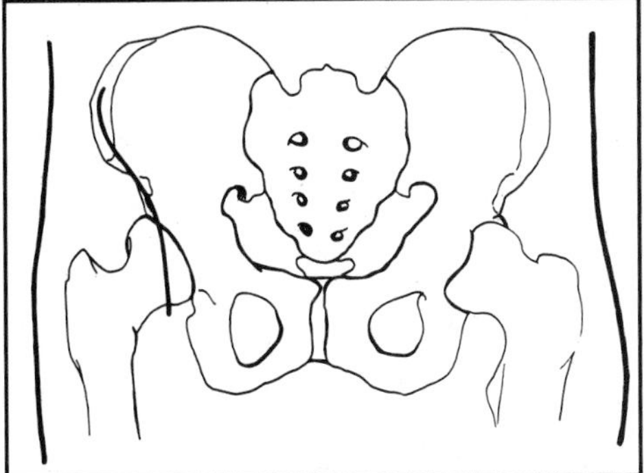

Figure 7-7A. Cutaneous incision.

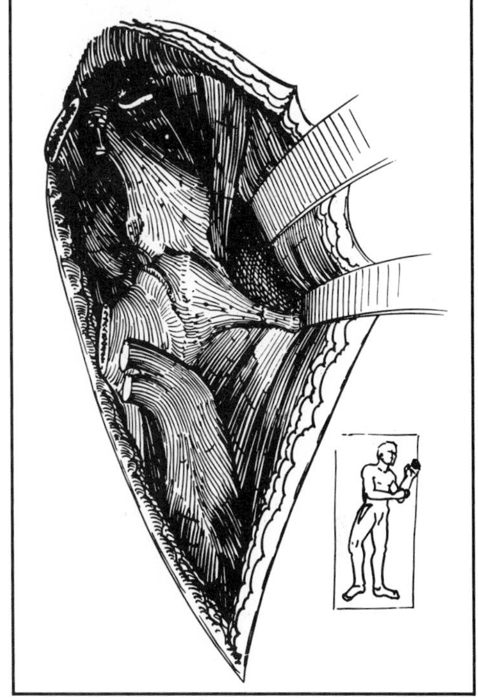

Figure 7-7B. Upon release of the sartorius, rectus femoris, and iliopsoas with medial retraction of the iliacus, the anterior aspect of the hip joint is visualized.

renamed it the iliofemoral approach (Figure 7-7). Here, the inferior extent of the incision from the level of the anterior superior iliac spine follows the sartorius along its medial border while the musculature on the external face of the iliac wing is preserved. The anterior abdominal musculature is incised from the iliac crest and the iliac fossa is exposed by elevation of the iliacus muscle. The cutaneous or external branch of the lateral femoral cutaneous nerve of the thigh is divided. To provide greater access to the anterior column, the iliopsoas tendon can be incised. In this way, the iliofemoral approach provides a visualization of the iliac crest, the superior portion of the anterior column and the superior pubic ramus, but not of the symphysis. Posteriorly, exposure of the ilium to the sacroiliac joint is possible, including a limited access to the inner wall of the true pelvis and the quadrilateral surface. During this exposure, the femoral nerve and vessels as well as the preserved branches of the lateral cutaneous nerve of the thigh are carefully protected. Subsequently, a routine anatomical closure is undertaken including, when necessary, a repair of the psoas musculature.

Finally, a similar exposure to the anterior column as in the iliofemoral approach can be obtained by the use of the anterior limb of the triradiate approach, which is discussed under *Extensile Exposures.* In this triradiate exposure, however, the lateral femoral cutaneous nerve of the thigh can be retracted. A curvilinear incision is made from the greater trochanter across the anterior superior spine. The muscular attachments on the anterior iliac crest including the origin of sartorius are incised. The myofascia of the tensor fascia is incised along the line of the cutaneous incision. The anterior border of the tensor fascia lata is incised from the adjacent fascia and reflected posteriorly along with the abductors after the trochanter is osteotomized. The direct head and, if necessary, the indirect head of rectus femoris are incised from the anterior inferior spine and the adjacent lateral ilium, and are reflected in an anterior direction. The musculature on the inner aspect of the ilium is elevated. When necessary the interval on the medial aspect of the iliopsoas can be developed to expose the superior pubic ramus. This extension of the incision is undertaken similarly to a comparable development of the ilioinguinal approach, although it does not permit a visualization of the symphysis. For the closure, the rectus femoris and sartorius are reattached to the pelvis by the use of large sutures inserted into 2-mm drill holes in the bone. The fascia of the tensor fascia lata is carefully repaired.

## Posterior Approach to the Acetabulum

Of the numerous posterior approaches previously utilized to expose a fracture of the acetabulum, the combination of a Langenbeck approach and a Kocher approach described as the Kocher-Langenbeck[3] approach provides adequate access for a wide variety of fractures of the posterior wall and posterior column (Figure 7-8). The operation is performed with the patient lying prone or preferably in a lateral position. If a fracture table is used in combination with a supracondylar traction pin, the knee is maintained in at least 45° of flexion to avoid excessive distraction on the sciatic nerve. The incision extends from the superior border of the greater trochanter toward the posterior superior iliac spine. While it usually terminates within 6cm to 8cm of the posterior superior spine, it can be continued directly to the spine. The incision can be extended distally along the outer surface of the thigh for approximately 6cm to 10cm.

The superficial fascia is divided in line with the cutaneous incision for the entire length of the incision. The gluteus maximus is bluntly split in line with its fibers. The branch of the inferior gluteal nerve to the upper part of the gluteus maximus is carefully protected to avoid paralysis of the corresponding part of the muscle. This hazard increases with more superior and medial extension of the dissection. Identification of the sciatic nerve is achieved by following the inferior border of the

Figure 7-8. The Kocher-Langenbeck posterior approach.

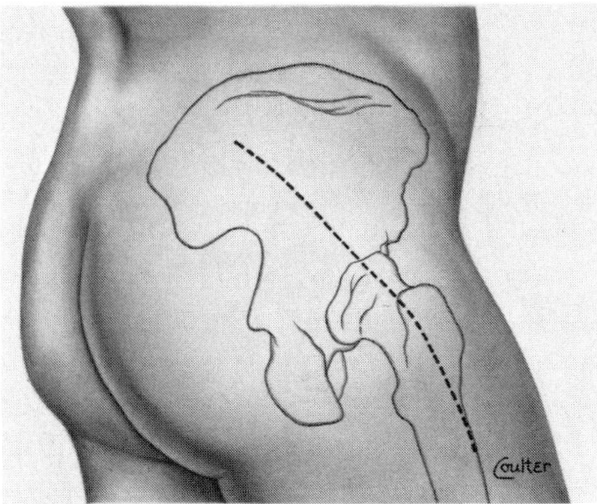

Figure 7-8A. Cutaneous incision.

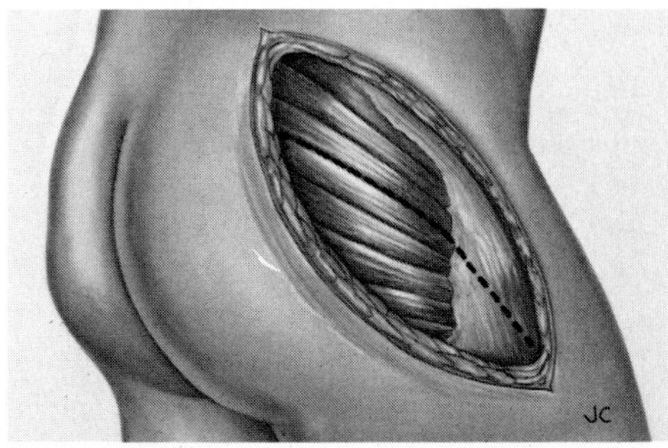

Figure 7-8B. The line of incision of the fascia lata and of the splitting of the gluteus maximus muscle is shown.

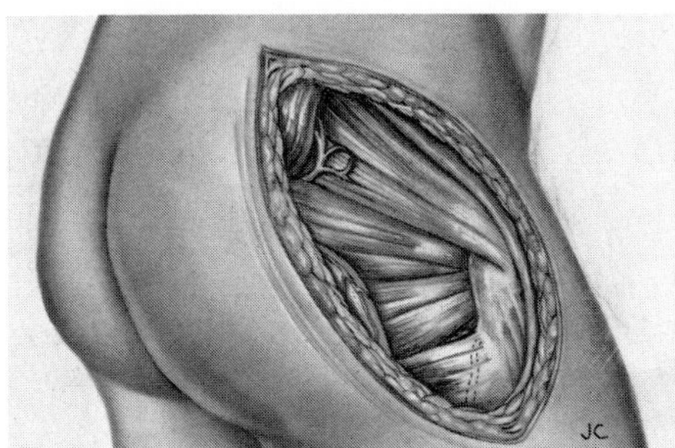

Figure 7-8C. Upon retraction of the gluteus maximus, the short externalrotators of the hip along with the sciatic nerve and gluteal vessels are revealed.

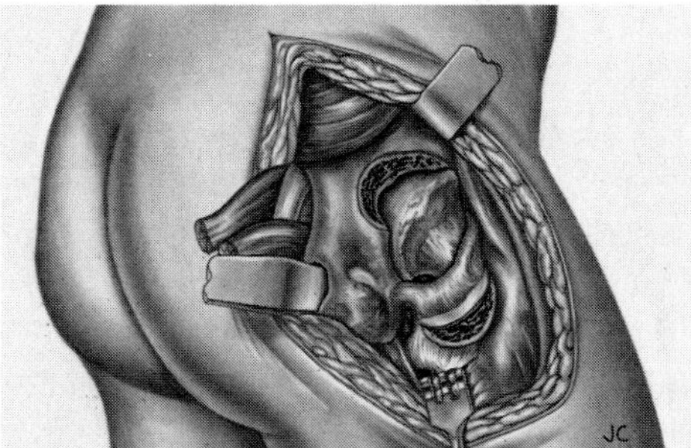

Figure 7-8D. Incision of the tendinous insertions of the piriformis and gemellae with posterior reflection of the short external rotators permits visualization of the posterior column and the capsule of the hip joint. Here, the capsule with the adjacent posterior wall fragment has been detached from the acetabular rim to permit a view of the acetabulum and femoral head.

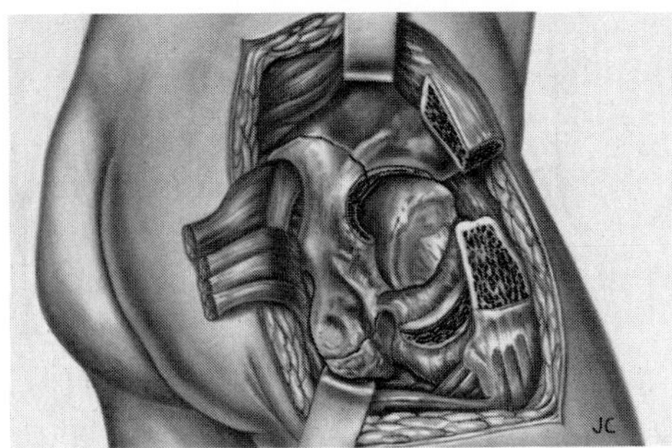

Figure 7-8E. The exposure is substantially enlarged by ostectomy of the greater trochanter and reflection of the origins of the hamstrings from the ischial tuberosity.

the quadratus femoris muscle in a medial direction. When necessary, removal of impaling bone fragments or a neurolysis of the sciatic nerve is performed. Occasionally the tendinous insertion of the gluteus maximus on the femur is incised to facilitate exposure of the inferior pubic ramus distal to the ischial tuberosity. The piriformis, obturator internus, and gemellae are incised from the greater trochanter and retracted medially where they provide protection for the sciatic nerve. The posterior column is visualized to the ischial tuberosity where the origin of semimembranosus is sharply elevated. Subperiosteal elevation of the gluteus minimus and medius is undertaken on the posterior and lateral ilium. The muscles can be retracted by the insertion of smooth Steinmann pins in the ilium 2cm and 5cm respectively above the roof of the greater sciatic notch. At the level of the greater sciatic notch, the superior gluteal nerve and gluteal vessels are identified and carefully protected. The exposure provides access to the whole posterior column medial to the greater and lesser sciatic notches, the ischial spine, and, by finger dissection, the inner wall of the pelvis. Incision of the sacrospinous ligament or osteotomy of its adjacent osseous insertion on the ischial spine augments the exposure of the inner wall of the pelvis although it compromises a substantial pelvic ligamentous support. By inferior dissection the ischiopubic ramus can be followed for at least 5cm beyond the ischial tuberosity. Further lateral extension of the incision can be achieved by osteotomy and elevation of the greater trochanter. Prior to a closure of the incision, a drain is inserted into the posterior wound adjacent to the bone. The short external rotators are reattached to their insertions on the posterior trochanteric crest. Finally the myofascia and subcutaneous tissues are closed. If the greater trochanter is osteotomized, it is reattached with two 6.5mm long-threaded cancellous lag screws anchored into the calcar femoralis.

## Extensile Acetabular Approaches

If there is involvement of both the anterior and posterior columns, a transverse acetabular fracture, or a "T" fracture, a more extensive visualization of the lateral ilium, rami, and acetabulum generally is required. Previously, various authors have employed separate anterior and posterior approaches to permit complete visualization of the fracture. An example is the use of a Kocher-Langenbeck posterior approach with an iliofemoral or ilioinguinal anterior approach. Whether the two approaches were performed at one operation or

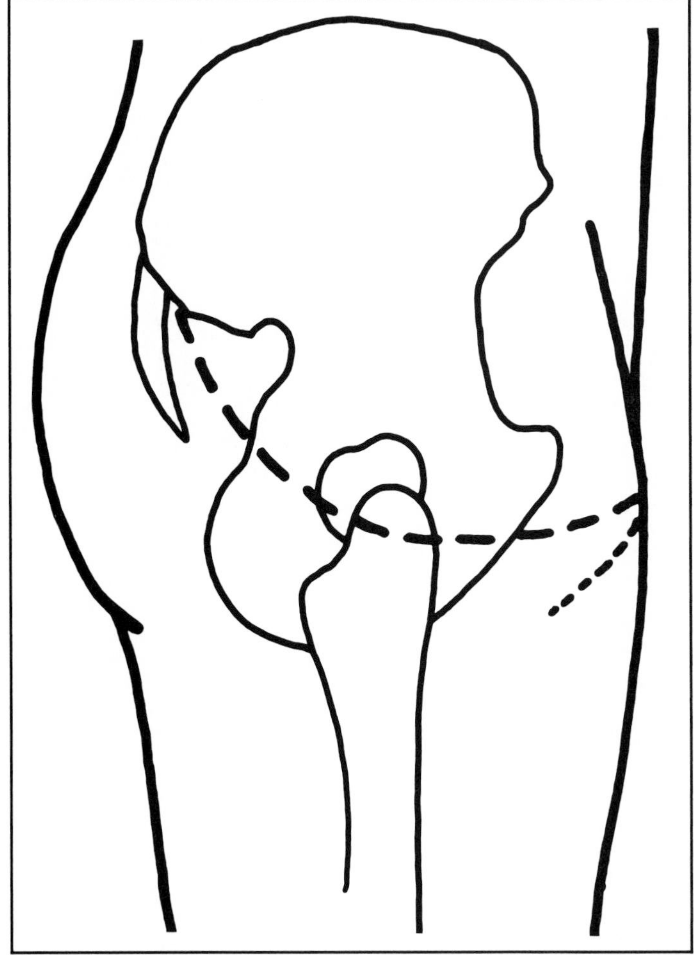

Figure 7-9. The Senegas extensile approach.

sequentially with a few intervening days, this method possesses considerable shortcomings. Frequently, the reduction and fixation of one portion of the fracture greatly complicates the later attempt to reduce and stabilize the other part of the fracture. Subsequently, several workers developed truly extensile approaches to the acetabulum, most of which are transtrochanteric routes.

## Senegas Approach

Senegas[2] has popularized a modified Ollier approach. The surgical incision extends from the posterior superior iliac spine to the midportion of the greater trochanter anteriorly around the anterior and medial aspect of the thigh and inferior to the middle of the superior pubic ramus (Figure 7-9). The posterior incision splits the gluteus maximus muscle, osteotomizes the greater trochanter, and proceeds anteriorly to transect the tensor fascia lata to the level of the femoral sheath. The superior portion of this flap is extended to expose the superior

Figure 7-10. The transtrochanteric lateral approach.

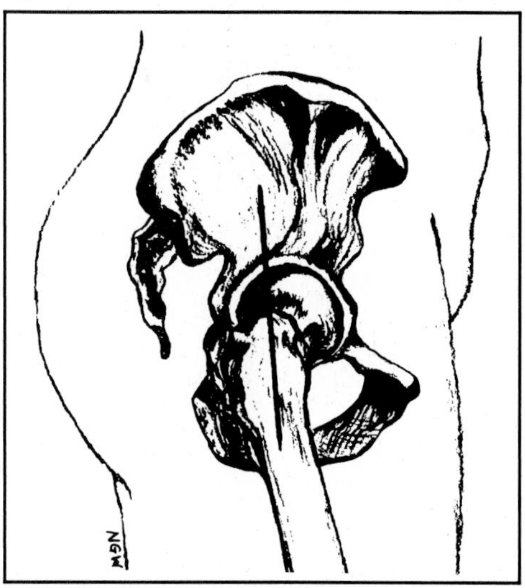

Figure 7-10A. Cutaneous incision. A more proximal straight or curved extension may be needed in some cases.

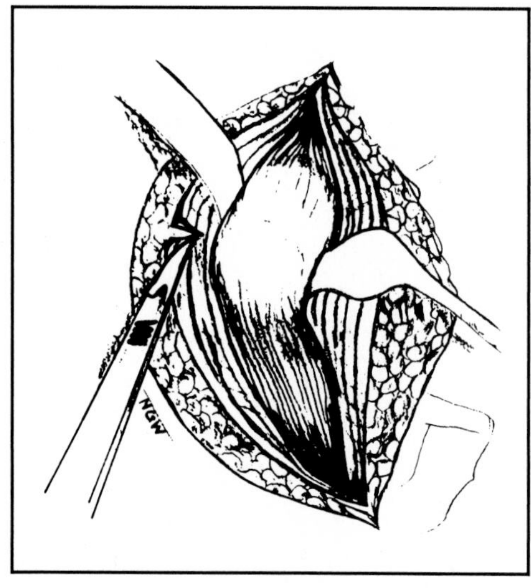

Figure 7-10B. Incision and reflection of the tensor fascia, fascia lata, and myofascia of the gluteus maximus. A posterior release of the fascia lata, shown here, greatly augments the exposure.

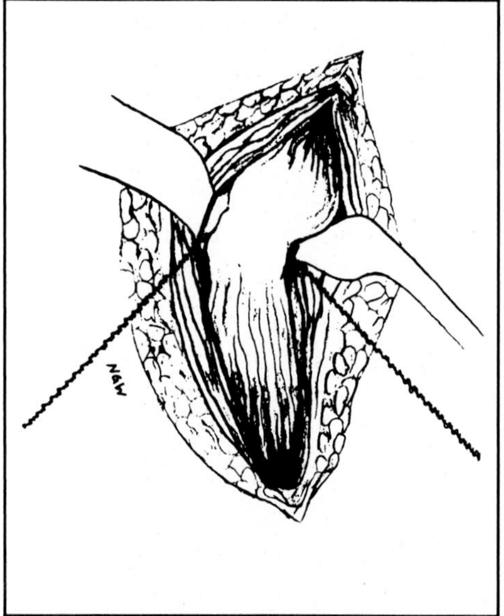

Figure 7-10C. Osteotomy of the greater trochanter with a gigli saw, or an osteotome.

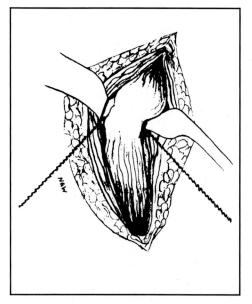

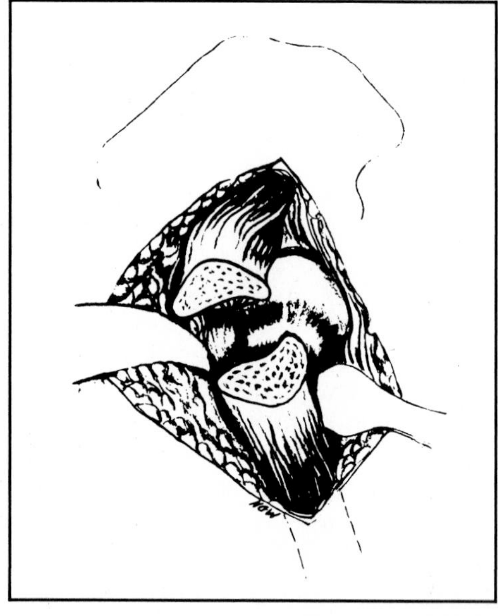

Figure 7-10D. Upon superior traction of the greater trochanter the capsule of the hip joint is incised around the acetabular rim. Once the capsule is reflected distally, the femoral head and adjacent acetabulum can be visualized.

aspect of the acetabulum. Next, the short external rotators are detached from their insertions on the greater trochanter. Sufficient exposure of the posterior column is undertaken to provide a complete visualization of the fracture. In addition, detachment of the rectus femoris both from the anterior inferior iliac spine and the superior acetabulum is undertaken to expose the origin of the superior ramus. This exposure is hampered by its limited access to the anterior column, which impedes attempts to reduce and stabilize those fractures that violate this region.

### Transtrochanteric Lateral Approach

A second transtrochanteric lateral approach employs a straight lateral longitudinal incision extending distally from the superior iliac crest across the midpoint of the greater trochanter to a variable level on the lateral aspect of the femur (Figure 7-10). The tensor fascia and the myofascia of gluteus maximus are split in line with the incision. The greater trochanter is osteotomized for proximal reflection of the gluteus minimus and medius. To augment the anterior visualization, the tensor fascia lata and gluteus minimus are sharply incised from their origins on the iliac crest in line with the incision. While this extension inevitably violates the nerve supply to the tensor fascia lata, it provides exposure of a fracture of the anterior iliac crest. Posterior exposure is enchanced by splitting the gluteus maximus muscle in line with its fibers and sharply reflecting the short external rotators from the proximal femur. Supplementary posterior exposure is comparable to that described for the Kocher-Langenbeck approach. This exposure also provides an inadequate visualization of a complex acetabular fracture that violates both the posterior and anterior columns.

## The Extended Iliofemoral Approach

Contributed by Joel M. Matta, MD.

This approach was developed by Letournel[3] as a technique to provide the maximum exposure of both the anterior and posterior columns, particularly of their external aspects through a single surgical incision. While it provides sufficient exposure for a wide variety of difficult fractures involving both the anterior and posterior columns, it is an anatomical approach that follows logical neurovascular planes. The muscles innervated by the superior and inferior gluteal nerves are reflected posteriorly as a unit without injury to their posterior neurovascular pedicles.

Indications for the approach include a both column fracture of the acetabulum, particularly a comminuted variant with posterior involvement of the iliac wing or disruption of the ipsilateral sacroiliac joint, or a simpler fracture more than ten days old that generally requires a more extensile exposure. This approach also is useful to expose a minority of T-shaped, transverse, and associated transverse and posterior wall fractures, particularly when the transverse component is a

Figure 7-11. The extended iliofemoral approach.

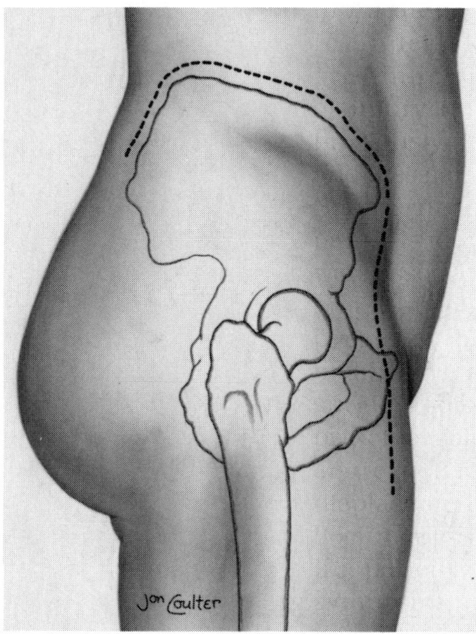


Figure 7-11A. Cutaneous incision.

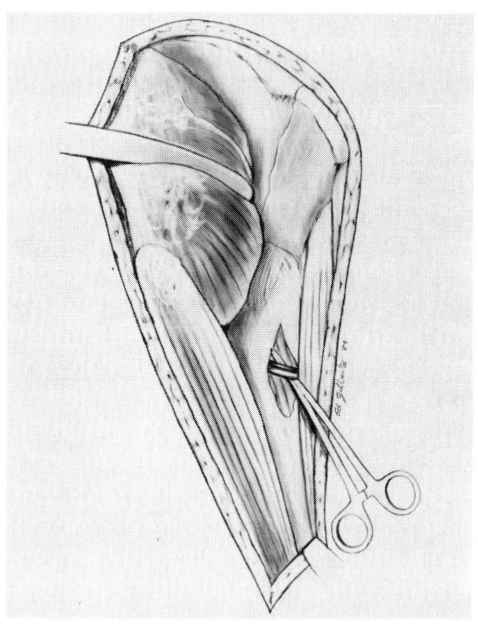

Figure 7-11B. Initial elevation and posterior retraction of tensor fascia lata and gluteal muscles. The lateral femoral circumflex vessels are seen through the incision in overlying fascia.

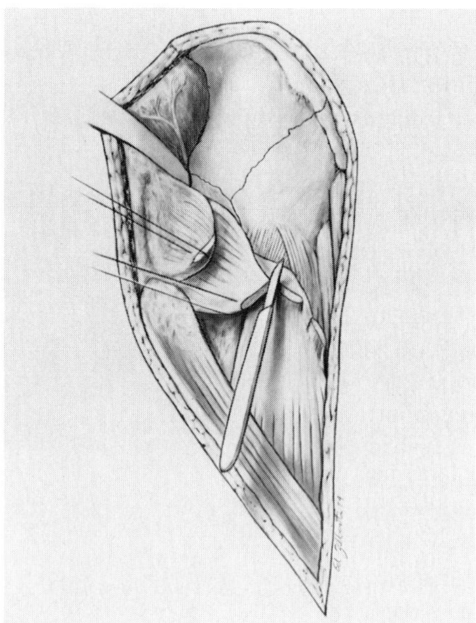

Figure 7-11C. The gluteus minimus tendon has been completely transected and the medius tendon partly transected. Posterior dissection along the iliac wing has reached the greater sciatic notch.

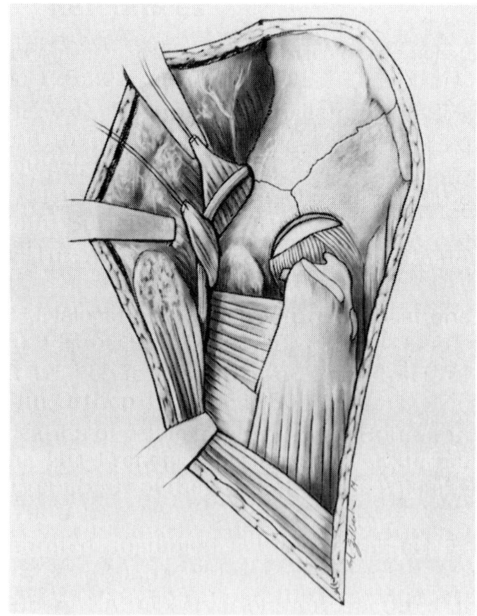

Figure 7-11D. The exposure of the external aspect of the innominate bone is now complete.

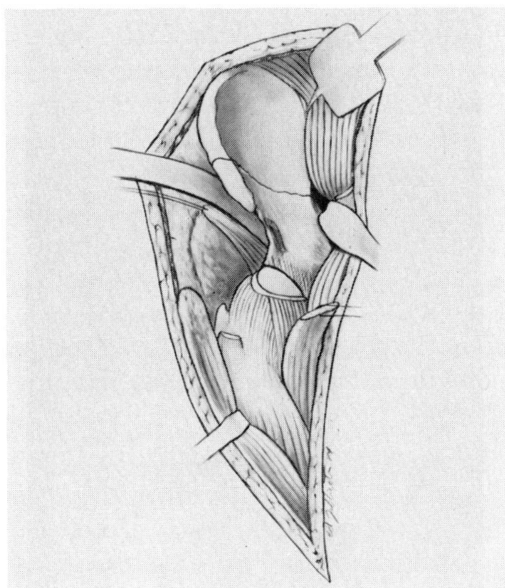

Figure 7-11E. Exposure of the internal iliac fossa pelvic brim and anterior rim of acetabulum.

transtectal pattern. Lastly, it is appropriate for fractures involving both the anterior and posterior column that are over three weeks old and require the removal of fracture callus prior to an open reduction. This approach provides access to the entire external aspect of the iliac wing and the external aspect of the posterior column distal to the ischial tuberosity. It can be extended to include the inner aspect of the iliac wing, as well as the anterior column as far distally as the pectineal eminence.

The patient is placed on the operating table in a lateral position. The patient can be maintained in skeletal traction applied by the use of a distal femoral pin if he is placed on the fracture table with a perineal post. A fracture table with a movable support underneath the injured thigh for the lateral displacement of the thigh and corresponding disimpaction of the femoral head from the acetabulum is preferred. A contrainidication to use of the fracture table is the presence of contralateral superior and inferior pubic ramus fractures. In such cases force imposed by the perineal post on the symphysis pubis can provoke a deformity of the lower part of the pelvic ring. If a standard operating table is used the leg is freely draped. The knee is maintained in a flexed position throughout the entire operation to avoid excessive tension of the sciatic nerve.

The incision extends anteriorly from the posterior superior iliac spine along the iliac crest to the anterior superior iliac spine. The incision continues anterolaterally about half way down the thigh (Figure 7-11). The periosteum of the superior edge of the iliac crest is sharply incised. The origins of the gluteal muscles and tensor fascia lata are elevated from the iliac crest and the external aspect of the iliac wing in a subperiosteal plane. This area is provisionally packed with a sponge.

The fascia of the tensor fascia lata is sharply incised distally from the anterior superior iliac spine. Dissection deep to this fascial layer minimizes the injury to the lateral cutaneous nerve of the thigh, although a division of some of its posterior branches with a corresponding loss of cutaneous sensation is almost inevitable. Posterior retraction of the tensor fascia lata permits visualization of the internal fascial sheath of the tensor fascia lata muscle, which is incised longitudinally to expose the vastus lateralis and the adjacent greater trochanter. Deep to this fascial sheath, the lateral femoral circumflex artery is identified, clamped, ligated, and divided (Figure 7-11B).

Elevation of the tensor fascia lata and gluteal muscles from the iliac wing progresses anteriorly to the reflected head of the rectus femoris and hip capsule. Posteriorly, a comparable dissection continues to the greater sciatic notch where the superior gluteal vessels and nerve are carefully identified. Frequently, neurovascular structures are identified within the fracture gap of the posterior column adjacent to the greater sciatic notch.

On the anterior aspect of the greater trochanter, the tendon of the gluteus minimus is divided in its midsubstance. A suture is placed on the incised end of the tendon near its musculotendinous junction. Both the tendons of the gluteus minimus and medius are sharply elevated from the hip capsule.

The strongest posterior superior portion of the tendon of the gluteus medius, its posterior superior attached, is optimally visualized by internal rotation of the hip. The tendon, 15mm in length, is divided and tagged with sutures to facilitate the subsequent repair (Figure 7-11C).

The piriformis and obturator externus tendons are divided and tagged with sutures adjacent to their insertions on the greater trochanter. Elevation of the piriformis and obturator internus muscles from the hip capsule permits exposure of the retroacetabular surface of the posterior column. The piriformis and the obturator internus progress to the greater and lesser sciatic notches, respectively. Underlying the tendon of the obturator internus where it exits the lesser sciatic notch, a bursa provides a suitable site for the insertion of a retractor to expose the posterior column distally to the ischial tuberosity. Another retractor can be placed in the greater sciatic notch. Gentle retraction affords adequate visualization of the posterior column provided that a sufficiently posterior incision is made along the iliac crest. Gentle retraction is crucial to avoid a traction injury to the sciatic nerve and the adjacent muscles. The intact femoral attachment of the quadratus femoris muscle protects the ascending branch of the medial femoral circumflex artery. At this stage, the fracture lines in the iliac wing, the posterior column and the posterior acetabular wall are evident. The inner aspect of the joint may be inspected. An extensive capsulotomy around the acetabular rim permits visualization of the articular surface (Figure 7-11D). Rim fragments are displaced in continuity with the hip capsule. The acetabular labrum is carefully preserved around the acetabular rim.

To expose the internal aspect of the iliac wing, the attachments of the abdominal muscles and the iliacus are elevated from the iliac crest and the internal aspect of the ilium, respectively (Figure 7-11E). The origins of the sartorius and inguinal ligament are incised subperiosteally from the anterior superior iliac spine. Further anterior exposure is achieved by incising the origins of the direct and indirect heads of the rectus femoris and by elevating the iliacus distally to the pectineal eminence. The hip capsule is incised from the acetabular rim almost circumferentially to facilitate visualization of the articular surface. Especially in the presence of a both-column fracture or other comminuted fracture variant where the anterior column fracture propagates to the iliac crest, a muscular attachment to each principal fracture fragment is carefully preserved to maintain the viability of the bone. The origins of the rectus femoris muscle, anterior hip capsule, and iliacus are appropriate vascular conduits for the anterior column. In contrast the superior iliac portion of a T-shaped or transverse fracture is not at risk of devascularization, even when complete anterior dissection is undertaken.

At the completion of the operation, a suction drainage tube is inserted along the external aspect of the iliac wing posteriorly to the retroacetabular surface. If the internal iliac fossa is exposed, a second drain is inserted along the inner pelvic wall. The hip capsule is repaired with interrupted sutures. The tendons of the obturator internus and piriformis are reattached to the greater trochanter. The obturator internus muscle provides a muscular barrier between the sciatic nerve and the fixation plates applied along the posterior column. The tendons of the gluteus medius and minimus are repaired anatomically by the use of tagging sutures. The rectus femoris is reattached to the anterior inferior spine with a transosseous suture that is inserted through a small drill hole. The fascial layers of the abductor musculature and tensor fascia lata are sutured to the iliac wing by the use of a few transosseous sutures. The origins of the sartorius and inguinal ligament are repaired in a similar way. Reattachment of the muscles to the pelvis is greatly facilitated by appropriate positioning of the lower extremity. Reattachment of the rectus femoris and sartorius is facilitated by flexion of the hip and extension of the knee. A repair of the fascia lata to the abdominal fascia is facilitated by abduction of the hip. Upon closure of the fascia in the distal portion of the incision, the subcutaneous and cutaneous repairs are completed. Postoperatively, the suction drains are removed 48 hours after surgery. Active flexion exercises of the hip are encouraged on the first postoperative day. Between the second and fifth days a partial weightbearing gait with the use of crutches is initiated.

Contribution concludes.

## The Triradiate Extensile Approach

The triradiate incision[4] is a modification of a surgical approach that Charnley initially employed for total hip joint replacement. This approach provides access for appropriate dissection to the greater trochanter, acetabulum (both extraarticular and intraarticular), anterior and posterior pelvic columns, sacroiliac joint, and inner wall of the pelvis. It is designed to provide a comparable visualization of the lateral aspect of the innominate bone as the extended iliofemoral approach without limiting the blood supply of the glutei, the principal hip abductors, to the superior gluteal vessels. With the extended iliofemoral approach, if the inferior gluteal bundle is injured traumatically or iatrogenically, ischemic necrosis of the massive abductor muscle flap creates a formidable complication. The triradiate concept also provides a way in which an initial exposure with the posterior and distal limbs of the incision can be enhanced rapidly if the initial visualization proves to be inadequate. Furthermore, the triradiate incision is appropriate for a subsequent total hip joint replacement by a posterior or anterior exposure.

Under general anesthesia, the patient is placed in a full lateral position on a conventional operating table. Routine preparation and draping is undertaken from the anterior to the posterior midlines, including the ipsilateral extremity. The extremity is fully exposed to permit intraoperative manipulation. The superficial landmarks for the incision are the anterior superior iliac spine, the posterior superior iliac spine, and the greater trochanter (Figure 7-12). The longitudinal limb of the triradiate incision extends distally from the greater trochanter for a distance of about 6cm to 8cm. The proximal extensions of the incision course in the anterosuperior and posterosuperior directions. The angle formed by the superior limbs is about 120°. The anterosuperior limb continues across the anterior superior iliac spine while the posterosuperior limb projects toward the posterior superior iliac spine. The distal longitudinal limb of the incision is extended down to the fascia lata, which is divided longitudinally. This fascial incision continues parallel to the anterior and posterior cutaneous incisions.

For exposure of the anterior column the fascia lata and myofascia of the tensor fascia lata are incised from the anterior superior spine to the greater trochanter. The anterior border of the tensor fascia lata muscle is sharply incised from its fascia so that the entire muscle can be retracted superiorly and posteriorly along with the cutaneous flap. The origins of the tensor fascia lata and the gluteus medius and minimus are incised from the iliac crest. Subperiosteal elevation of the gluteus medius and minimus is undertaken from anterior to posterior and distally to the capsule of the hip joint.

Through the posterior limb of the incision proximal to the greater trochanter, following the incision of the myofascia of the gluteus maximus, the muscle is bluntly split in line with its fibers. On the lateral aspect of the proximal femur the interval between the gluteus medius and the vastus lateralis is identified and a transverse incision is made in the periosteum. With an osteotome or an oscillating saw the greater trochanter with the attached gluteus medius and minimus is osteotomized and reflected craniad. With curved heavy scissors working from proximal to distal and anterior to posterior, the gluteus medius and minimus are sharply elevated from the capsule of the hip joint. The capsule is carefully preserved. The dissection continues to the greater sciatic notch where the superior gluteal vessels are identified. Next the short external rotators of the hip are incised from their insertions to the proximal femur, distal to the midportion of the quadratus femoris. These muscles are reflected posteriorly to visualize the underlying posterior column and the adjacent capsule of the hip joint. With the gluteus medius and minimus reflected superiorly, the lateral pelvis and roof of the acetabulum are approached by elevation of the periosteum. By the use of sharp and blunt dissection, the posterior column is exposed from the greater sciatic notch to the ischial tuberosity. Blunt Hohmann retractors are carefully inserted into the greater and lesser sciatic notches to maintain the exposure of the posterior column. The abductor muscle mass is anchored superiorly and posteriorly by the use of two Steinmann pins inserted into the ilium 2.5cm and 5.0cm above the roof of the greater sciatic notch. The distal portion of the posterior column is observed to the level of the ischial tuberosity

Figure 7-12. The triradiate extensile approach.

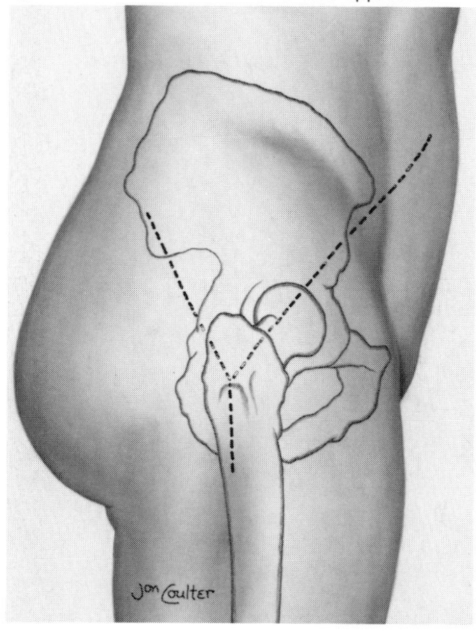


Figure 7-12A. Cutaneous incision.

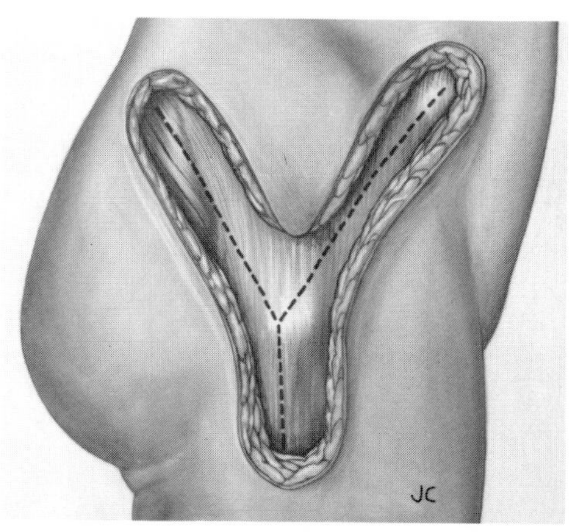


Figure 7-12B. Fascial incision superficial to the tensor fascia lata, gluteus maximus and fascia lata.

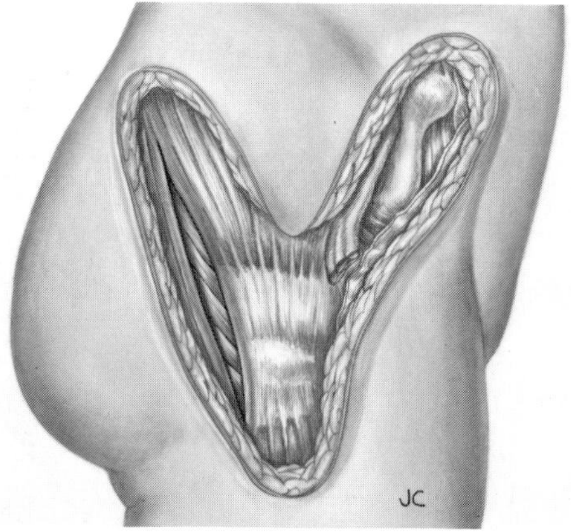


Figure 7-12C. Upon elevation of the myofascia from the anterior border of the tensor muscle and incision of the origin of the tensor from the anterior iliac crest, the anterior border of the lateral ilium is evident. Also the gluteus maximus has been split in line with the fibers up to the inferior gluteal neurovascular bundle.

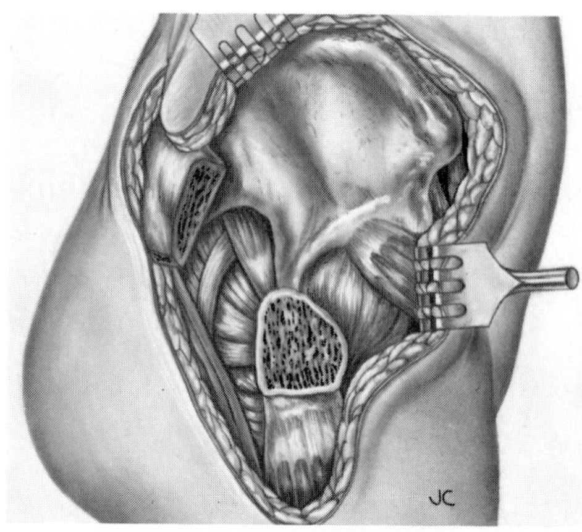


Figure 7-12D. The greater trochanter is osteotomized. The glutei and tensor muscles are elevated from the lateral ilium and the hip capsule and reflected posteriorly.

by sharp incision of the origin of the hamstring muscles. The ridge on the ischial tuberosity may be trimmed with a rongeur to facilitate the application of a plate along the posterior column. The sacrospinous ligament can be incised to facilitate palpation of the inner wall of the ilium. This maneuver is discouraged as it compromises one of the few stabilizing elements that is undamaged in many acetabular fractures.

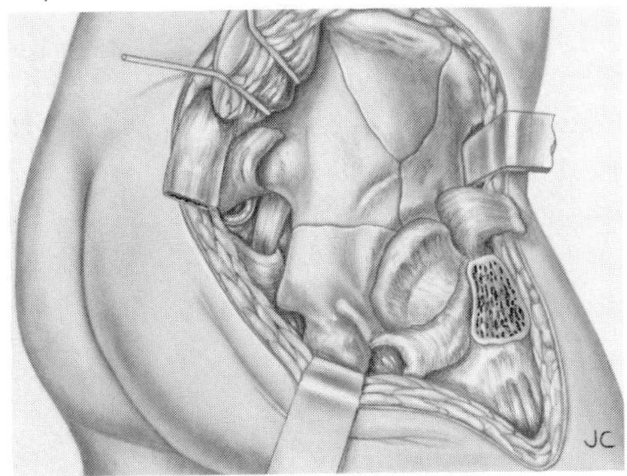


Figure 7-12E. The tendinous insertions of the piriformis gemelli and obturator externus are incised from the greater trochanter. The glutei and tensor muscles are reflected superiorly to expose the posterior column. The capsular origin is incised with Steinmann pins from the acetabular rim.

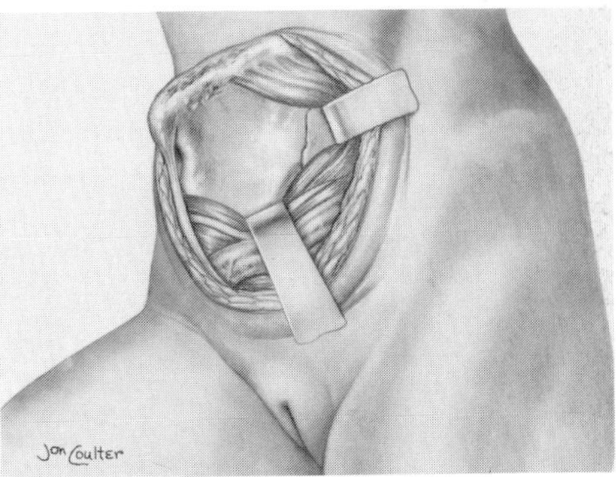

Figure 7-12F. Anterior exposure of the inner pelvic wall is achieved by incision of the abdominal muscles from the iliac crest, subperiosteal elevation of the iliacus, and incision of the origins of the sartorius, inguinal ligament and rectus femoris from the anterior superior and anterior inferior spines, respectively.

As part of the exposure of the anterior column, often it is necessary to extend the dissection medially to the iliopectineal eminence and posteriorly to the sacroiliac joint (Figure 7-12F). The anterior limb of the cutaneous incision is continued 6cm to 8cm medial to the anterior superior iliac crest. The insertion of the abdominal musculature on the anterior iliac crest is sharply incised. The iliacus muscle is elevated subperiosteally from the inner table of the ilium and retracted medially. The exposure continues posteriorly to visualize the anterior aspect of the sacroiliac joint. In addition to exposure of the sacroiliac joint, the inner wall of the ilium and the superior pubic ramus to within 2cm of the symphysis can be visualized.

To augment the anterior exposure, the origins of the sartorius and the direct and indirect heads of rectus femoris are incised from the anterior superior and anterior inferior spines and the hip capsule, respectively. The aponeurosis of the external oblique and the inguinal ligament are incised as previously described under the ilioinguinal approach. The interval between the psoas muscle and the external iliac vessels is developed. After adequate identification of the external iliac vessels, the interval between them and the spermatic cord or round ligament and the rectus abdominus is developed. Subperiosteal elevation is undertaken along the superior pubic ramus by the use of each of these longitudinal intervals. By medial or lateral retraction of the iliopsoas, external iliac vessels, and rectus abdominus virtually the entire length of the anterior column can be visualized and the quadrilateral surface can be palpated.

Especially when extensive visualization of the inner and outer pelvic surfaces is needed, great care is taken to preserve a muscular attachment as a blood supply to each major osseous fragment. Particularly for a both-column fracture, with segmental comminution of the anterior column and extension of the fracture to the iliac crest, the iliac fragments are maintained in continuity with a major muscle group. In the last example, the origins of the rectus femoris and the sartorius are preserved to the anterior iliac fragment. Visualization of the inner pelvic wall is achieved by a rotational displacement of the anterior iliac fragment. The mobility of the fragment is realized by a soft-tissue release of its iliac crest and inner pelvic surface.

When the capsule is intact it is incised sharply from its origin around the acetabular rim to permit access to the hip joint. In the presence of a posterior wall fracture, the osteochondral fragment with its adjacent capsule is reflected to expose the hip joint. If necessary, the adjacent intact capsule is incised from its origin until sufficient exposure of the hip joint is achieved. Following the exposure of the adjacent parts of the pelvis, visualization of the hip joint is necessary in order to identify and remove loose interposed osteochondral fragments, to verify the presence of an anatomical reduction and to observe and remove misdirected screws that violate the joint.

For closure of the triradiate incision a suction drain is inserted along the outer pelvic wall. If the inner pelvic wall is exposed, a second drain is employed. The lower extremity is positioned on a stand with about 30° of abduction of the hip joint. If an extensive intrapelvic dissection is performed, this phase of the repair is undertaken as described under the ilioinguinal approach. The two Steinmann pins are removed from the ilium to permit reattachment of the origins of the glutei and the tensor fascia lata to the iliac crest. The capsule of the hip joint is reattached to the origin of the indirect head of rectus femoris and to the ilium. Both of the previous repairs may be facilitated by the use of sutures inserted through 2mm drill holes in the ilium. The greater trochanter is accurately reduced and temporarily immobilized with a tenaculum forceps. Two 6.5mm long-threaded cancellous screws with washers are used to secure the greater trochanter. In the presence of mildly osteoporotic bone a supplementary figure-of-eight 18 gauge tension band wire is employed. If the bone is moderately osteoporotic, a hook plate (Synthes Ltd. (USA), Wayne, Pennsylvania) is used to reattach the greater trochanter. An apical stitch is used to reconstruct the three fascial edges superficial to the greater trochanter. Then the three fascial limbs of the incision are repaired, followed by the closure of the subcutaneous and cutaneous layers.

## References

1. Tile M: Fractures of the Pelvis and Acetabulum. Baltimore, Williams and Wilkins, 1984, p 234.
2. Senegas J, Liorzou G, Yates M: Complex acetabular fractures: A transtrochanteric lateral surgical approach. Clin Orthop 151:107, 1980.
3. Letournel E, Judet R: Fractures of the Acetabulum. New York, Springer-Verlag, 1981, p 232.
4. Mears DC, Rubash HE: Extensile exposure of the pelvis. Contemp Orthop 6:21, 1983.

# CHAPTER 8

# Techniques of Reduction

## Introduction

Of the several challenging aspects of pelvic and acetabular reconstruction, including the specific diagnosis, surgical exposure, and stabilization, until recently the least understood aspect remained the techniques of fracture reduction. After a presentation of the various surgical exposures, a typical fracture manual refers to the technique for stabilization but fails to mention the crucial method to achieve an anatomical reduction. Even experienced pelvic surgeons encounter formidable difficulties in the realization of a precise anatomical open reduction, especially in the presence of marked comminution, osteoporosis, and late presentation. In parallel with other pelvic surgeons[1,2] in our laboratory and clinical studies,[3,4] we have assessed the application of various reduction tools and especially the preferred sequence of reduction of comminuted fractures, topics which are now reviewed.

## Closed Reduction of the Pelvis

### Indications

With the recent acceptance of the role of external fixation for the stabilization of a broad spectrum of pelvic disruptions, the role of closed reduction techniques has grown considerably. A closed reduction can also be used in those uncommon cases where skeletal traction is employed as the definitive technique of immobilization or, particularly in children, when cast immobilization with a double hip spica is utilized. A closed reduction can be undertaken prior to an open reduction particularly when longitudinal traction is needed to correct superior migration of a hemipelvis. The foremost indication for a closed reduction remains a diastasis of the symphysis. Rotational deviation and superior displacement of a hemipelvis provide other indications. In the presence of marked displacement of an unstable hemipelvis, particularly with posterior migration documented on an inlet radiograph and superior migration on the anteroposterior view, the application of a closed reduction is unlikely to provide a sufficiently accurate reduction.[5] In the presence of a comminuted pelvic ring with bilateral sacroiliac disruptions, other comparable posterior injuries, or displaced comminuted anterior injuries such as bilateral ramus fractures, the application of various techniques of closed reduction is most unlikely to succeed. Similarly in the presence of a pelvic ring disruption and an acetabular fracture, such a complex injury necessitates an open reduction with internal fixation of the several disrupted sites. When a late presentation more than two to three weeks after the time of the injury is encountered, an accurate closed reduction of an unstable hemipelvis is unlikely to succeed. For the management of a malunion or a nonunion of the pelvis, an open reduction with internal fixation is required.

## Techniques

### *Closed Reduction of a Diastasis of the Symphysis Pubis*

When this method is employed in conjunction with the use of external fixation, the half pins are inserted into the pelvis with a conventional sterile technique. After the wounds have been closed and dressed, the external frame is provisionally assembled. Prior to tightening the frame, the patient is turned from a supine to a full lateral position to rest on the uninvolved hemipelvis. Approximation of the pins, which project from the two hemipelves, assisted by the favorable influence of gravity, readily provides a reduction of the diastasis. Once the frame has been tightened, radiographic confirmation of the reduction is attained. If an imperfect reduction is documented, the frame is loosened so that the reduction can be corrected.

### *Correction of Rotational Deviation of a Hemipelvis*

In the presence of a lateral compression injury with rotation of a hemipelvis, a closed manipulation under general anesthesia may correct the typical inward and upward rotation of the hemipelvis with apparent foreshortening of the ipsilateral lower extremity.[6] With the patient in a supine position, the ipsilateral lower extremity is positioned in external rotation with sufficient flexion of the knee so that the foot can be placed on the opposite knee. A downward pressure is applied to the ipsilateral distal femur, which thereby acts as a lever to reduce the fracture. Generally, this method is employed in conjunction with the use of external pelvic fixation. The maneuver is performed immediately prior to final tightening of the frame. During the reduction a downward force is applied to the affected anterior superior spine, while an assistant stabilizes the contralateral anterior superior spine to prevent rotation of the uninvolved hemipelvis.

Another method suitable for application to a lateral compression injury with upward and inward rotation of the hemipelvis employs the protruding external fixation pins (Figure 8-1), an AO femoral distractor pin (Synthes Ltd. (USA), Wayne, Pennsylvania), or a Steinmann pin inserted in the anterior superior spine. With both the Hoffmann instrumentation (Howmedica, Inc., Rutherford, New Jersey) and the femoral distractor, a handle is available that clamps to the relevant pin and augments the mechanical advantage available to the surgeon. Upon scrutiny of the radiograph of a lateral compression injury, frequently an apparent superior migration of the affected hemipelvis is evident. Upon closer study, this deformity can be recognized as a rotational deviation with anterior and superior displacement of the acetabulum and rami. Once the rotational correction of the hemipelvis has been confirmed, in suitable cases external pelvic fixation can be applied. Subsequently, inlet, outlet, and anteroposterior radiographs are taken to confirm the adequacy of the reduction.

### Correction of Vertical Displacement of a Hemipelvis

In the presence of superior migration of a hemipelvis following a vertical shear injury, longitudinal traction can be applied by resort to a skeletal traction pin or a fracture table (Figure 8-2). Frequently, this method is used in conjunction with the application of external pelvic fixation. Following the closed reduction and stabilization, an anteroposterior radiograph confirms whether sufficient inferior manipulation of the hemipelvis has been undertaken. A supplementary inlet radiograph and generally one or two cuts of a computed scan confirm whether reapproximation of the sacroiliac joint has occurred. Usually a supplementary open reduction and

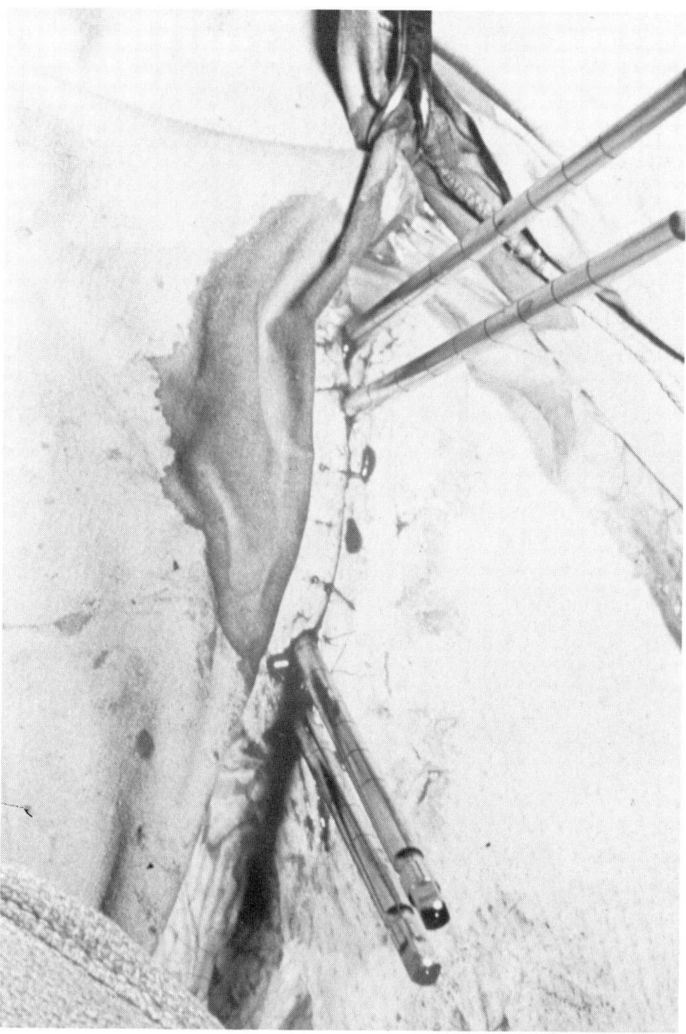

Figure 8-1. The protruding 5mm half pins permit the application of a rotational force to a hemipelvis prior to assembly of a triangular frame.

internal fixation of the sacroiliac joint is needed to correct the inadequate closed reduction. Immediately prior to an open reduction of the sacroiliac joint, longitudinal traction can be applied to a vertical shear injury to minimize the amount of correction that is needed at the time of the open reduction.

## Open Reduction of the Pelvis

### Indications

An open pelvic reduction is indicated when an attempted reduction fails and provides unacceptable correction of a rotational deviation, vertical or other displacement of the involved hemipelvis. Typically within a week after the time of the injury, the correction of rotational deviation and vertical displacement becomes much more difficult than an acute reduction. In the

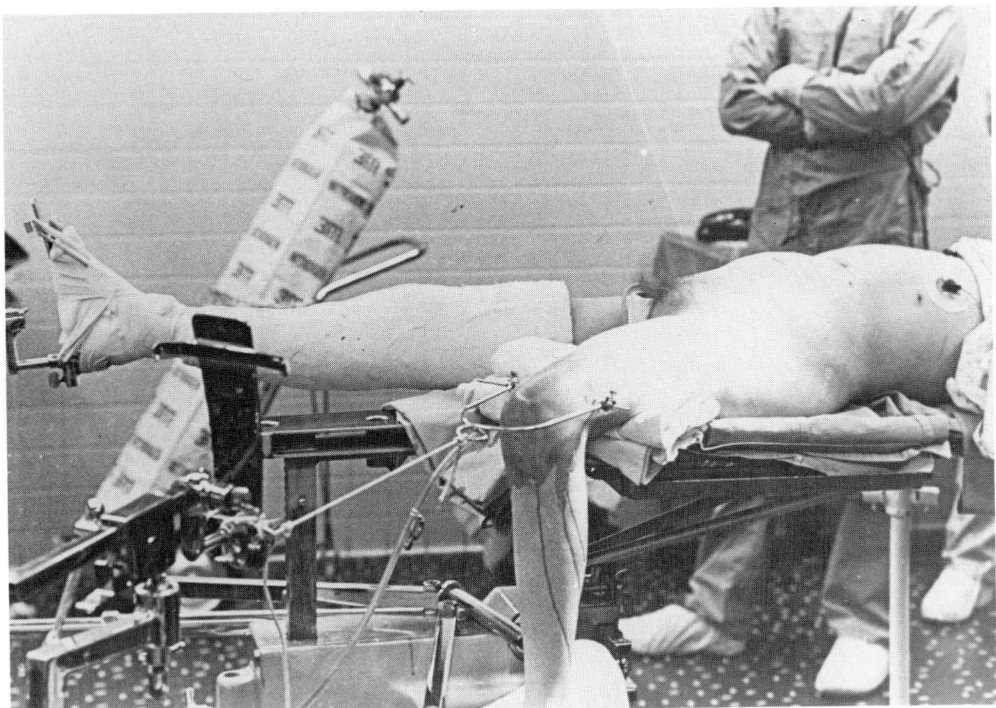

Figure 8-2. The application of longitudinal traction to the distal femur permits the correction of superior migration of the left hemipelvis.

presence of a complex pelvic fracture with bilateral unstable sacroiliac joints, a central or anterior iliac fracture and/or an acetabular fracture, generally the use of closed methods is contraindicated and an open reduction with internal fixation is needed. For virtually all nonunions and malunions with significant displacement, an open reduction is required.

## Contraindications and Limitations

Once the degree of pelvic displacement is categorized as unacceptable and a closed reduction has failed or is recognized as an inappropriate method, there are few if any absolute contraindications for the use of an open reduction. When the patient is hemodynamically or otherwise unstable, or when the patient possesses an open wound superficial to the displaced pelvic fracture site, a temporary deferral of the open reduction is indicated. With an open fracture, the open wound is debrided promptly. In the presence of an open ramus fracture, generally external fixation is preferred to minimize the soft tissue stripping that would be needed for the application of a plate. In the presence of an open sacroiliac fracture/dislocation, generally the debridement is notable for an extraordinary degree of instability of the sacroiliac joint. Once the debridement is completed an open reduction with lag screw fixation is undertaken.

Figure 8-3. A: The Lambotte-Farabeuf forceps, AO reduction forceps, and tenaculum forceps are demonstrated (left to right). B: The AO pelvic reduction forceps.

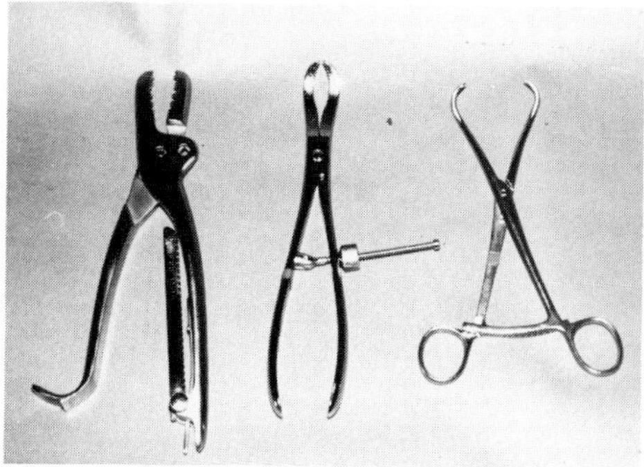

Figure 8-3A.

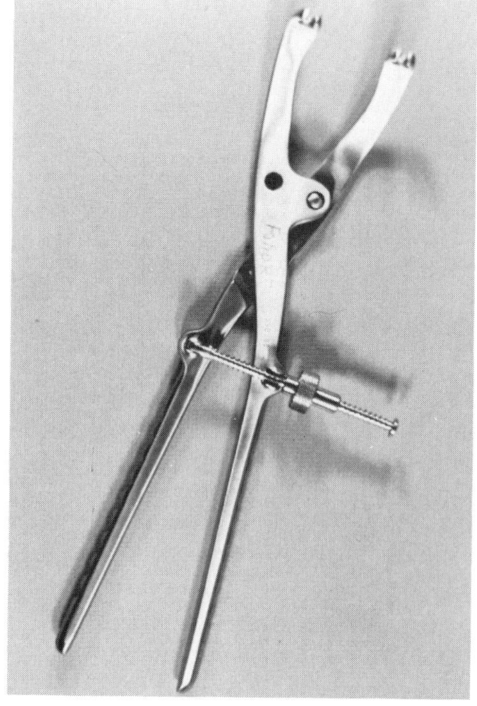

Figure 8-3B.

## Techniques of Open Reduction

A variety of bone holding forceps is available that provides the most widely employed instrument for open reduction (Figure 8-3). In the simplest technique, tenaculum bone holding forceps (Synthes Ltd. (USA), Wayne, Pennsylvania) of various sizes with the jaws embedded in 3.2mm unicortical drill holes (Figure 8-4) are anchored around stable bony projections. For example, with a diastasis of the symphysis pubis the jaws can be inserted into the opposing obturator foramen. For the reduction of a widened sacroiliac joint, one jaw is placed in a unicortical drill hole on the outer surface of the ilium, while the other is placed around the spinous process of the sacrum or within a unicortical drill hole in the sacrum. Frequently, to correct a concomitant vertical displacement of the ilium referable to the sacrum, a second tenaculum forceps is inserted into comparable drill holes prepared in the iliac crest and the adjacent sacrum. Occasionally, the use of the regular AO bone holding forceps is preferred for the correction of a vertical displacement of a symphysis or a diastasis, although this forceps is prone to spontaneous disengagement from the surface of the bone. Either the regular AO bone holding forceps (Synthes Ltd. (USA), Wayne,

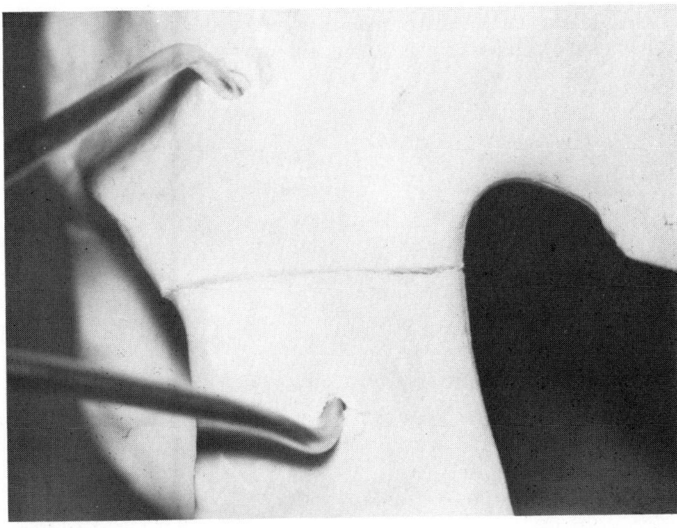

Figure 8-4. Application of tenaculum forceps by insertion of the jaws into 3.2mm unicortical drill holes.

Pennsylvania) or preferably the Lambotte-Farabeuf model (Zimmer, Warsaw, Indiana) can be applied to the protruding heads of 4.5mm cortical or 6.5mm cancellous screws (Figure 8-5). This method provides the optimal means to afford mechanical force for the reduction provided that the screws are anchored into solid bone. The method is not suitable for application to markedly osteoporotic bone. It requires somewhat more time to apply than the use of the tenaculum bone holding forceps. If the screws are inserted inappropriately so that the optimal vector of correction cannot be applied, the method requires a greater period of time to change the position of the screw than the comparable alteration needed to adjust the position of the tenaculum bone holding forceps. Another model, the AO pelvic forceps (Synthes Ltd. (USA), Wayne, Pennsylvania), also attaches to protruding screw heads (Figure 8-6). With its large size, it provides the optimal mechanical advantage to achieve a reduction. For typical cases its large size is a considerable disadvantage. Also, with the position of the jaws, frequently it is difficult to manipulate the bone in three planes. It can be difficult to insert a screw in the optimal direction to allow simple apposition of the fracture site. As the jaws are closed they follow a curved pathway (Figure 8-6b and 8-6c). With the widespread availability of the Lambotte-Farabeuf and AO tenaculum bone holding forceps, the AO pelvic forceps is rarely employed.

The AO femoral distractor (Figure 8-7) provides a means to afford considerable mechanical force to a reduction particularly to correct a longitudinal or vertical displacement of a sacroiliac joint. Fixation pins are inserted in 4.5mm drill holes. The device can be used for distraction or compression.

Figure 8-5. The application of a Lambotte-Farabeuf forceps to a posterior column fracture. A: Opposing 6.5mm cancellous screws. B: Reduction of the fracture with the Lambotte-Farabeuf forceps.

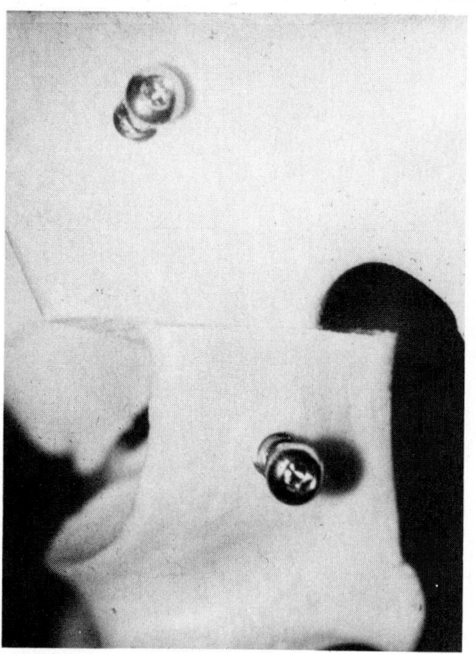

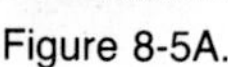

Figure 8-5A.

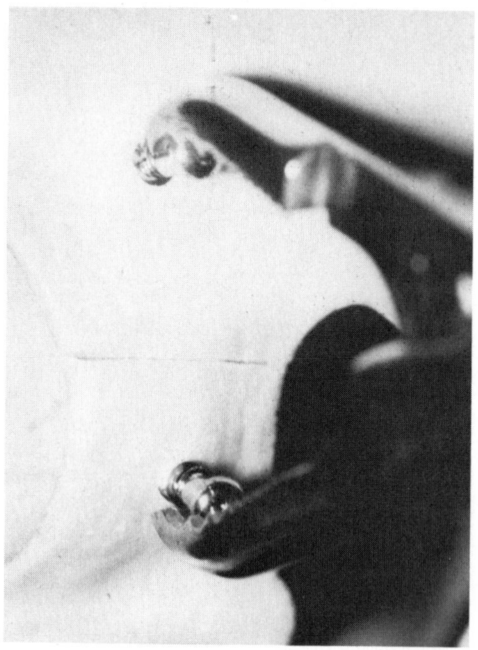

Figure 8-5B.

Particularly for application on the lateral ilium when one side of a fracture is displaced deep to the other side, a 3.5mm DC plate (Synthes Ltd. (USA), Wayne, Pennsylvania) can be used as a reduction tool. The plate is anchored with 3.5mm cortical screws to the more superficial bone fragment. Then screws are inserted through the plate into the deeper bone fragment. As the latter screws are tightened, the fragment is retracted to the level of the superficial bone fragment for realization of an anatomical reduction. Frequently, two or three four- to six-hole plates are used to immobilize the broad surface of the lateral ilium. In a somewhat similar way for rigorous apposition of the unstable sacroiliac joint, two 6.5mm cancellous lag screws are inserted from the lateral ilium into the ala and the adjacent portion of the first sacral body (Figure 8-8). By the use of the screws the sacroiliac joint is reduced and stabilized.

### *Specific Sites for the Application of Reduction Forceps*

For the reduction of a diastasis of the symphysis pubis through a Pfannenstiel or a vertical midline approach, generally a tenaculum forceps is applied into the medial aspects of the opposing obturator foramen. The adjacent rami are slowly approximated at the midline. Periodically, the most inferior aspects of the opposing rami are palpated to ensure that the Foley catheter and the

Figure 8-6. A: The AO pelvic forceps applied to a posterior column fracture. B and C: During approximation of the jaws, the obligatory curved pathway of the AO pelvic forceps prevents a direct reapproximation of opposing fragments. This liability of the forceps is evident on a reduction of the symphysis.

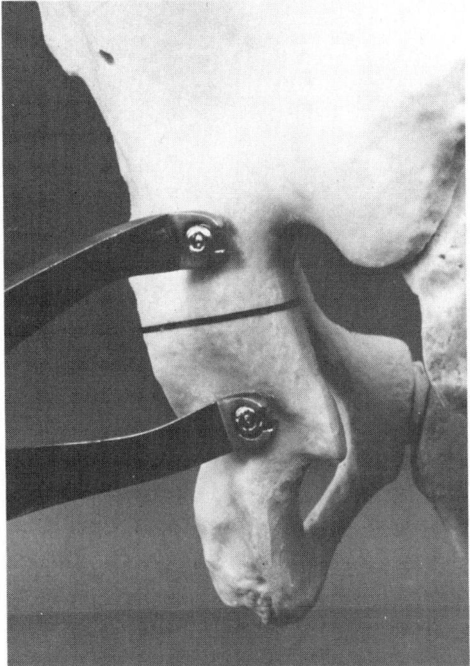

Figure 8-6A.

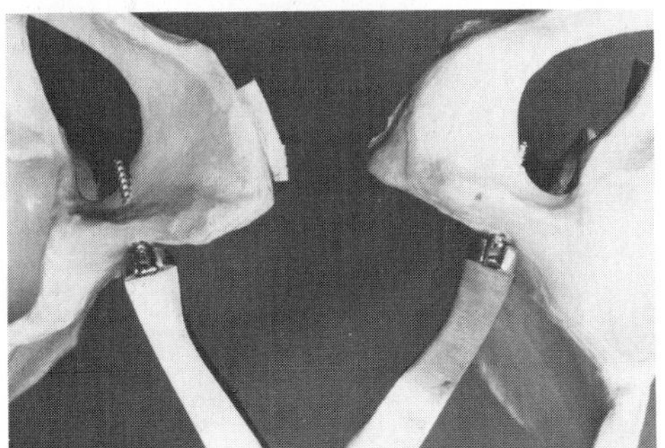

Figure 8-6B.

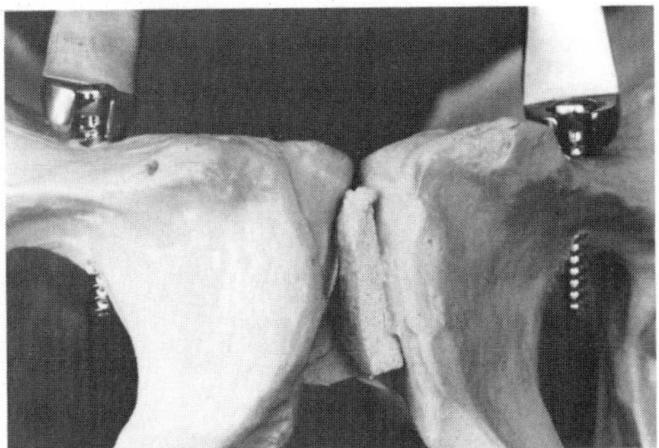

Figure 8-6C.

surrounding urethra are not trapped between the rami. Upon scrutiny of the superior aspect of the symphysis, an associated vertical or rotational displacement may be evident. To correct this deformity a second tenaculum forceps is placed from the inferior aspect of one superior ramus to the superior aspect of the other. If the anterior injury involves the rami instead of the symphysis, comparable techniques of reduction are employed, especially by resort to the tenaculum forceps inserted in 3.2mm drill holes. The drill holes are prepared in the anterior or superior surfaces of the disrupted superior pubic ramus.

Figure 8-7. A: The AO femoral distractor with straight and bent pins. B: Distraction of the femoral head from the acetabulum with the femoral distractor.

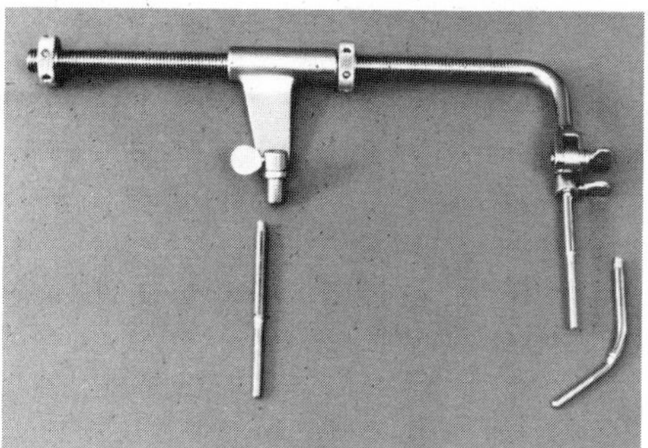

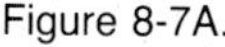

Figure 8-7A.

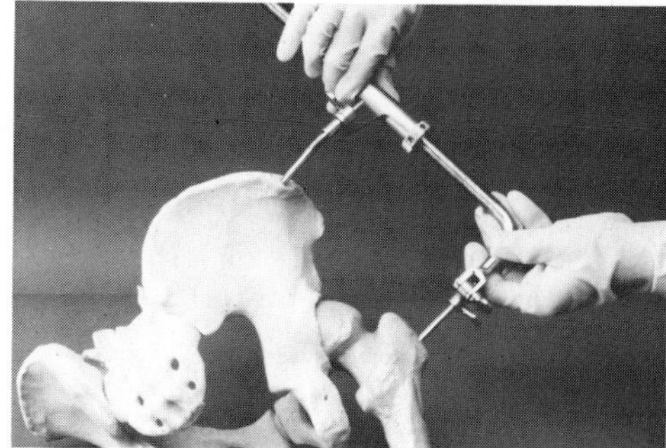

Figure 8-7B.

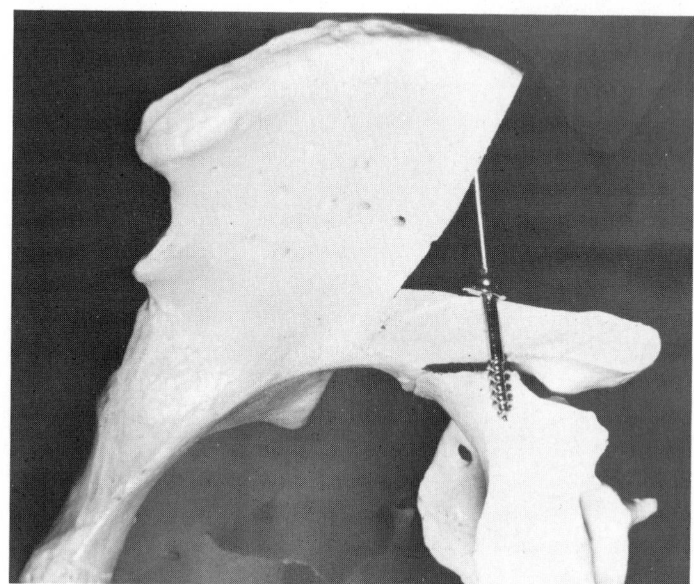

Figure 8-8. Approximation of the posterior ilium to the sacrum by the insertion of a cancellous lag screw.

To correct the displacement of a sacroiliac joint, usually tenaculum bone holding forceps are employed. Two or three forceps are needed to correct multiple planes of deformity. During the approximation of the sacroiliac joint, the reduction is monitored by inspection of the opposing sacrum and ilium at the posterior margin of the greater sciatic notch (Figure 8-9). Also, a finger can be used to palpate the inferior margin of the sacroiliac joint deep to the sciatic nerve as it exits from the pelvis. The adjacent flat surfaces of the ilium and sacrum provide a good indication of the accuracy of the reduction. When rotation deviation of the hemipelvis accompanies the

Figure 8-9. Confirmation of the accuracy of a sacroiliac reduction. A: The posterior portion of the greater sciatic notch. Also within the sciatic notch the flat articulation of the sacrum and ilium can be palpated. B: With appropriate surgical exposures, the anterior portion of the sacroiliac joint provides the most accurate estimate of the accuracy of the reduction.

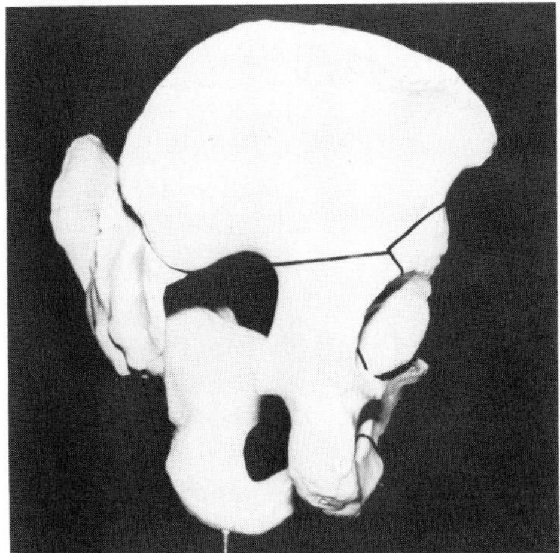

Figure 8-9A.

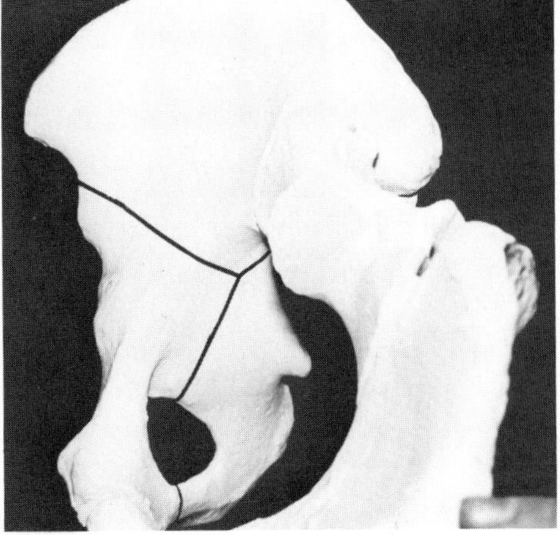

Figure 8-9B.

displacement, supplementary tools such as a Steinmann pin or particularly a femoral distractor pin are needed. The pin is inserted into the posterior ilium between the posterior superior and posterior inferior spines. When the posterior disruption violates the ilium or the adjacent sacrum, adjacent to the sacroiliac joint to achieve the reduction, the use of multiple tenaculum bone holding forceps is preferred.

In the presence of an iliac fracture, either tenaculum or Lambotte-Farabeuf bone holding forceps are applied to the iliac crest and the lateral ilium. The forceps are appropriately spaced so that the fracture surfaces can be symmetrically reapproximated. Many of these fractures course obliquely across the outer and inner tables of the pelvis. As they are reduced such unstable oblique surfaces tend to override with an unacceptable malalignment. To prevent the overriding, prior to the final reduction, one or two 3.5mm DC plates are attached to the more superficial iliac fragment. When the iliac fracture is reduced the plates inhibit a malreduction. Generally, an attempt is made to anatomically reduce all of the iliac fragments so that the most stable anatomical reduction is achieved. In the presence of marked iliac comminution, the extraordinarily thin midportion of the lateral ilium may preclude assembly of the fragile thin fragments. Also, where comminution of the inner wall of the pelvis creates numerous free fragments that are inaccessible from the outer aspect of the ilium, the comminuted fragments are not subject to stabilization.

# Closed Reduction of the Acetabulum

## Indications

While in the previous chapter the indications for an open reduction of the acetabulum were examined rigorously, the present account outlines briefly the role of closed and open methods for particular fracture patterns.

A closed reduction of the acetabulum with or without an associated fracture-dislocation of the femoral head can be undertaken as a definitive therapeutic method or in conjunction with a surgical reconstruction of the acetabulum. For a posterior fracture-dislocation or an isolated traumatic dislocation of the femoral head, a closed reduction is indicated to reposition the femoral head and, in appropriate cases, to reduce the posterior wall or column of the acetabulum. Particularly in the presence of a low or infratectal pattern of a transverse or a certain minimally displaced associated or complex acetabular fracture, a satisfactory closed reduction can be attained by the use of skeletal traction. In a highly comminuted both-column fracture, or especially in the presence of osteoporosis and a late presentation for definitive management, more than three weeks after the time of the injury, technical difficulties are likely to thwart the realization of an accurate anatomical open reduction and stable internal fixation. With the need for extensive visualization of the comminuted fracture fragments, such cases are prone to postoperative ectopic bone formation. If there are radiographic features of so-called secondary congruence of the acetabulum with the femoral head, whereby the displaced acetabular fragments are congruent with the femoral head, nonoperative methods are preferred.

A preliminary closed reduction also can be undertaken to simplify a subsequent surgical reconstruction. The Judet Orthopaedic Table (Tasserit SA, Collemiers-89930, Gron, France) permits the application of skeletal traction via the greater trochanter for lateral displacement of the proximal femur along with conventional longitudinal traction. When the ilioinguinal approach is undertaken, whereby a limited exposure of the articular surface of the acetabulum is realized, a closed reduction of the femoral head greatly facilitates the subsequent open reduction of the acetabular fragments.

In the presence of a typical displaced associated fracture such as a "T" type, both-column, or an anterior column, posterior hemitransverse fracture, a closed reduction is unlikely to provide an accurate anatomical restoration of the acetabulum. Also, the method is unlikely to facilitate open reduction and internal fixation. Most displaced posterior column or anterior column fractures are not amenable to a closed reduction. A displaced acetabular fracture in a skeletally immature individual with disassociation of the triradiate cartilage merits consideration for an open reduction and internal fixation. Certain displaced and comminuted fractures, particularly in osteoporotic individuals of more than 70 years of age, especially in the presence of other major medical problems, merit consideration for a closed reduction when in the absence of such complicating factors an open reduction of a comparably displaced fracture would be recommended.

## Techniques of Closed Reduction

The most widely employed technique of closed reduction is the application of longitudinal skeletal traction by resort to a distal femoral or proximal tibial pin. While this method corrects superior migration of the femoral head, it does not correct medial displacement. A wide variety of designs of greater trochanteric pins have been inserted to provide traction along the orientation of the femoral neck.[4] While this method has theoretical attractions a traction pin inserted into the trochanteric cancellous bone inevitably undergoes premature loosening with a predilection for a pin tract infection. Once such an infection arises, then a surgical reconstruction of the acetabulum undertaken to correct persistent unacceptable displacement of the fracture is prone to major postoperative wound infection. The use of a greater trochanteric pin as a definitive source of skeletal traction is strongly discouraged. When the Judet Orthopaedic Table is used in conjunction with an ilioinguinal incision, the intraoperative application of lateral and supplementary longitudinal traction provides a closed reduction of the femoral head and simplifies the open reduction of the acetabulum.

For a minimally displaced acetabular fracture, the application of a continuous passive motion machine such as the Kinetec Design (Richards Manufacturing Co., Inc., Memphis, Tennessee) provides a way to immobilize the hip and to maintain a limited degree of traction with sufficient immobilization of the patient. For three years, this method has been utilized in our clinic as a way to permit a rapid discharge from the hospital for appropriate acetabular fracture victims. When a minimially displaced fracture of a potentially unstable fracture pattern is documented, the continuous passive motion machine is applied to the relevant lower extremity. One week later serial radiographs of the pelvis are undertaken. Provided that there has been no further displacement of the fracture, the patient is discharged

Figure 8-10. A: "Pitons" and "lifesavers" with an appropriate 4.5mm cortical screw. B: Reduction of a lateral iliac fracture with the use of a "piton" and a "lifesaver."

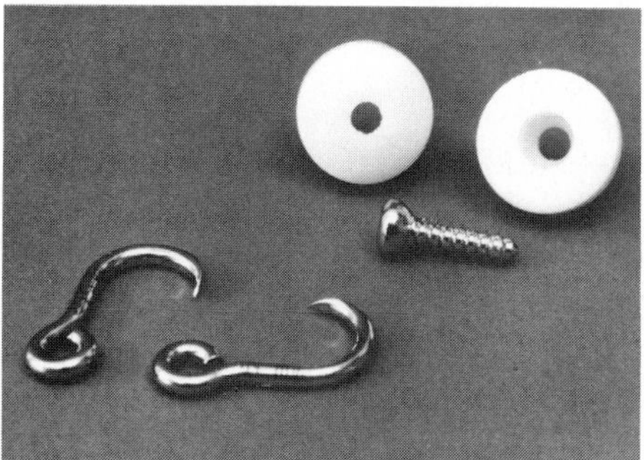

Figure 8-10A.

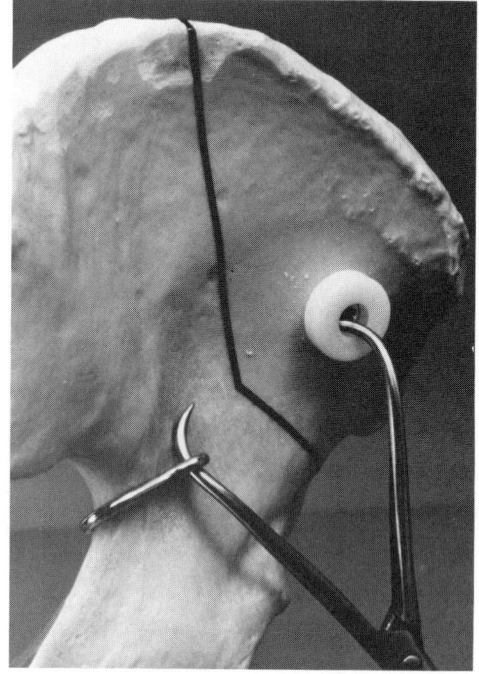

Figure 8-10B.

in the continuous passive motion machine, which is employed for a total of six weeks.

# Open Reduction of the Acetabulum

## Indications

An open reduction of the acetabulum is indicated when a concentric surface of the acetabulum, especially of the principal weightbearing portion, cannot be established by closed methods to within an accuracy of 1mm to 3mm. For a simple fracture such as a displaced posterior wall or a posterior column injury or a transtectal or supratectal transverse fracture, generally an open reduction is indicated. Most displaced associated fractures necessitate an open reduction. While hemodynamic instability or other medical problems, or the presence of an adjacent open wound, temporarily contraindicates open reduction, the principal absolute contraindication to surgical reconstruction of a displaced fracture is excessive comminution and/or osteoporosis that precludes the realization of an effective stabilization.

## Techniques

The most versatile tool for acetabular reduction is the tenaculum forceps. Recently in an attempt to improve

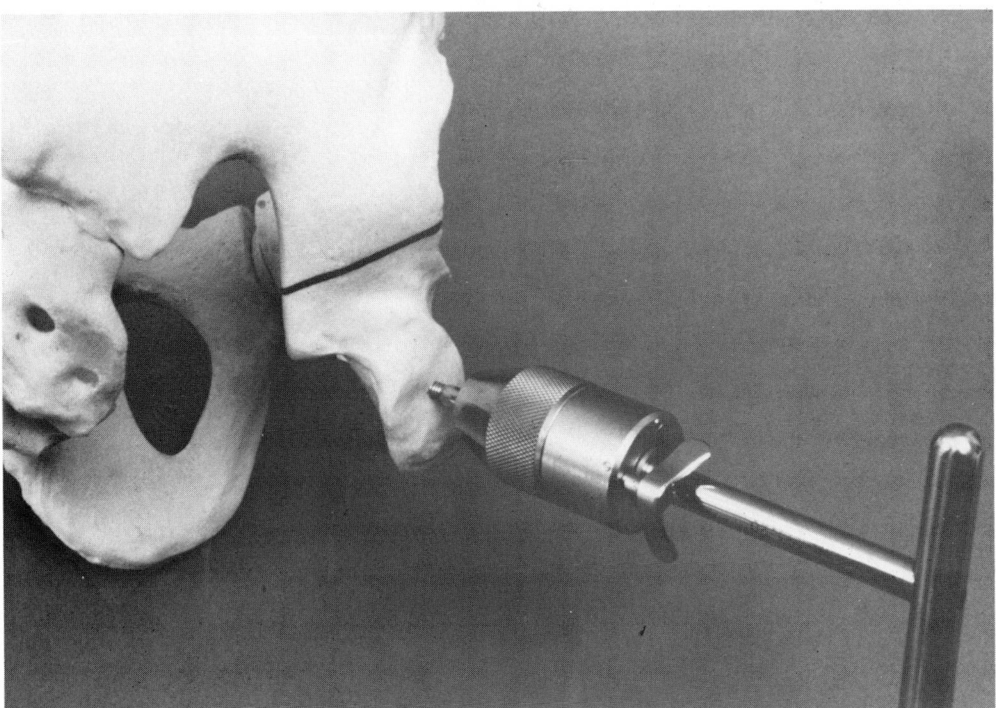

Figure 8-11. The application of a femoral distractor pin with a T-handle chuck into the ischial tuberosity to reduce a low posterior column fracture.

the anchorage of the forceps to bone, Mast[7] has devised "lifesavers" and "pitons" (Synthes, Ltd. (USA), Wayne, Pennsylvania) (Figure 8-10). A "lifesaver" is a thickened plastic washer that is anchored to bone by the use of a 4.5mm cortical screw. Its thickened rim provides a suitable site for attachment of a tenaculum forceps. A "piton" is a stainless steel hook with an eye. The hook is applied to a suitable recess, such as the greater or lesser sciatic notch, while the eye is used to anchor the tenaculum forceps. These tools not only augment the sites for attachment of the forceps to bone, but also extend the direction of the force that can be effectively applied to reduce a fracture.

As supplementary reduction forceps, the Lambotte-Farabeuf, conventional AO, and pelvic reduction clamps are available. Rotational correction of a displaced column can be corrected by the insertion of a femoral distractor pin or other comparable pin or femoral head extractor into the displaced segment. A T-handle chuck is applied to the femoral distractor pin for manipulation of the bone fragment (Figure 8-11).

The 3.5mm reconstruction plate (Synthes, Ltd. (USA), Wayne, Pennsylvania) is a highly effective reduction tool particularly for application to a low posterior column disruption (Figure 8-12). The plate is contoured and applied to the inferior fracture fragment, on the ischial

Figure 8-12. The use of a 3.5mm reconstruction plate as a reduction tool. A: The jaw of an ancillary tenaculum forceps is embedded in a drill hole. B: The jaw of the forceps is applied around the iliac crest.

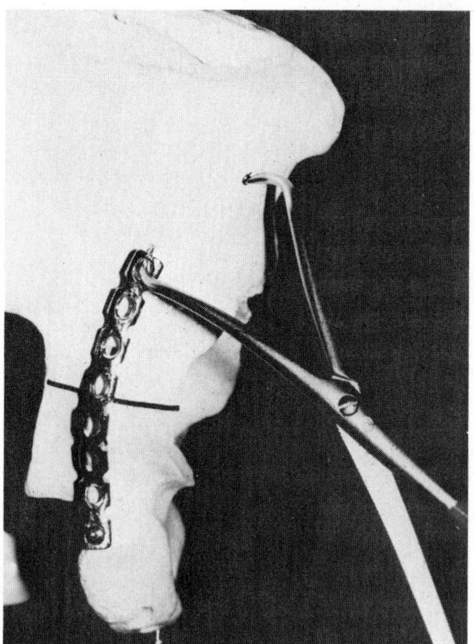

Figure 8-12A.

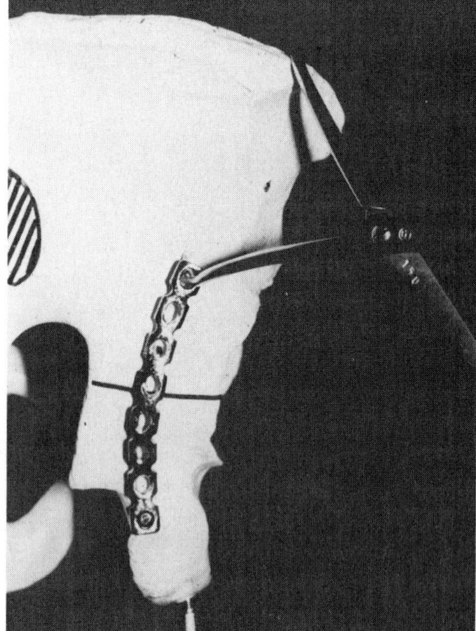

Figure 8-12B.

tuberosity. Then a tenaculum bone holding forceps is applied to the upper end of the plate and to a 3.2mm unicortical drill hole in the lateral ilium or to a "lifesaver" or around the iliac crest. Once the fracture is reduced, the residual screws are inserted into the plate. Even though the plate cannot be perfectly contoured to the bone prior to its application, as the screws are tightened the malleable plate rigorously coadapts to the bone and buttresses the anatomical reduction.

A low anterior column disruption such as the relevant portion of a "T" fracture frequently provides a considerable difficulty in correction of the posterior and medial displacement. An attempt to correct simultaneously the two vectors of displacement and achieve an anatomical reduction is greatly simplified if a Kirschner wire is employed as a trunnion (Figure 8-13). Initially, the exposed anterior column fracture fragment is manipulated with a bone hook applied around the superior surface of the superior pubic ramus and into the obturator foramen. Once the posterior displacement has been eliminated, any supplementary rotational deviation also is corrected. Next, a Kirschner wire is inserted across the fracture site by the use of a power tool. The wire is introduced along the superior gluteal ridge about 2.5cm superior to the acetabular rim. Once the fracture has been immobilized, although

Figure 8-13. The use of a Kirschner wire to facilitate reduction of a low anterior column fracture. A: A model of a "T" fracture with the Kirschner wire advanced to the disruption site in the anterior column. B: Upon reduction of the fracture with a bone hook the Kirschner wire is advanced. While it rotates in a drill, a tenaculum forceps is applied to approximate the fracture surfaces.

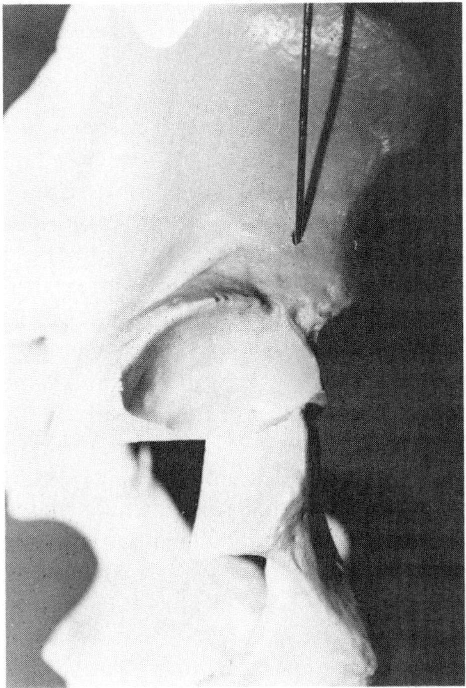

Figure 8-13A.

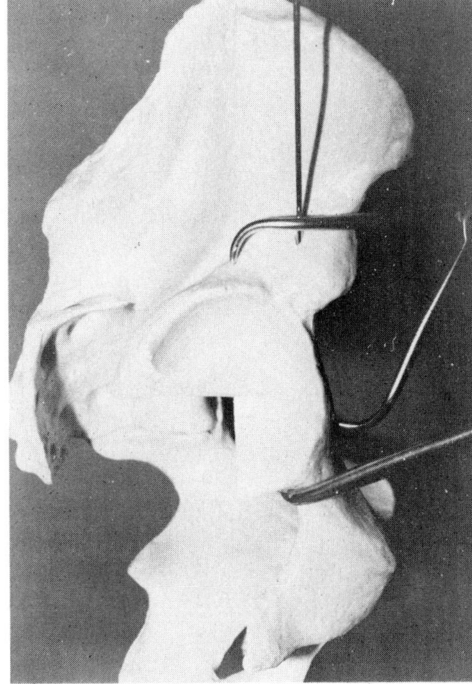

Figure 8-13B.

with a persistent fracture gap, the wire is rotated in the power drill. A tenaculum bone holding forceps is applied across the anterior column disruption. While the Kirschner wire rotates as a trunnion, the fracture fragments are approximated.

## Specific Fracture Pattern

Both with respect to the sequence of reduction of multiple fracture fragments and the selection of the optimal tools and reduction techniques, particular fracture patterns are optimally reassembled by the use of highly defined protocols. Prior to the reduction of a posterior wall fragment, a drill hole is prepared in the wall fragment in a retrograde fashion. Generally a 4.5mm cortical screw is employed. By the preparation of the 4.5mm gliding hole in a retrograde fashion, its orientation adjacent to the articular surface of the acetabulum is carefully directed. A 3.2mm drill sleeve is inserted into the drill hole in the fragment in an antegrade manner. Then the wall fragment is anatomically reduced by the use of tenaculum bone holding forceps. The 3.2mm thread hole is made in the principal iliac portion of the posterior column. After the use of a depth gauge and 4.5mm tap, the lag screw is inserted. Generally to buttress the fracture a supplementary 3.5mm reconstruction plate is applied.

## Posterior Wall with Posterior Column or Transverse Fracture

After the appropriate surgical exposure has been completed, the posterior wall fragment and its capsular attachment are sufficiently displaced to provide the optimal visualization of the posterior column or transverse fracture. The posterior column or transverse fracture is reduced and stabilized with a 4.5mm cortical screw and buttressed with a 3.5mm reconstruction plate prior to the reduction of the posterior wall disruption (Figure 8-14). Once the wall fragment is reduced, its capsular attachment precludes adequate visualization of the posterior column or transverse disruption.

A high posterior column fracture that violates the roof of the greater sciatic notch provides a particular hazard to the superior gluteal vessels during the reduction phase of management (Figure 8-15). The vessels are subject to impalement by the sharp fracture fragments in the notch. Generally, a tenaculum bone holding forceps is applied around the notch with or without the use of the piton. While the fracture is cautiously reduced, the gluteal vessels are gently displaced with a blunt instrument. In contrast an inferior type of posterior column fracture is optimally managed by the use of a reconstruction plate as a reduction tool. The plate is provisionally applied to the inferior portion of the posterior column immediately prior to the reduction. In this way, the relatively inaccessible fracture fragment is readily controlled.

As a general rule, most comminuted acetabular fractures or acetabular disruptions with an associated injury to the ipsilateral sacroiliac joint and/or involvement of the lateral ilium are reduced by progression from the anatomically situated pelvis to more remote sites of displacement. For example, in the presence of an ipsilateral sacroiliac disruption, the sacrum represents the anatomical base for the reconstruction (Figure 8-16). First, the posterior ilium is anatomically reduced with respect to the sacrum. Next, comminution of the lateral ilium is reconstructed starting from the most posterior site and progressing anteriorly and inferiorly. In this way, a portion of the adjacent acetabulum is anatomically reduced. In contrast, when the sacroiliac disruption is a contralateral injury, this problem is addressed after the acetabular reconstruction has been completed. When the acetabular fracture is accompanied by multiple posterior injuries and a diastasis of the symphysis pubis, consideration is given to the use of

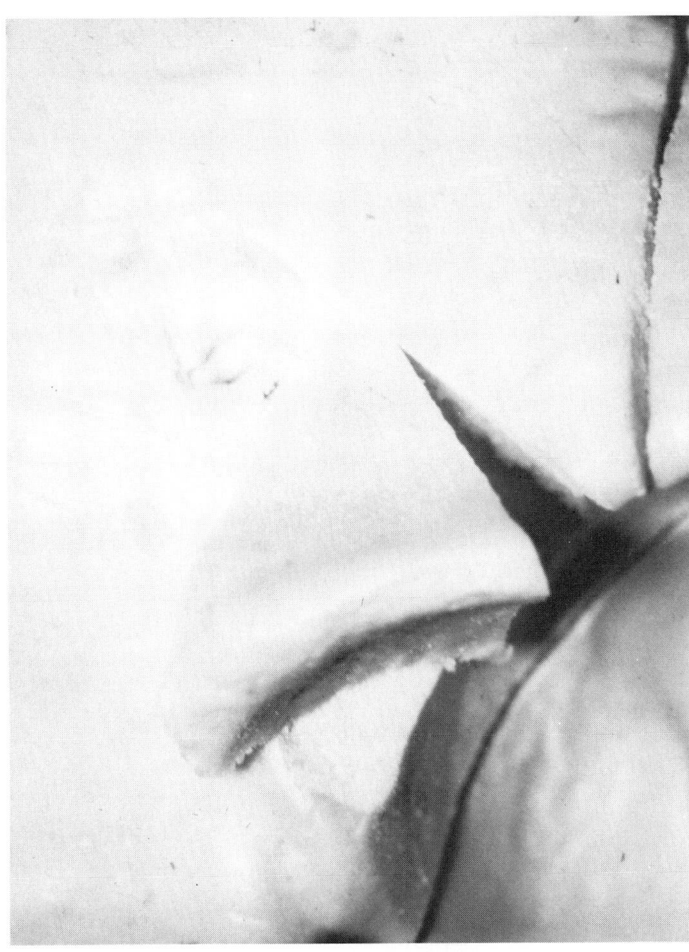

Figure 8-14. A "T" fracture with a posterior wall fragment. Initially, the wall fragment is displaced to facilitate the reduction of the posterior column.

an ilioinguinal incision, which permits an open reduction of the anterior column and the symphysis.

With the ilioinguinal incision, however, fixation of the sacroiliac joint and open reduction of the posterior wall and column becomes difficult or impossible. If the anterior column fracture exits through the posterior portion of the iliac crest, exaggeration of the displacement of the lateral ilium provides access to the outer table of the posterior iliac fragment adjacent to the sacroiliac joint.

Elevation of the gluteal muscular origins on the posterior iliac fragment permits an adequate exposure superior to the roof of the greater sciatic notch, so that two cancellous lag screws can be inserted in a typical fashion to immobilize the sacroiliac joint. A subperiosteal exposure of the adjacent posterior column provides limited access for reduction and stabilization of the posterior part of the acetabulum. If the posterior column and wall are markedly displaced and comminuted, then this extended form of ilioinguinal approach does not provide adequate visualization. In such a case either a

Figure 8-15. A and B: An inlet radiograph and a 3D computed scan that show a high posterior column fracture as part of a both-column injury. During the reduction of the displaced posterior column fragment in the greater sciatic notch, the superior gluteal vessels are carefully protected from the sharp beak of the column fragment.

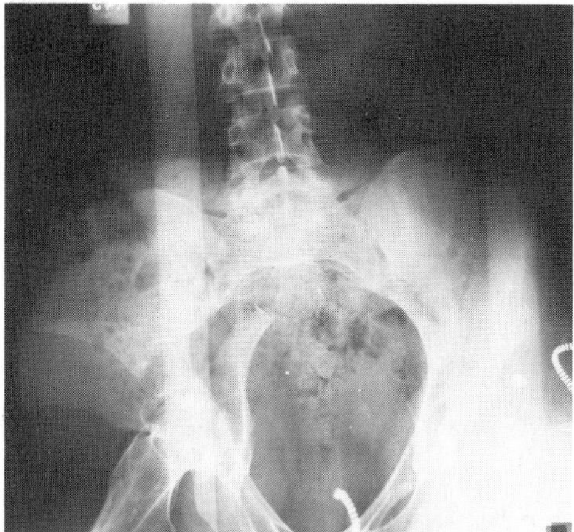

Figure 8-15A.

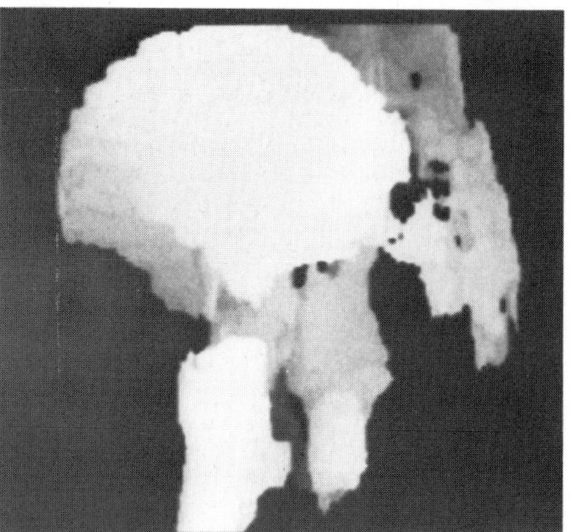

Figure 8-15B.

Figure 8-16. The sequential reduction technique applied to a transverse fracture with iliac comminution and subluxation of the sacroiliac joint. Despite the application of longitudinal and lateral skeletal traction to reduce the femoral head, the acetabular fragments remain widely displaced. For the subsequent open reduction the preferred sequence is the sacroiliac joint, the lateral ilium, and the transverse fracture. A: Preoperative anteroposterior view. B: Preoperative inlet view. C: Preoperative computed scan of the sacroiliac joint. D: Postoperative anteroposterior radiograph.

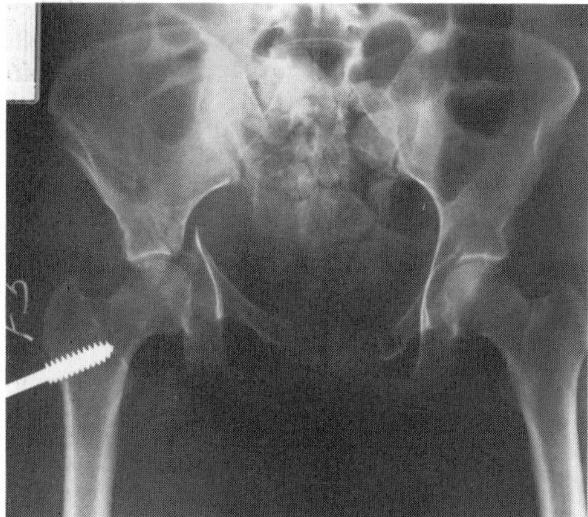

Figure 8-16A.

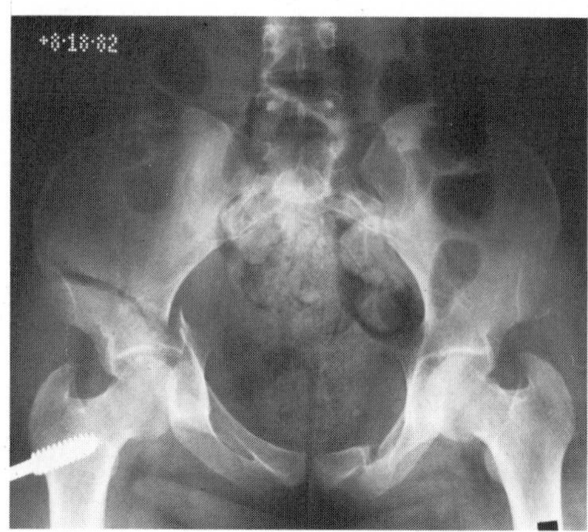

Figure 8-16B.

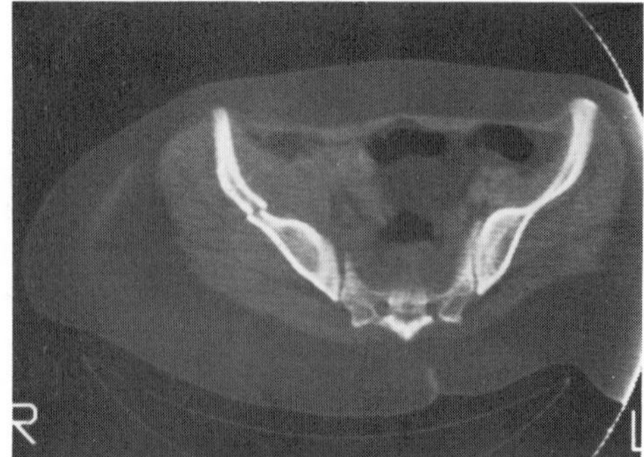


Figure 8-16C.

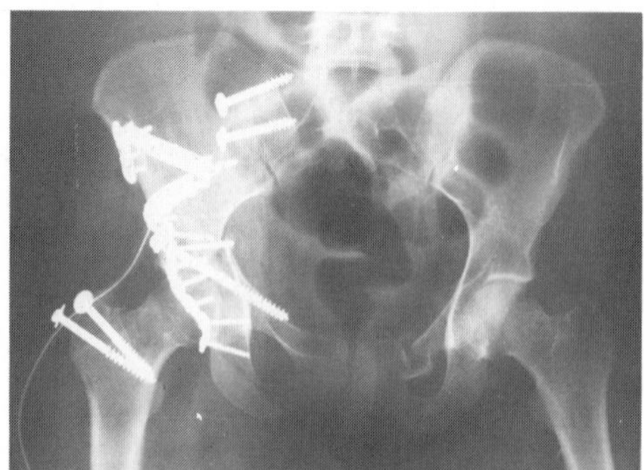

Figure 8-16D.

Figure 8-17. The reduction of a "T" fracture. A: Manipulation of the posterior column fragment with a bone hook. B: With the reduction achieved by compression of the superior fracture lines, a small separation of the base of the "T" fracture inevitably occurs.

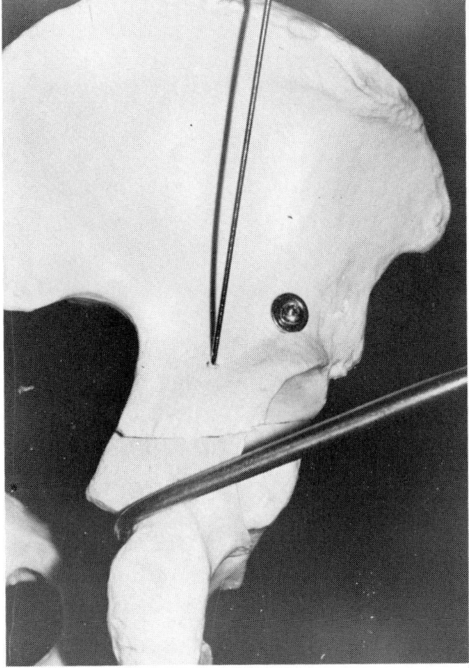

Figure 8-17A.

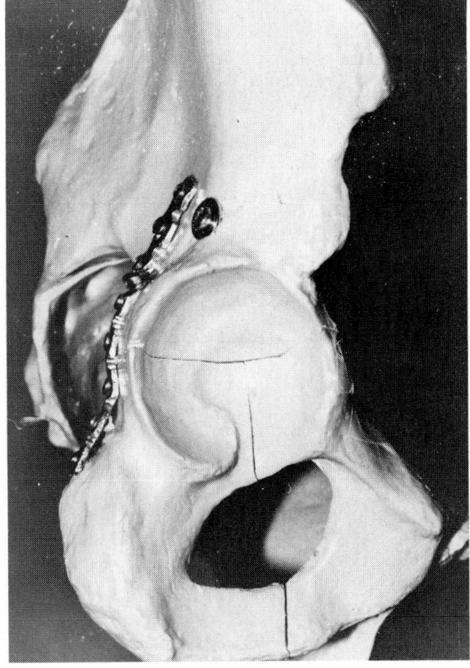

Figure 8-17B.

triradiate or extended iliofemoral approach is utilized for the acetabular exposure, and a Pfannenstiel approach is used to visualize the symphysis.

For the reduction of a "T" fracture, where the anterior and posterior column fragments are both displaced, first the anterior column is reduced with respect to the ilium and provisionally stabilized with a Kirschner wire (Figure 8-13). Then the posterior column fragment is reduced with respect to its posterior surface and with supplementary palpation of the adjacent quadrilateral surface (Figure 8-17). The acetabular surface is inspected while the final approximation of the anterior and posterior column fragments is undertaken. Since the inferior margins of the fracture line between the anterior and posterior fragments cannot be visualized and the compressive force realized by the application of the reduction forceps is imparted strictly to the superior portions of the fracture lines, the inferior portion of the acetabulum tends to yawn apart. For this reason, a typical reduction of a "T" fracture is notable for a slight enlargement of the acetabulum, mainly evident in its inferior equator. Theoretically, a 4.0mm cancellous lag screw can be inserted across the base of the acetabulum, with its insertion into the anterior surface of the superior pubic ramus; the screw courses parallel and immediately

Figure 8-18. Preoperative 3D computed scans (A and B) and a postoperative radiograph (C) illustrate the preferred sequence of reduction for a both-column fracture with segmental comminution of the anterior column. Initially the large anterior iliac fragment is displaced to permit visualization of the inferior portion of the anterior column and the posterior column. Subsequently, the inferior half of the acetabulum is reassembled to the superior half.

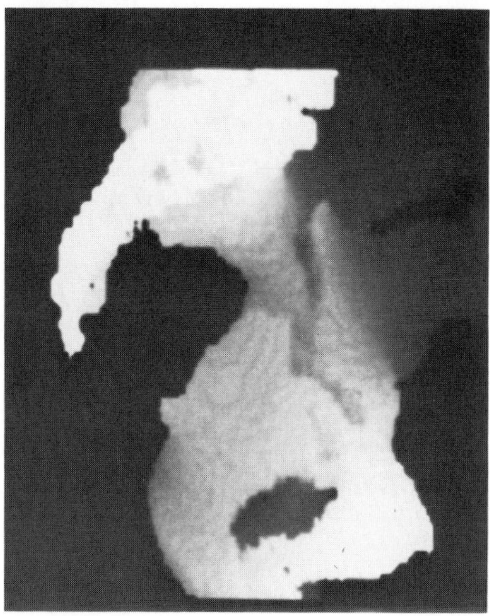

Figure 8-18A.

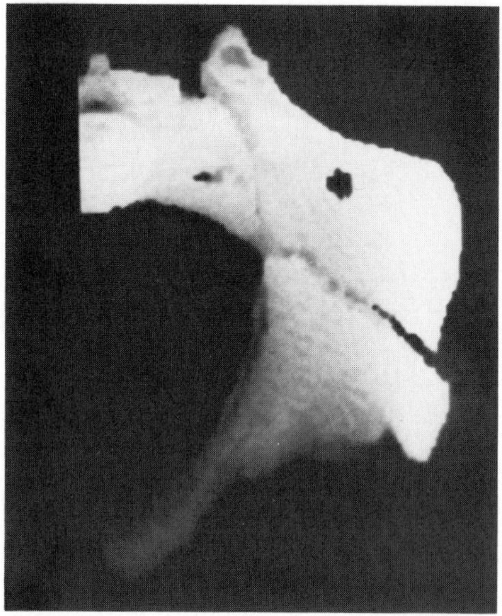

Figure 8-18B.

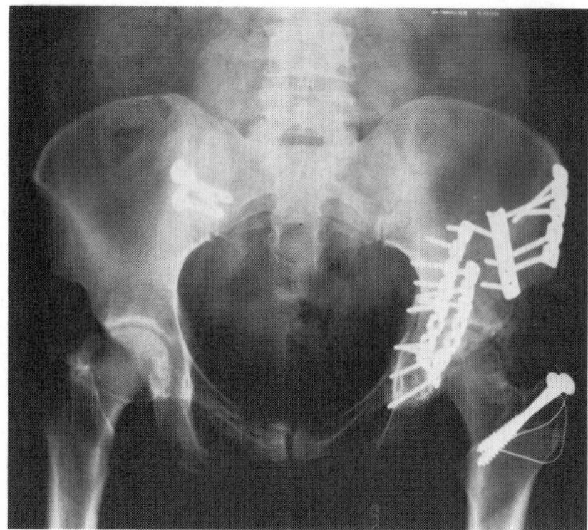

Figure 8-18C.

superior to the roof of the obturator foramen. With the necessary extension of the exposure for adequate visualization of the superior pubic ramus and the limited amount of bone available for the insertion of one perfectly positioned screw, this method is rarely used. Also, this type of acetabular deformity is minimal in the superior weightbearing portion and appears to be consistent with a favorable prognosis.

Another peculiar associated fracture problem is the reduction of a both-column fracture with a segmental disruption of the anterior column (Figure 8-18). This pattern probably accounts for at least half of the both-column fracture variants. In an empirical fashion, the optimal reduction technique elucidated to date and used in conjunction with a triradiate exposure involves an initial rotational displacement of the superior anterior column fragment that includes the anterior superior spine. Upon a surgical release of the insertions of the abdominal muscles, as well as the origins of tensor and the adjacent glutei, the anterior iliac fragment is rotated inwardly by at least 60°. Once it is sufficiently displaced, the articular surfaces of the principal posterior column fragment and the middle fragment of the anterior column are visualized. Then the posterior column is reduced with respect to the inferior half of the anterior column. A 4.0mm cancellous lag screw or a 4.5mm cortical screw is inserted with a lag technique to rigorously approximate these two fragments. By the use of tenaculum bone holding forceps, the inferior half of the acetabulum is reattached to the superior portion of the posterior column. Finally the surgically displaced superior anterior column fragment is reduced. Supplementary lag screws and buttress plates are applied as necessary. This method permits the optimal visualization of the crucial inferior half of the acetabulum. In contrast, when the fracture is sequentially manipulated in the more conventional sequence, working from the anatomically situated ilium to the adjacent displaced fragments and ultimately to the inferior portion of the anterior column, the inferior fragments are largely obscured by the superior ones.

## Late Presentations and Nonunion/Malunion

In these instances the reduction is complicated by the presence of granulation tissue and callus, as well as possible contractures of adjacent soft tissues. Prior to the reduction, a rigorous debridement of all of the displaced fracture surfaces including adjacent ectopic bone is essential. In the presence of posterior column displacement, consideration is given to a releasing incision of the sacrospinous and sacrotuberous ligaments as a way to mobilize the posterior column fragment. Usually these techniques are associated with considerable hemorrhage from the denuded osseous surfaces. Nevertheless, unless the debridement is meticulously performed, an accurate reduction cannot be achieved.

## References

1. Letournel E, Judet R: Fractures of the Acetabulum. New York, Springer-Verlag, 1981, p 247.
2. Tile M: Fractures of the Pelvis and Acetabulum. Baltimore, Williams and Wilkins, 1984, p 223.

3. Mears DC, Rubash HE: External and internal fixation of the pelvic ring, in: AAOS Instructional Course Lectures. St. Louis, Mosby, 33:144, 1984.
4. Mears DC, Rubash HE, Sawaguchi T: Fractures of the acetabulum, in: The Hip, The Proceedings of the Thirteenth Open Meeting of the Hip Society. vol 13, in Press, 1985.
5. Bucholz RW: The pathological anatomy of Malgaigne fracture-dislocations of the pelvis. J Bone Joint Surg 63A:400, 1981.
6. Tile M, Pennal GF: Pelvic disruption: Principles of management. Clin Orthop 151:56, 1980.
7. Mast JW: in Letournel E, ed: Fractures of the Acetabulum and Pelvis, Second Course and Workshop. Paris, 1985, p 50.

# CHAPTER 9

# Techniques of Internal Fixation

## Introduction

Historically the internal fixation devices widely available for use on the long bones of the lower extremity were used to immobilize pelvic and acetabular fractures. The extraordinarily strong and rigid plates designed for use on the femur and tibia were difficult to contour to fit accurately against the irregular pelvic surface. During the past decade several unique designs of plate have been adapted for use on the pelvis. Perhaps the optimal design for widespread application is the 3.5mm reconstruction plate. With the allied bending tools this extraordinarily malleable plate can be contoured to coadapt to virtually all portions of the pelvis. Even when the plate is imperfectly contoured it approximates the reduced fracture fragments. Unlike previous stiffer plates, as the adjacent screws are tightened approximation of the plate to the bone does not provoke deformity of the fracture. This malleability permits the plate to be employed as a reduction tool. With the advent of novel implants such as the Double Cobra plate, combined with biomechanical data[1] on the optimal configuration of the existing implants such as bone screws, most patterns of pelvic and acetabular fracture can be effectively immobilized with stable internal fixation.

For the optimal stabilization of an unstable pelvic or acetabular disruption, generally each anterior, posterior and/or lateral site of involvement is immobilized. Where the pelvic ring is not restored as a stable unit, a late failure of the fixation is likely to occur.

In the following discussion, techniques applicable to specific regions of the pelvis and the acetabulum are reviewed. In many instances for the management of a particular case, multiple techniques are required.

## Internal Fixation of the Pelvis

### Anterior Stabilization

Internal fixation of the symphysis is generally achieved by application of a five or six hole 3.5mm reconstruction plate on the superior aspect of the adjacent superior pubic rami (Figure 9-1). Prior to its application the plate is meticulously contoured with the bending instrumentation. If the screws are carefully directed along the length of the principal thickness of the rami adjacent to the symphysis, they approximate 36mm to 40mm in length and thereby obtain a solid purchase. In younger individuals who possess dense bone, either 3.5mm cortical or cancellous screws are used. In somewhat older individuals with mild osteoporosis or who weigh more than 220 pounds, the 4.5mm reconstruction plate with 4.5mm cortical screws is preferred. To immobilize a nonunion or a malunion where a more prolonged healing period is anticipated, the plate is supplemented by a transverse lag screw or by a second plate applied to the front of the symphysis (Figure 9-2).

When the diastasis of the symphysis is accompanied by a fracture of either superior pubic ramus, then a more extensive exposure is required to permit the application of a longer plate, which courses across the symphysis and the "floating" segment of ramus to the adjacent portions of superior intact pubic rami. Similarly if both superior pubic rami are fractured with or without a diastasis of the symphysis, they are stabilized by resort to a substantially longer 4.5mm reconstruction plate, generally of 10 or 12 holes, which bridges the comminuted zone to the intact pelvic ring (Figure 9-3). A unilateral or bilateral ilioinguinal exposure is needed to provide adequate visualization for the two latter cases. When a screw is inserted into the lateral end of the superior pubic ramus adjacent to the acetabulum, it is carefully oriented parallel to the iliopectineal line so that the risk of inadvertent penetration of the hip joint is minimized. The plate is accurately contoured to fit along the iliopectineal line. When the plate requires a more acute curvature to approximate the iliopectineal line, it is bent

Figure 9-1. Application of a 3.5mm reconstruction plate to the symphysis.

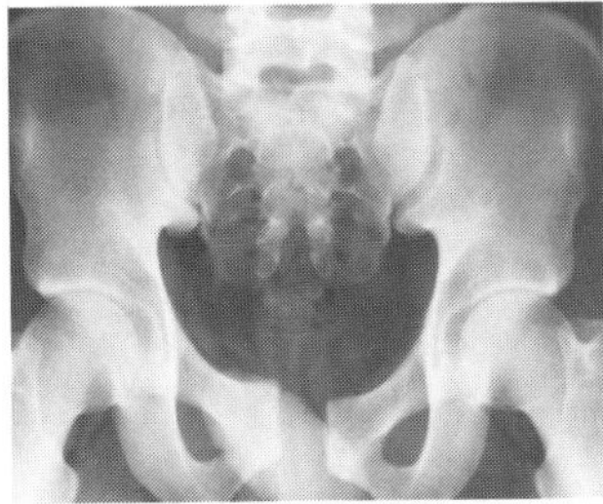
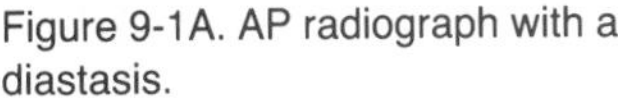

Figure 9-1A. AP radiograph with a diastasis.

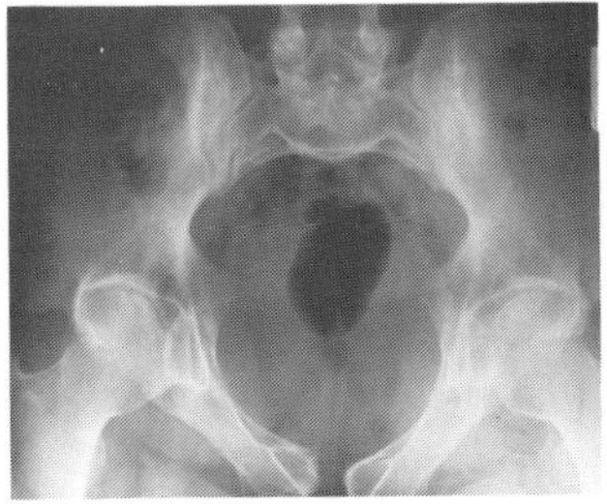

Figure 9-1B. Inlet view.

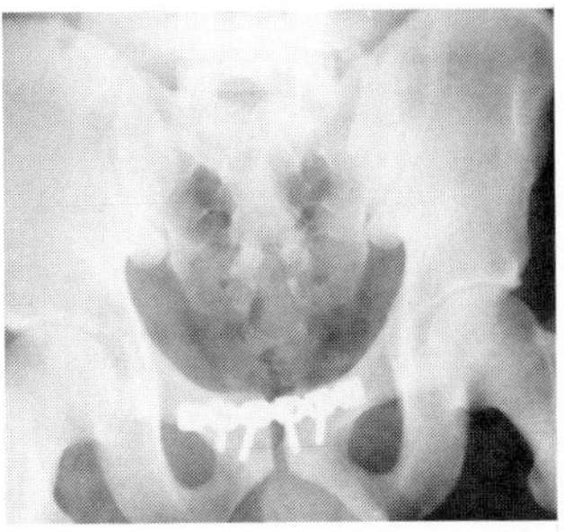

Figure 9-1C. Postoperative AP view.

Figure 9-2. Supplementary anterior fixation. A: AP view of a wide diastasis and unstable left hemipelvis. B: Postoperative AP view after stabilization with 3.5mm anterior reconstruction plate, 4.5mm malleolar screw, and supplementary sacroiliac lag screws. C: Postoperative outlet view after alternative fixation technique with two plates across the symphysis. D: Preoperative AP view of diastasis with right ramus fracture. E: Postoperative view after fixation with a plate.

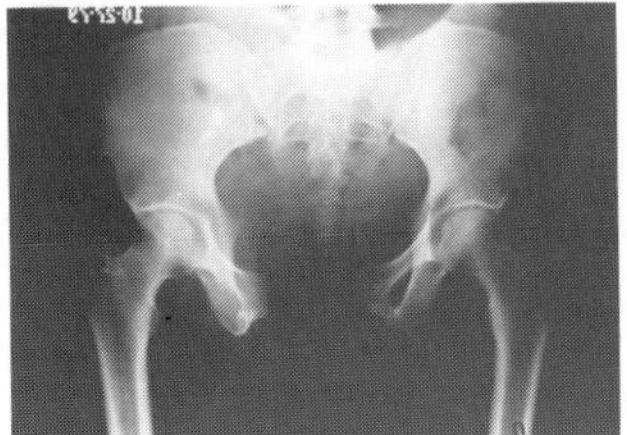

Figure 9-2A.

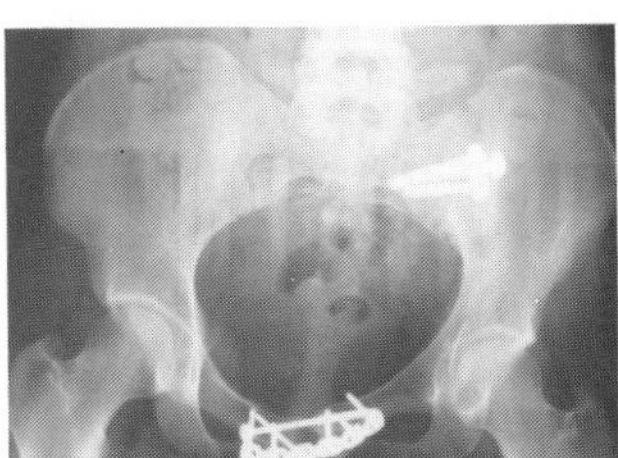

Figure 9-2B.

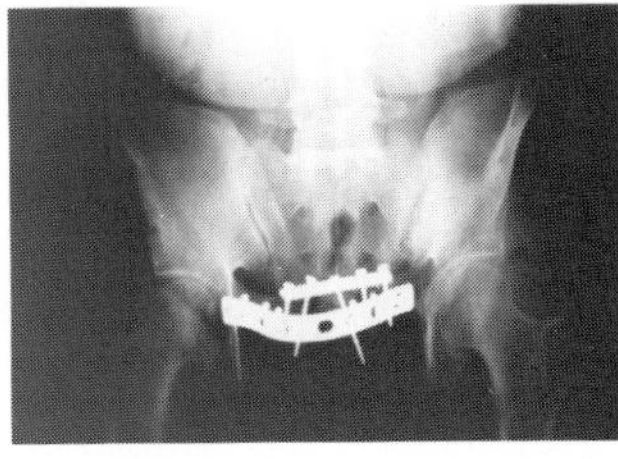

Figure 9-2C.

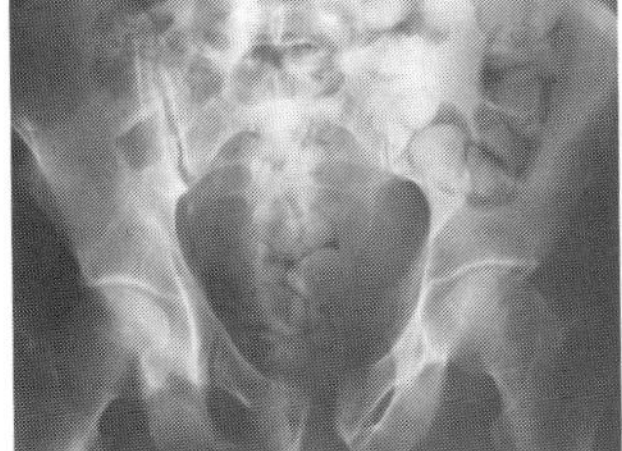

Figure 9-2D.

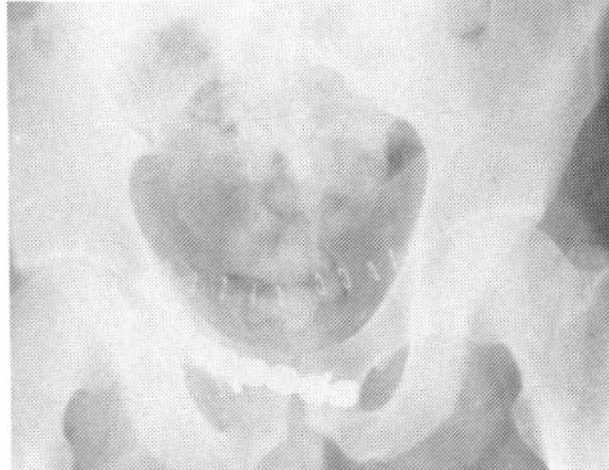

Figure 9-2E.

in the large AO plate bender. Usually repeated alterations in the curavture and trial fittings of the plate are required to prepare an exact replica of the contour. The plate is most easily introduced into the wound through the central aperture achieved by incision of the insertion of one or both heads of the rectus abdominus.

## Posterior Stabilization

A unilateral sacroiliac disruption is immobilized by the insertion of 6.5mm cancellous lag screws from the lateral ilium, which course into the sacral ala or the first sacral vertebral body (Figure 9-4). Generally two screws

Figure 9-3. A 23-year-old woman with a four-part ramus fracture, an unstable right sacroiliac dislocation, and a left-sided sacral fracture. A: Preoperative AP view. B: Postoperative inlet view after internal fixation of the ramic and right SI joint, and external fixation of the sacrum. C: One year later, AP view after removal of anterior plate and the external frame.

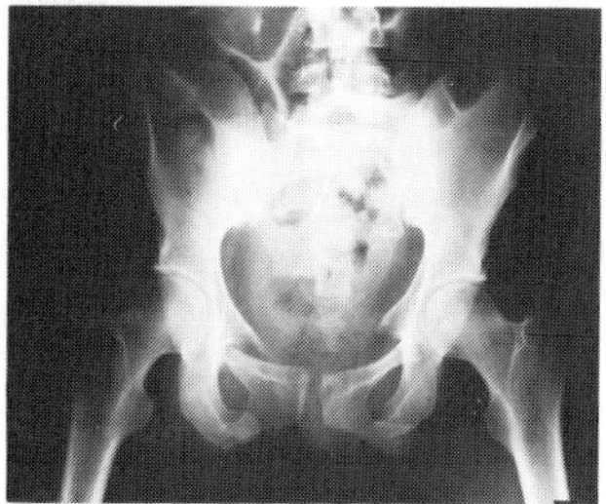

Figure 9-3A.

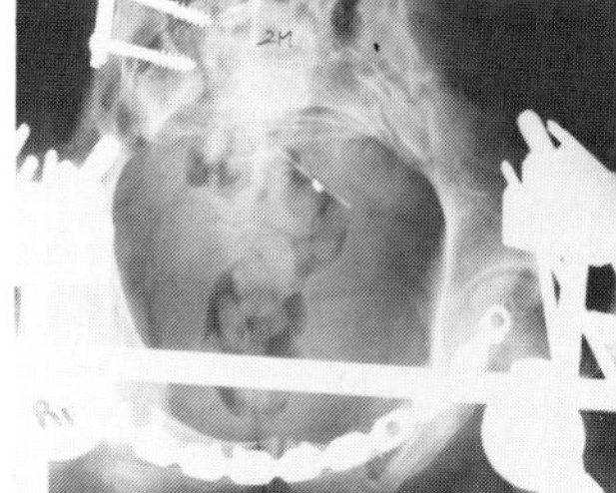

Figure 9-3B.

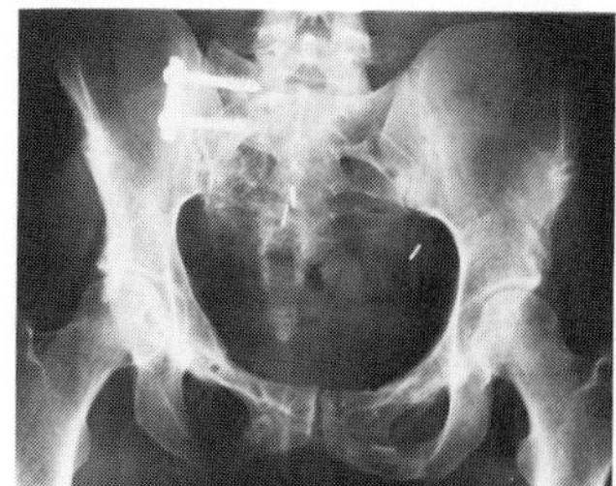

Figure 9-3C.

Figure 9-4. Lag screw fixation of a sacroiliac joint. A: Initial AP view of a vertical shear injury and dislocated right sacroiliac joint. B: Postoperative view with mulitple lag screws. C: Postoperative computed scan of the SI joints with correctly oriented lag screw. D: Postoperative computed scan of the SI joints with technical failure. The screw is directed posteriorly into the neural foramen, fortunately without neurological compromise.

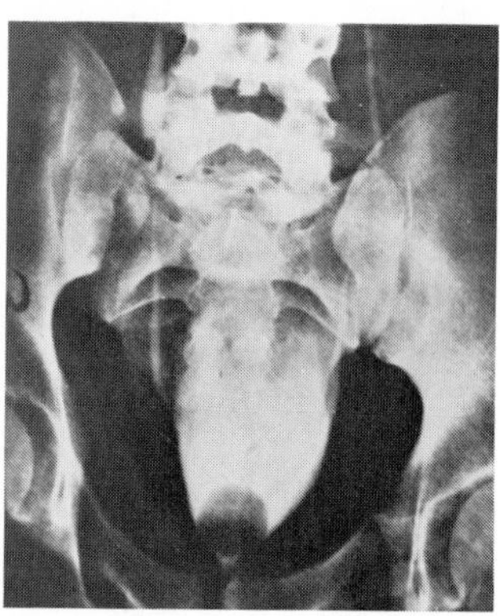

Figure 9-4A.

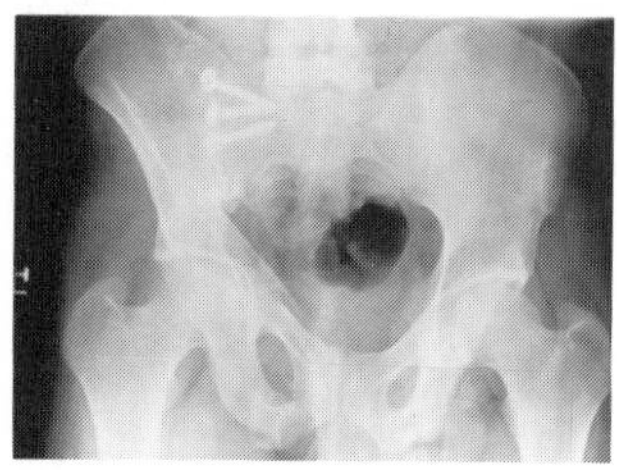

Figure 9-4B.

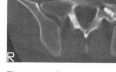

Figure 9-4C.

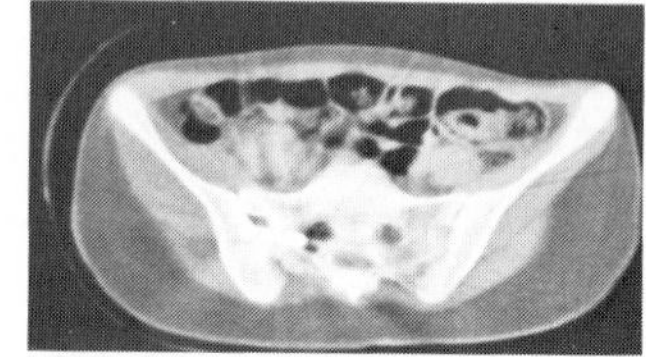

Figure 9-4D.

suffice, although three are used in particularly large individuals. For optimal fixation the screws are inserted through a two or three hole plate, which serves as an extended washer to augment the rotational stability of the fixation[2]; otherwise, a conventional washer is employed with each screw. The first screw is inserted 2.5cm superior and posterior to the roof of the greater sciatic notch (Figure 9-5). The second screw is inserted 2.5cm superior and posterior to the first screw along an imaginary line that courses parallel to a line drawn from the posterior superior spine to the posterior inferior spine. For an isolated internal fixation of the sacroiliac joint, the procedure is undertaken with the patient mounted in a position that is halfway between prone and lateral so that the lateral ilium is parallel to the floor. Through a posterior longitudinal incision superficial to the posterior superior spine and with a reflection of the superior portion of the origin of gluteus maximus, the sacroiliac joint and the adjacent lateral ilium are approached. Otherwise, the procedure can be undertaken as a part of an acetabular exposure that visualizes the posterior column and greater sciatic notch. Once the sacroiliac joint has been satisfactorily reduced, the lag screws are inserted using 3.2mm drill holes. A 3.2mm drill bit is inserted at a right angle to the ilium. The advancement of the drill through the superficial and deep iliac cortices is noted. In typical cases where the posterior sacroiliac ligaments are wholly disrupted, the advancement of the drill bit into the sacral ala is monitored by a fingertip inserted into the sacroiliac joint. After the drill bit has been inserted through the superficial cortex of the sacrum, it is advanced slowly and cautiously. It is not permitted to exit through the deep sacral cortex with the obvious risk to various soft tissues. Typically, the drill bit is inserted for a length of 50mm, although 45mm to 60mm lengths may be employed in smaller or larger individuals respectively. Ideally a depth marker is applied to the drill bit to inhibit the likelihood for excessive insertion. After the use of a depth gauge and appropriate tap, the screw is inserted. To realize a lag effect the 45mm screw possesses a short thread of 16mm. When a 50mm or longer screw is employed, the 32mm thread length is suitable and provides a superior fixation. The screws are tightened until the ilium approximates the sacrum.

While the first posterior sacral foramen is palpated, a 3.2mm drill bit is applied to the lateral ilium and aimed superior to the foramen to minimize the likelihood of a nerve root injury.

When the sacrum is fractured through the lateral sacrum or neural foramina, lag screw fixation can be employed, although much greater care is required for the insertion of lengthy screws into the sacral bodies without violation of the neural canal and foramina (Figure 9-6). While the insertion of the longer screw into the first sacral body can be undertaken as previously described, the insertion of the screw into the second sacral body is more hazardous. The position of the sacral foramina is so variable that image intensification is needed to identify the appropriate site for the insertion. With a technique of biplane image intensification described by Matta,[3] an anteroposterior and an oblique view equivalent to a Fergusson radiographic view are obtained. As an alternative, the use of a Double Cobra

Figure 9-5. A model pelvis with sacroiliac fixation.

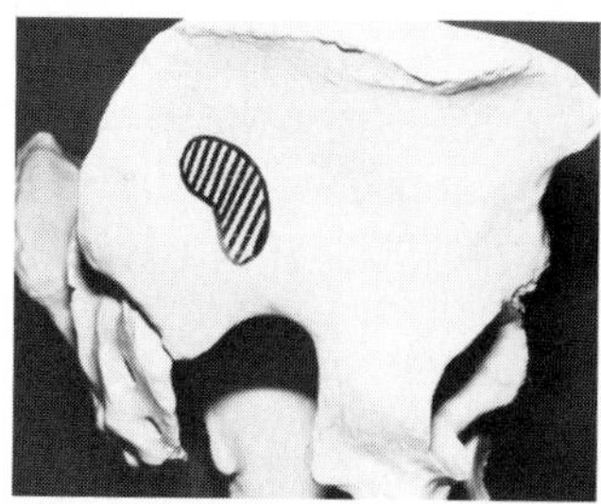

Figure 9-5A. Insertion site on lateral ilium.

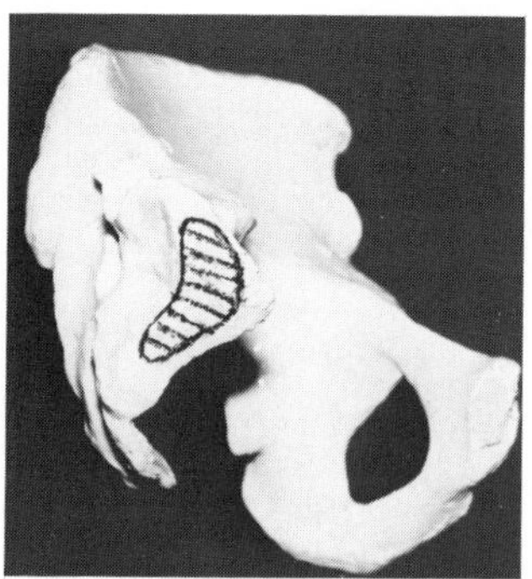

Figure 9-5B. Insertion site on sacral ala.

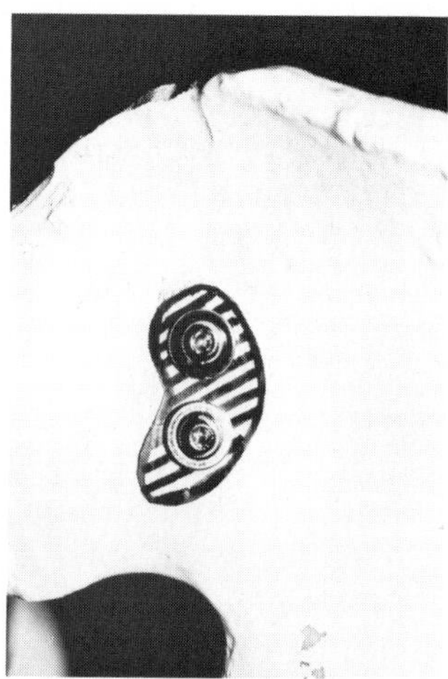

Figure 9-5C. Close-up of screws on lateral ilium.

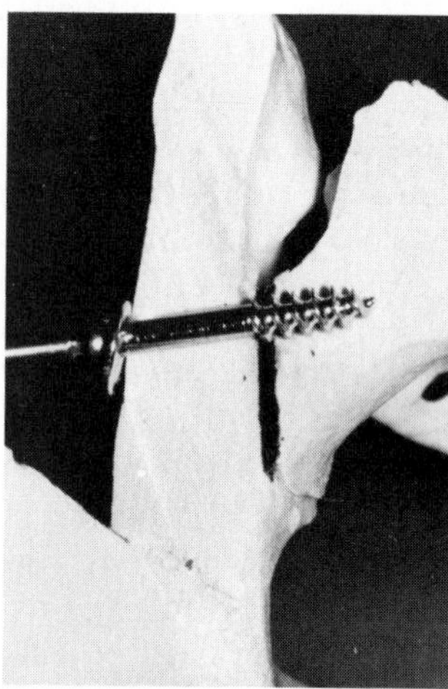

Figure 9-5D. Cross-section, with properly oriented screw.

Figure 9-6. Sacral fracture stabilized with three lengthy lag screws and a plate that serves as a washer. A simple external frame supplemented the posterior internal fixation. A: Preoperative AP view with a right-sided vertical shear injury through the neural foramina. B: Postoperative AP view.

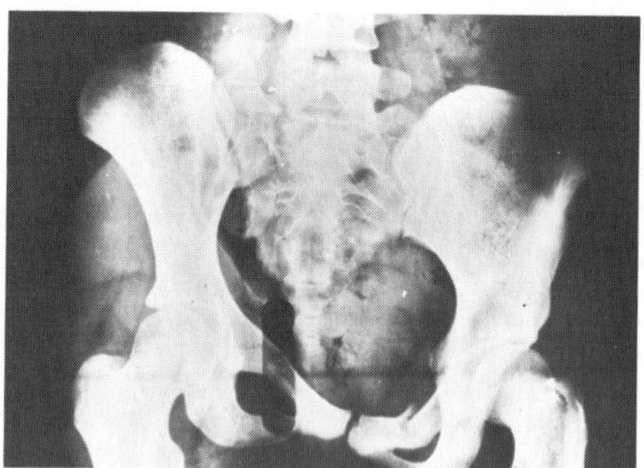

Figure 9-6A.

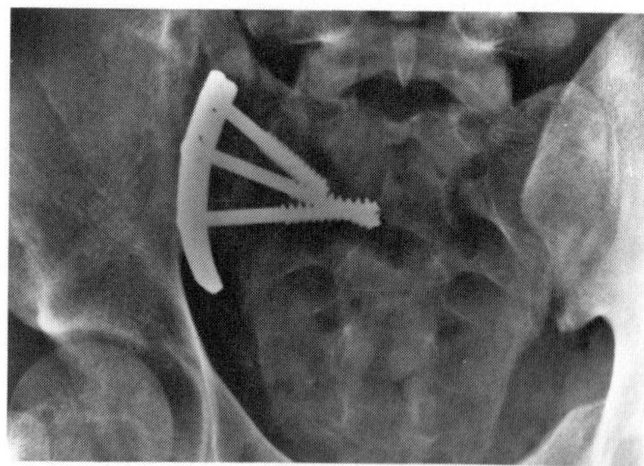

Figure 9-6B.

plate[4] provides a way to stabilize the fracture with a substantially lower risk to the adjacent neurological structures. For most displaced fractures of the sacral body, the latter method is preferred.

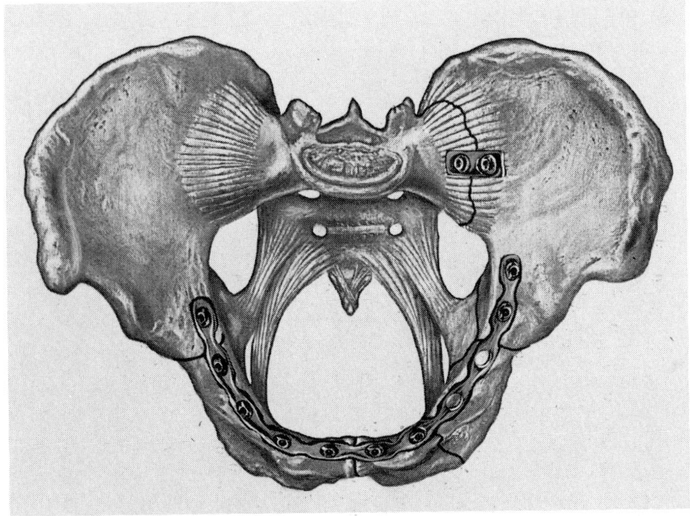

Figure 9-7. Anterior fixation of a sacroiliac joint with a two-hole plate combined with a Letournel plate for the contralateral ramus fractures, performed through an extended ilioinguinal incision.

For a posterior iliac fracture adjacent to the sacrum or a fracture/dislocation extending from the sacroiliac joint into the posterior ilium, comparable techniques of exposure equivalent to that described for immobilization of a sacroiliac joint are employed. Typically, the posterior iliac fragment is displaced and tethered by the intact posterior sacroiliac ligament (Figure 9-5C). The fragment is reduced by the use of tenaculum bone holding forceps. Then, two or three 6.5mm long-threaded cancellous lag screws are inserted into the posterior iliac crest between the posterior superior and inferior spines. The screws provide highly effective fixation of the ilium without the need to immobilize or fuse the sacroiliac joint. Occasionally, in more comminuted examples a supplementary buttress plate is applied to the lateral ilium or along the iliac crest. For a highly unstable fracture dislocation, lag screws across the sacroiliac joint complement the reconstruction of the posterior ilium.

As part of an anterior pelvic or acetabular reconstruction, stabilization of the sacroiliac joint can be undertaken. By the use of the AO flexible drilling instrumentation, lag screws can be inserted into the sacral ala that secure the posterior ilium. During the procedure, the fifth lumbar nerve root is carefully protected. In the absence of the flexible instrumentation, a two-hole plate can be applied to the sacroiliac joint (Figure 9-7). From a biomechanical consideration, the fixation is less effective than the use of lag screws, although satisfactory clinical results have been documented. In many of the cases where an anterior exposure of an associated acetabular fracture with a sacroiliac dislocation is performed, a supplementary

Figure 9-8. Stabilization of a sacroiliac joint by resort to an ilioinguinal approach to a both-column fracture with marked comminution of the lateral ilium and anterior column. The iliac fracture was displaced to permit the insertion of the sacroiliac lag screws.

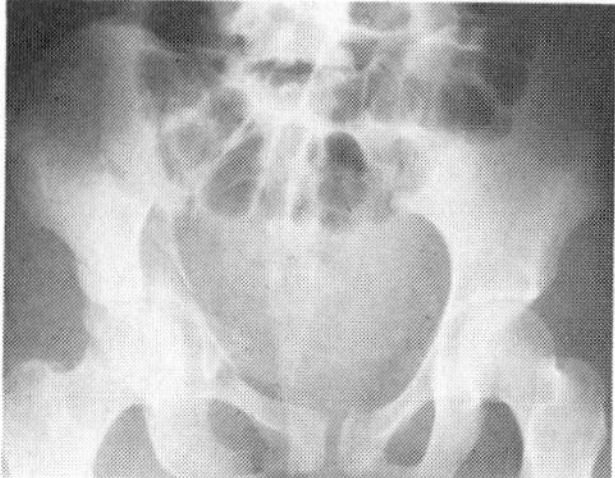

Figure 9-8A. AP view.

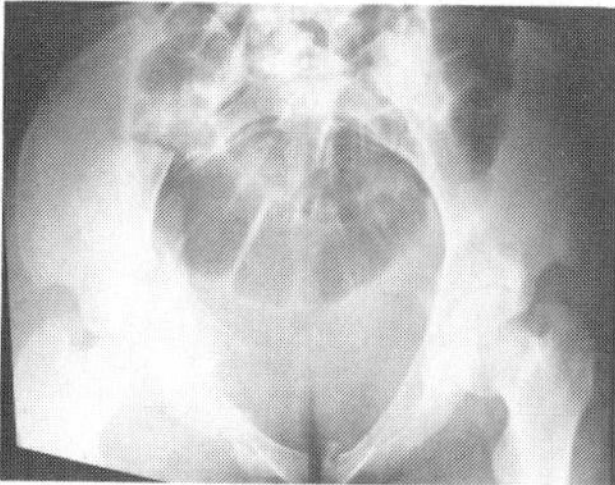

Figure 9-8B. Inlet view.

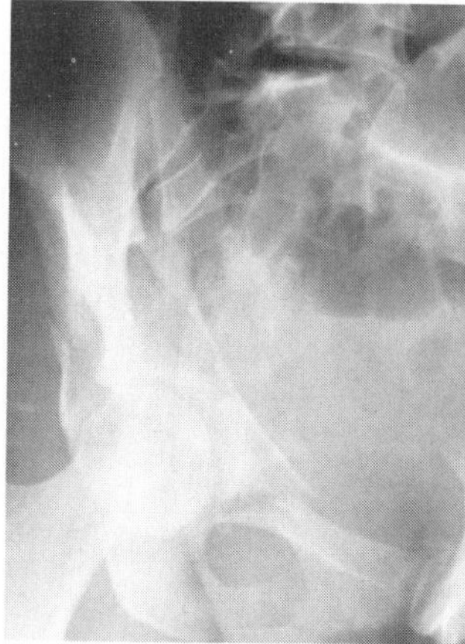

Figure 9-8C. Obturator oblique view.

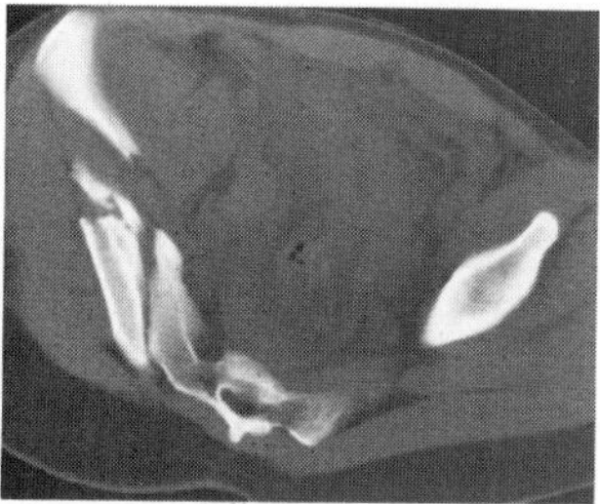

Figure 9-8D. Computed scan, SI and iliac disruption.

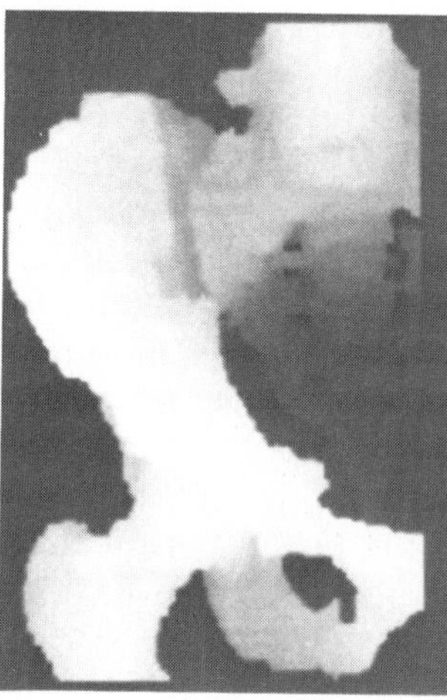

Figure 9-8E. 3D anterior view.

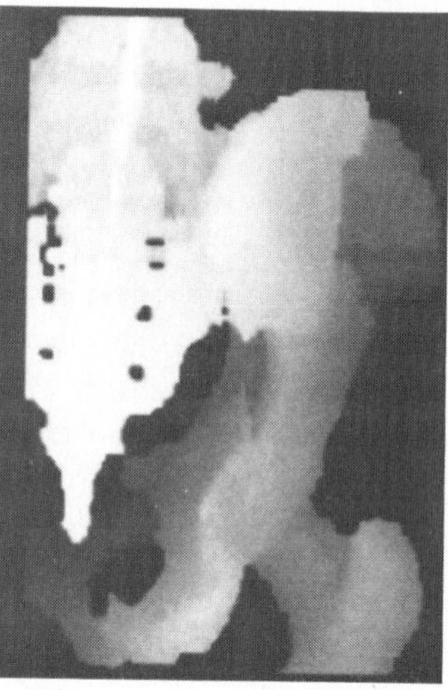

Figure 9-8F. 3D posterior view.

fracture line transgresses the posterior ilium (Figure 9-8). After the sacroiliac joint is reduced, possibly through an ilioinguinal incision, the iliac fracture is deliberately displaced to provide access to the outer surface of the posterior iliac fragment. Two or three cancellous lag screws are inserted across the sacroiliac joint in a conventional manner.

For immobilization of bilateral unstable sacroiliac dislocations or a comminuted sacral fracture, two types of immobilization are available. A threaded sacral bar can be inserted with a transverse orientation through the portions of the posterior ilia that project beyond the sacroiliac joints. In the case of bilateral sacroiliac disruptions, supplementary cancellous lag screws are

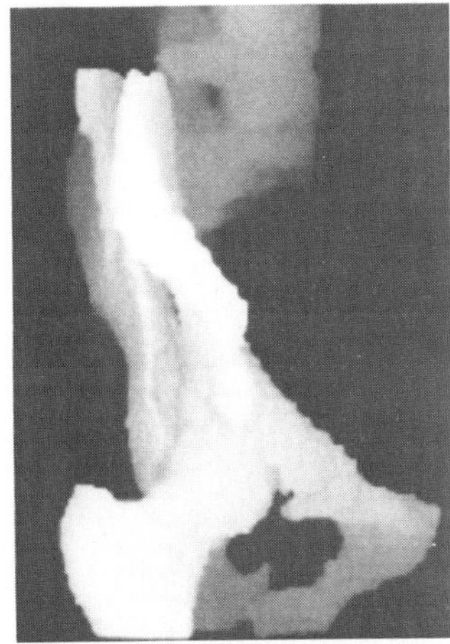

Figure 9-8G. 3D obturator oblique view.

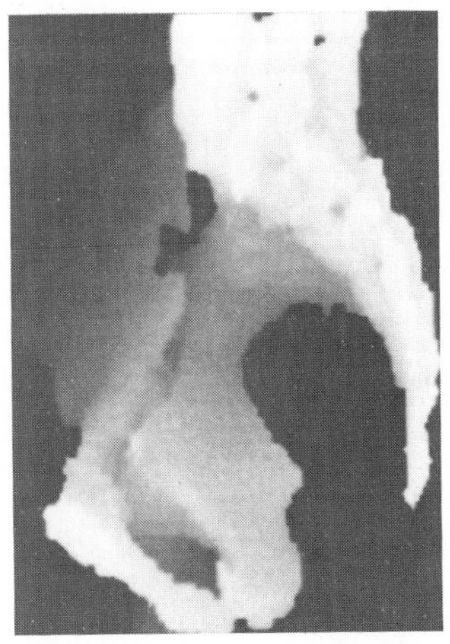

Figure 9-8H. 3D inner view.

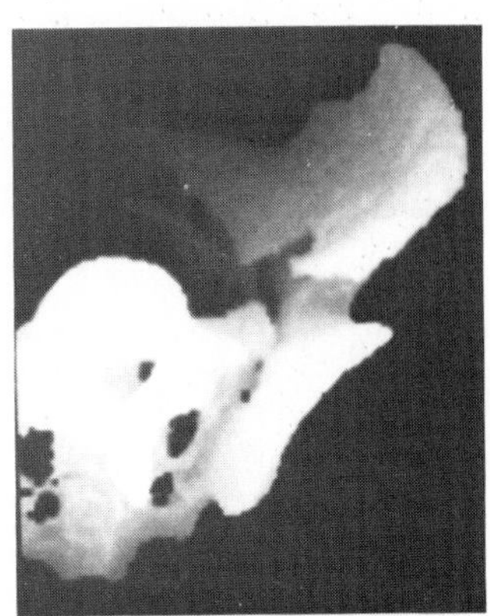

Figure 9-8I. 3D superior view.

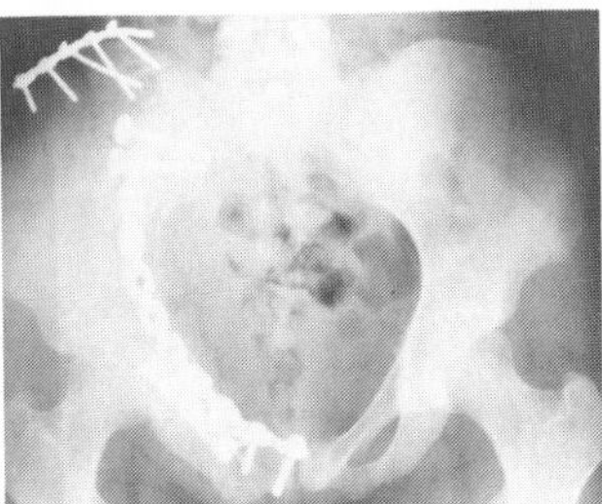

Figure 9-8J. Postoperative AP view.

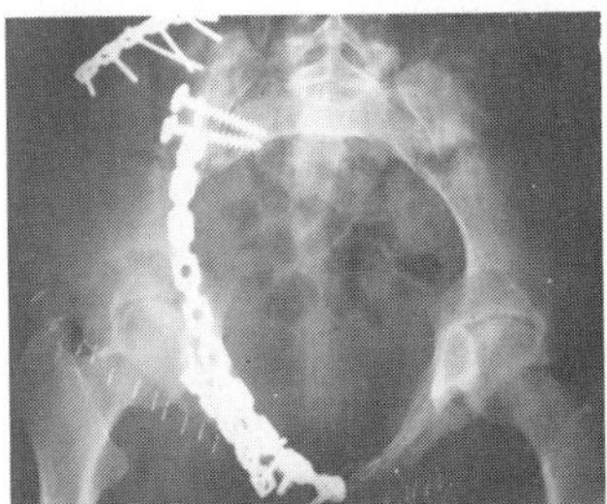

Figure 9-8K. Postoperative inlet view.

used to immobilize the sacroiliac joints.[5] In the absence of such screws, the sacral bar itself does not afford stability of the sacroiliac joints so that the sacrum displaces anteriorly and inferiorly with respect to the opposing posterior ilia. More recently, special washer-plates have been devised that attach to the sacral bar. Sacroiliac lag screws are inserted through the washer-plates to provide fixation of the posterior pelvic ring.

In an effort to develop a more effective technique applicable to both bilateral sacroiliac disruptions and comminuted sacral fractures, the Double Cobra plate was devised[4] (Figure 9-9). It is available in multiple sizes for application to individuals of differing weights. The width of the plate is referable to the width of the posterior pelvis at the level of the posterior superior spines. This measurement can be documented by scrutiny of the appropriate section of a computed scan. The plate is inserted into to a tunnel below the paraspinous muscles with the osteotomized spinous processes. The portion of the posterior iliac crest and the spines that protrude beyond the back of the sacrum are osteotomized. Once the plate has been inserted into the tunnel, two screws

Figure 9-9. Radiographic and computed views of a farmer of 35 years and 360 pounds, who overturned his tractor, which landed upon him. His bilateral unstable sacroiliac joints and diastasis were immobilized with a Double Cobra plate and a plate across the symphysis. He returned to work about four months later.

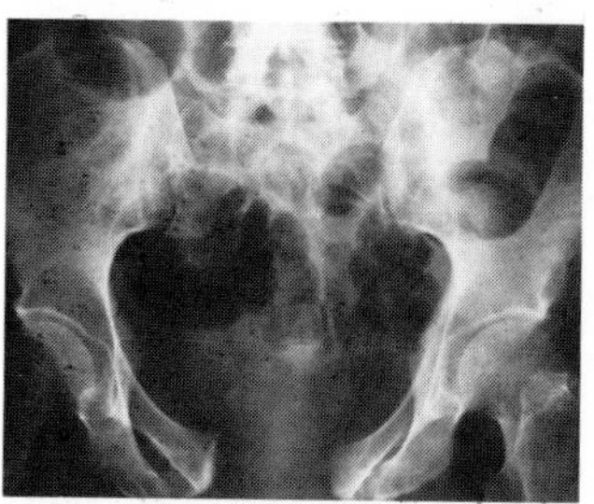

Figure 9-9A. Preoperative AP view.

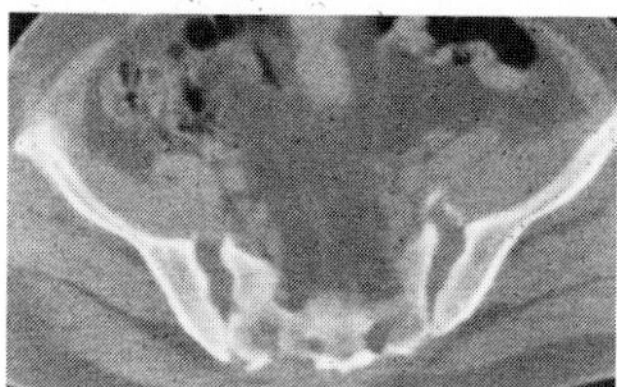

Figure 9-9B. Computed scan, posterior pelvis.

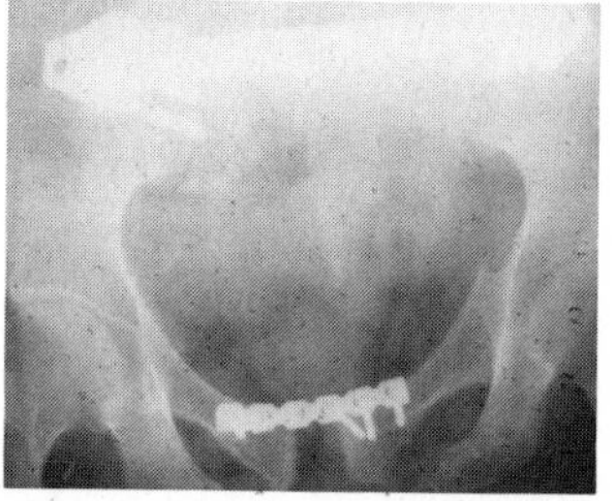

Figure 9-9C. Postoperative AP view.

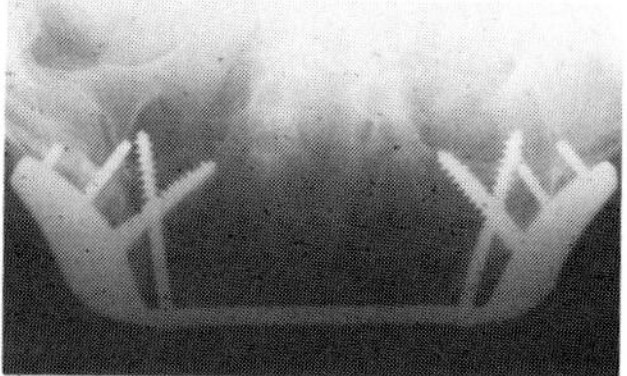

Figure 9-9D. Fergusson view, four months postoperative.

are inserted through the drill holes in the principal part of the plate. The screws are directed between the tables of the ilia and permit approximation of the plate to the ilia and, thereby, to the back of the sacrum. With the obliquity of the ends of the plate during the insertion of the screws, the fracture surfaces are rigorously approximated. Supplementary screws are inserted into the ends of the plate, which provide both lag screw fixation of the sacroiliac joints and rotational stability for the posterior pelvic ring.

In a smaller individual who presents with bilateral sacroiliac disruptions or a comminuted sacral fracture, a 4.5mm reconstruction plate is used instead of the Double Cobra plate (Figure 9-10). The posterior superior spines are osteotomized to provide a flat surface across the back of the pelvic ring. The plate is contoured to fit this surface so that two or three holes at either end of the plate fit against the lateral ilia.

## Stabilization of the Lateral Ilium

In most instances stabilization of the lateral ilium is undertaken as part of the reconstruction of an associated acetabular fracture or multiple pelvic ring disruptions. For a minimally comminuted fracture, lag screw fixation is preferred to minimize the devascularization of the broad iliac surface that inevitably follows the application of multiple plates. Both the iliac crest and the acetabular roof are amenable to lag screw fixation in an approximately anteroposterior plane. Generally, 6.5mm long-threaded cancellous lag screws, 4.5mm cortical

Figure 9-10. Techniques of fixation of bilateral unstable sacroiliac joints or a sacral fracture in a smaller individual. A: Diagram of bilateral fixation of the SI joints with lag screws combined with a plate across the symphysis. B: Alternatively, with an unstable sacral fracture a 4.5 reconstruction plate can be employed: (i) initial AP view with left-sided sacral fracture and multiple ramus disruption; (ii) initial inlet view; (iii) postoperative AP view; (iv) postoperative inlet view; (v) postoperative Fergusson view.

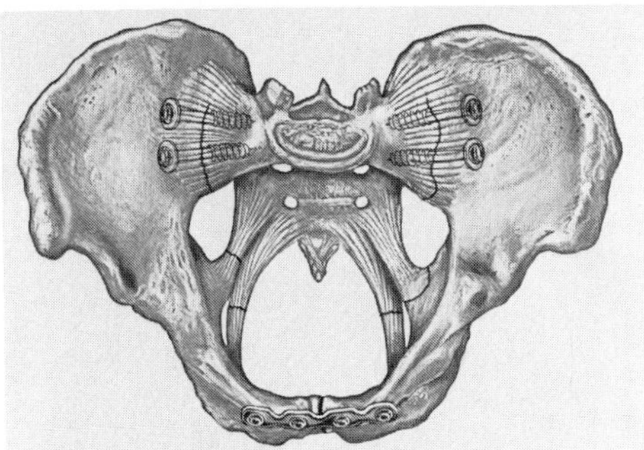

Figure 9-10A.

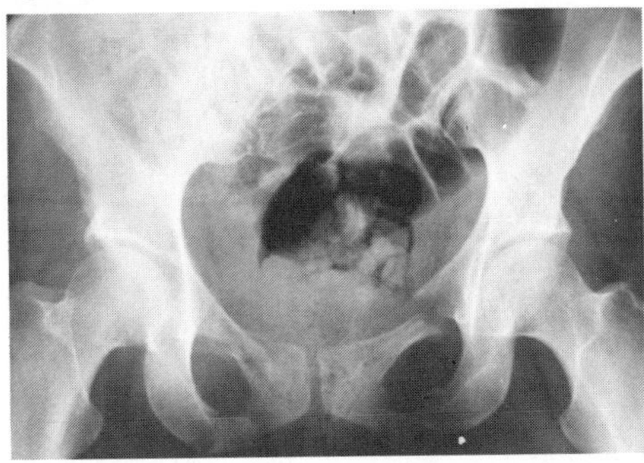

Figure 9-10B i.

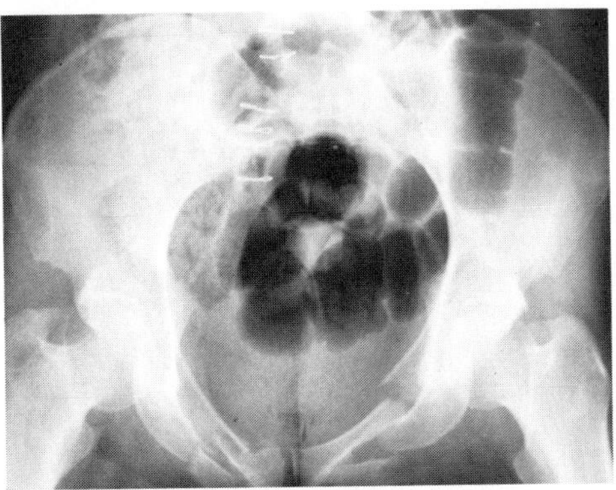

Figure 9-10B ii.

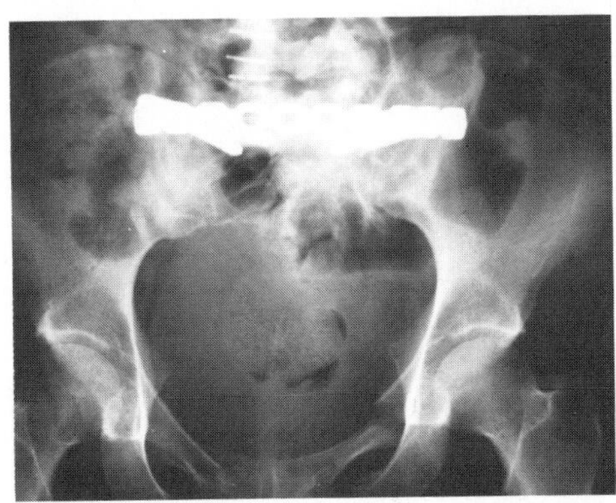

Figure 9-10B iii.

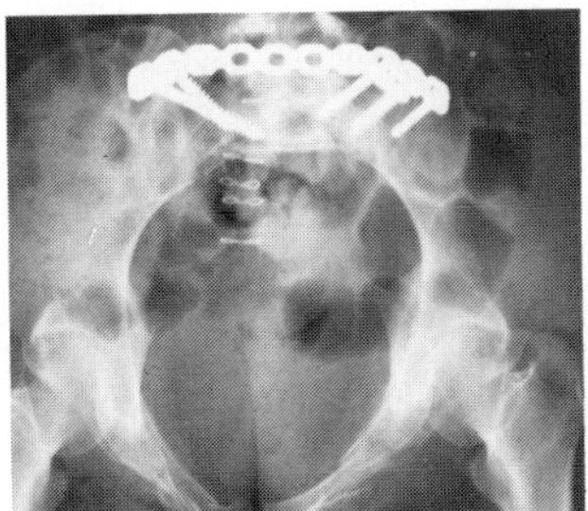

Figure 9-10B iv.

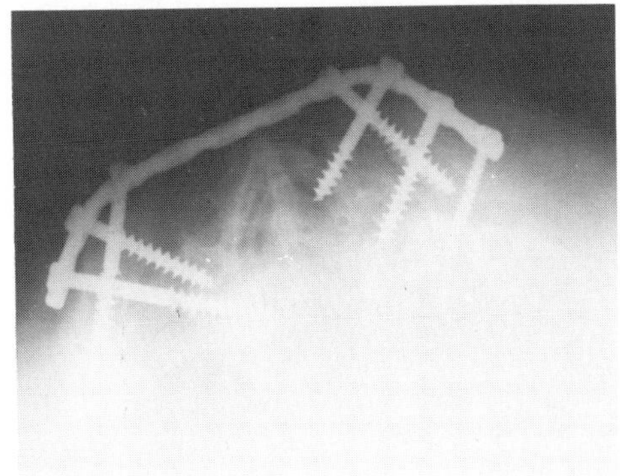

Figure 9-10B v.

screws inserted with a lag technique, or 4.5mm malleolar screws are preferred. Rarely, in smaller individuals 4.0 cancellous screws are used. The use of particularly long screws greatly augments the stability of the fixation.[1] As the degree of comminution of the bone increases,

Figure 9-11. Vertical shear injury with a diastasis and a left iliac fracture in an 18-year-old motorcyclist with a right distal tibial fracture and a left femoral fracture. With the bilateral lower extremity fractures and the initial nonweightbearing status, only the ilium was reconstructed.

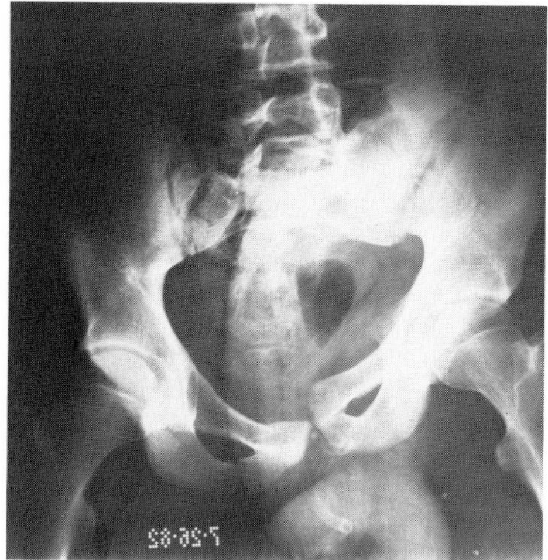
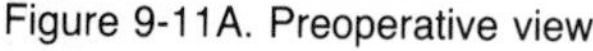

Figure 9-11A. Preoperative view.

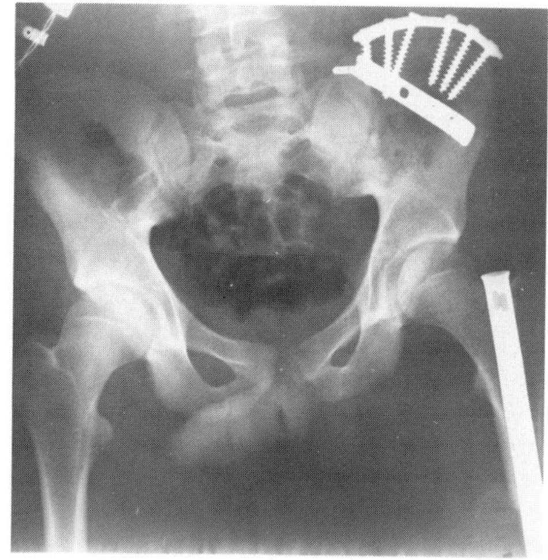

Figure 9-11B. Postoperative view.

Figure 9-12. A comminuted right iliac fracture with bilateral sacroiliac disruptions and four-part ramus fractures. A: Preoperative inlet view. B: Preoperative 3D scan. C: Preoperative computed scan of posterior pelvis. D: Postoperative AP view with buttress plates and supplementary lag screws.

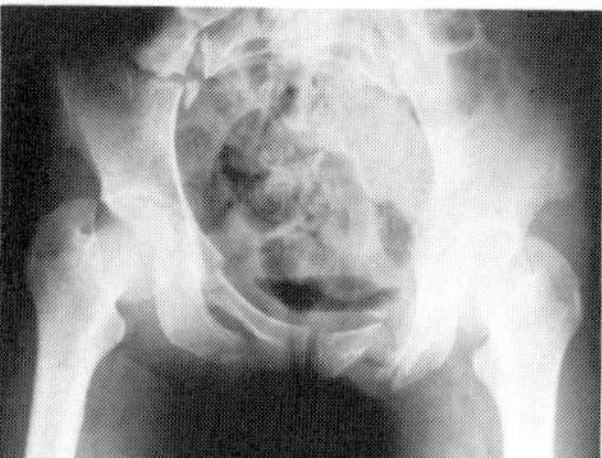

Figure 9-12A.

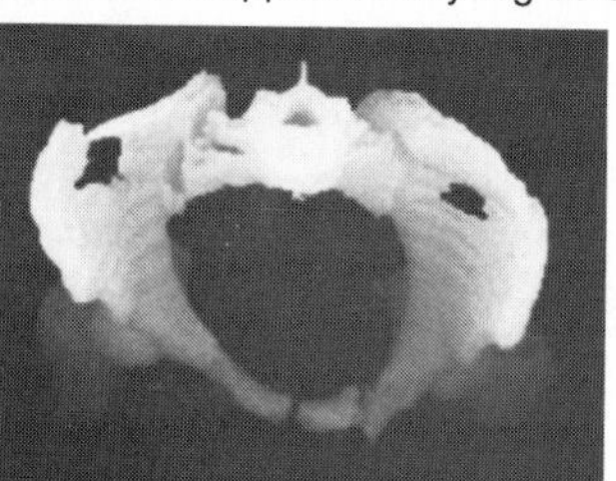

Figure 9-12B.

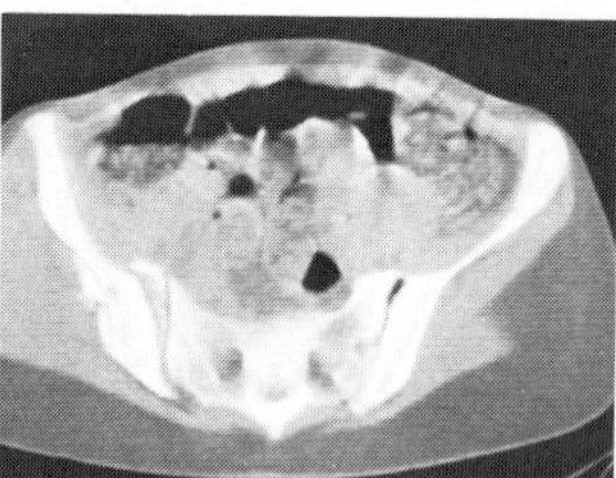

Figure 9-12C.

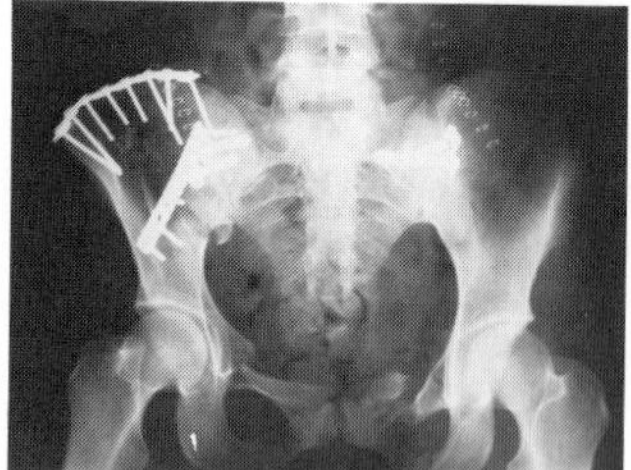

Figure 9-12D.

the role of buttress plates grows progressively (Figures 9-11 and 9-12). Generally, 3.5mm DC plates are applied to the inner or outer table depending upon the type of surgical exposure. In most other portions of the pelvis, 3.5mm reconstruction plates are preferred so that the plates contour spontaneously to the bone to minimize malalignment of the fracture. In contrast with the thin

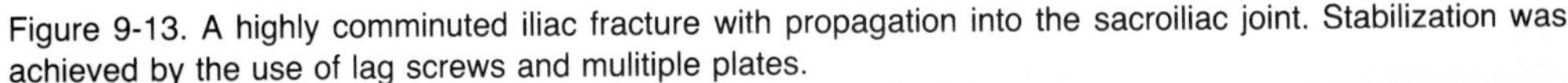

Figure 9-13. A highly comminuted iliac fracture with propagation into the sacroiliac joint. Stabilization was achieved by the use of lag screws and mulitiple plates.

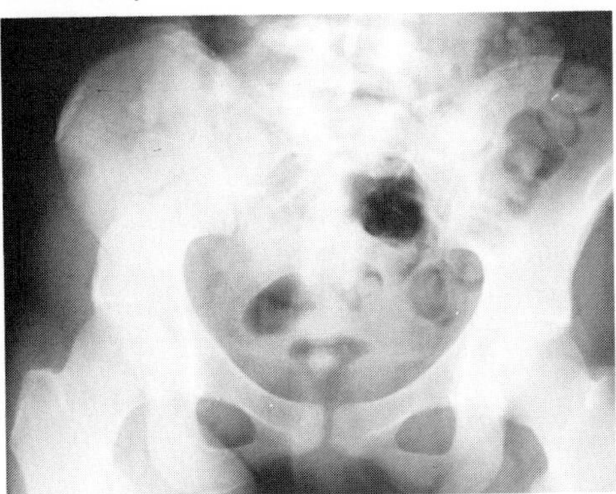

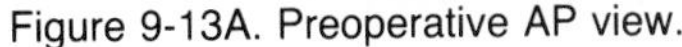

Figure 9-13A. Preoperative AP view.

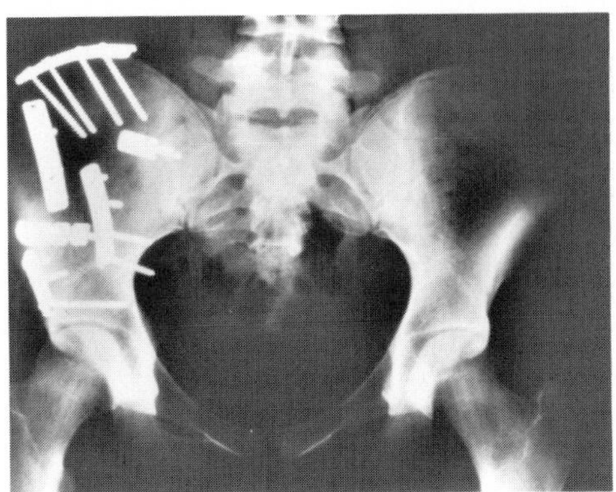

Figure 9-13B. Postoperative AP view.

segment of available ilium apart from the crest or acetabular roof, a more rigid plate is preferred to buttress the bone and prevent instability. Also, the more rigid plate is employed partly as a reduction tool when one major fragment is displaced deep to the other. Initially the plate is anchored to the more superficial bone fragment. Then supplementary screws are inserted into the deeper fragment. As the latter screws are tightened, the fragment is elevated to the level of the adjacent bone. If the more flexible reconstruction plate is used, the plate coadapts to the displaced osseous fragment. In the most comminuted fractures, a supplementary reconstruction plate is applied around the iliac crest to provide fixation at 90° to the buttress plates applied to the lateral ilium or the inner table. With the extraordinarily thin nature of the central portion of the bone, effective stabilization of the typical highly comminuted fracture necessitates the application of multiple plates (Figure 9-13).

When the lateral iliac fracture represents a propagation of an acetabular fracture, a lengthy plate is used to buttress both the ilium and the relevant portion of acetabulum. For example, a straight plate can be applied along the posterior column and the adjacent ilium, or a curved plate can be contoured to the posterior wall and the acetabular rim with extension to the superior gluteal ridge (Figure 9-14). When an ilioinguinal incision is employed to approach a comminuted anterior column disruption (Figures 9-8 and 9-15), the plate extends from the lateral ilium along the superior pubic ramus to or across the symphysis pubis. Whenever the longer plates are used to bridge from the posterior or anterior column to the ilium, the screws inserted into the midportion require careful orientation away from the articular surface of the hip joint. In such a high risk zone frequently one

Figure 9-14. A highly comminuted both-column fracture with anterior extension into the lateral ilium. By the use of an extended iliofemoral approach, a long plate was applied from the posterior column to the lateral ilium along with a supplementary iliac plate. A: Preoperative AP view. B: Inlet view. C: Obturator oblique view. D: Iliac oblique view. E: Computed scan with iliac fracture and propagation into the SI joint. F: Postoperative inlet view. G: Postoperative outlet view. H: AP view at 12 weeks with small amount of ectopic bone.

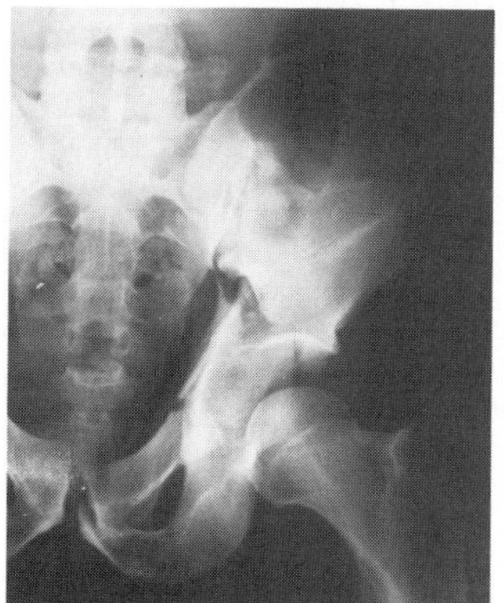

Figure 9-14A.

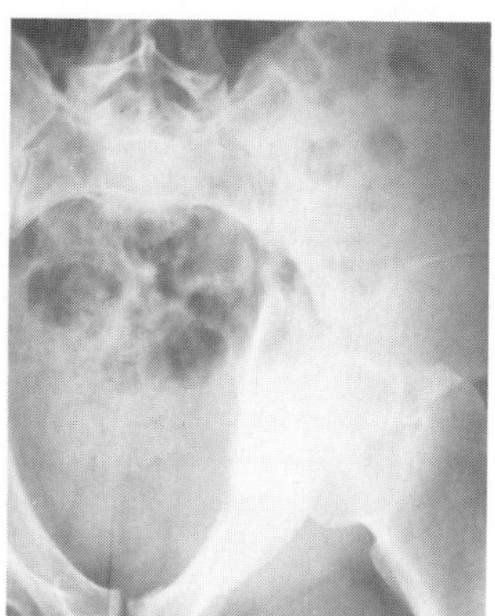

Figure 9-14B.

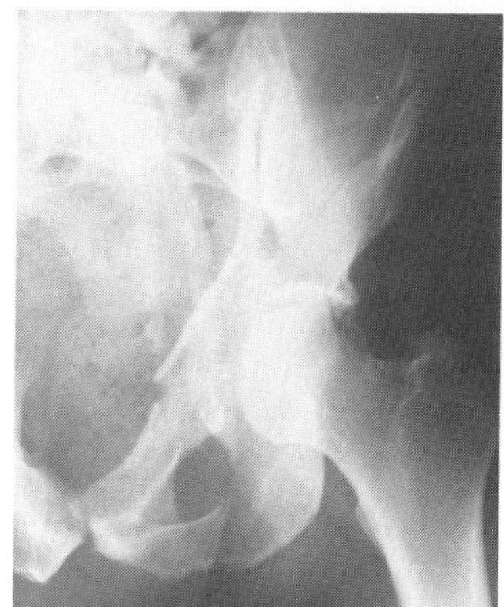

Figure 9-14C.

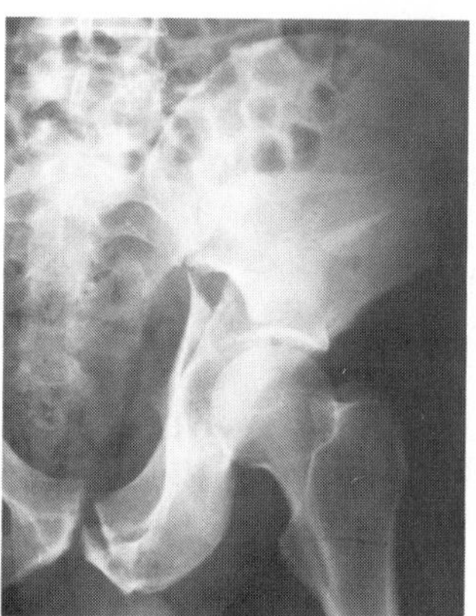

Figure 9-14D.

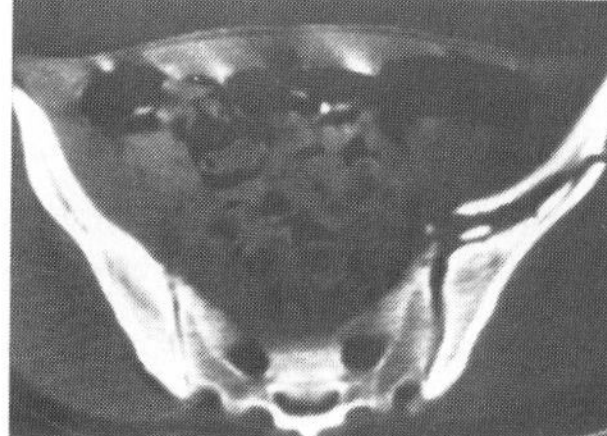

Figure 9-14E.

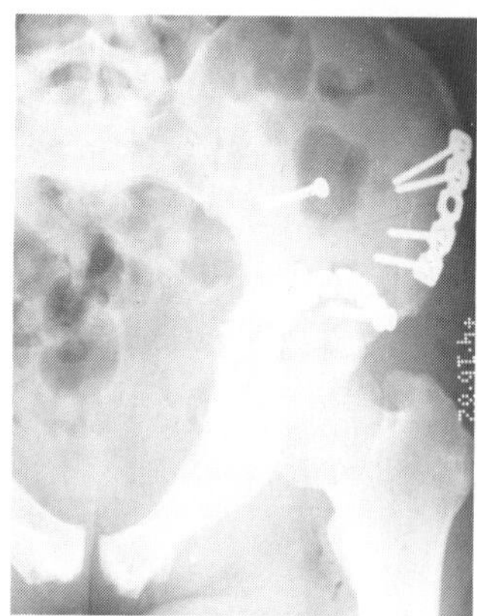

Figure 9-14F.

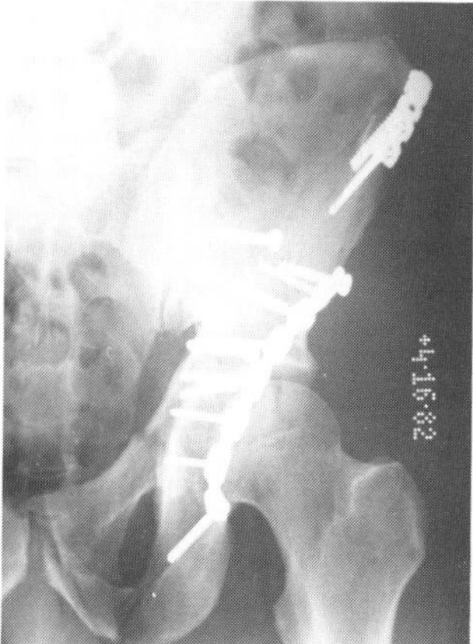

Figure 9-14G.

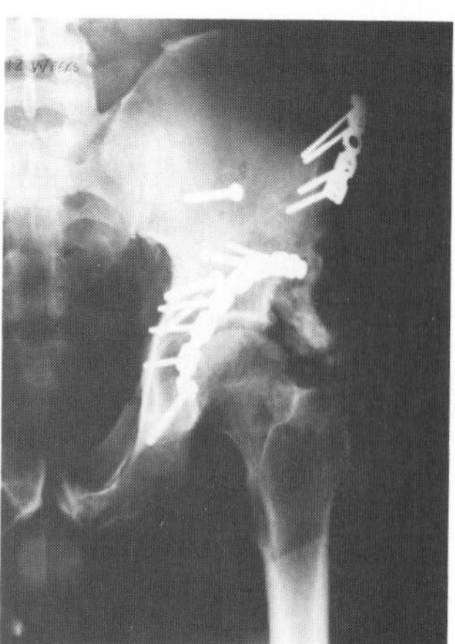

Figure 9-14H.

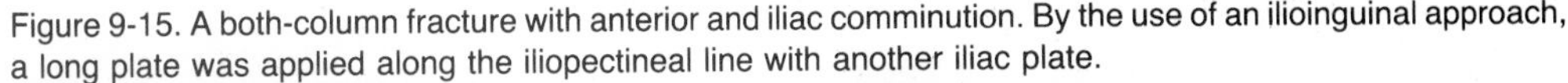
Figure 9-15. A both-column fracture with anterior and iliac comminution. By the use of an ilioinguinal approach, a long plate was applied along the iliopectineal line with another iliac plate.

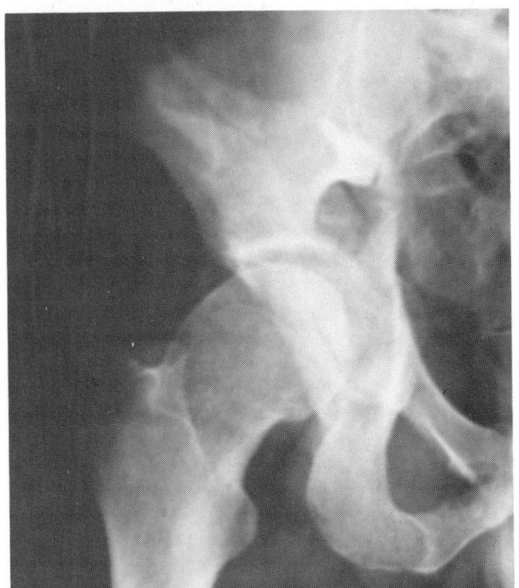

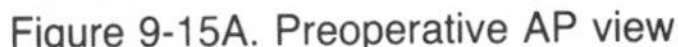
Figure 9-15A. Preoperative AP view.

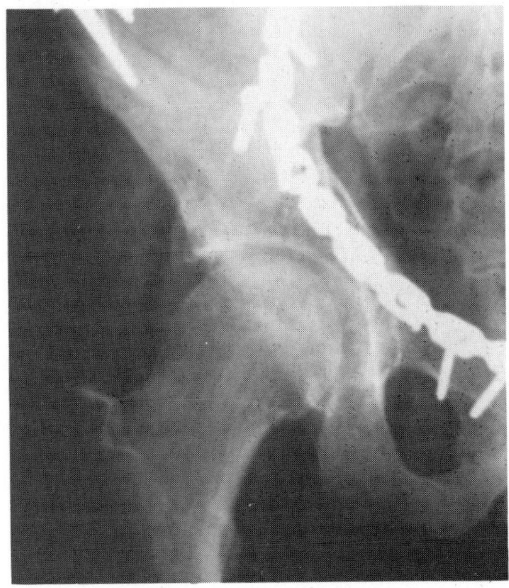

Figure 9-15B. Postoperative AP view.

or two of the screw holes are not employed in view of the inordinate risk of penetration of the joint.

# Acetabular Fixation

## Fixation of the Posterior Wall and Column

Stabilization of the posterior wall and posterior column is undertaken for a wide variety of simple and associated fracture patterns, including isolated disruptions of the posterior wall and column and transverse fractures. Various associated injuries, including fractures of the posterior wall and posterior column, posterior wall and transverse, anterior column or wall with posterior hemitransverse, "T" fractures and both-column injuries, all require some type of posterior fixation. A variety of examples is given that provides the general principles of fixation for virtually all of these injuries.

To stabilize an isolated posterior wall fracture, generally a combination of lag screws and a buttress plate is employed (Figures 9-16 and 9-17). While isolated lag screw fixation has been utilized historically, in a substantial number of cases the screws disengaged spontaneously with the loss of the reduction. In view of the catastrophic nature of this problem and the relative ease and low morbidity for the application of a buttress plate, generally the combined fixation is now employed. Prior to the reduction of the posterior wall fracture and after the joint has been thoroughly inspected and

Figure 9-16. Fixation of the posterior wall with lag screws. A comminuted posterior wall fracture in a man of 41 years managed some years ago with two lag screws. The apparently simple injury documented in the conventional radiographs actually is quite involved. A: Preoperative AP view with the presence of three small fragments. B: Preoperative obturator oblique view with the principal wall fragment. C: Preoperative iliac oblique view with evidence of a fracture or impacted zone on the superior portion of the femoral head. D: Initial computed scan with dislocated femoral head. E: Computed scan after the closed reduction to show the large wall fragment adjacent to the dome. F: Comminuted posterior wall at the level of the quadrilateral surface. Currently this finding is an indication to employ a buttress plate. G: An inferior scan provides an indication of the extensive region of involvement. H: Initial postoperative AP view. I: Late AP view two years later, with narrowing of hip joint and ectopic bone. J: Late computed scan at two years shows the orientation of the screw and the irregularity of the joint.

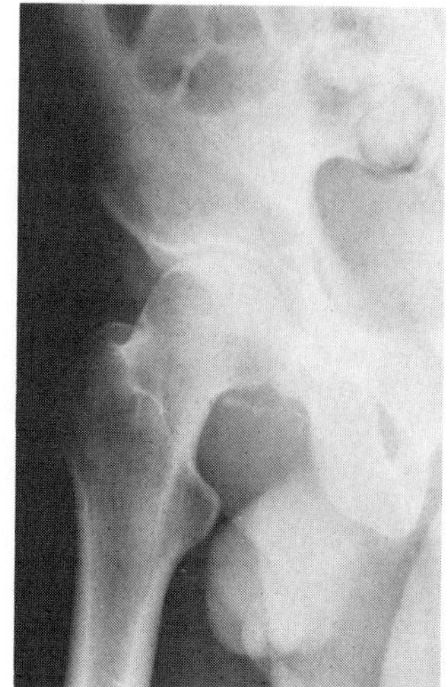

Figure 9-16A.

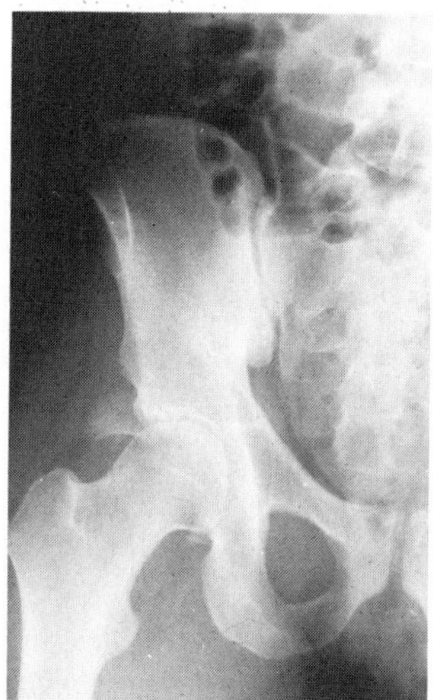

Figure 9-16B.

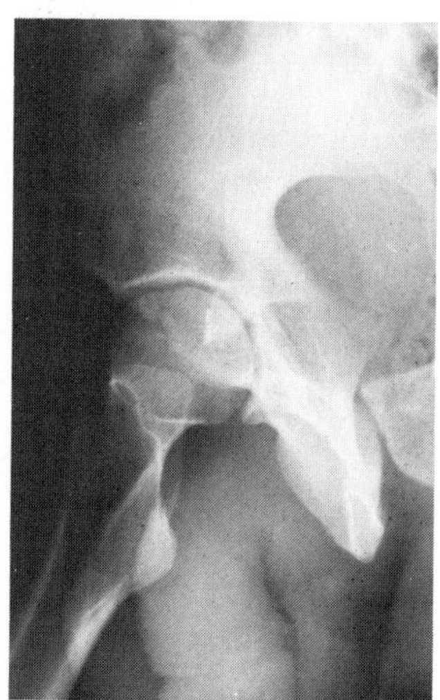

Figure 9-16C.

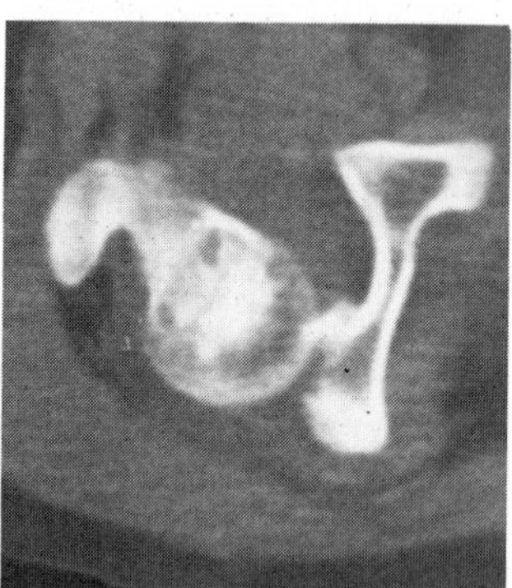

Figure 9-16D.

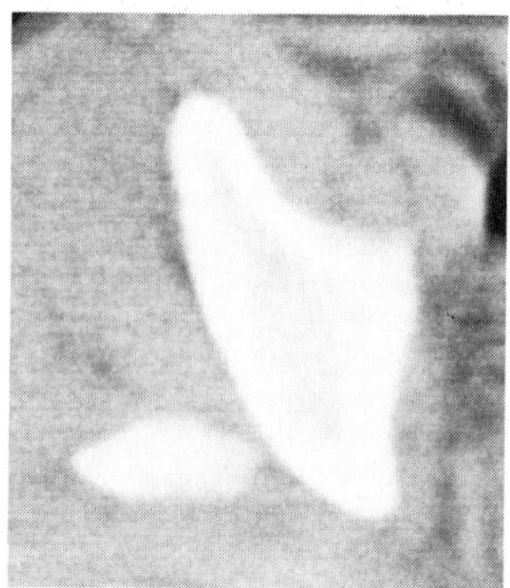

Figure 9-16E.

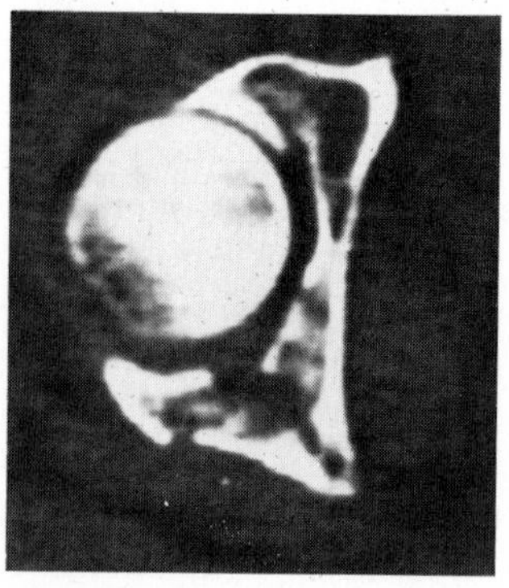

Figure 9-16F.

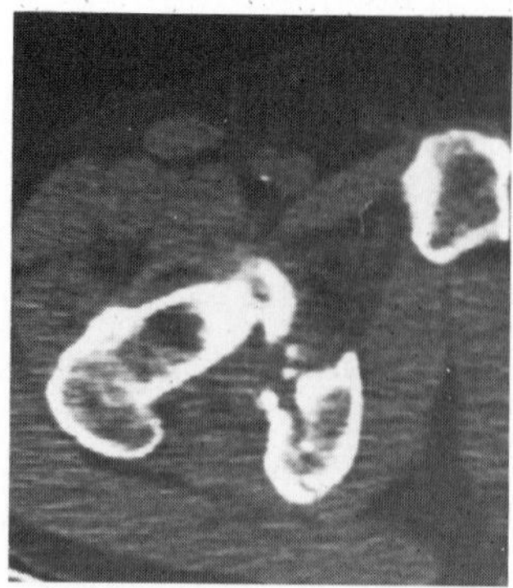

Figure 9-16G.

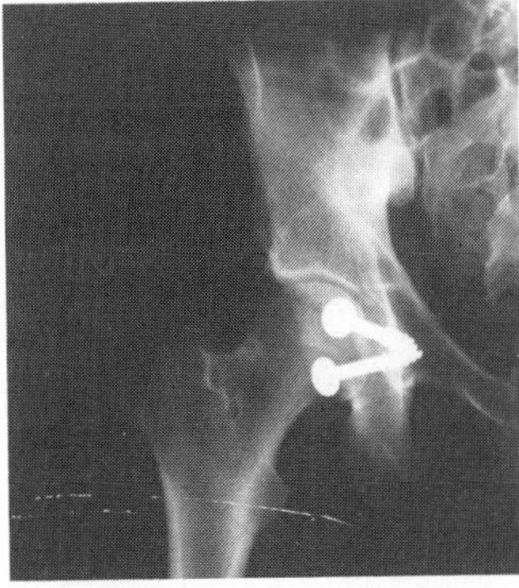

Figure 9-16H.

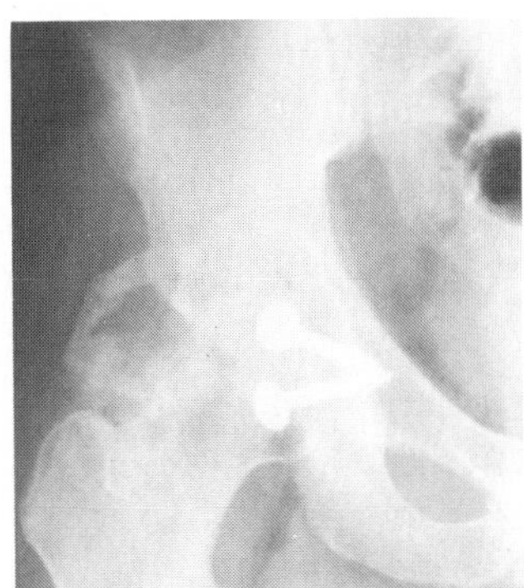

Figure 9-16I.

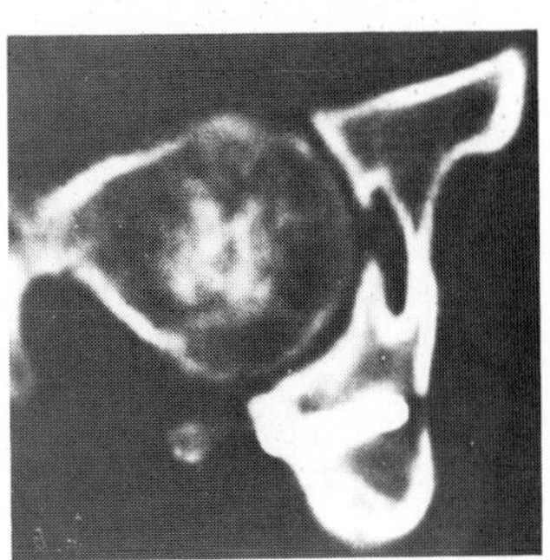

Figure 9-16J.

debrided, the articular surface is scrutinized for possible marginal impaction.[6] If such impacted fragments are identified they are reduced by elevation and derotation. The void thereby created in the impacted cancellous bone at the base of the impacted articular fragment is obliterated with cancellous bone graft harvested from the iliac crest, ischial tuberosity, or the greater trochanter. Immediately prior to the reduction of the wall fragment, gliding holes of appropriate diameter are made in the wall fragment by the use of a retrograde drilling technique from the fracture surface to the outer cortex. A suitable drill sleeve is inserted into the holes on the superficial cortex. The hip is positioned in abduction, generally by elevation of the limb on a stand. The posterior wall fragment is anatomically reduced and provisionally stabilized with tenaculum bone holding forceps or a supplementary Kirschner wire. The thread holes are drilled through the drill sleeves into the principal portion of the posterior column. For the conventional 4.5mm cortical screw the gliding hole is 4.5mm and the thread hole is 3.2mm in diameter. In the presence of a smaller fragment, 4.0mm cancellous screws are inserted into 2mm drill holes. Once the lag screws have been inserted and tightened, a 3.5mm reconstruction plate generally of six holes is applied to buttress the posterior column. In the superior portion of the wall where penetration of the hip joint by an excessively lengthy screw is particularly likely to occur, either unicortical screws are employed or the holes in the plate are left vacant.

From the mechanical point of view stabilization of the posterior column is optimally achieved by resort to lag screws and a buttress plate (Figure 9-18). While isolated application of appropriately directed lag screws suffices, unless a retrograde drilling technique is carefully applied, the precise orientation of the screws across the fracture is unknown. When the conventional Kocher-Langenbeck

Figure 9-17. Reconstruction of a posterior wall fracture with the use of a buttress plate. A: Initial AP view. B: Outer view, 3D scan, with wall fragment on top of the dislocated femoral head. C: Inner view, 3D scan. D: Superior view, 3D scan. E: Inferior view, 3D scan, with a hint of irregularity of the acetabular articular surface. F: Computed scan through dome and wall fragment. G: Computed scan through femoral head with marginal impaction of a posterior wall fragment that is malrotated by 90°. H: Drawing of a large posterior wall fragment stabilized with a buttress plate. I: Postoperative AP view of lag screw and buttress plate after the open reduction and application of bone graft to realign the impacted wall fragment.

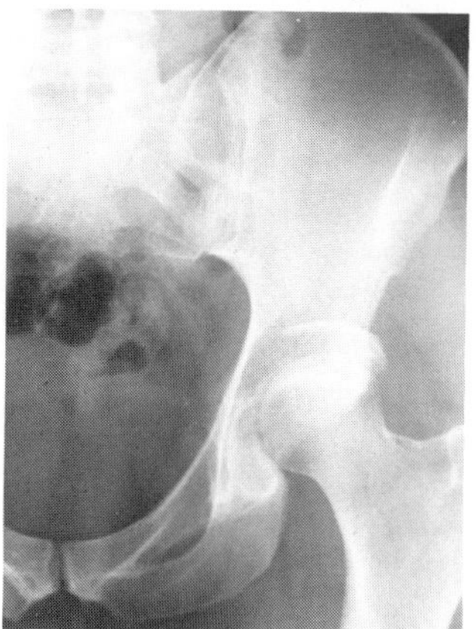

Figure 9-17A.

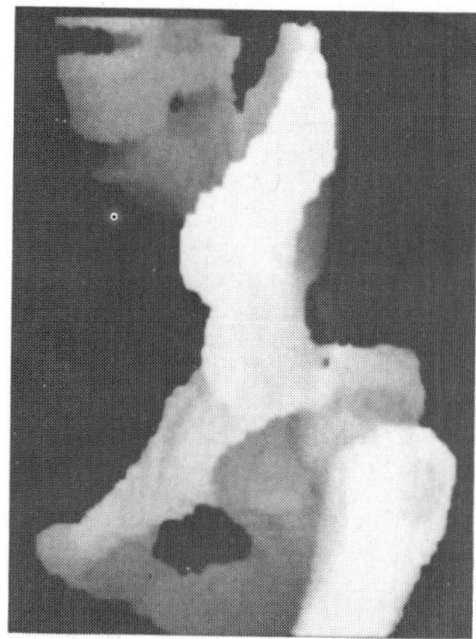

Figure 9-17B.

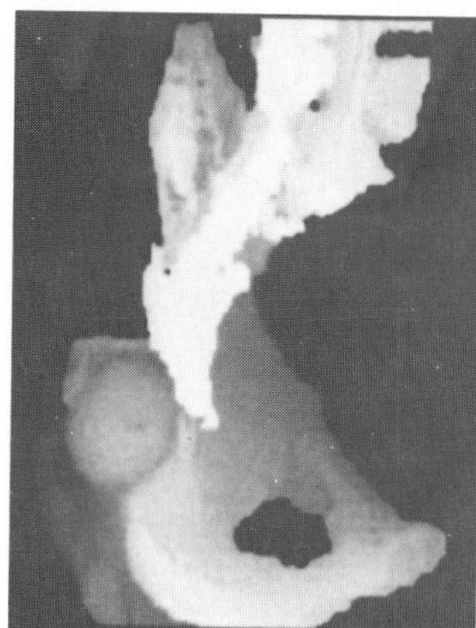

Figure 9-17C.

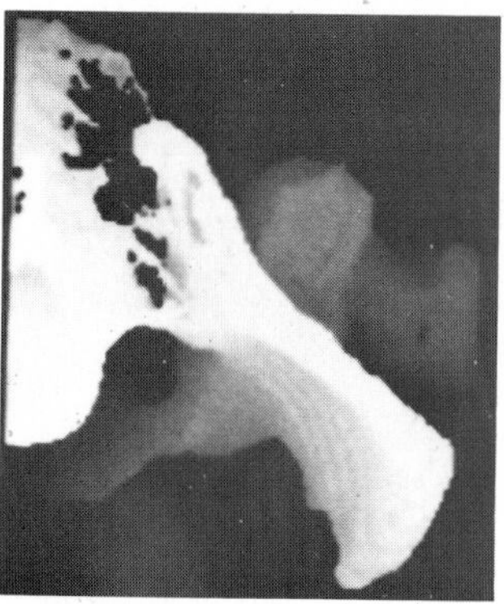

Figure 9-17D.

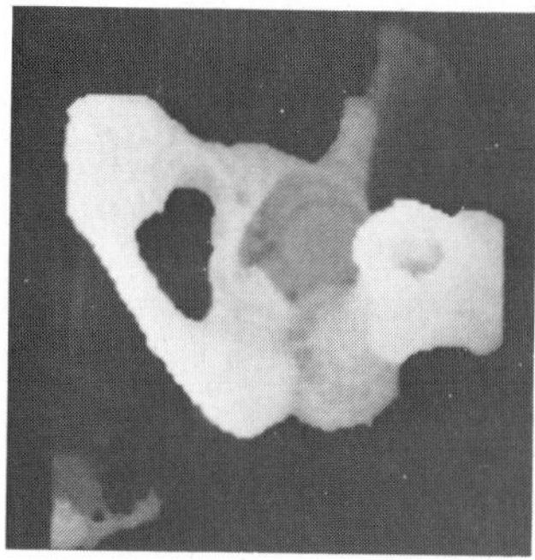

Figure 9-17E.

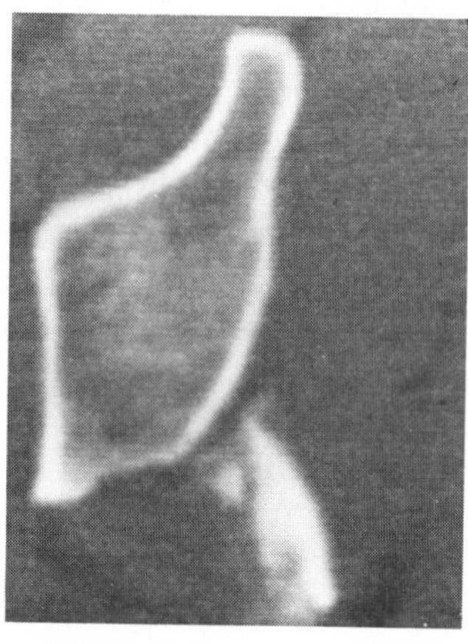

Figure 9-17F.

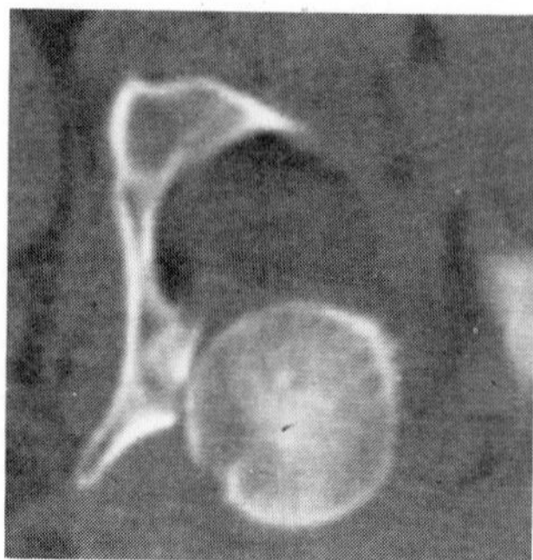

Figure 9-17G.

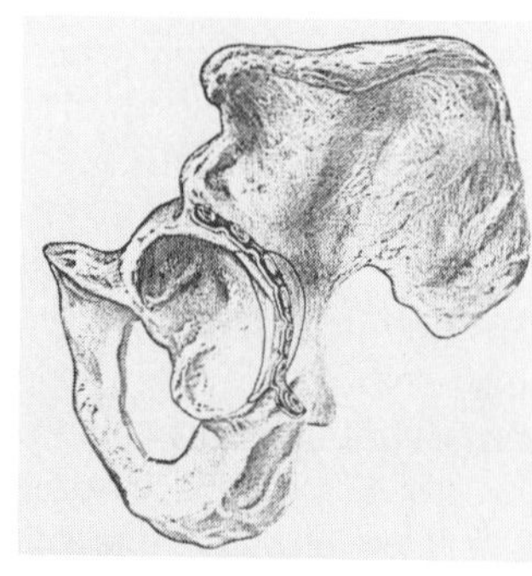

Figure 9-17H.

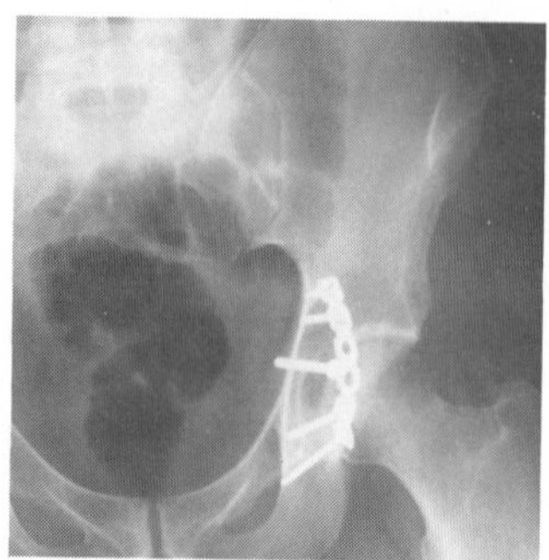

Figure 9-17I.

Figure 9-18. Reconstruction of a posterior column fracture stabilized with a lag screw and a buttress plate. A: Initial AP view with deceptive appearance of minimal displacement. B: Iliac oblique view with posterior displacement. C: Drawing of typical method of fixation. D: Late AP view, one year after surgery. E: Late iliac oblique view.

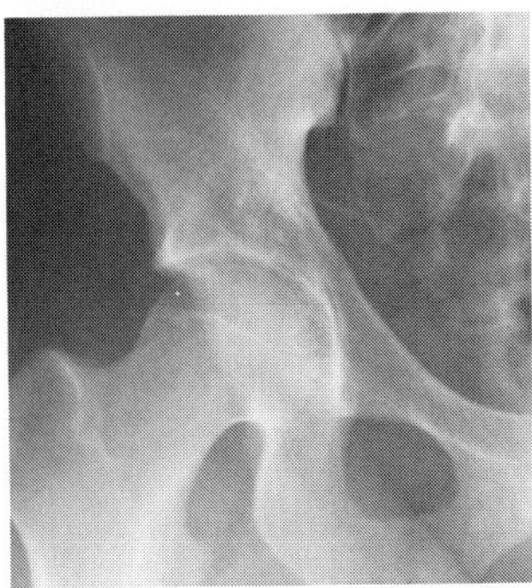

Figure 9-18A.

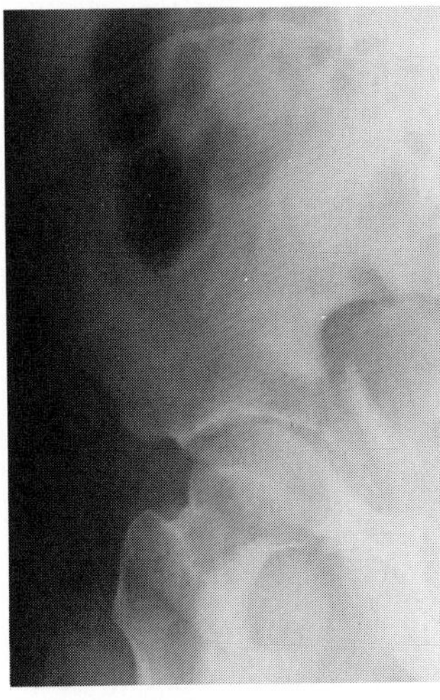

Figure 9-18B.

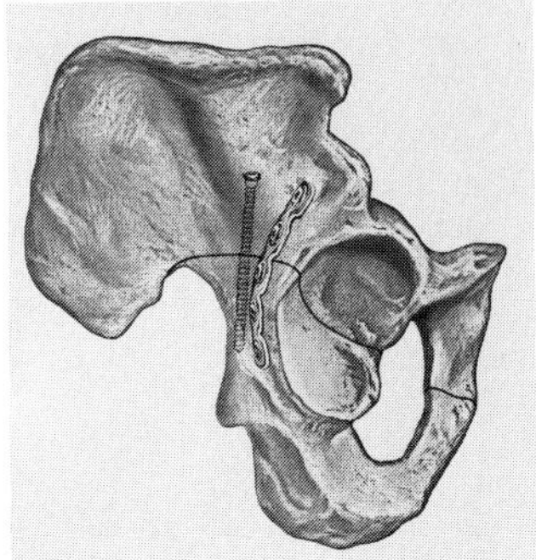

Figure 9-18C.

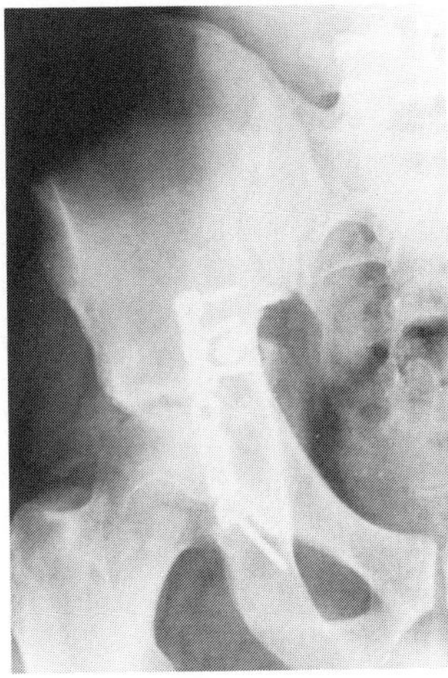

Figure 9-18D.

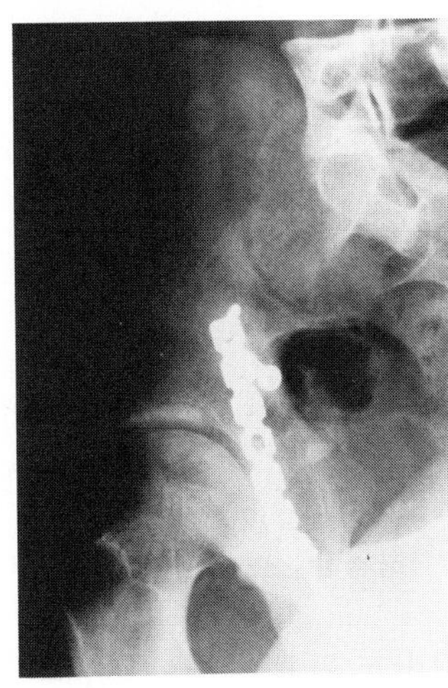

Figure 9-18E.

incision is used to approach an inferior or distal pattern of a posterior column disruption, the exposure does not provide appropriate access to permit the insertion of the screws unless the AO flexible instrumentation is available to prepare and tap the holes. With certain oblique fracture lines the insertion of a lag screw produces overriding of the fracture fragments. Also, more comminuted injuries cannot be adequately stabilized solely by the use of lag screws. For all of these reasons the supplementary application of a buttress plate frequently is undertaken. A simple fracture generally is stabilized by the use of a 3.5mm reconstruction plate, while a comminuted fracture encountered in a individual

Figure 9-19. A posterior column with an associated posterior wall fracture, with preliminary reconstruction of the posterior column by the use of one plate and a subsequent repair of the posterior wall with a second plate. A: Initial obturator oblique view. B: Initial iliac oblique view. C: Superior view, 3D scan. D: Computed scan with displaced posterior column, posterior wall, and femoral head. E: Drawing of the fixation, with two plates and a supplementary posterior column lag screw. F: Postoperative AP view.

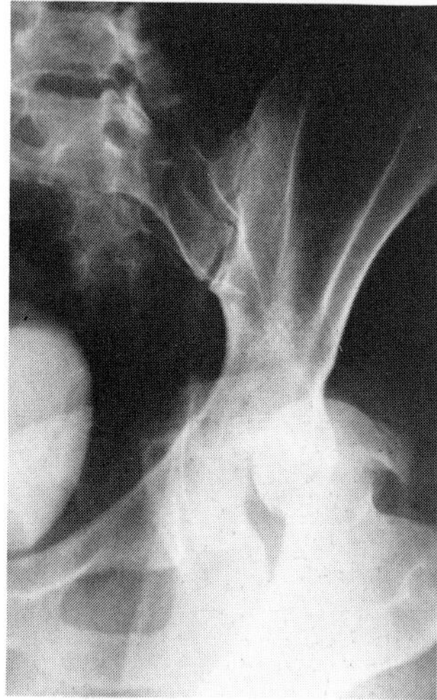

Figure 9-19A.

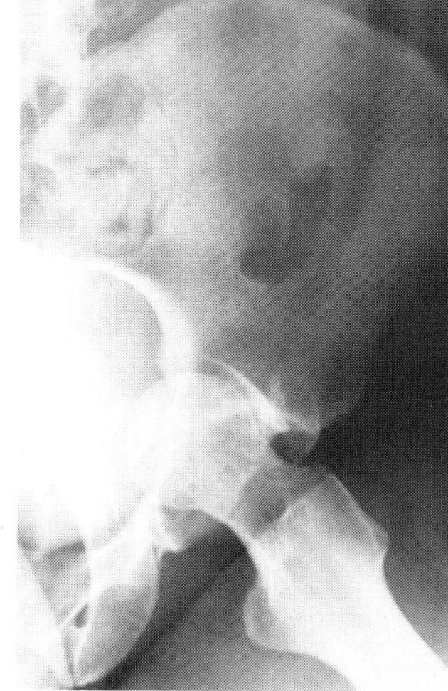

Figure 9-19B.

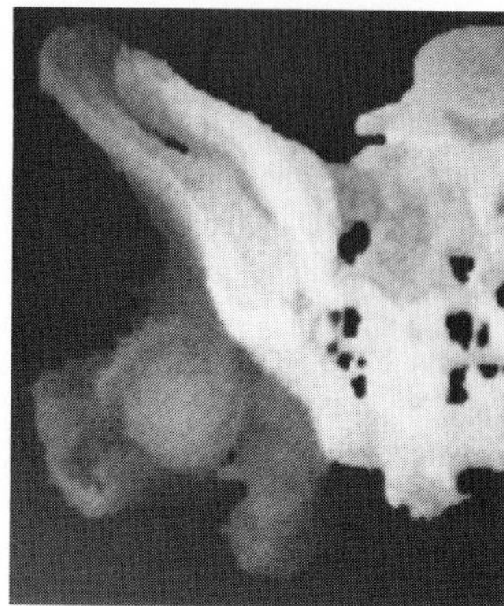

Figure 9-19C.

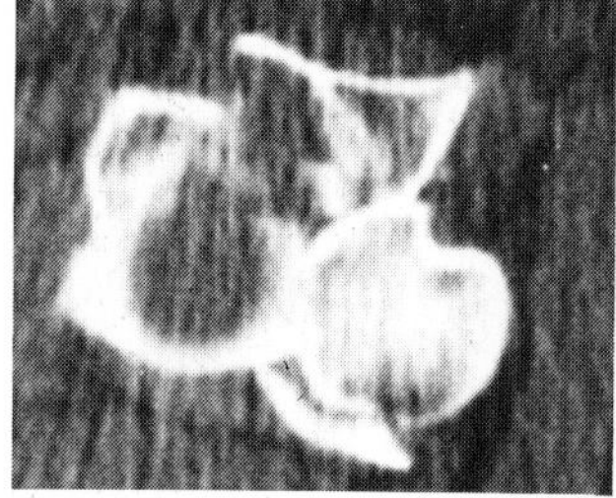

Figure 9-19D.

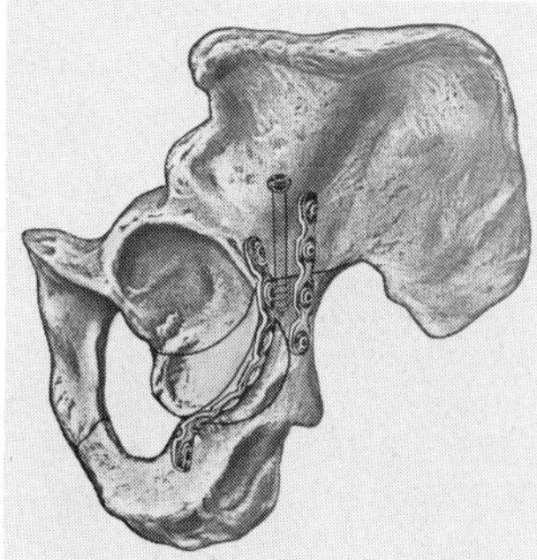

Figure 9-19E.

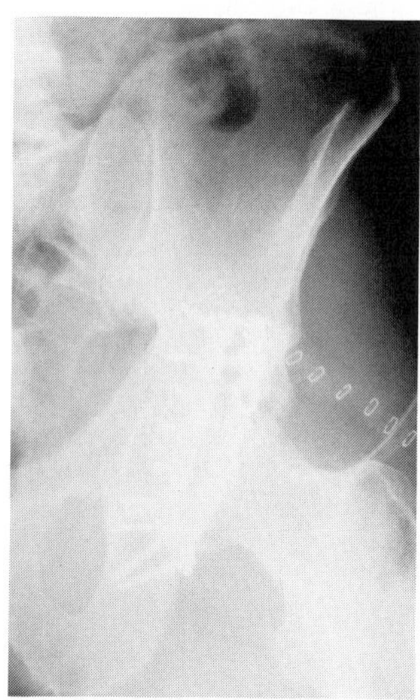

Figure 9-19F.

who weighs more than 250 pounds is stabilized by resort to a 4.5mm reconstruction plate. Typically, the plate courses from the superior aspect of the ischial tuberosity to the lateral ilium at or above the roof of the greater sciatic notch. The precise site is selected according to the level of the posterior column disruption. For a particularly high injury that extends into the greater sciatic notch, a somewhat more superior application of the plate is undertaken. For a distal injury that extends from the inferior aspect of the ischial spine immediately

Figure 9-20. Posterior column associated with a posterior wall fracture. With the large size of the posterior wall and the inferior nature of the posterior column, initally the latter is repaired with lag screws. Then the wall is buttressed with a plate. A: Initial AP view. B: Initial obturator oblique view, with displaced wall fragment. C: Inlet view, with low posterior column facture. D: 3D obtruator oblique view. E: 3D iliac oblique view with comminution of posterior wall. F: Postoperative AP view. G: Postoperative iliac oblique view. H: Postoperative obturator oblique view.

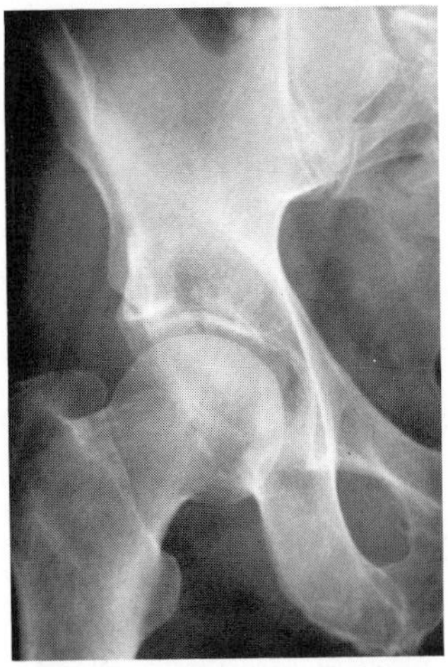

Figure 9-20A.

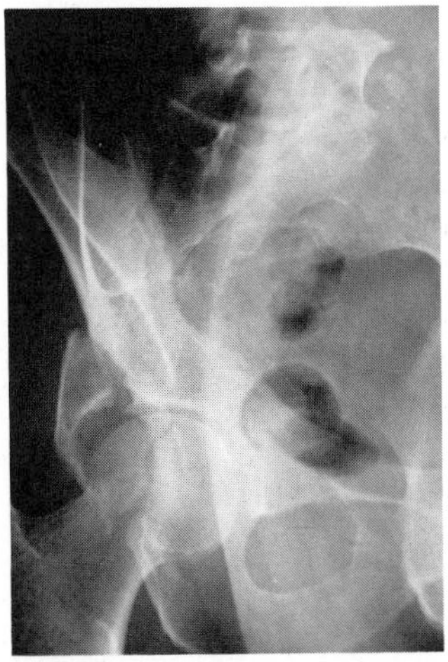

Figure 9-20B.

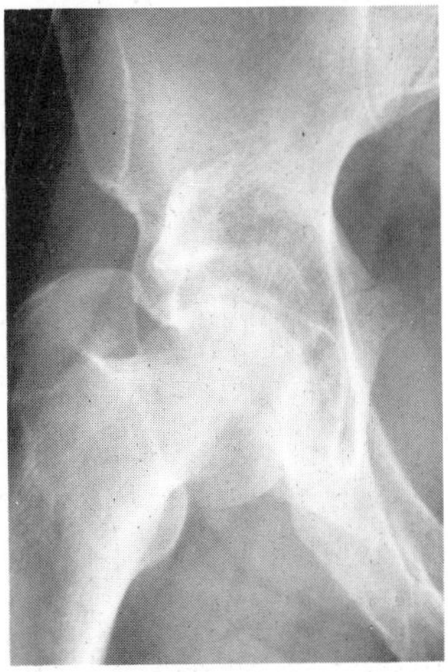

Figure 9-20C.

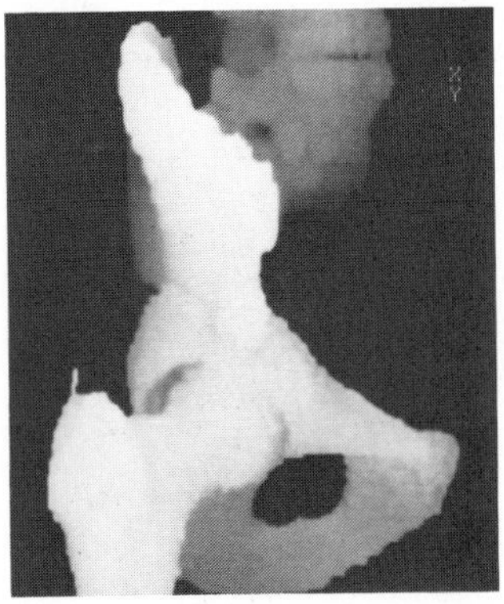

Figure 9-20D.

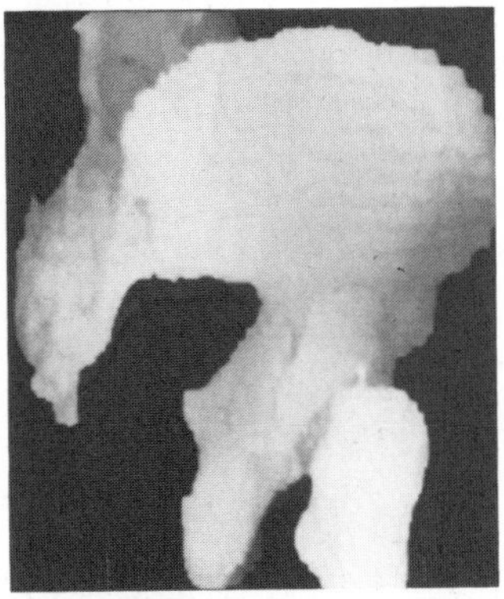

Figure 9-20E.

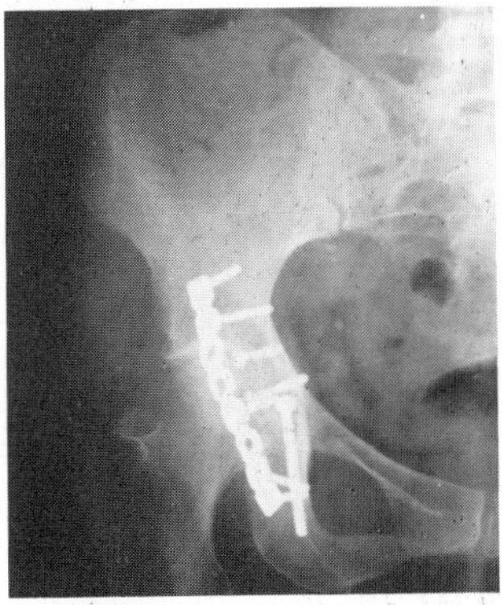

Figure 9-20F.

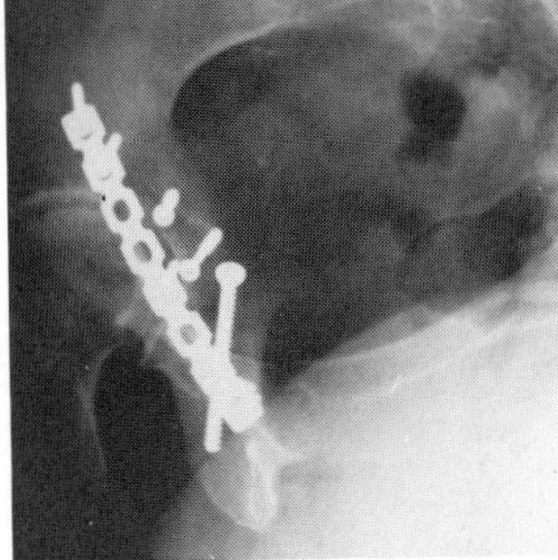

Figure 9-20G.

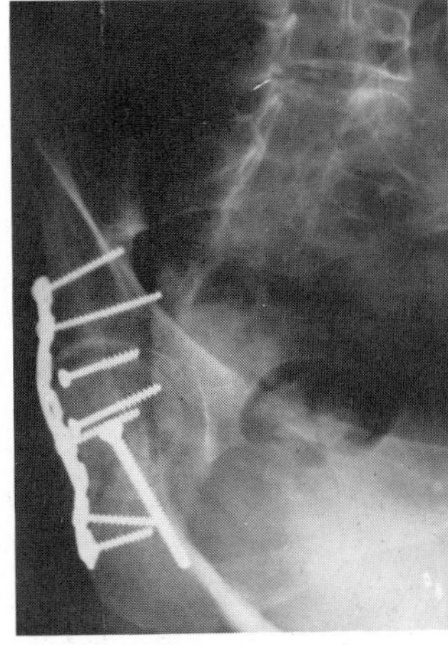

Figure 9-20H.

Figure 9-21. A high posterior column associated with a posterior wall fracture and propagation across the ilium into the sacroiliac joint. A Kocher-Langenbeck approach with osteotomy of the greater trochanter was used, with the wall fragment displaced to facilitate the reduction. The sacroiliac joint, ilium, and posterior column are repaired, then the wall fragment is replaced and a posterior buttress plate is applied. A: Initial AP view. B: Obturator oblique view. C: Outlet view. D: Sagittal computed scan. E: Computed scan through SI joint and ilium. F: Computed scan through displaced posterior wall and column. G: Postoperative AP view. H: Postoperative iliac oblique view. I: Postoperative obturator oblique view.

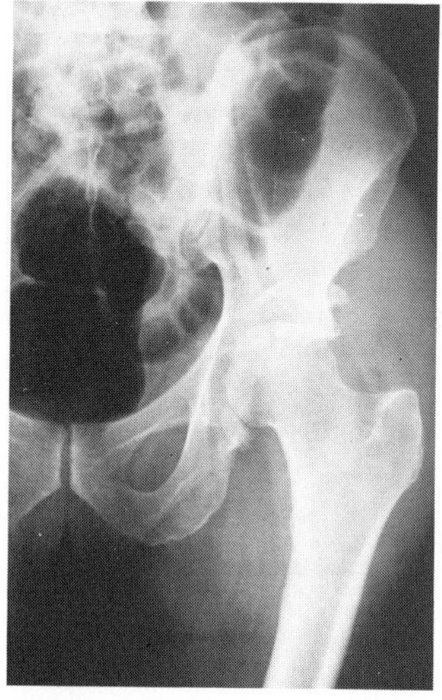

Figure 9-21A.

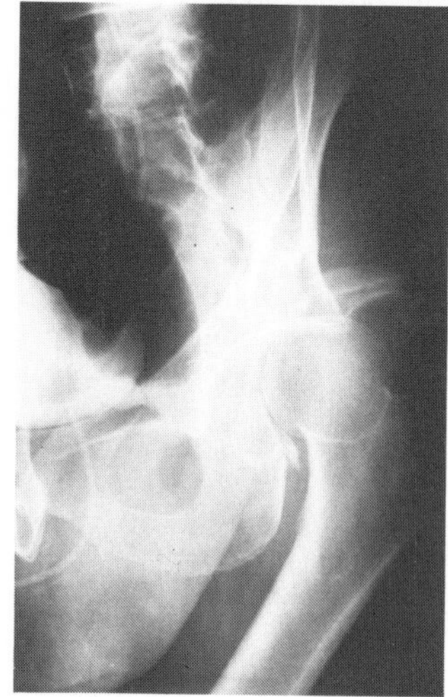

Figure 9-21B.

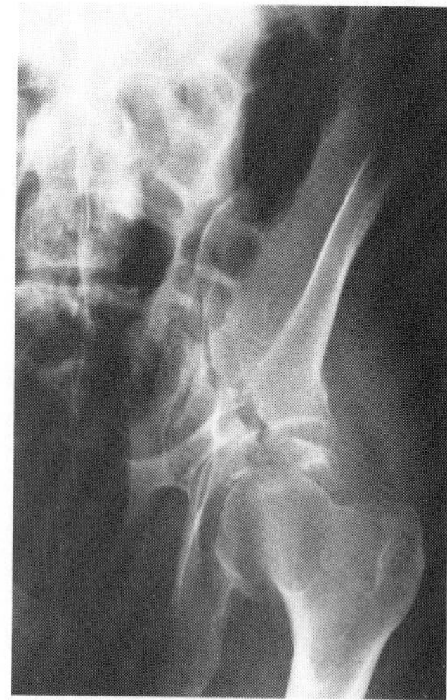

Figure 9-21C.

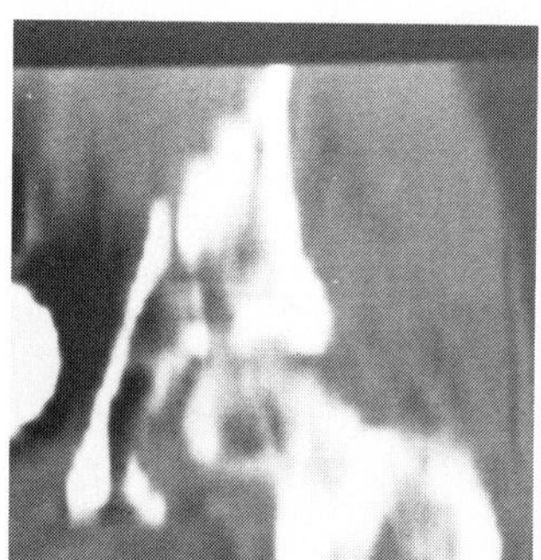

Figure 9-21D.

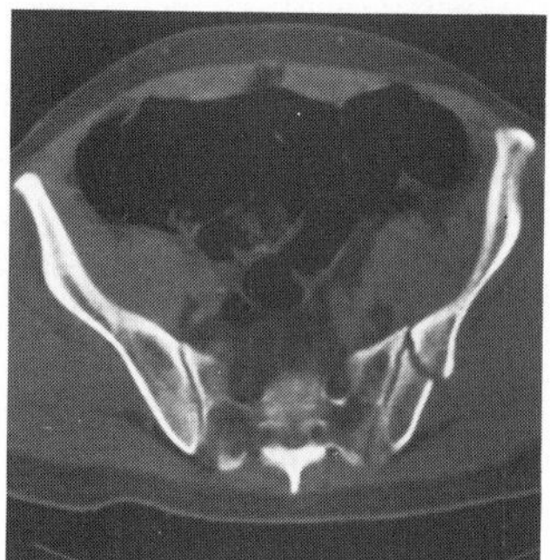

Figure 9-21E.

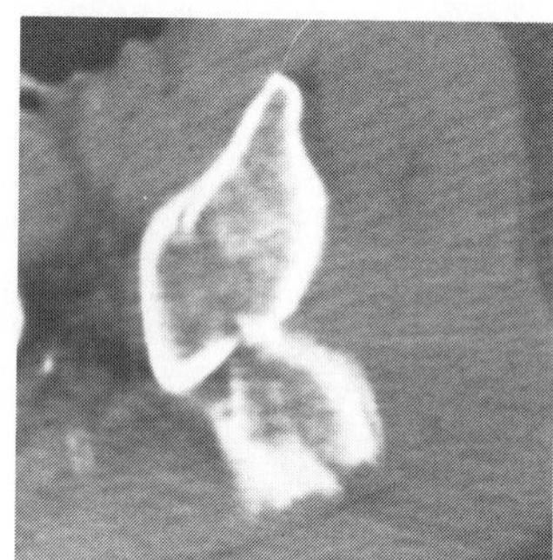

Figure 9-21F.

superior to the ischial tuberosity, a more inferior application of the plate is undertaken. To avoid inadvertent penetration of the acetabulum with the screws, the plate is positioned on the medial half of the posterior column near the posterior border of the greater sciatic notch. The plate is most easily applied after the fracture is anatomically reduced. A plate simulator is applied at the appropriate site on the posterior column and a plate of appropriate length is contoured meticulously in three planes. To secure it to the bone the drill holes are angled away from the articular surface of the posterior acetabulum. Periodically during the insertion of the drill holes and insertion of the screws, the articular surface of the acetabulum is inspected to

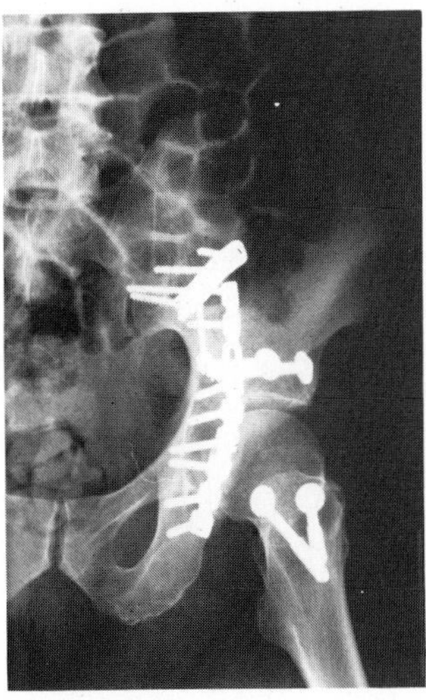

Figure 9-21G.

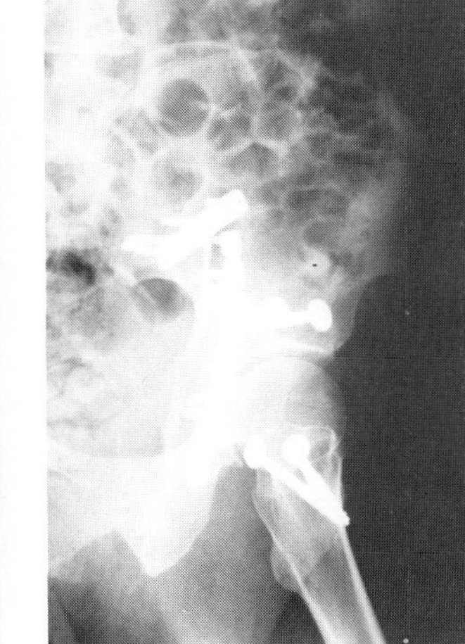

Figure 9-21H.

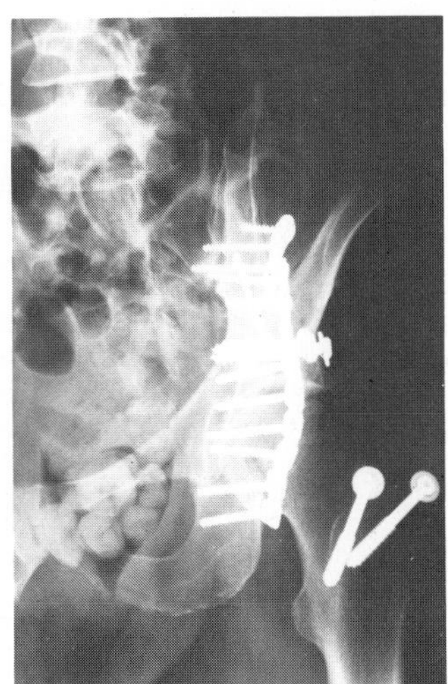

Figure 9-21I.

confirm the accuracy of the reduction and the absence of an errantly directed screw. A distal fracture pattern of the posterior column provides an especially difficult reduction adjacent to the ischial tuberosity. An inordinate amount of release of the origin of the hamstrings is needed to permit the application of a typical bone holding forceps to the inferior fracture fragment. The use of the 3.5mm reconstruction plate considerably facilitates the reduction. The plate is approximately contoured and anchored to the inferior fracture fragment. A tenaculum bone holding forceps is applied from the superior end of the plate into a 3.2mm drill hole on the lateral ilium, possibly with the use of a "life-saver" or around the iliac crest. The fracture is reduced and the residual screws are inserted through the plate and into the bone.

The associated fracture pattern with a posterior column and a posterior wall fracture is stabilized in one of two ways. Where the posterior wall fragment possesses a width of less than 50% of the posterior column, the posterior column is anatomically reduced and stabilized with a combination of lag screws and a buttress plate (Figure 9-19). After a final inspection of the joint has been undertaken, the wall fragment is reduced and stabilized with a lag screw and the application of a second 3.5mm reconstruction plate. In this way, the initially displaced wall fragment facilitates the accurate reduction of the posterior column. Once the posterior wall fragment is substantially wider than 50% of the posterior column, a plate cannot be applied to the posterior column until the wall fragment has been reduced. In this instance the posterior column is provisionally stabilized by the application of a cancellous lag screw (Figures 9-20 and 9-21). Upon a final inspection of the hip joint, the wall fragment is reduced and a single buttress plate is applied to immobilize both the posterior wall and column. Generally, one or two screw holes adjacent to the superior wall region is left vacant so that the risk of inadvertent penetration of the hip joint by a screw is minimized. Again with the latter technique, lag screw fixation of the wall is undertaken by resort to a retrograde drilling technique prior to the reduction of the wall fragment.

Several associated fracture patterns are encountered where a minimally or undisplaced posterior column disruption is encountered by substantial displacement of the anterior column or wall. Examples include an anterior column or wall with a posterior hemitransverse fracture, a "T" fracture, and a both-column fracture. The ideal exposure for these injuries is an ilioinguinal approach, which facilitates the careful open reduction and internal fixation of the anterior column or wall with the application of a buttress plate around the iliopectineal line. The posterior column is stabilized by the insertion of a lag screw near the iliopectineal line, which is directed inferiorly into the posterior column itself (Figure 9-22). The screw is carefully oriented away from the posterior articular surface of the acetabulum.

## Stabilization of the Anterior Column and Wall

The techniques of fixation of the anterior column and wall correspond to the relative position of the fracture along the anterior column. High, middle, and low variants are encountered along with segmental fractures that propagate into two or more adjacent regions. While isolated anterior wall and column disruptions are encountered (Figure 9-23), the vast majority of these cases accompany associated fractures, especially anterior wall or column with posterior hemitransverse, "T," and both-column injuries.

High fractures of the anterior column possess a large iliac fragment extending from the iliac crest and anterior superior spine into the roof of the acetabulum. The open reduction is largely an extraarticular procedure whereby confirmation of the reduction is achieved by a scrutiny of the iliac crest itself along with the acetabular rim. For a simple stable fracture, fixation is realized by the application of 6.5mm cancellous lag screws or 4.5mm cortical screws inserted with a lag technique adjacent to the iliac crest and superior to the rim of the acetabulum (Figure 9-24). The screws are inserted into the anterior superior or inferior spine or the adjacent anterior iliac crest. The comminuted variants are stabilized by resort to 3.5mm reconstruction plates applied to the iliac crest and lateral ilium. For a plate situated on the iliac crest, lengthy 3.5mm cancellous screws up to 40mm in length

Figure 9-22. An anterior column with associated posterior hemitransverse fracture, with primarily anterior displacement. By the use of an ilioinguinal incision the fracture is reduced. The posterior column is immobilized with a lag screw, while a buttress plate is applied to the anterior column.

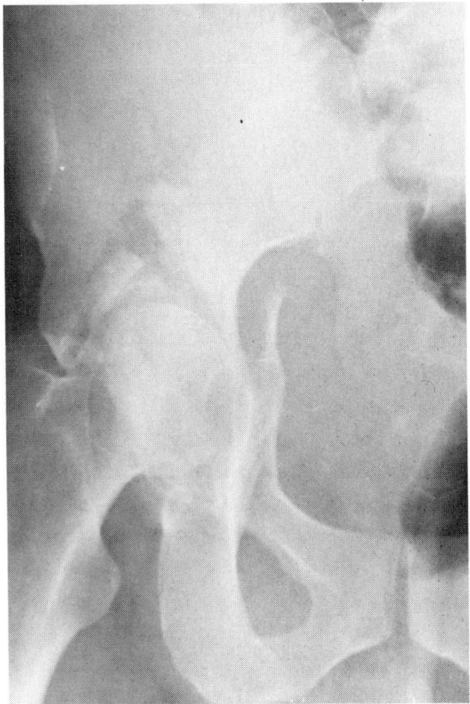

Figure 9-22A. Initial AP view.

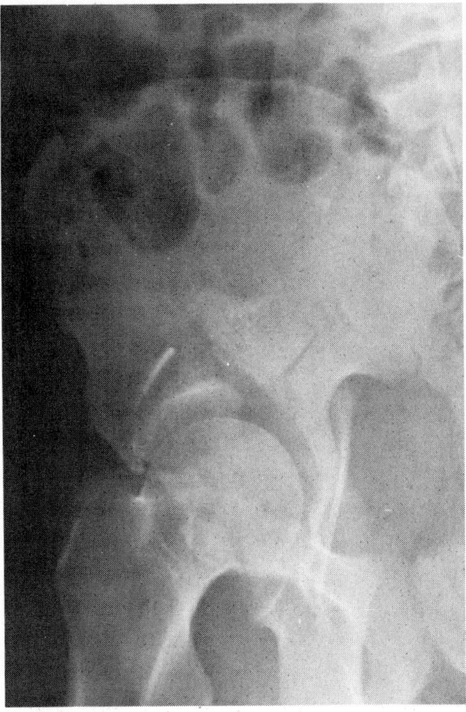

Figure 9-22B. Iliac oblique view.

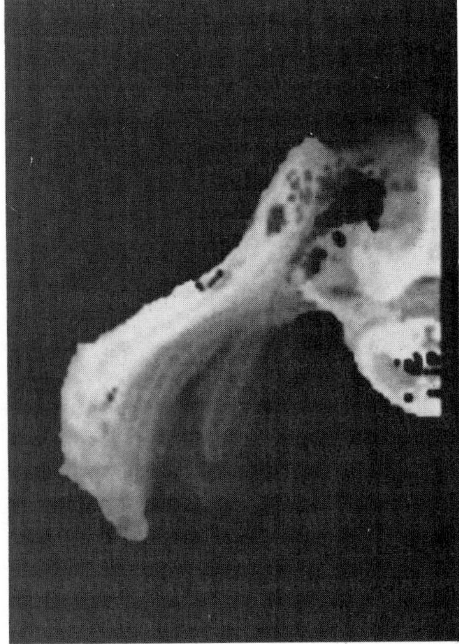

Figure 9-22C. Superior view, 3D scan.

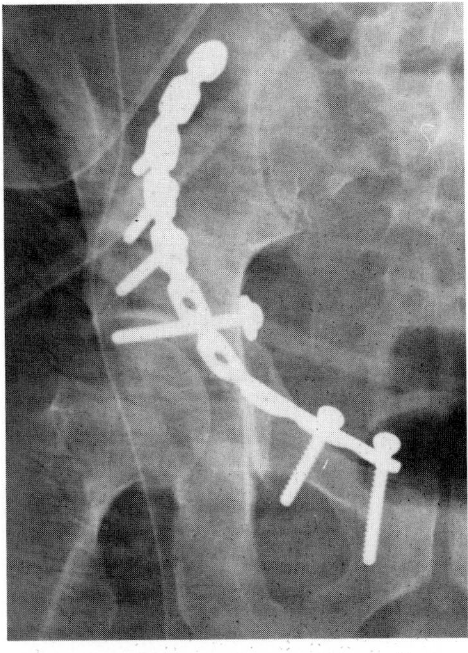

Figure 9-22D. Postoperative AP view.

Figure 9-23. Techniques for the repair of an isolated anterior wall disruption. While an isolated fragment is restored with lag screws, a comminuted fracture or the presence of osteoporosis may indicate the use of a buttress plate.

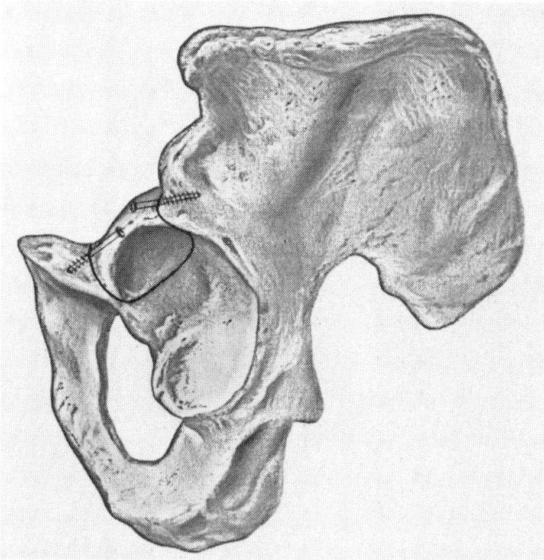

Figure 9-23A i. Outer view, lag screw fixation.

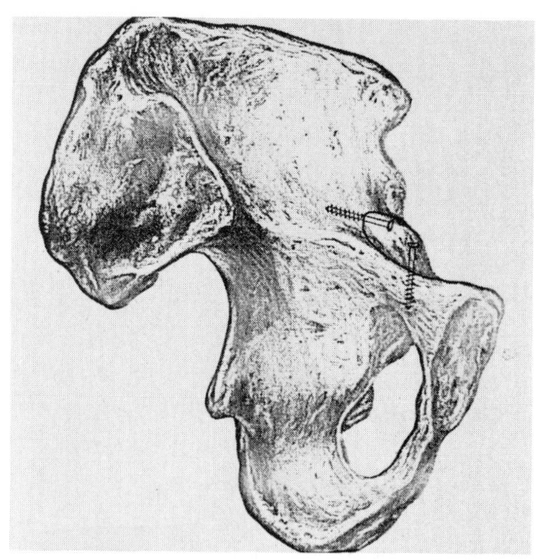

Figure 9-23A ii. Inner view, lag screw fixation.

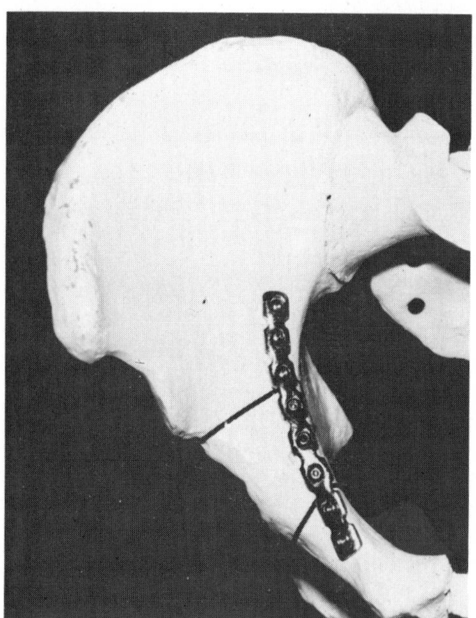

Figure 9-23B i. Inlet view, buttress plate.

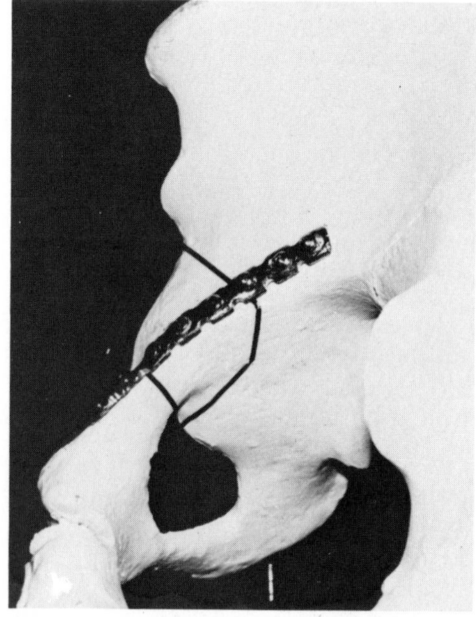

Figure 9-23B ii. Superior view, buttress plate.

are used. For a lateral iliac plate generally of six holes, 3.5mm cortical screws are preferred.

A fracture of the midportion of the anterior column requires an extensive visualization to achieve an accurate reduction and to confirm that the fixation screws do not penetrate the hip joint. A simple fracture of the midportion is satisfactorily immobilized by the insertion of a lengthy screw directed from the superior gluteal ridge into the superior pubic ramus (Figures 9-25 and

Figure 9-24. Repair of a high anterior column fracture. A (i, ii): Preferred method, primarily with lag screw fixation. B: Alternative method for comminuted injuries, with plate fixation.

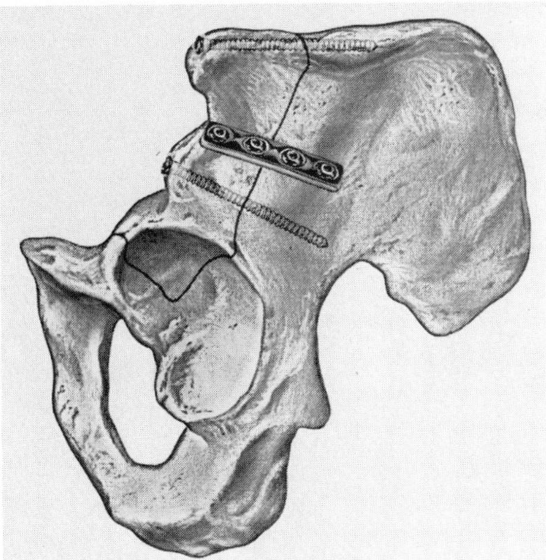

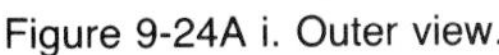

Figure 9-24A i. Outer view.

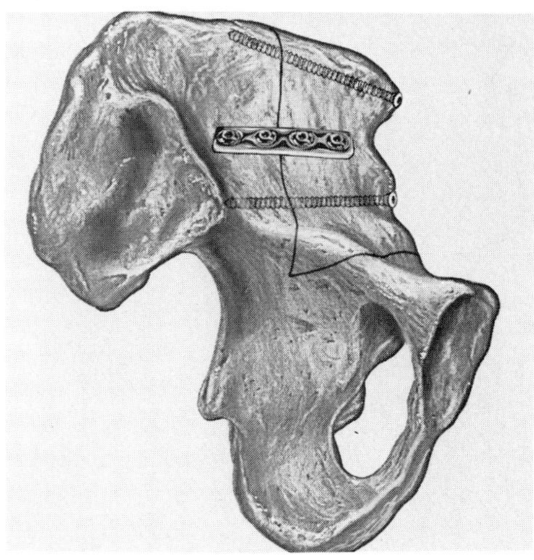

Figure 9-24A ii. Inner view.

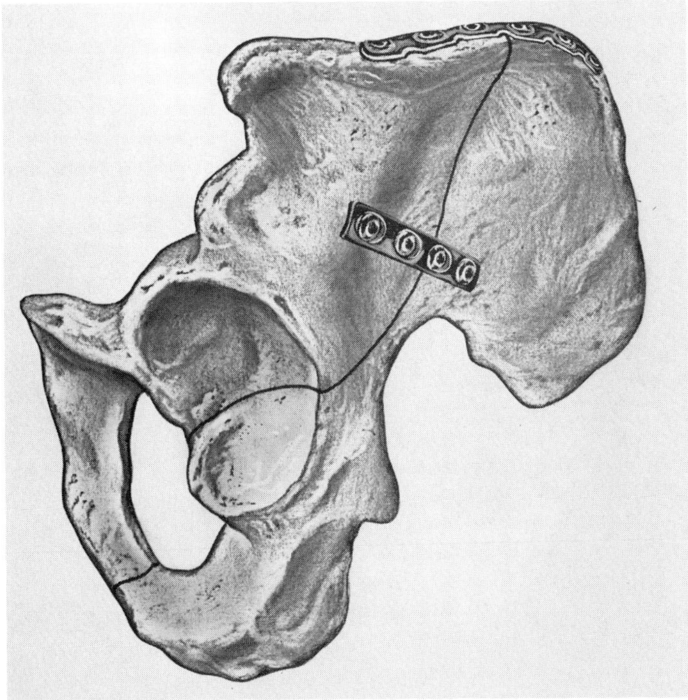

Figure 9-24B.

9-26). A 6.5mm cancellous screw or 4.5mm cortical screw is inserted about 2.5cm superior to the acetabular rim. An index finger is inserted inferior to the anterior inferior spine and around the superior border of the superior pubic ramus. Both the roof of the acetabulum and the adjacent quadrilateral surface are palpated while the drill hole is made. When a cortical screw is employed the gliding hole is prepared prior to the reduction of the fracture. When a 6.5mm long-threaded cancellous screw

Figure 9-25. An anterior column disruption involving stabilization of the midportion. A (i, ii): The use of lag screws inserted into the anterior inferior spine. B: The use of a short plate for a comminuted injury. The method is also suitable as part of the fixation of certain transverse and "T" fractures. C (i, ii, iii): Use of an anterior cruciate-type guide to facilitate the proper orientation of the anterior column lag screw.

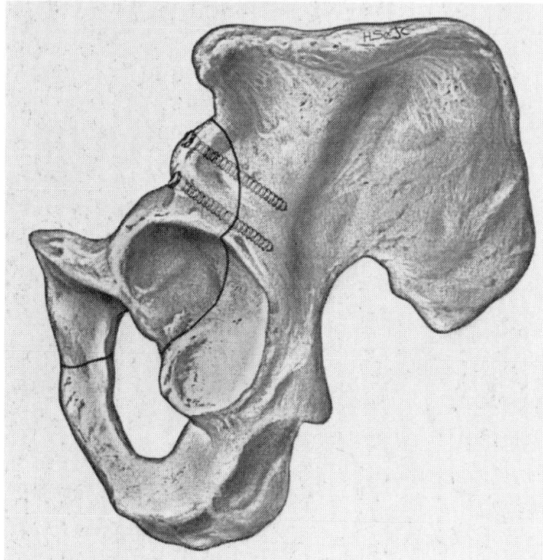

Figure 9-25A i. Outer view.

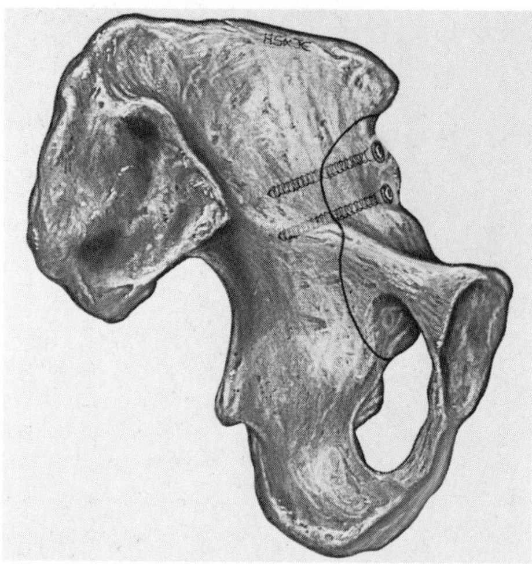

Figure 9-25A ii. Inner view.

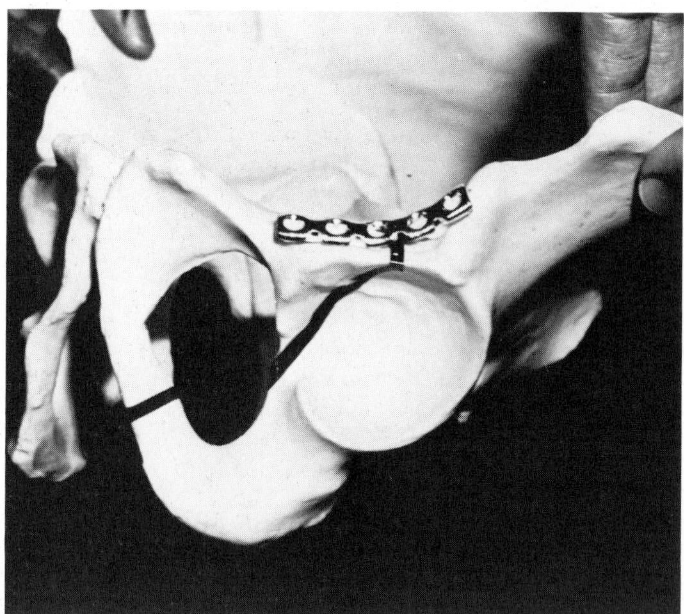

Figure 9-25B.

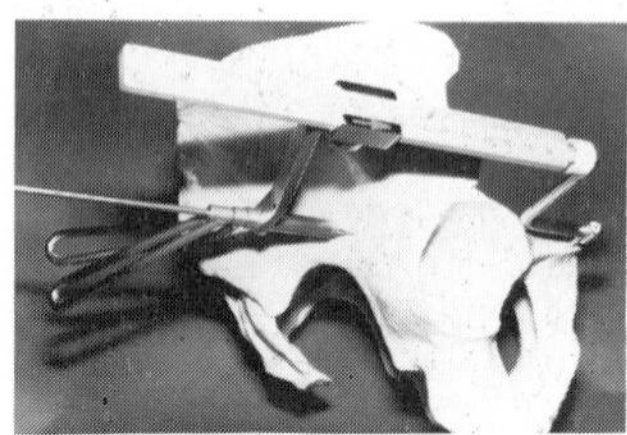

Figure 9-25C i. Lateral view.

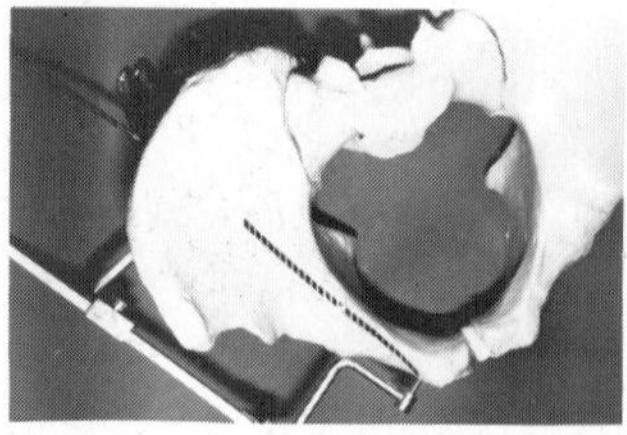

Figure 9-25C ii. Superior view.

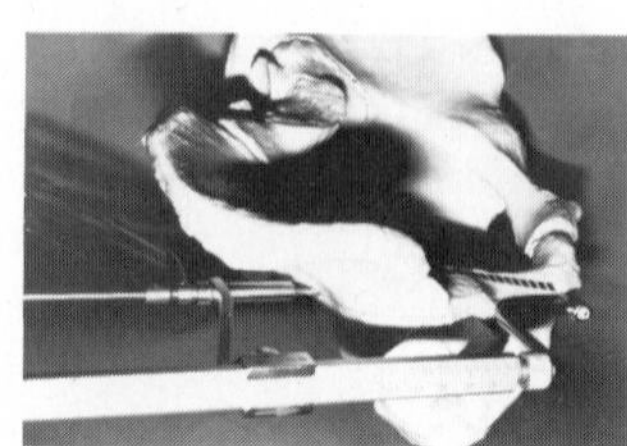

Figure 9-25C iii. Oblique view.

Figure 9-26. A comminuted fracture of the high and midportions of the anterior column. While an anatomical reduction is evident, the 4.5mm plate is poorly contoured. With the difficulties in obtaining an accurate fit with this plate, the use of a more pliable 3.5 reconstruction plate would have been preferred.

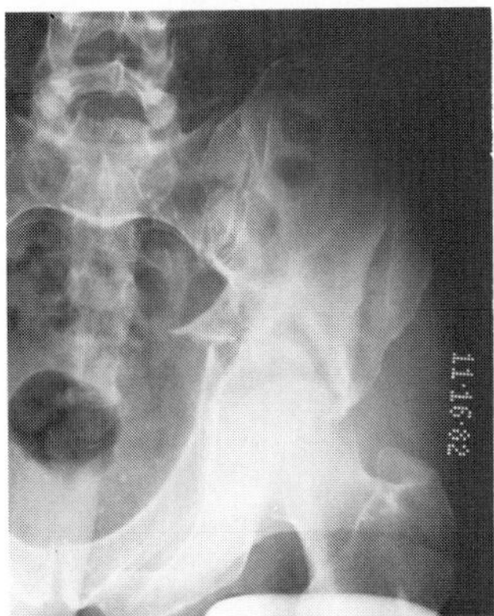


Figure 9-26A. Initial inlet view.

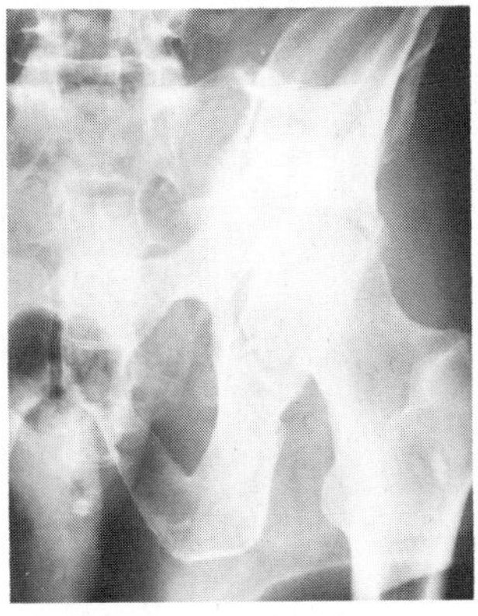

Figure 9-26B. Outlet view.

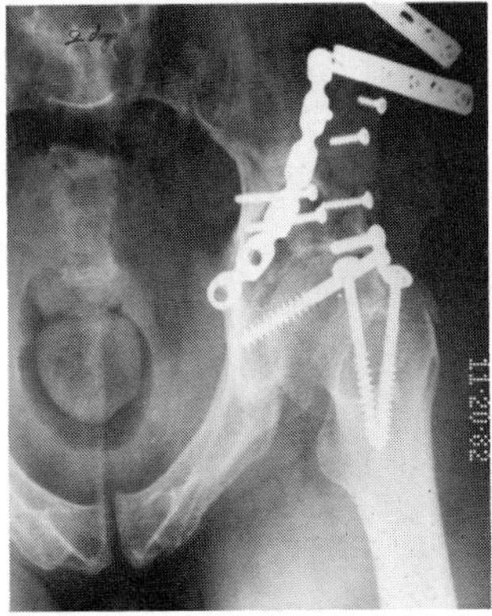


Figure 9-26C. Postoperative inlet view.

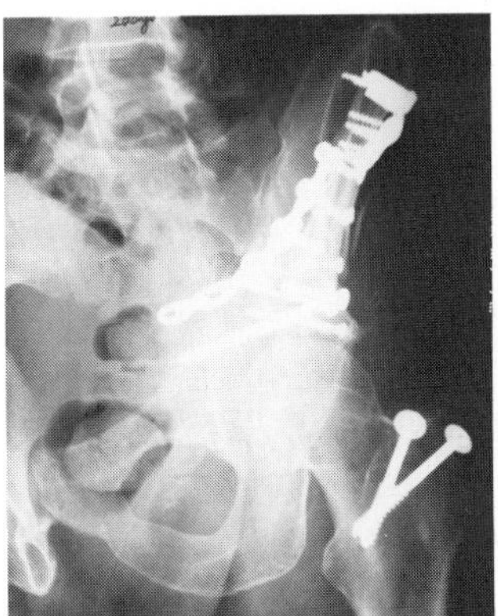

Figure 9-26D. Postoperative obturator oblique view.

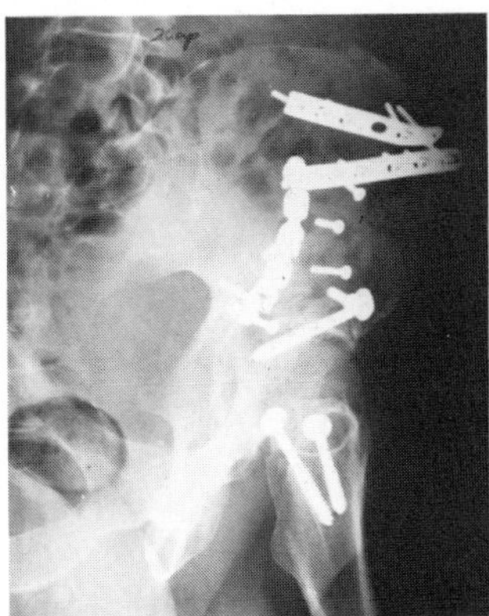

Figure 9-26E. Postoperative iliac oblique view.

is selected, the drill hole is made after the fracture has been reduced. Since the target zone in the superior pubic ramus is about 8.0mm in its minor axis, proper orientation of the pilot hole and the screw is essential. Several techniques have been devised in an effort to simplify the insertion of the screw. A modified version of an anterior cruciate guide is applied from the superior gluteal ridge to the pubic tubercle. Another technique employs one of the several available forms of cannulated screw. A guide wire is inserted into the superior gluteal ridge under image intensification. Once the appropriate orientation is confirmed, the screw is inserted over the guide wire. A typical length of screw is 80mm to 120mm. More comminuted fracture variants necessitate an extensive exposure of the inner table of the ilium, the acetabular roof, and the superior pubic ramus. A 3.5mm or 4.5mm reconstruction plate is applied along the

Figure 9-27. Stabilization of a low anterior column fracture with a lag screw. In the typical case illustrated here, the anterior column fracture follows a lateral compression fracture of the pelvic ring. In this instance the pelvic disruption was managed by the use of an external pelvic frame. A: Initial obturator oblique view, with disruption of the anterior column and the ipsilateral sacroiliac joint. B (i, ii): Lag screw fixation of the anterior column, with insertion of the screw along the superior gluteal ridge. C: Postoperative outlet view, with external frame. D: Six months later, AP view. E: Late inlet view.

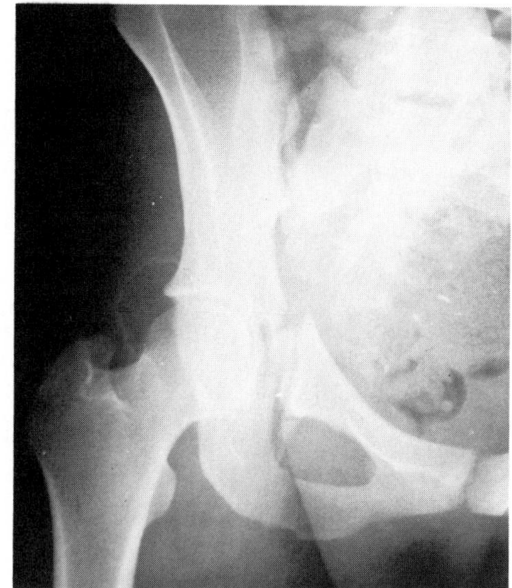

Figure 9-27A.

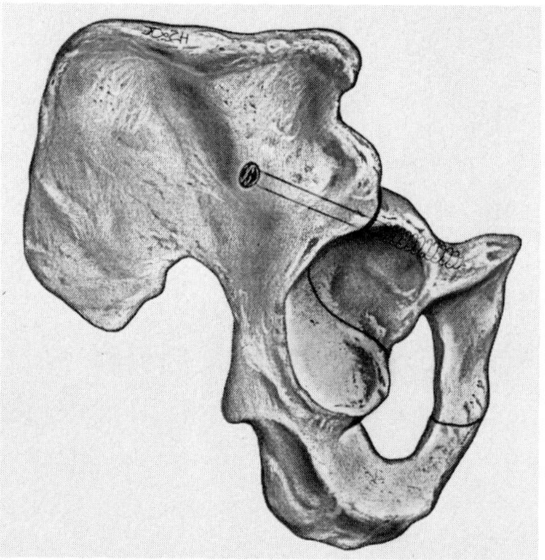

Figure 9-27B i. Outer view.

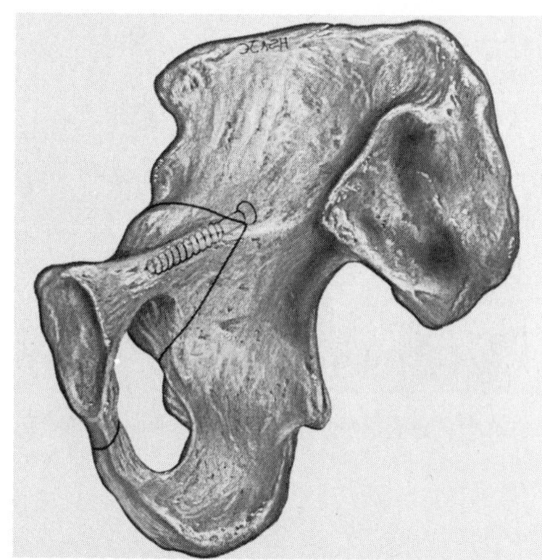

Figure 9-27B ii. Inner view.

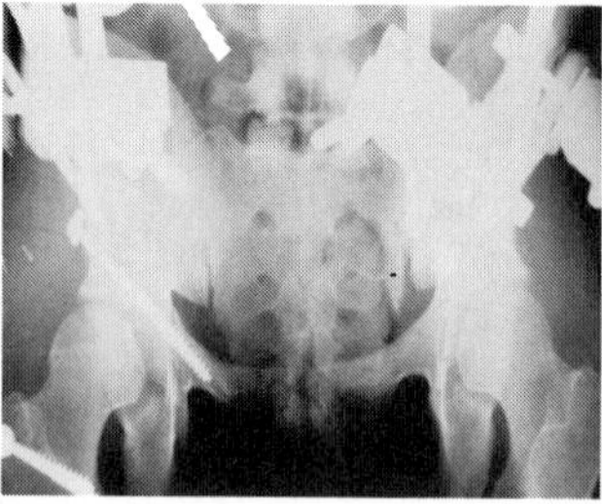

Figure 9-27C.

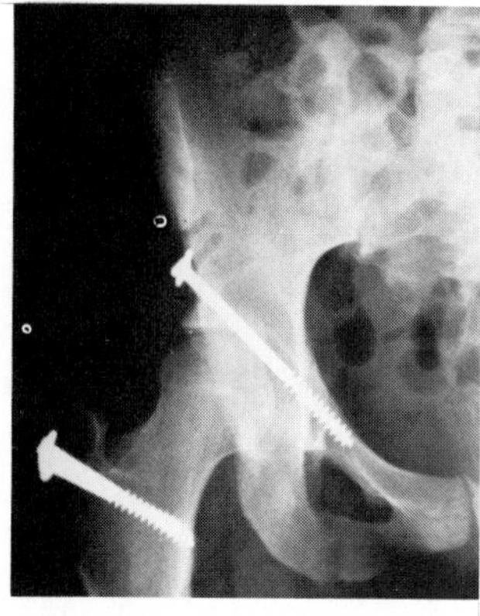

Figure 9-27D.

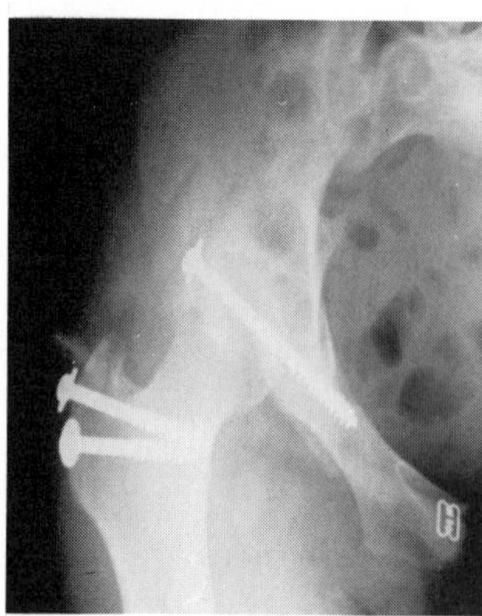

Figure 9-27E.

Figure 9-28. A both-column fracture with primary involvement of the anterior column. By resort to an ilioinguinal incision, the posterior column is repaired with a lag screw. A lengthy anterior column buttress plate is applied, along with shorter plates for the immobilization of the ilium. In 9-28F, some persistent displacement of the posterior column is evident.

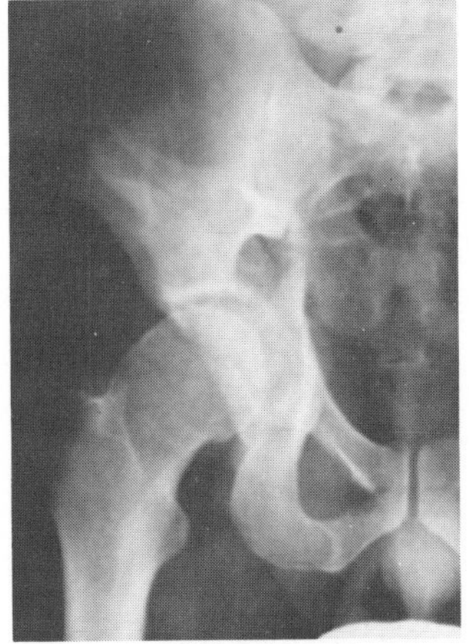

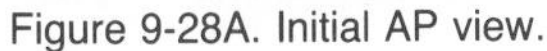

Figure 9-28A. Initial AP view.

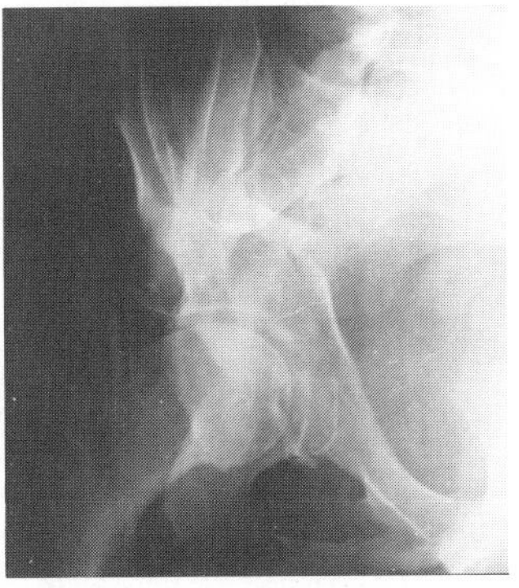

Figure 9-28B. Initial obturator oblique view.

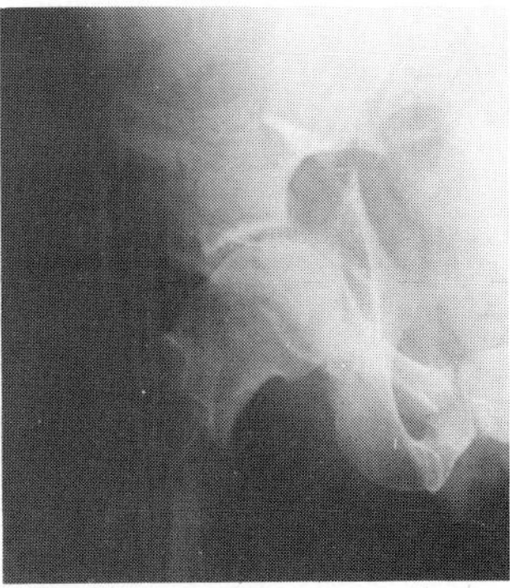

Figure 9-28C. Initial iliac oblique view.

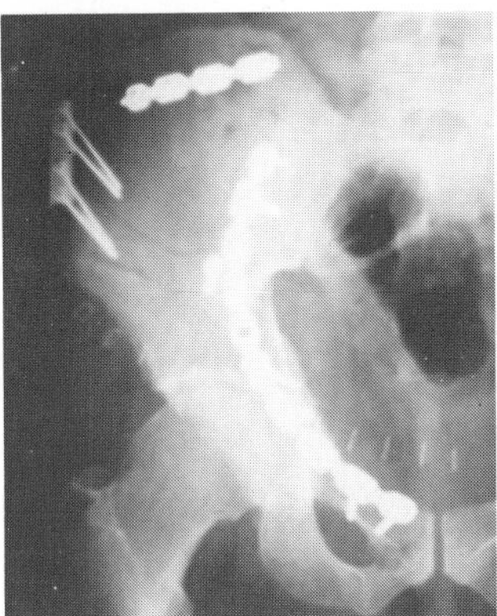

Figure 9-28D. Postoperative AP view.

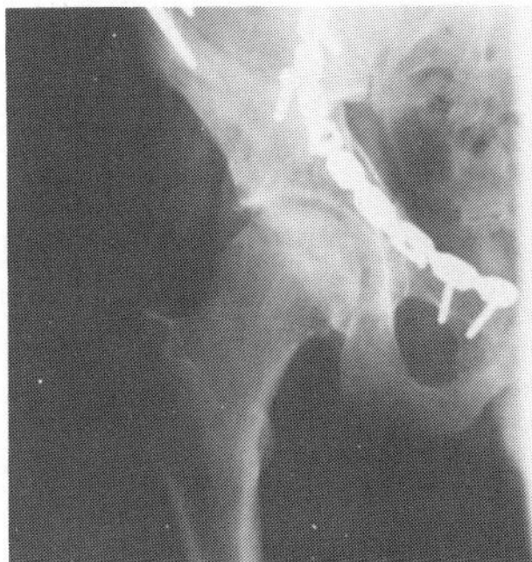

Figure 9-28E. Postoperative obturator oblique view.

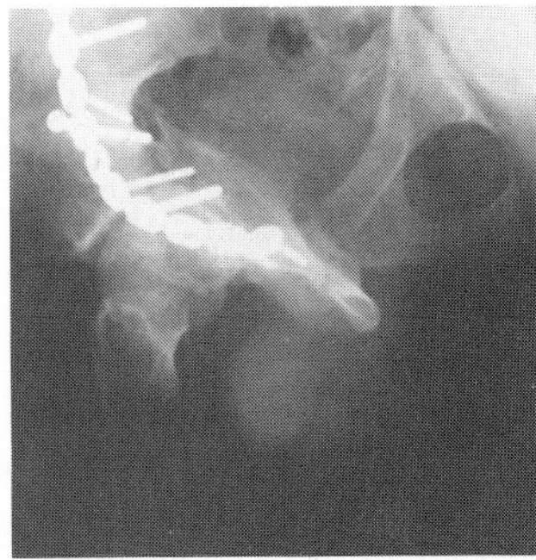

Figure 9-28F. Postoperative iliac oblique view.

iliopectineal line. Unless the articular surface of the acetabulum can be thoroughly inspected, the screw holes superficial to the roof are not utilized. Otherwise the screws are directed away from the hip joint.

Inferior disruptions of the anterior column are rarely approached surgically unless they are associated with a disruption of the symphysis or the ipsilateral ilium and adjacent acetabulum. In such cases, an anterior column lag screw is suitable for fixation (Figure 9-27). More typically, with an anterior column or anterior wall with a posterior hemitransverse fracture, supplementary lag screw fixation of the posterior column is needed. Usually a buttress plate is applied along the iliopectineal line from the posterior intact ilium to the stable portion of superior pubic ramus or, in appropriate cases, across

Figure 9-29. A left "T" fracture with primarily anterior column displacement and a right low anterior column fracture and ipsilateral sacroiliac dislocation. By resort to a bilateral ilioinguinal incision, the fractures were reduced and immobilized by a lengthy Letournel plate and a supplementary lag screw for the posterior column of the "T" fracture. Through a separate exposure, the right sacroiliac joint was stabilized with lag screws. Incidentally, a highly comminuted fracture of the left femoral shaft was repaired with a static locking nail.

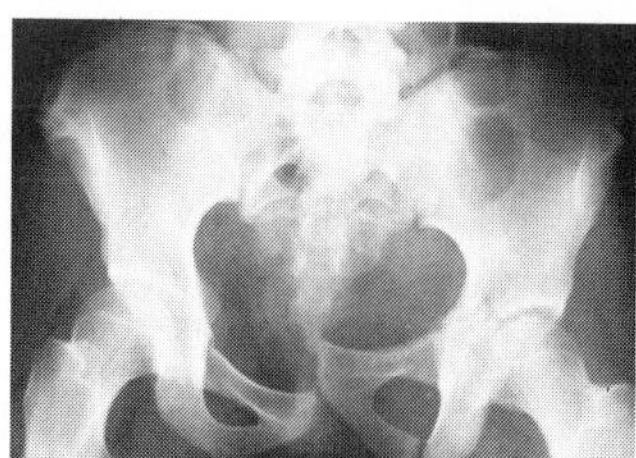

Figure 9-29A. Initial AP view.

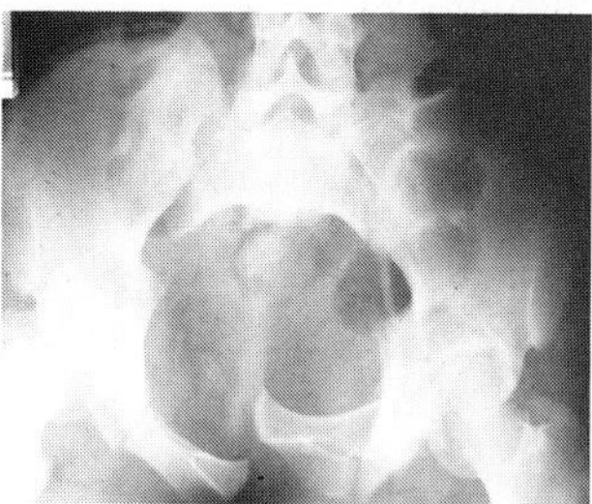

Figure 9-29B. Inlet view.

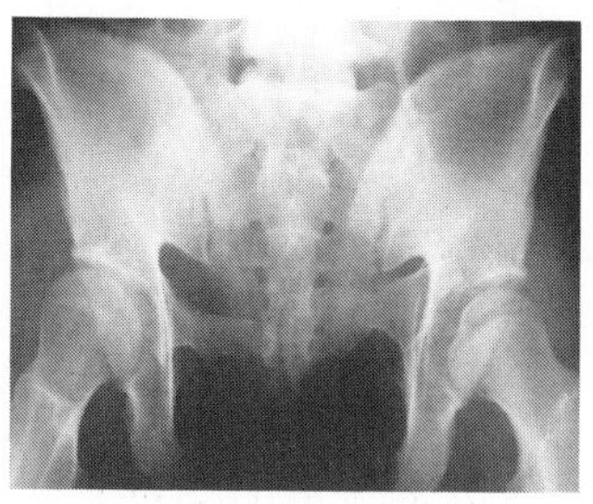

Figure 9-29C. Outlet view.

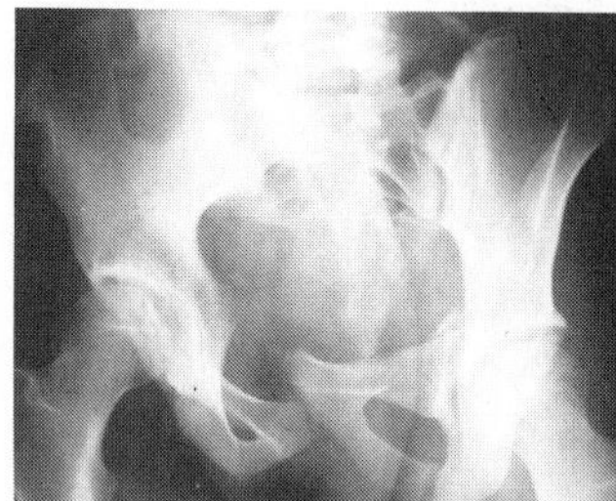

Figure 9-29D. Obturator oblique view, left hip.

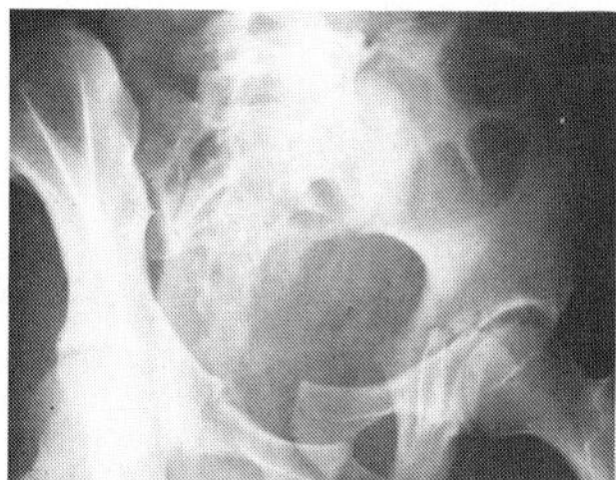

Figure 9-29E. Iliac oblique view, left hip.

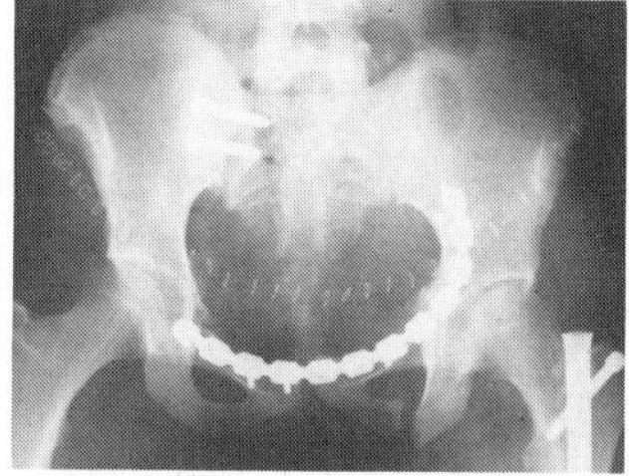

Figure 9-29F. Initial postoperative AP view.

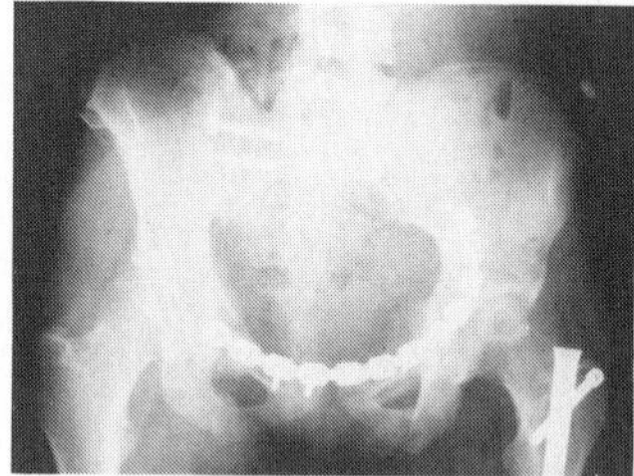

Figure 9-29G. Followup at six months.

the disrupted symphysis to the contralateral superior pubic ramus (Figures 9-22, 9-28, and 9-29). While absolutely essential, accurate contouring of the plate is greatly hampered by the presence of the external iliac vessels and the femoral nerve, which cross the surgical field.

## Transverse Fractures

Stabilization of a transverse fracture or the transverse element of a "T" fracture is readily accomplished by resort to fixation methods previously described for the posterior and anterior columns. Usually the extension of the fracture across the anterior column is immobilized with a lengthy lag screw inserted from the lateral ilium about 2.5cm above the roof of the acetabulum into the superior pubic ramus (Figures 9-30 and 9-31). The posterior column is stabilized by a lag screw directed from superior to inferior parallel to the medial border of the posterior column. A supplementary 3.5mm reconstruction plate

Figure 9-30. Techniques of lag screw fixation with a supplementary buttress plate for the posterior column, for a typical transverse fracture. A: Diagram of a high transverse fracture, using 6.5mm cancellous lag screws. B: Diagram of a midtransverse fracture with 4.5mm cortical screws inserted with a lag technique. While predrilling of the gliding holes prior to the reduction of the fracture is necessary, this method provides a more reliable orientation of the screws and a greater margin for error. C: Orientation of the posterior column lag screw. D: Orientation of the anterior column lag screw. E: Cross-section of the anterior column to show the site for the lag screw. Ideally the screw is inserted more posterior and parallel to the iliopectineal line.

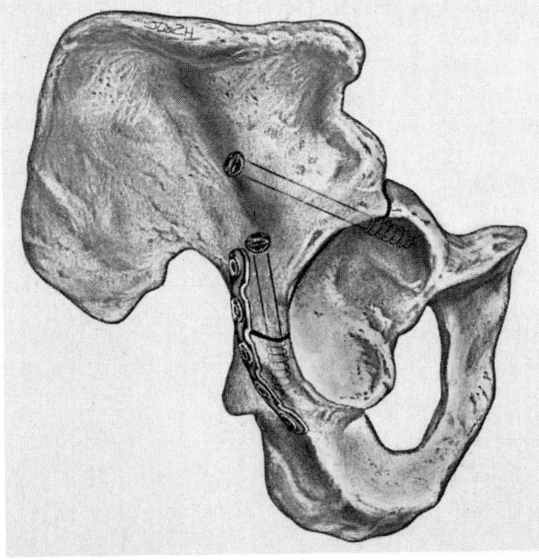

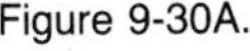

Figure 9-30A.

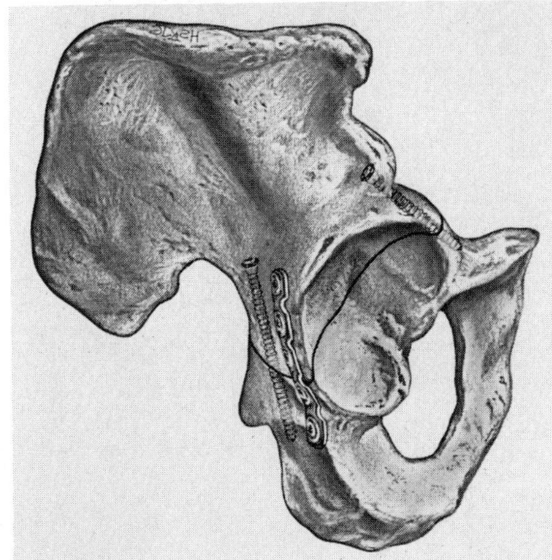

Figure 9-30B.

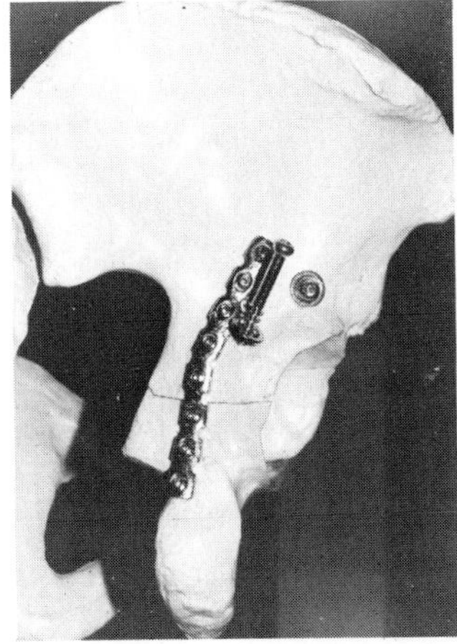

Figure 9-30C.

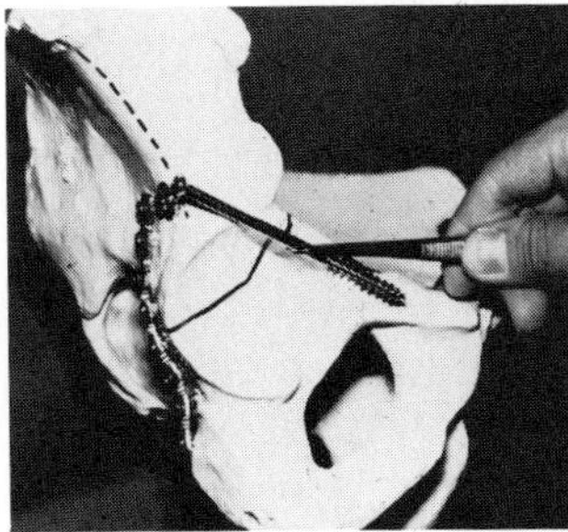

Figure 9-30D.

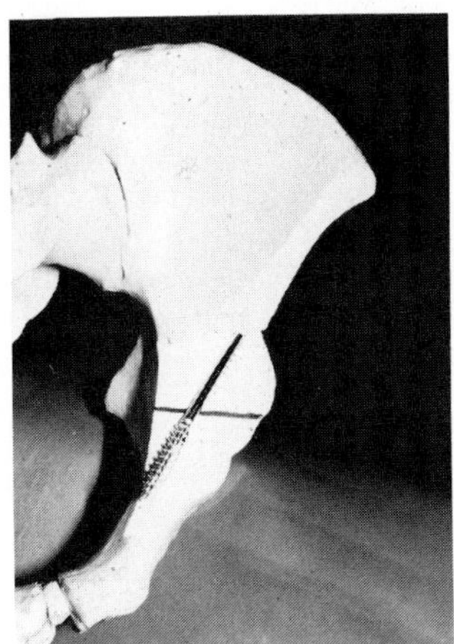

Figure 9-30E.

is used to buttress the posterior column. A low transverse fracture or an oblique variant that exits low anteriorly requires the use of a supplementary anterior plate (Figure 9-32). Many transverse fractures involve the posterior wall, whereupon the technique of reduction is similar to a posterior column associated with a posterior wall fracture. Initially, the transverse portion of the injury is realigned and at least provisionally stabilized. Exaggerated intraoperative displacement of the wall fragment augments the exposure of the articular surface

Figure 9-31. A simple transverse acetabular fracture stabilized with a posterior column plate and lag screw. The fracture is truly transverse across the midtectal portion. A: Initial AP view. B: Anterior view, 3D scan. C: Superior view, 3D scan, illustrates the primarily anterior displacement with hinging around the posterior column. D: Postoperative AP view. E: Postoperative iliac oblique view.

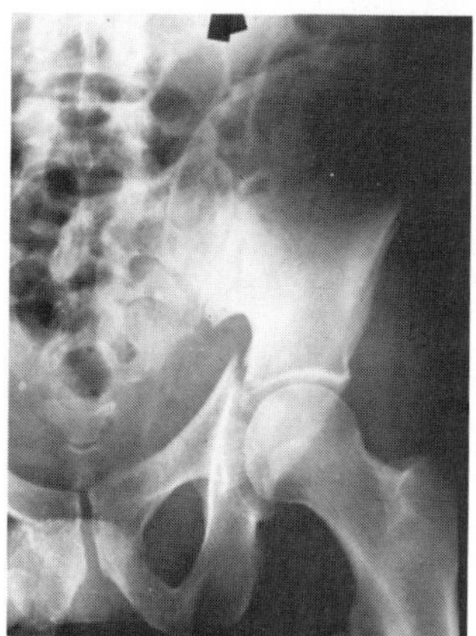

Figure 9-31A.

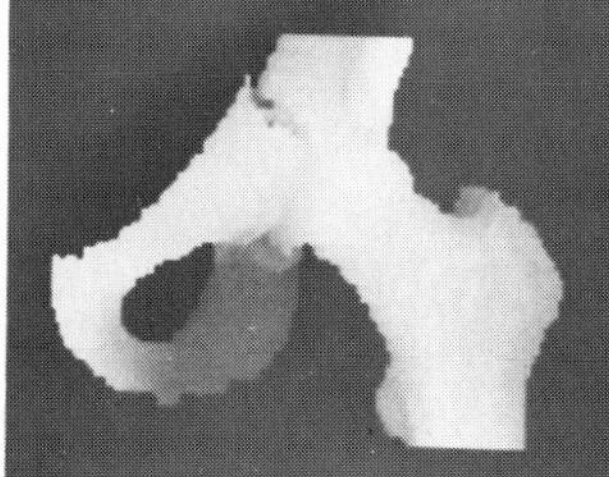

Figure 9-31B.

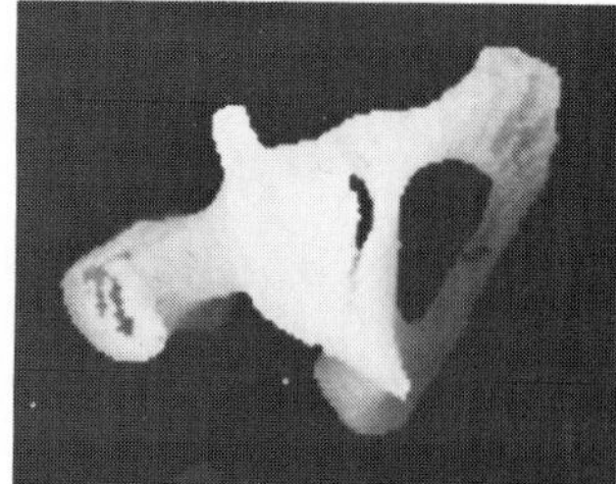

Figure 9-31C.

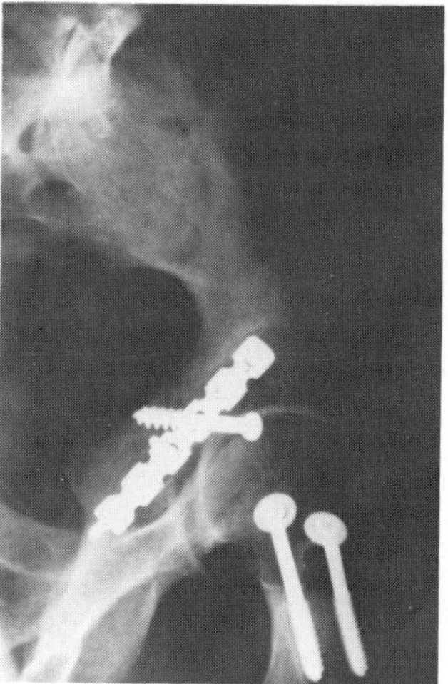

Figure 9-31D.

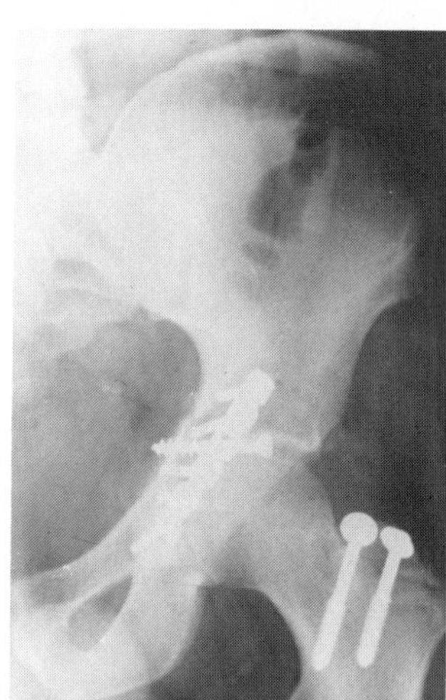

Figure 9-31E.

of the displaced transverse fracture. Then the wall fragment is reduced and stabilized (Figures 9-33 to 9-36). Still other transverse fractures possess marked iliac involvement, often with an associated ipsilateral subluxation of the sacroiliac joint (Figure 9-37). The complexity of the reconstruction mounts rapidly with the presence of comminution. Still other transverse fractures are of a bilateral nature, with associated dislocation of one or both sacroiliac joints (Figure 9-38). An arduous procedure involving one or more repositions in the operating room is needed to realize an accurate restoration of the several injuries.

A "T" fracture employs similiar general principles of stabilization. Inevitably, as the degree of comminution and displacement increases, the technical problems also grow (Figures 9-39 to 9-44). When this technique is employed to immobilize a "T" fracture, such lag fixation to the superior part of the acetabulum is accompanied by a minor separation of the base of the "T," in the most

Figure 9-32. For a low transverse fracture or as in the following clinical case, which has an oblique propagation from high in the posterior column to low in the anterior column, an anterior plate is needed to supplement the posterior fixation. A: AP view with right transverse acetabular fracture, along with a diastasis, contralateral ramus fractures, and unstable sacral fracture. B: Computed scan through sacral fracture. C: Schematic diagram of stabilization technique. D: Postoperative inlet view, with supplementary external pelvic frame to immobilize the pelvic ring. E: Six months later, AP view. F: Late outlet view with orientation of column screws.

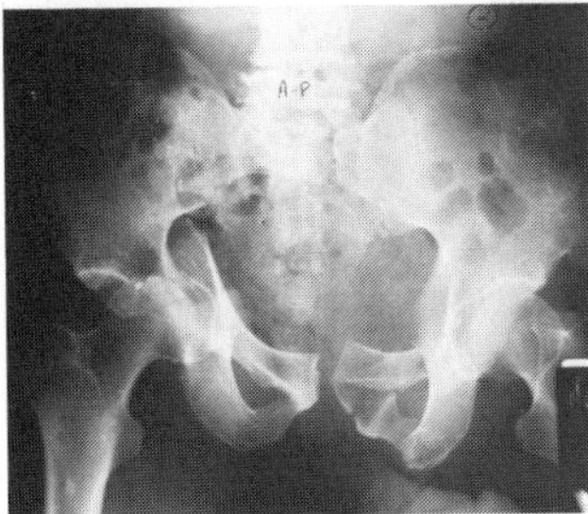

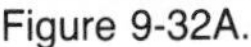

Figure 9-32A.

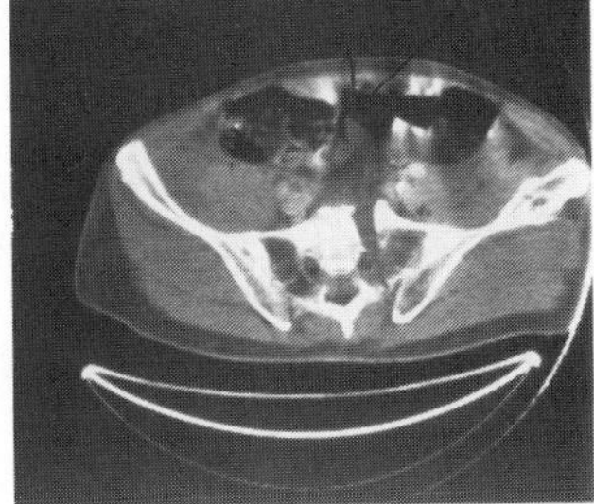

Figure 9-32B.

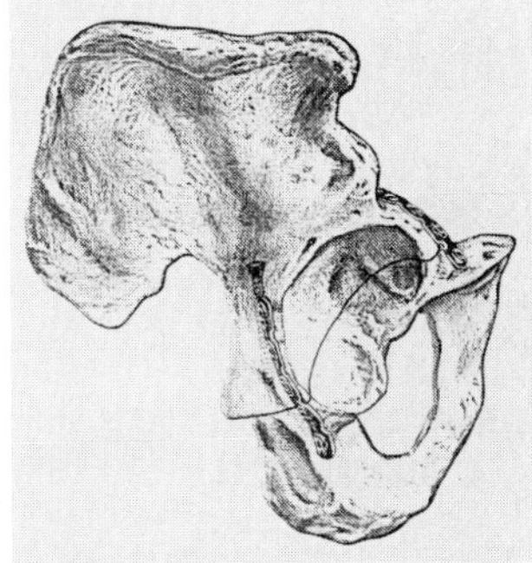

Figure 9-32C.

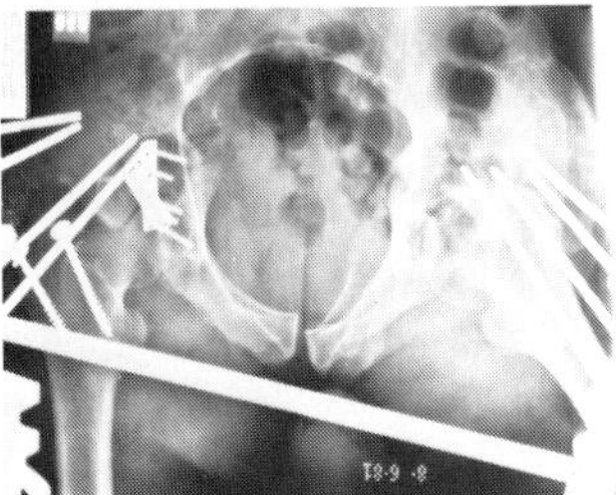

Figure 9-32D.

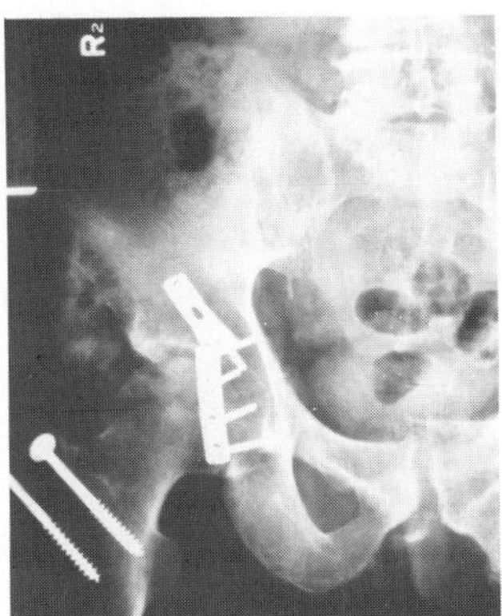

Figure 9-32E.

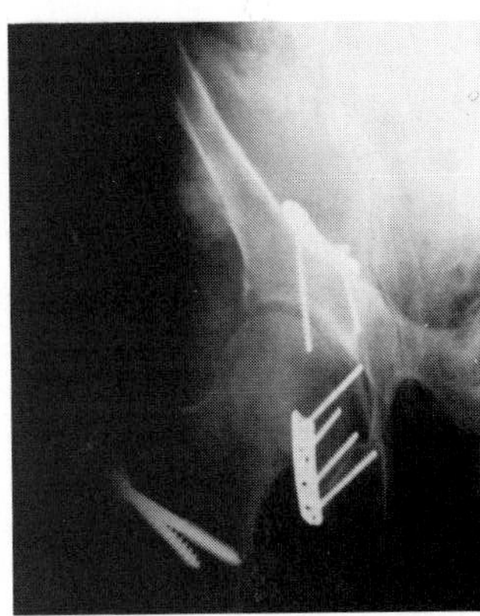

Figure 9-32F.

inferior portion of the acetabulum. Such a yawning apart of the two principal inferior fracture fragments can be prevented by the insertion of a 4.5mm malleolar screw or 4.0mm cancellous screw immediately superior to the roof of the obturator foramen. The screw is inserted through the relevant portion of the top of the superior pubic ramus and directed toward the posterior portion of the ischial tuberosity. Routine application of this screw is not undertaken since it necessitates a much greater exposure of the anterior column with its insertion immediately below the external iliac vessels. The available bone stock is excessively thin, so that the margins for error during the insertion of the screw are limited.

Anterior column with posterior hemitransverse injuries are a modification of a "T" fracture. They may possess primarily anterior or posterior column involvement and displacement. The preoperative evaluation focuses upon this feature to help define the optimal surgical exposure.

Figure 9-33. A minimally displaced transverse associated with a posterior wall fracture in a small woman is immobilized by intraoperative stabilization of the transverse element with a K-wire followed by a posterior buttress plate. Marginal impaction of the posterior wall required elevation and bone graft. A: Initial view. B: Computed scan with marginal impaction. C: Postoperative AP view. D: Late iliac oblique view with healing transverse fracture.

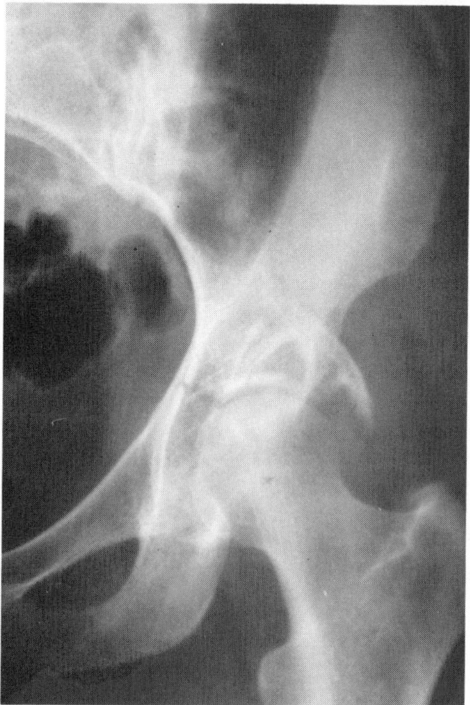

Figure 9-33A.

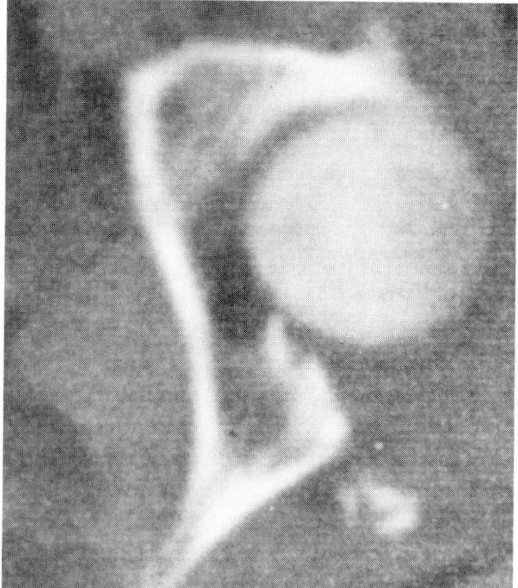

Figure 9-33B.

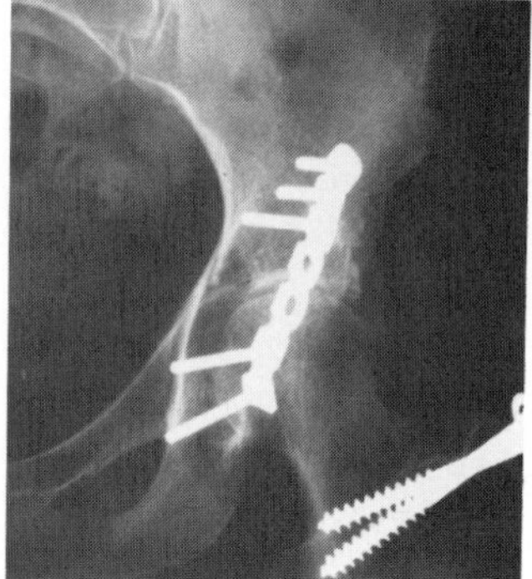

Figure 9-33C.

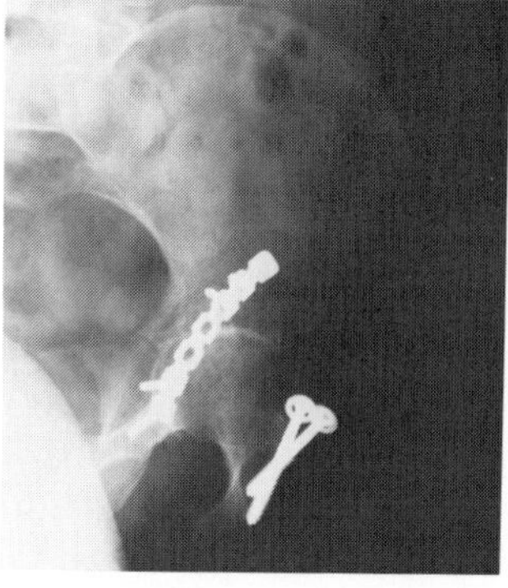

Figure 9-33D.

Figure 9-34. A transverse with associated posterior wall fracture stabilized initially with a posterior column plate and followed by a buttress plate for the posterior wall. A: Initial AP view. B: Anterior 3D scan. C: Iliac oblique 3D scan. D: Superior 3D scan. E: Drawing of fixation with lag screws in both columns and posterior plates in the posterior column and wall; some combination of these methods is used routinely. F: Postoperative AP view.

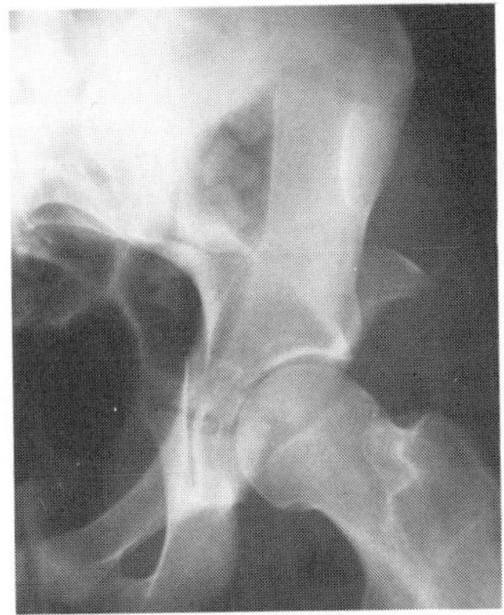

Figure 9-34A.

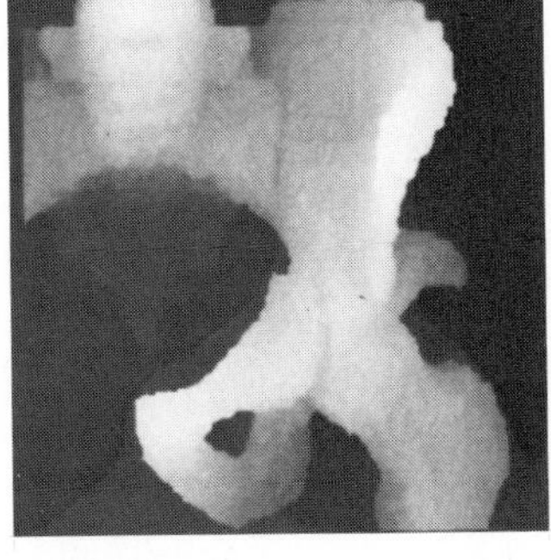

Figure 9-34B.

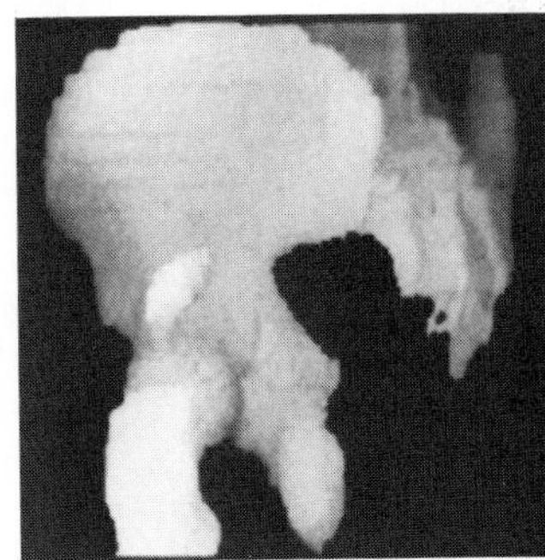

Figure 9-34C.

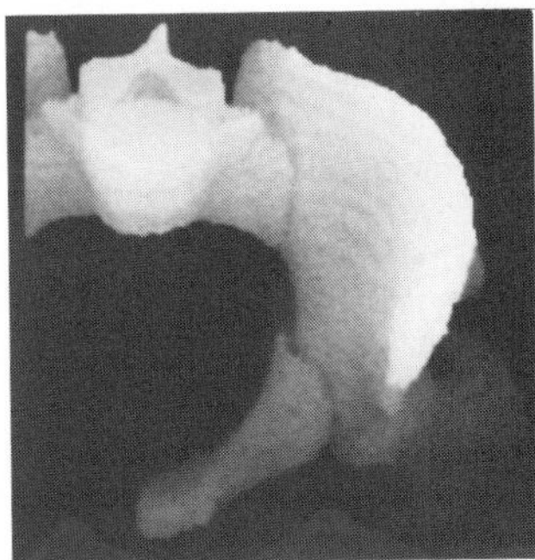

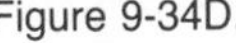

Figure 9-34D.

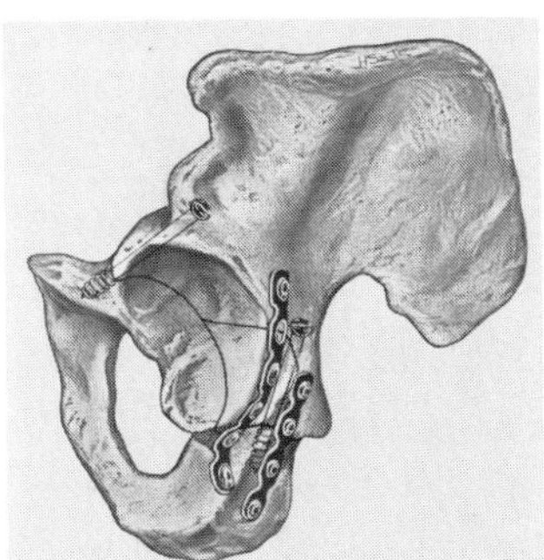

Figure 9-34E.

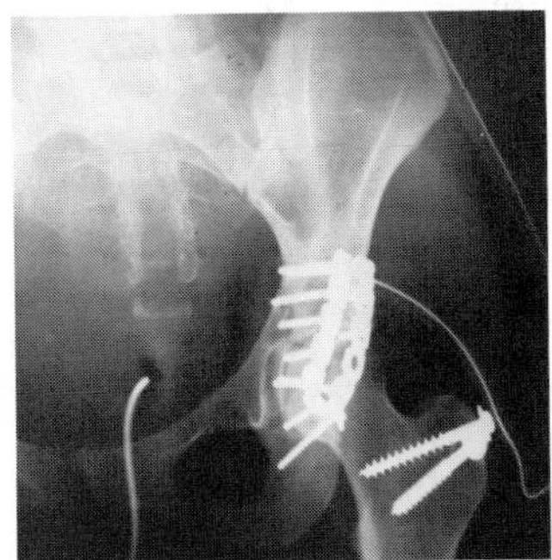

Figure 9-34F.

While such a fracture with marked posterior column displacement is approached with a posterior or extensile lateral exposure, a fracture with marked anterior column displacement is approached anteriorly (Figures 9-22, 9-45, and 9-46). Otherwise the techniques of stabilization are similar to those previously described for anterior column and "T" fractures.

The both-column fractures possess an enormous variety, with a highly varied pattern of comminution and displacement. One hallmark is the central displacement with a rotational deviation of the anterior and posterior column fragments to create a large defect in the center of the acetabulum. Unless this characteristic "bar-room door" deformity is fully appreciated, an accurate reduction is unlikely to be achieved. The three-dimensional scans are especially helpful to evaluate the deformity and facilitate the evolution of the surgical tactic.

The postoperative inlet view provides the best indication of the accuracy of the overall reduction and

Figure 9-35. A transverse associated with a posterior wall fracture stabilized with an anterior column lag screw and a posterior buttress plate. A: Initial AP view with malrotation of right iliac wing secondary to sacroiliac subluxation. B: Obturator oblique view. C: Computed scan through comminuted dome. D: Computed scan with involvement of medial wall and interposed fragment. E: Postoperative view at three months with minor ectopic bone but full hip motion. F: Late obturator oblique view with orientation of anterior column lag screw.

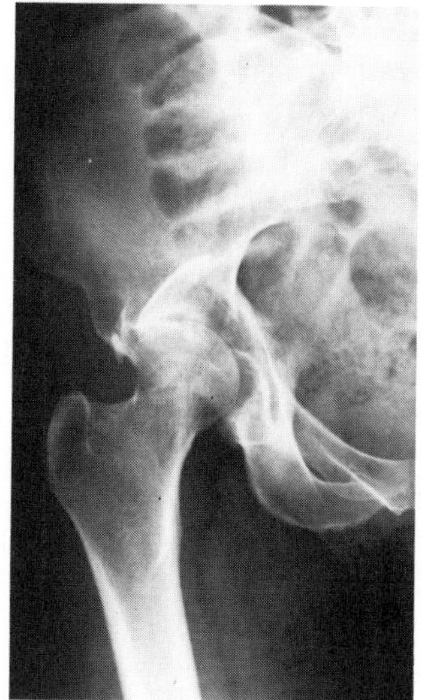

Figure 9-35A.

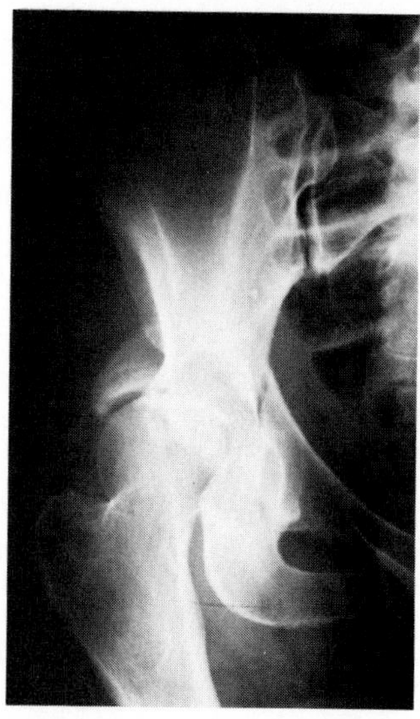

Figure 9-35B.

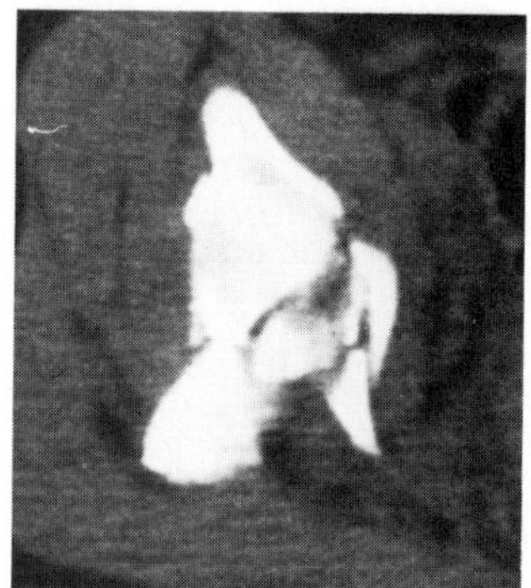

Figure 9-35C.

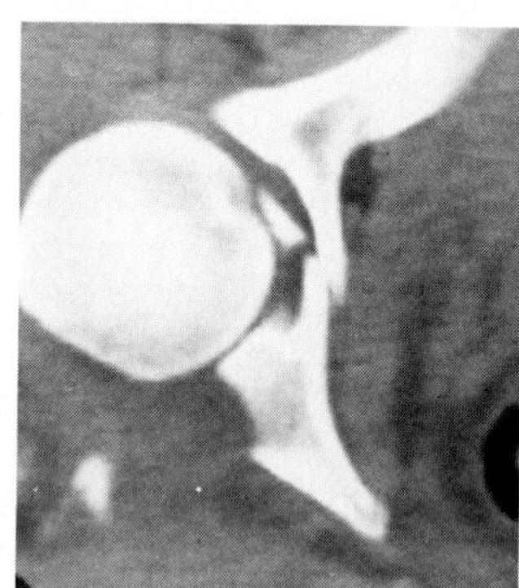

Figure 9-35D.

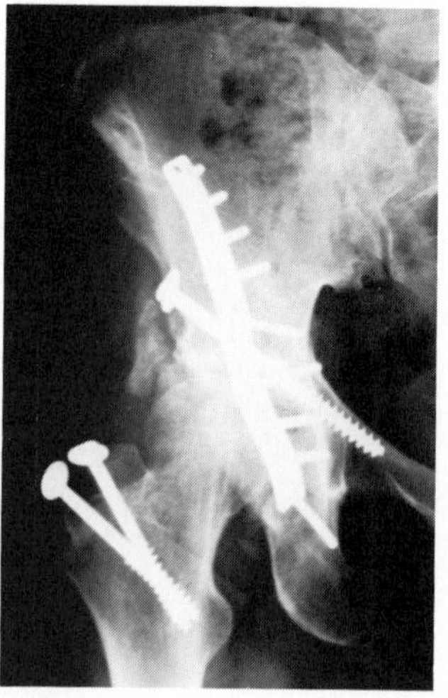

Figure 9-35E.

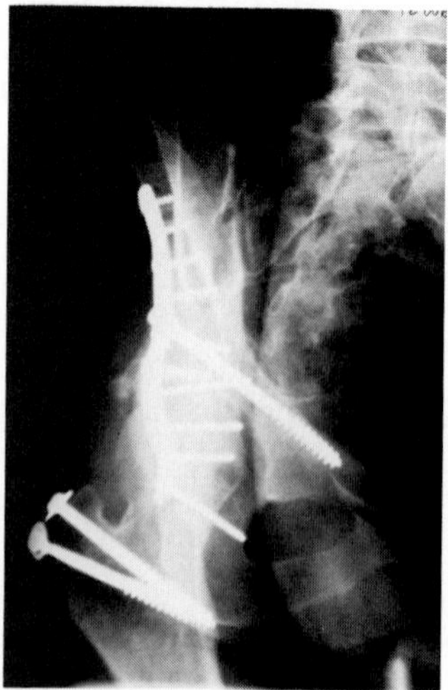

Figure 9-35F.

Figure 9-36. A comminuted transverse with associated posterior wall fracture, stabilized with a lag screw and plate for the transverse element and a buttress plate for the posterior wall.

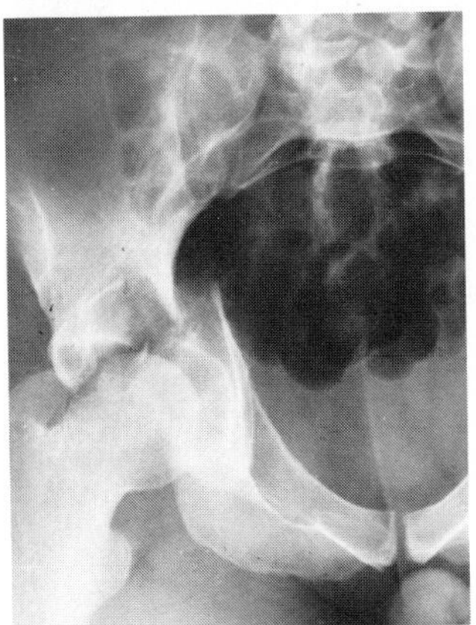

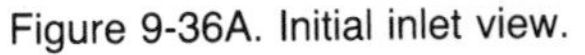
Figure 9-36A. Initial inlet view.

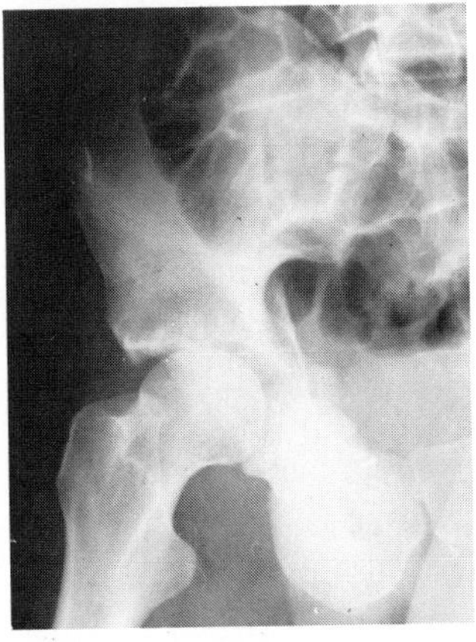
Figure 9-36B. Iliac oblique view.

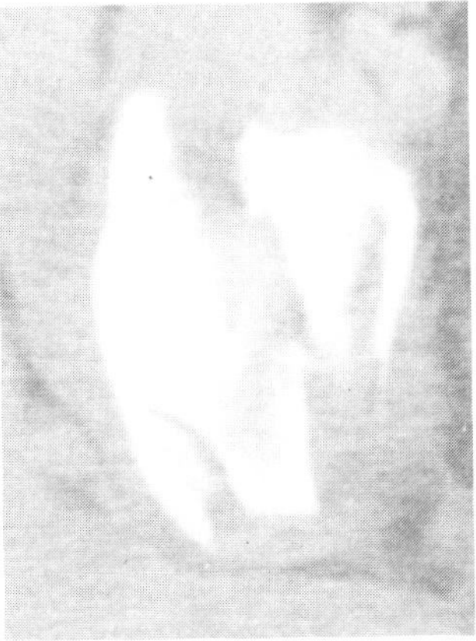
Figure 9-36C. Computed scan through comminuted dome.

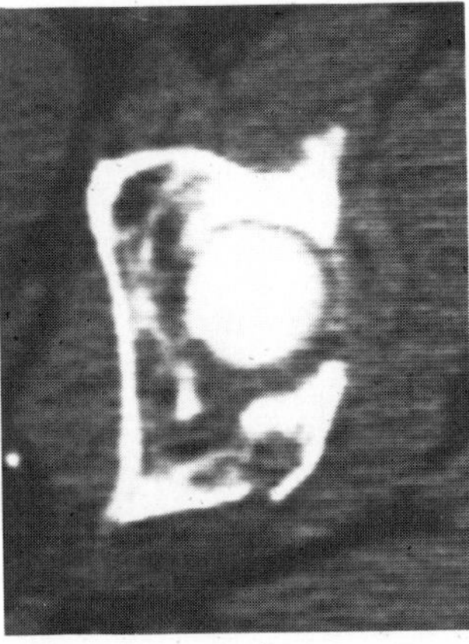
Figure 9-36D. Computed scan with posterior wall involvement.

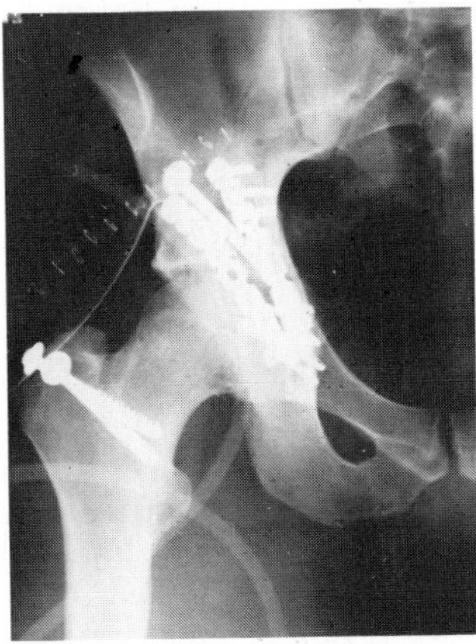
Figure 9-36E. Postoperative AP view.

correction of the central displacement. Irrespective of the approach, whenever possible lag screws are employed to secure larger fragments of dense bone. As the degree of comminution and osteoporosis increases, a conversion to plate fixation is needed to buttress the unstable segments. The ilioinguinal approach is preferred for the appropriate injuries with primarily anterior displacement. These typically comminuted fractures possess a predilection for ectopic bone formation, which is minimized by an extraarticular exposure. Also, the central deformity is much more readily apparent on the inner aspect of the innominate bone. Unless the approach is modified with a T-type extension across the anterior aspect of the hip joint, interposed fragments cannot be removed. Also, the intraarticular surface cannot be

Figure 9-37. A transverse fracture with comminution of the posterior wall and lateral ilium.

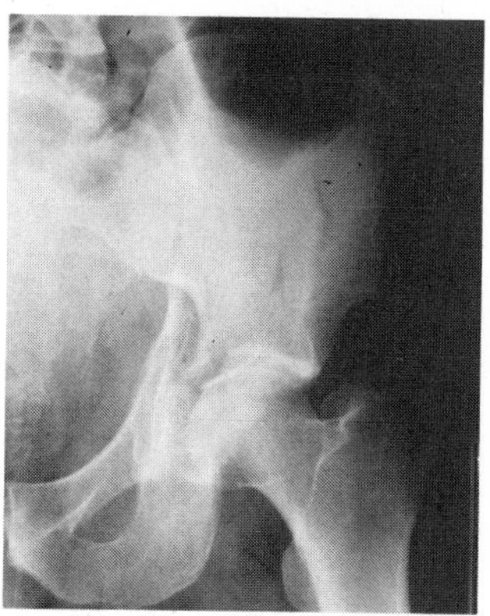

Figure 9-37A. Initial AP view.

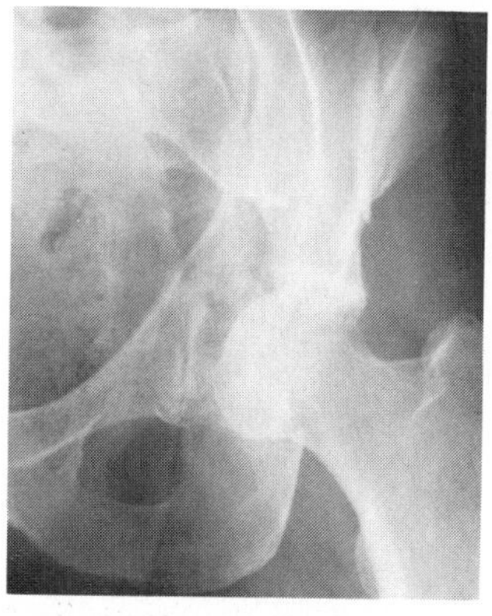

Figure 9-37B. Obturator oblique view.

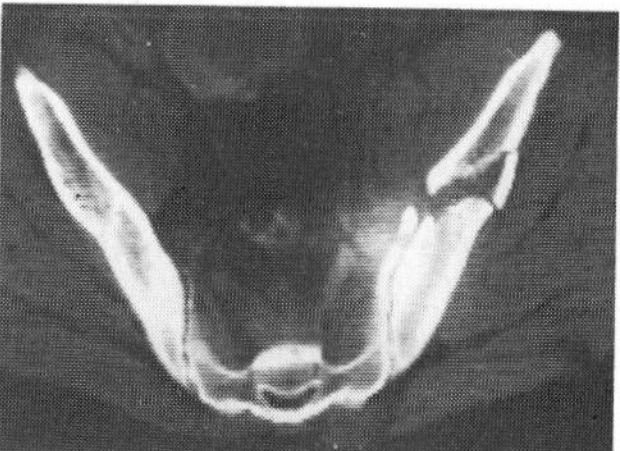

Figure 9-37C. Computed scan, comminuted ilium.

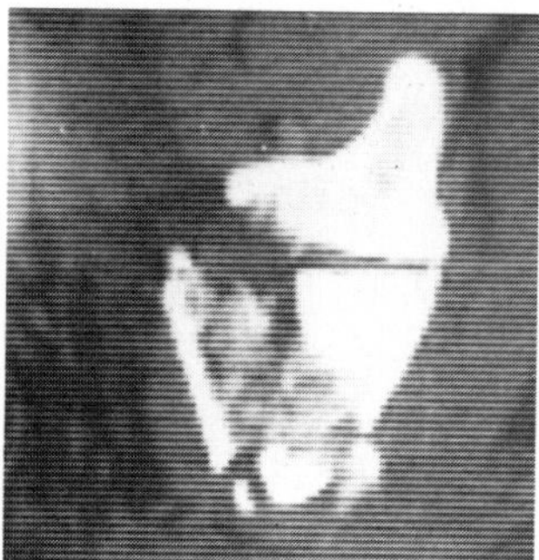

Figure 9-37D. Computed scan, comminuted dome.

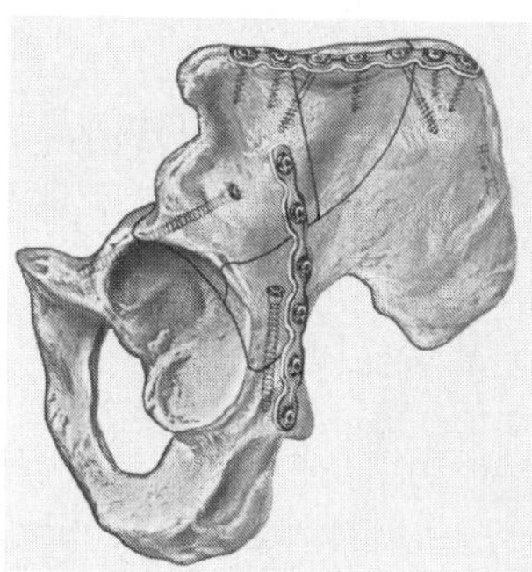

Figure 9-37E. Diagram of typical stabilization.

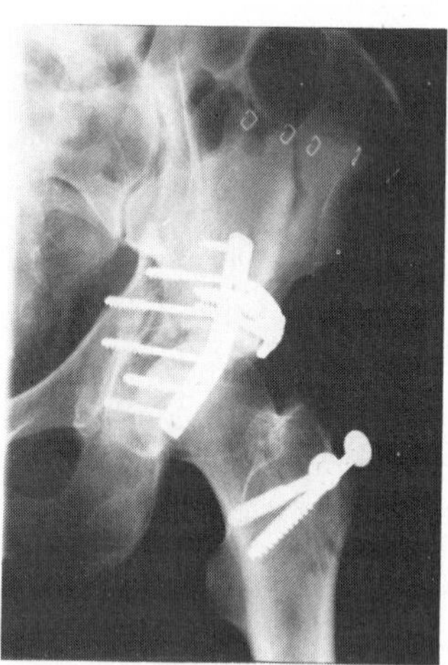

Figure 9-37F. Postoperative AP view.

examined to judge the accuracy of the reduction and the presence of a penetrating screw. A few examples of the anterior stabilization techique are shown in Figures 9-47 to 9-49.

Where an extensile lateral approach is employed, particular care is needed to ensure that the anterior and posterior columns are accurately realigned (Figures 9-50 to 9-52). Even though the outer fracture surfaces contact one another, a considerable rotational deformity of the columns can persist. For the fracture variants wth a segmental anterior column fracture, the superior iliac fragment is deliberately displaced so that the inferior half of the acetabulum is reduced (Figure 9-53). A 4.0mm cancellous screw is inserted across the inferior acetabulum. Ultimately, an accurate restoration of the pelvis is confirmed by scrutiny of the inlet view (Figure 9-54).

Figure 9-38. A bilateral transverse fracture with a dislocation of the left sacroiliac joint.

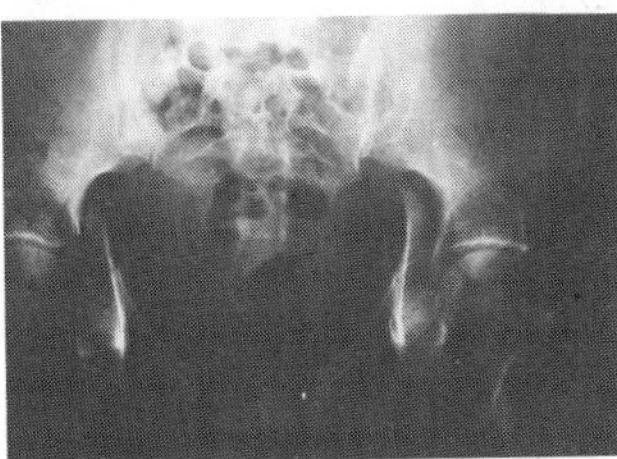
Figure 9-38A. Preoperative AP view.

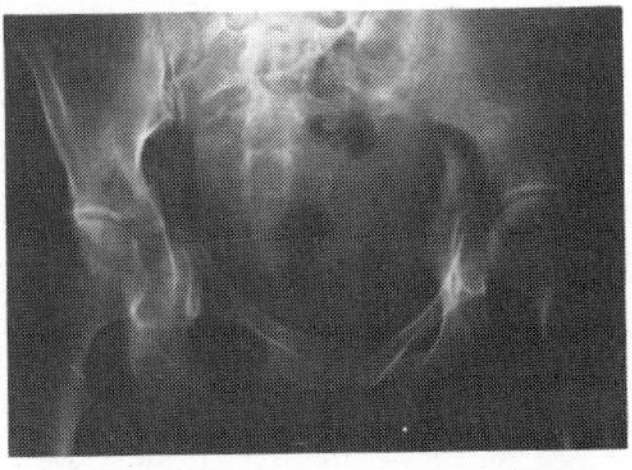
Figure 9-38B. Initial iliac oblique view, left hip.

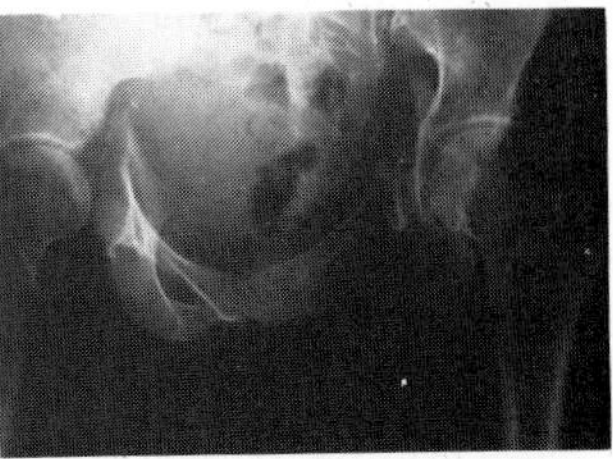
Figure 9-38C. Initial obturator oblique view, left hip.

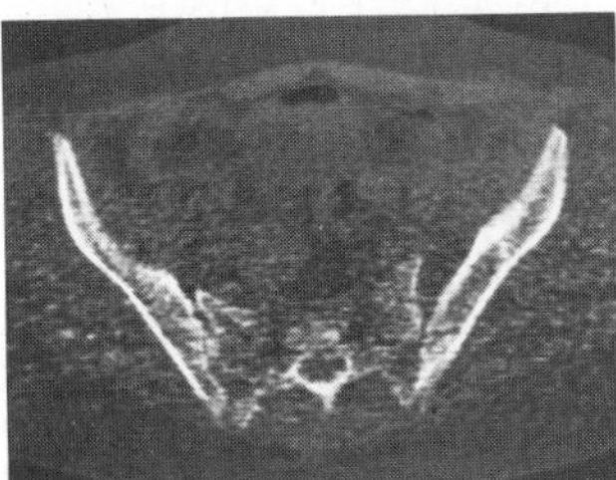
Figure 9-38D. Computed scan, dislocated SI joint.

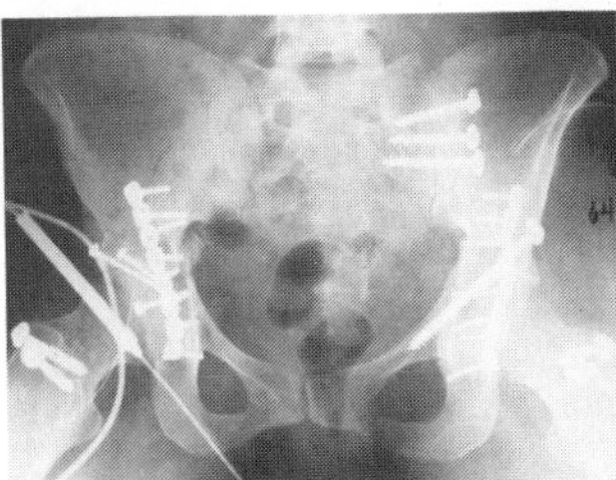
Figure 9-38E. Postoperative AP view.

## Stabilization of the Quadrilateral Surface

For the typical both-column fracture, the quadrilateral surface is displaced as a portion of the posterior column. With the reduction and fixation of the posterior column by the conventional methods, the quadrilateral surface is thereby immobilized to inhibit excessive medial migration or protrusio of the femoral head. Infrequently, a large rectangular fragment of the quadrilateral surface accompanies a both-column fracture (Figure 9-55). The fragment is hinged at its base and undergoes a marked medial displacement of its superior portion before the advancing femoral head. Once the femoral head has been reduced, the quadrilateral surface is reduced by resort to an ilioinguinal or occasionally a triradiate incision. Unless this wafer-like fragment of the inner cortical wall 2mm in thickness is stabilized, with sitting or standing the femoral head displaces the fragment to recreate the protrusio. To stabilize the quadrilateral surface a 3.5mm reconstruction plate is contoured so that it extends from the posterior surface of the posterior column, across the quadrilateral surface with progression across the iliopectineal line, to the superior pubic ramus or even the anterior inferior spine. The plate requires a peculiar bend at either end that is only possible with the 3.5mm reconstruction plate.

Figure 9-39. Techniques for stabilization of "T" fractures. A (i, ii): Both-column lag screws and a posterior column plate for a high "T" type. B: Similar method for a midtectal "T" type. C: Fixation of a low tectal "T" type. D: Fixation of a posterior "T" type.

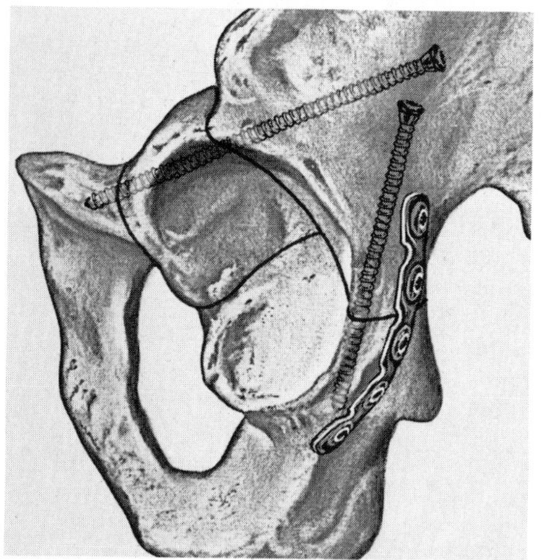

Figure 9-39A i. Outer view.

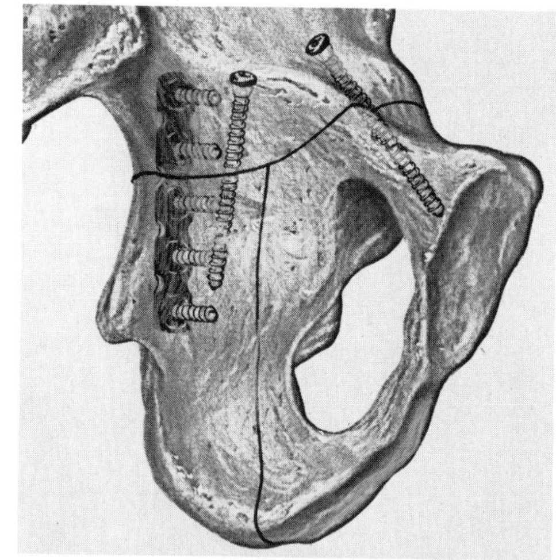

Figure 9-39A ii. Inner view.

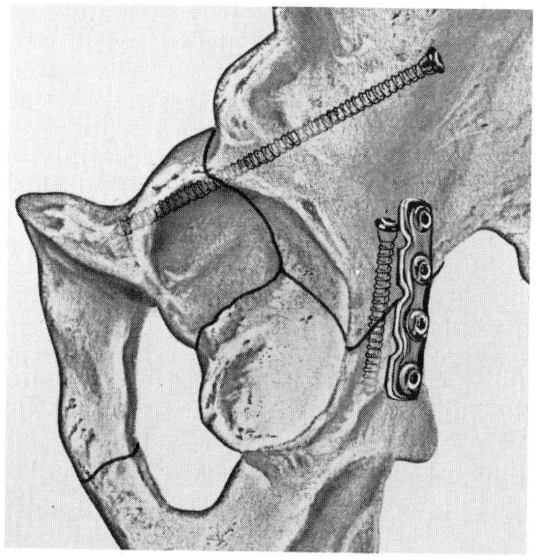

Figure 9-39B.

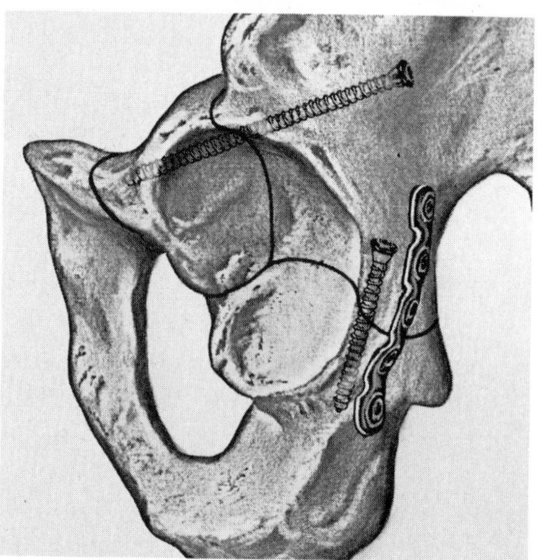

Figure 9-39C.

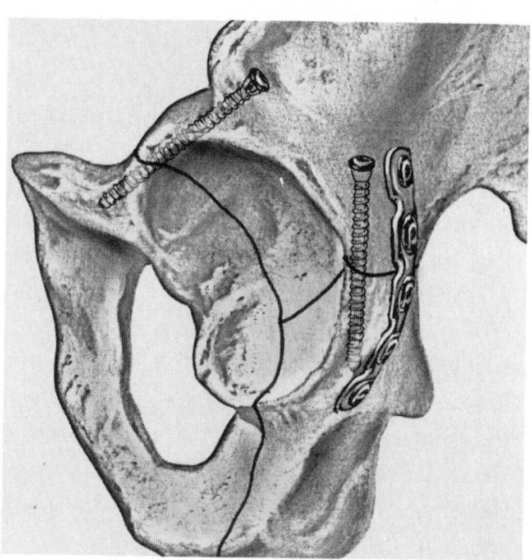

Figure 9-39D.

Figure 9-40. A posterior "T" fracture with minor displacement. After the anterior and posterior columns are reduced with tenaculum forceps, an anterior column lag screw and a posterior plate are applied.

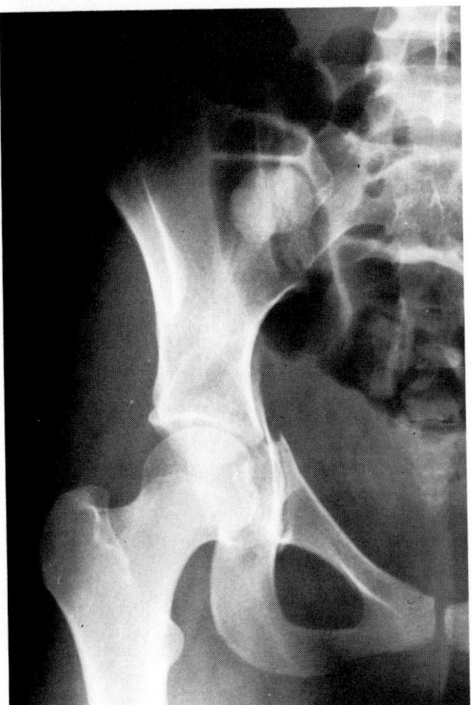

Figure 9-40A. Preoperative AP view.

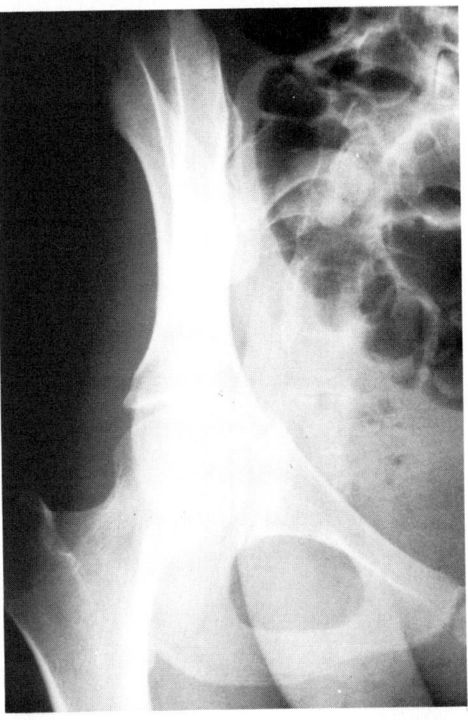

Figure 9-40B. Obturator oblique view indicative of posterior extent of the "T" element.

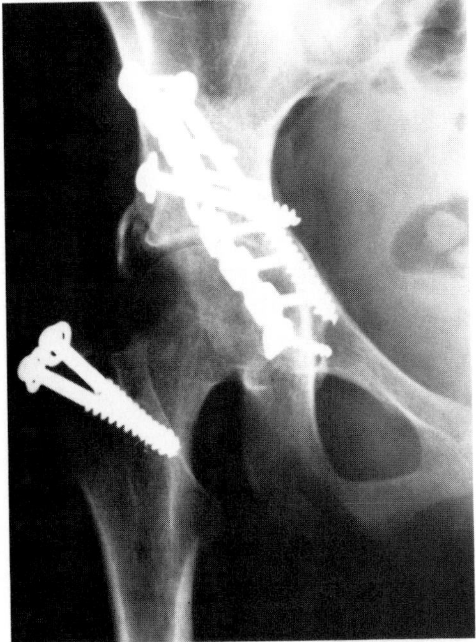

Figure 9-40C. Postoperative AP view at two years.

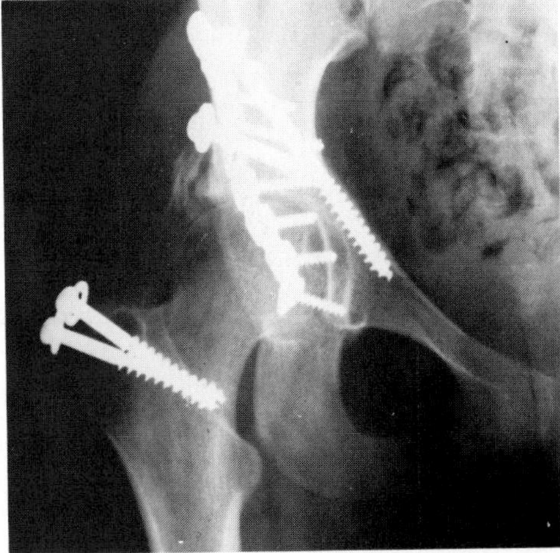

Figure 9-40D. Late obturator oblique view.

Figure 9-41. A "T" fracture in a 300-pound man of 40 years. While the reduction of the acetabulum is concentric with the femoral head, a careful scrutiny of the postoperative obturator oblique view indicates the typical separation of the inferior part of the reduction adjacent to the obturator foramen. This minor deformity arises from the absence of a reduction tool across the obturator ring during the fixation. A: Initial AP view. B: Outer view, 3D scan, with marked displacement of posterior scan. C: Inner view of anterior column with posterior "T" fracture. D: Inner view confirms the "T" pattern. E: Postoperative view at one year. F: Late obturator oblique view. G: Late iliac oblique view.

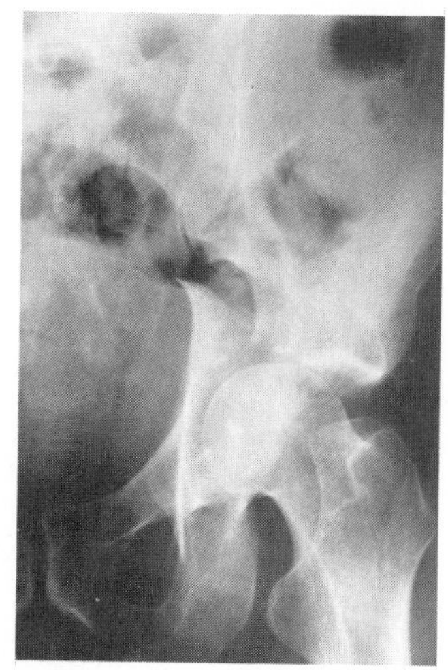

Figure 9-41A.

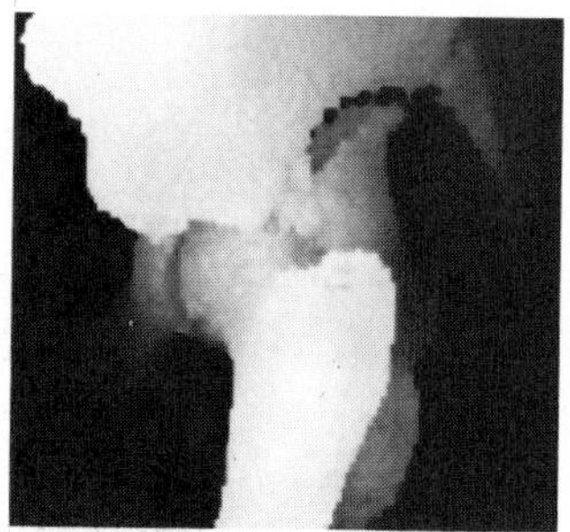

Figure 9-41B.

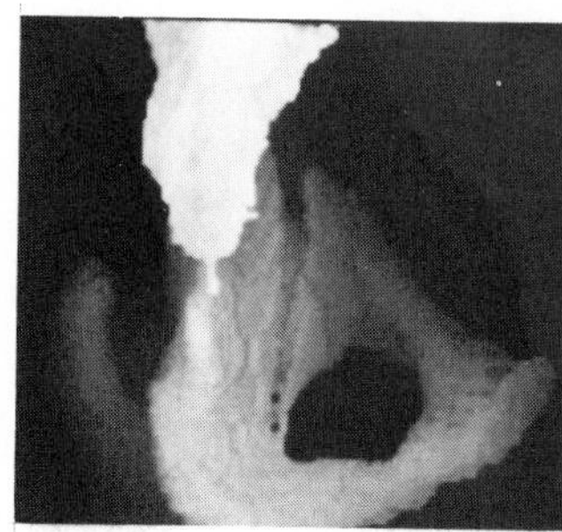

Figure 9-41C.

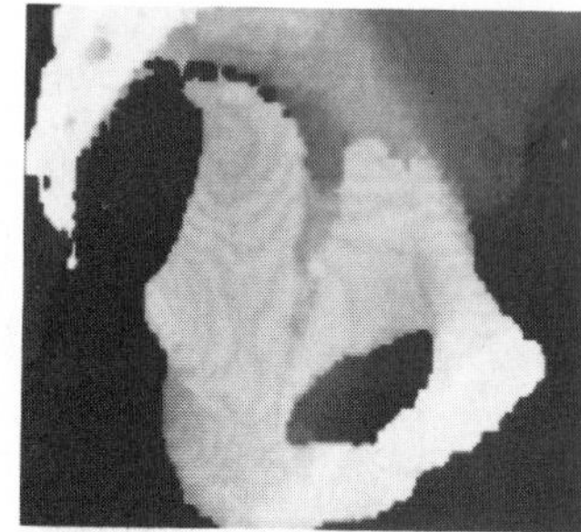

Figure 9-41D.

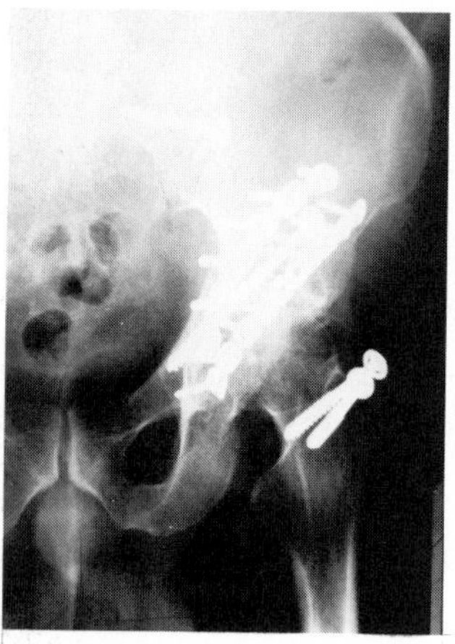

Figure 9-41E.

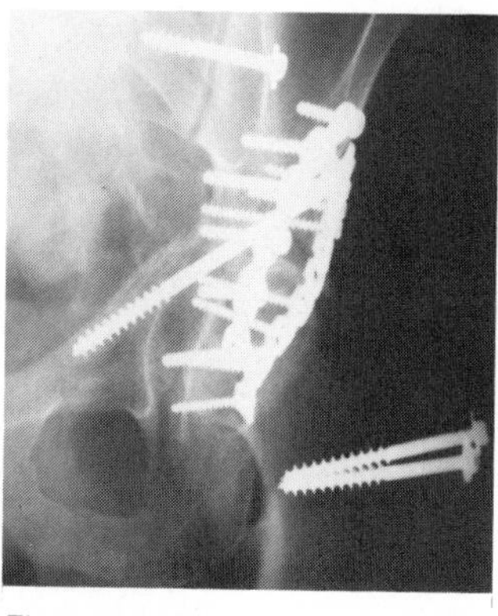

Figure 9-41F.

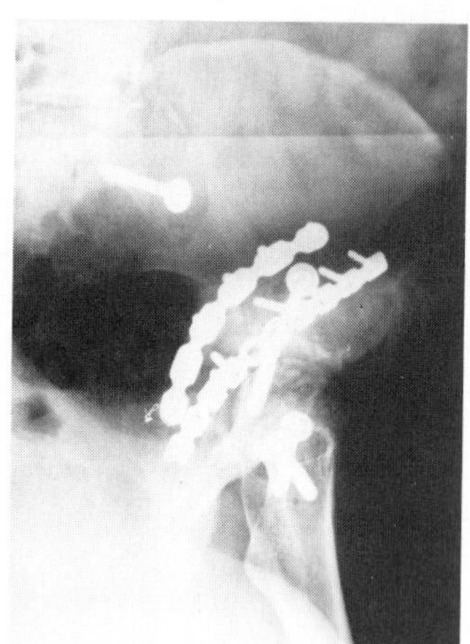

Figure 9-41G.

Figure 9-42. A comminuted "T" fracture with propagation across the dome to the sacroiliac joint.

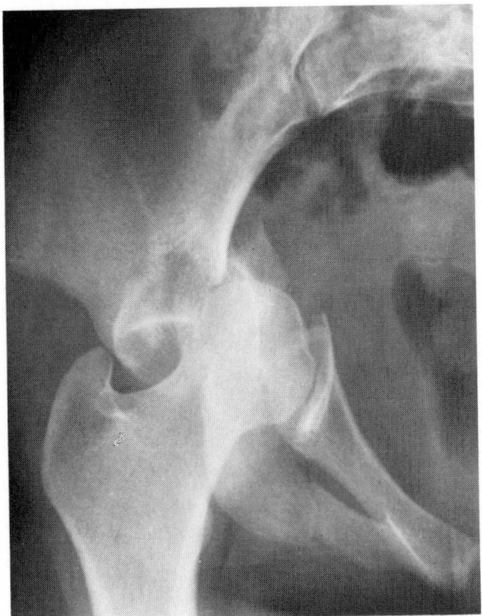

Figure 9-42A. Initial inlet view.

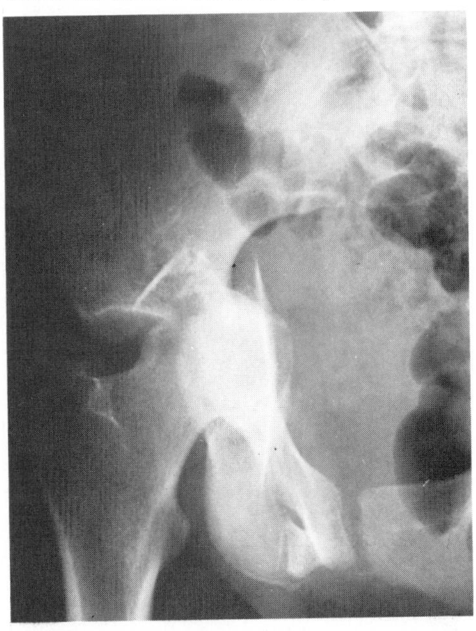

Figure 9-42B. Iliac oblique view.

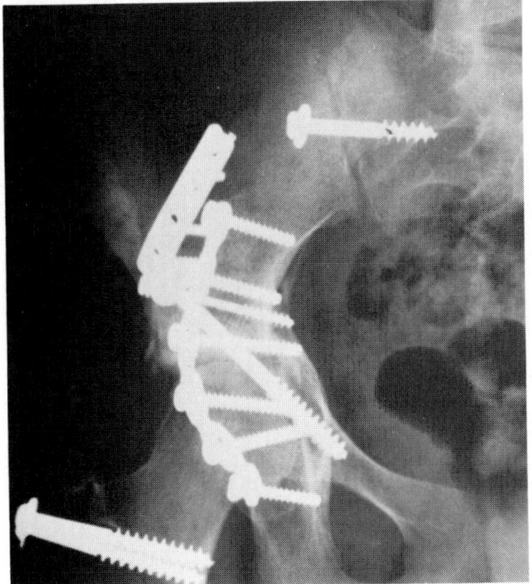

Figure 9-42C. AP view, two years postoperative.

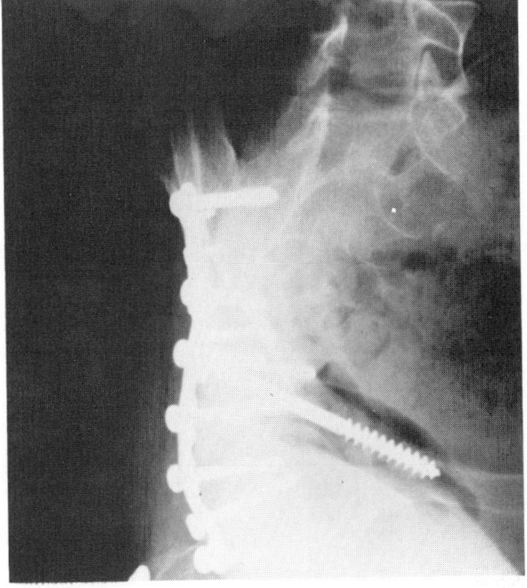

Figure 9-42D. Late obturator oblique view.

## Stabilization with Supplementary Bone Graft

With a wide variety of comminuted acetabular fractures, especially in the presence of osteoporosis and in late reconstruction, the use of autologous bone graft is needed to buttress articular fragments. For a posterior wall or column injury with marginal impaction, the anatomically reduced impacted fragment requires a

Figure 9-43. A high posterior and low anterior "T" fracture, with the use of a cannulated screw for the anterior column repair. Intraoperative use of an image intensifier permits accurate alignment of a guidewire in the anterior column as a cannula for the screw. A: Initial AP view. B: Anterior 3D computed scan of posterior "T" fracture. C: Inner iliac oblique view with posterior column displacement. D: Outer iliac oblique view with supplementary posterior wall fragment. E: Computed scan with central displacement. F: Intraoperative view with position of guidewire in anterior column. G: Late AP view at 18 months. H: Late obturator oblique view.

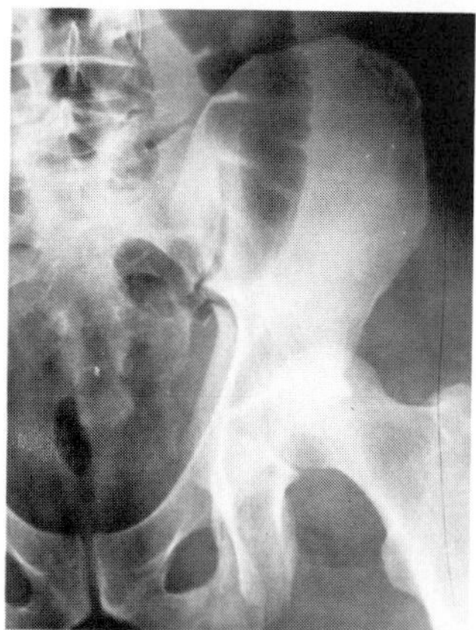
Figure 9-43A.

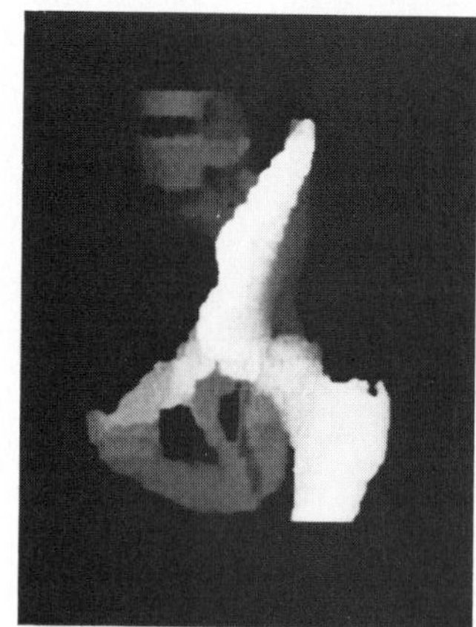
Figure 9-43B.

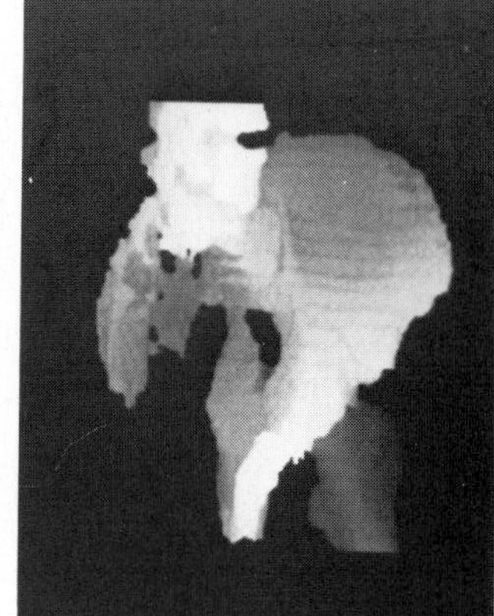
Figure 9-43C.

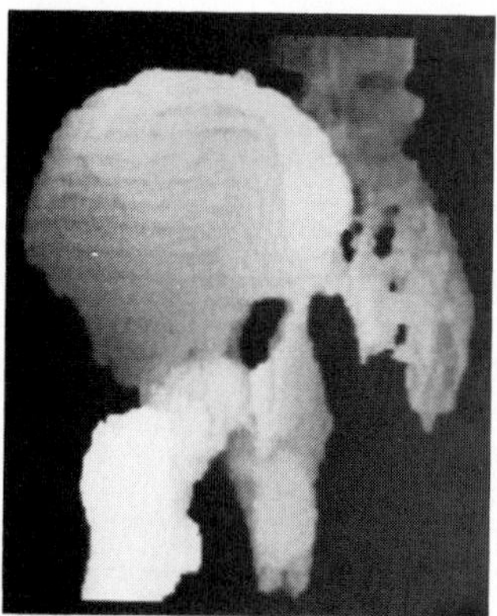
Figure 9-43D.

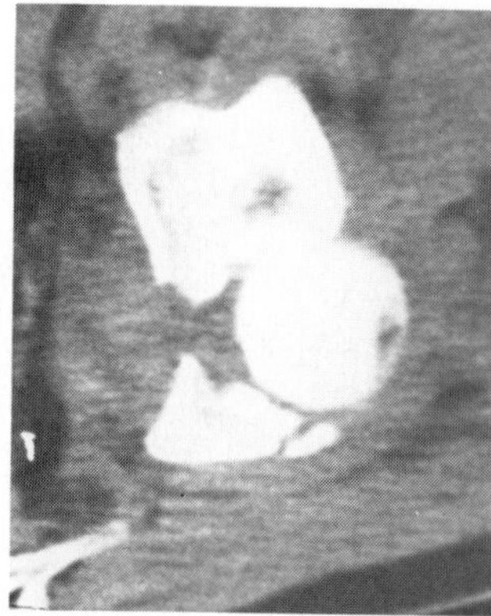
Figure 9-43E.

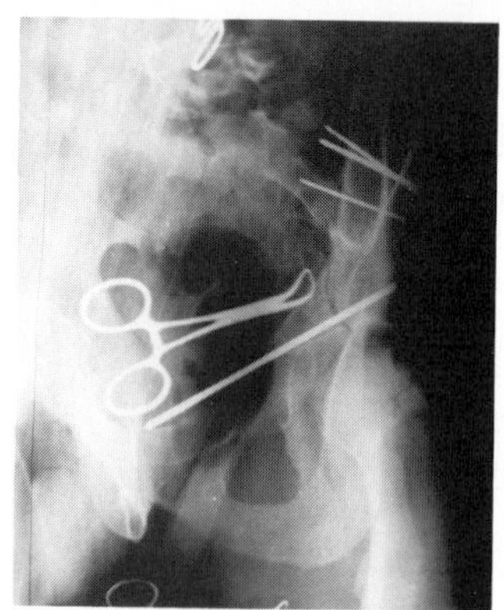
Figure 9-43F.

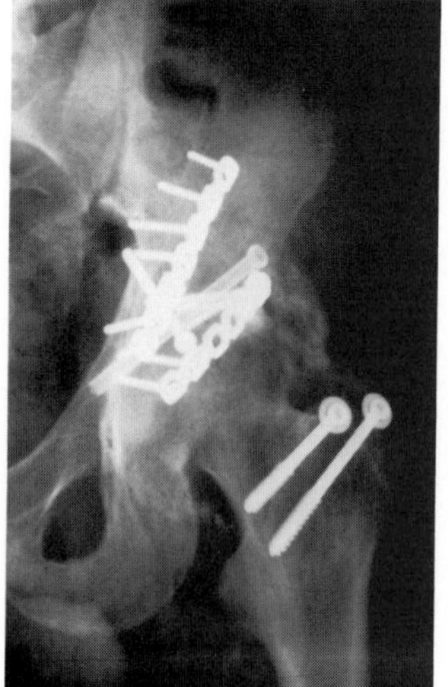
Figure 9-43G.

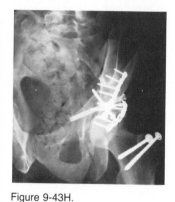

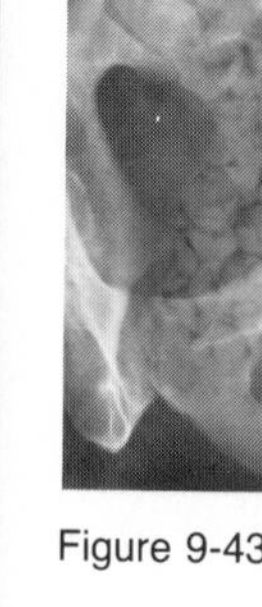
Figure 9-43H.

Figure 9-44. A highly comminuted "T" fracture with associated subluxation of the sacroiliac joint and ramus fractures. A: Initial AP view. B: Inlet view. C: Late AP view at two years. D: Late inlet view with highly symmetrical pelvic ring.

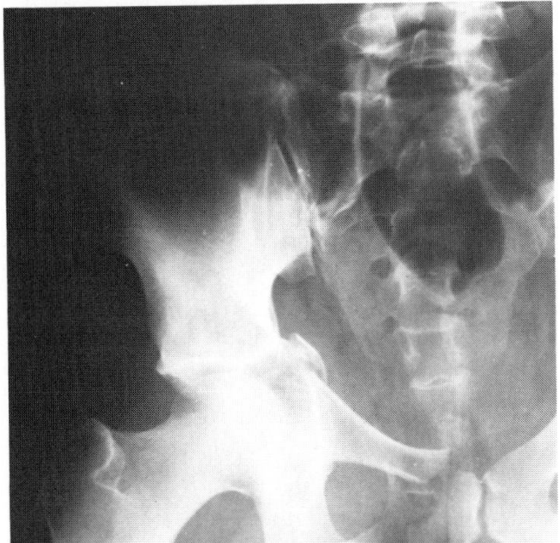

Figure 9-44A.

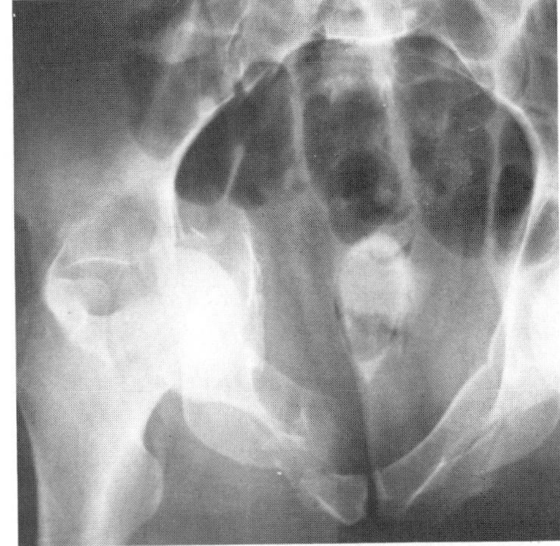

Figure 9-44B.

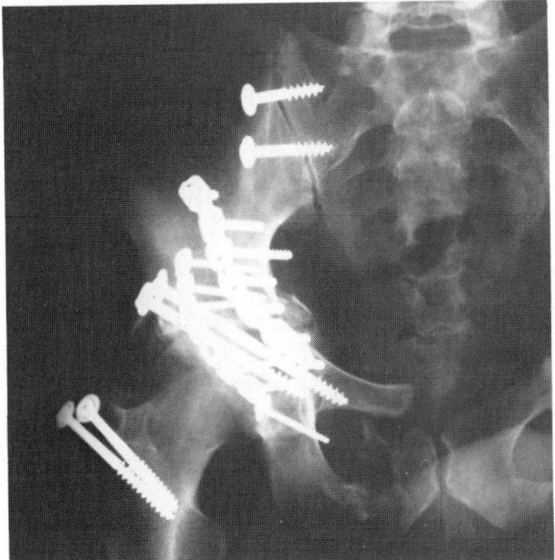

Figure 9-44C.

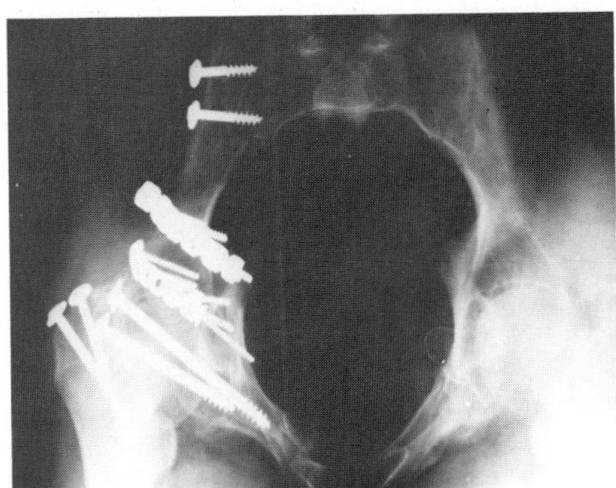

Figure 9-44D.

supportive bony bed to prevent a late subsidence with recurrent deformity. Many "T" and both-column fractures undergo comminution of the dome-region where the several fracture lines intersect. The dome fragments undergo a central migration with impaction of the cancellous bone between the inner table and the articular surface. In these and other cases, cancellous and corticocancellous bone graft is harvested and applied to the defect. The graft and supplementary articular fragments are impacted carefully so that they are unlikely to be dislodged after the femoral head has been reduced. Frequently, an area of regional impaction of the femoral head provoked by its forceful impaction against the

Figure 9-45. The general principles of stabilization of an anterior column with associated posterior hemitransverse fracture. Usually, supplementary lag screws are necessary. A: For a fracture with primarily posterior column displacement exposed from a lateral or posterior approach. B: For a variant with anterior column displacement visualized with an ilioinguinal exposure.

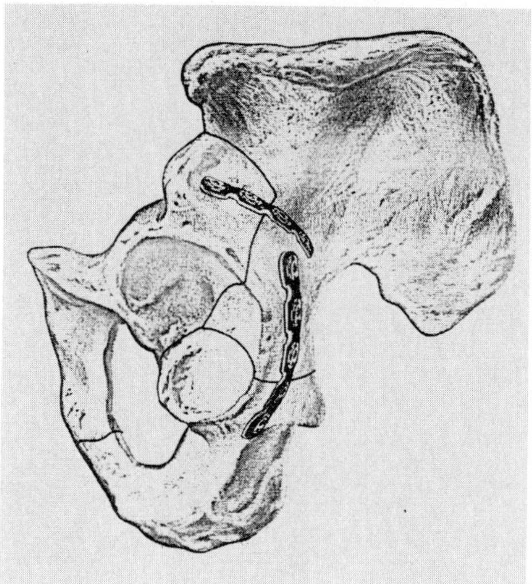

Figure 9-45A.

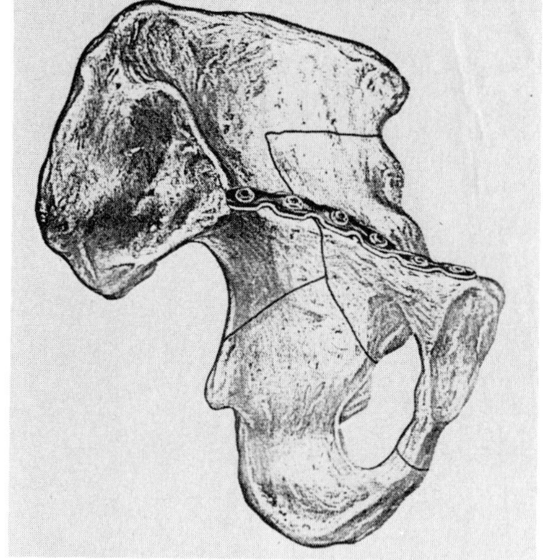

Figure 9-45B.

acetabulum is observed. Elevation of the articular cartilage by the application of cancellous bone graft to the subchondral defect permits a restoration of the normal curvature of the femoral head.

## References


1. Sawaguchi T, Brown TD, Rubash HE, Mears DC: Stability of acetabular fractures after internal fixation. Acta Orthop Scand 55:601, 1984.
2. Rubash HE, Mears DC: External fixation of the pelvis, in: AAOS Instructional Course Lectures. St. Louis, Mosby, 32:329, 1983.
3. Matta JM: The use of a computed scan to monitor sacral lag screw fixation, in Letournel E (ed): Fractures of the Acetabulum and Pelvis, Second Course. Paris, May 6-10, 1985.
4. Mears DC, Rubash HE: External and internal fixation of the pelvic ring, in: AAOS Instructional Course Lectures. St. Louis, Mosby, 33:144, 1984.
5. Tile M: Fractures of the Pelvis and Acetabulum. Baltimore, Williams and Wilkins, 1984, p 144.
6. Letournel E, Judet R: Fractures of the Acetabulum. New York, Springer-Verlag, 1981, p 33.

Figure 9-46. An anterior column with associated posterior hemitransverse fracture, with moderate anterior and minimal posterior displacements. An ilioinguinal incision was used to approach the fracture.

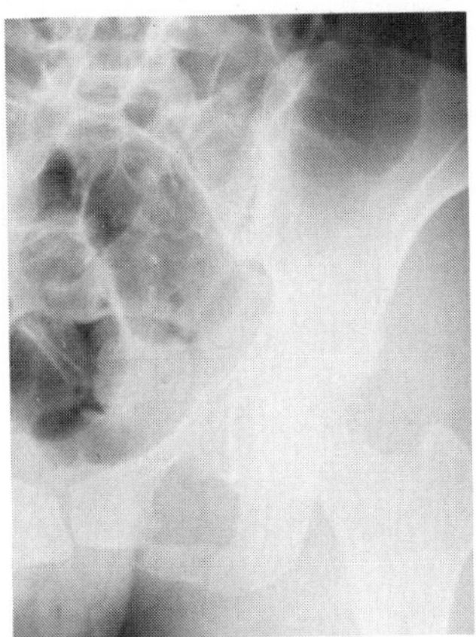

Figure 9-46A. Initial AP view.

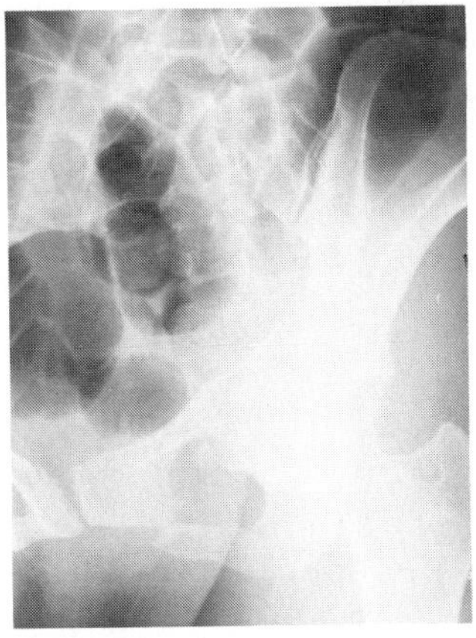

Figure 9-46B. Initial obturator oblique view.

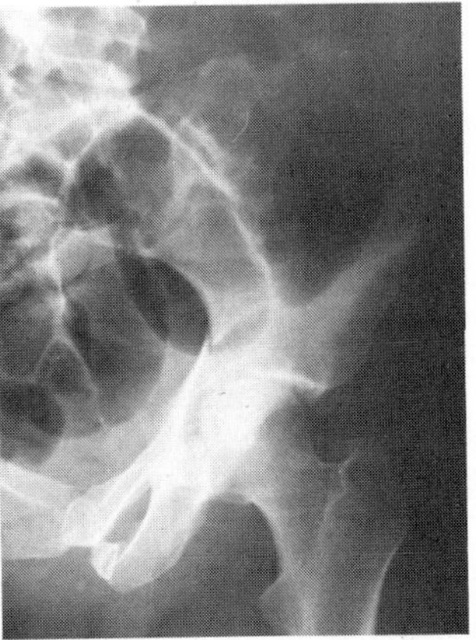

Figure 9-46C. Initial iliac oblique view.

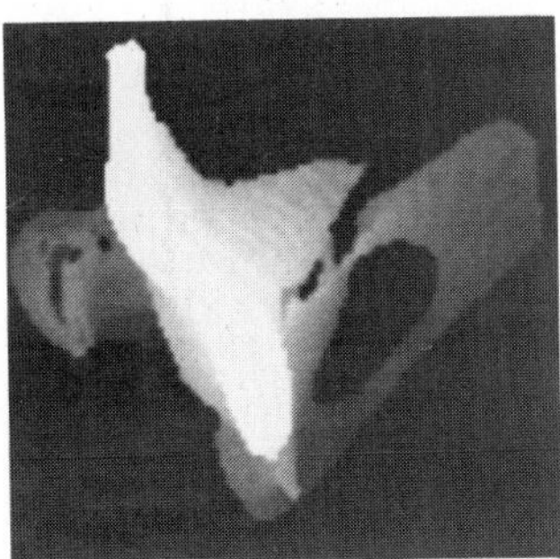

Figure 9-46D. 3D scan, superior view.

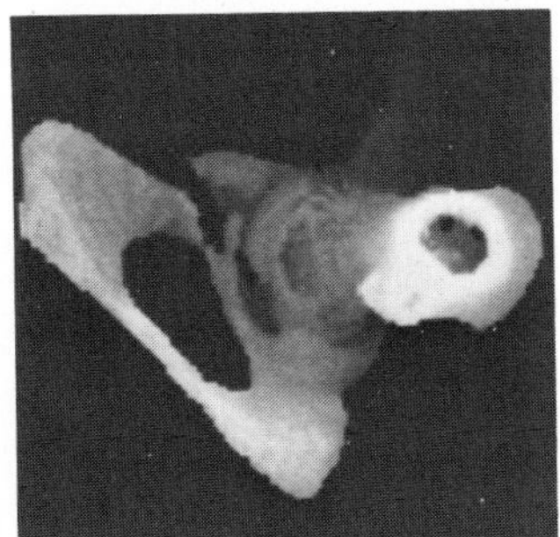

Figure 9-46E. 3D scan, inferior view.

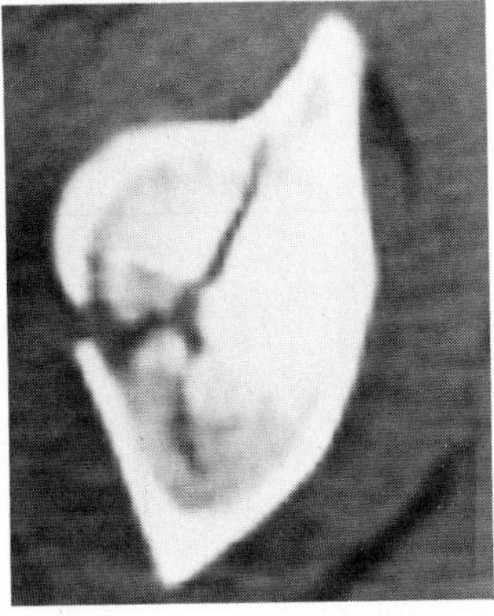

Figure 9-46F. Computed scan through dome.

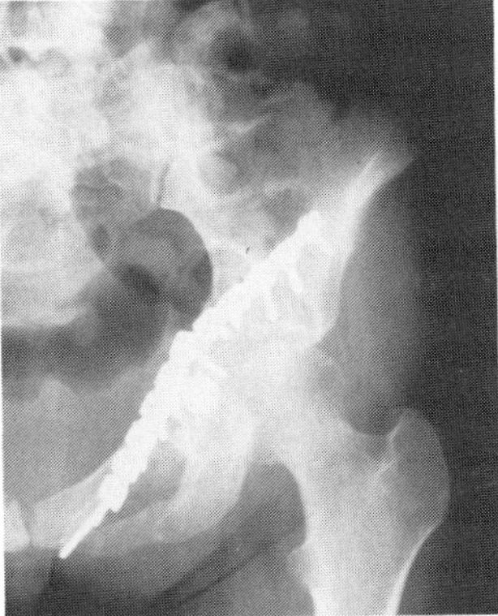

Figure 9-46G. Postoperative AP view.

Figure 9-47. Diagrams of the typical stabilization of a both-column fracture with primarily anterior displacement by the use of an ilioinguinal approach. A (i, ii): For a fracture with anterior iliac involvement where the fracture exits between the anterior inferior and anterior superior spines or, as evident here, posterior to the anterior superior spine, the iliac portion can be stabilized with a cancellous lag screw and/or plate along the iliac crest. The crucial anterior column plate is positioned along the iliopectineal line. The posterior screws are used to lag the posterior column, or separate lag screws are inserted. B: Where the iliac fracture propagates to the posterior iliac crest, usually with associated comminution, a plate is required along the iliac crest, as seen here, or along the inner aspect of the crest.

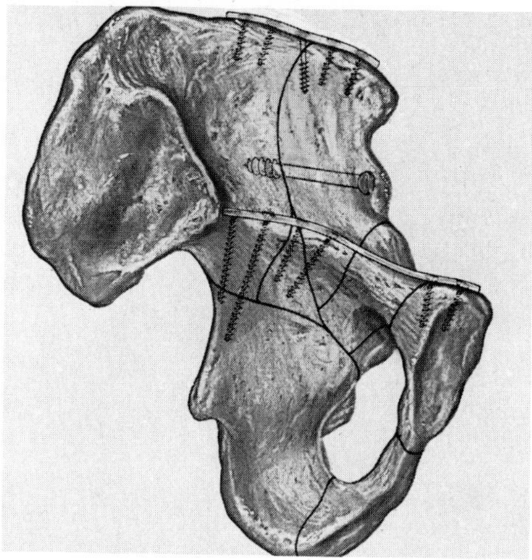

Figure 9-47A i. Inner view.

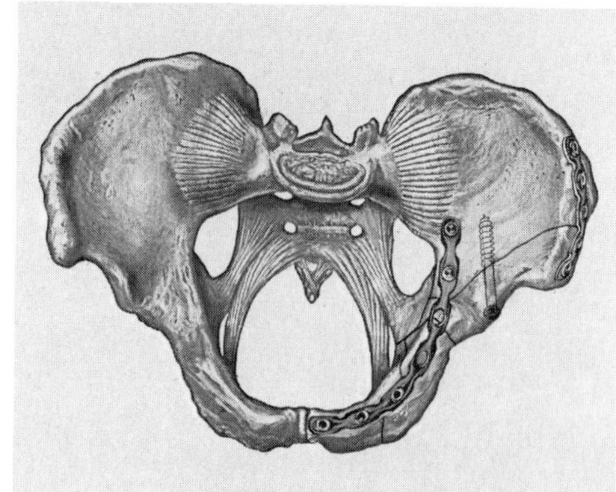

Figure 9-47A ii. Superior view.

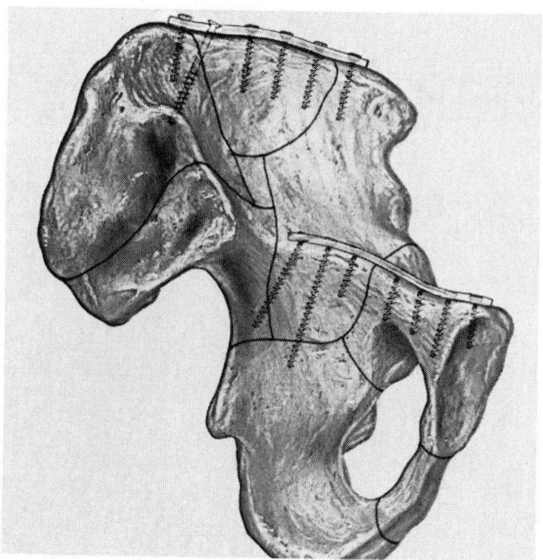

Figure 9-47B.

Figure 9-48. A both-column fracture with primarily anterior column displacement approached by an ilioinguinal incision. A: Initial obturator oblique view. B: Initial iliac oblique view. C: Anterior view, 3D scan. D: Outer iliac oblique view, 3D scan. E: Inner view, 3D scan. F: Superior view, 3D scan. G: Computed scan through quadrilateral surface with primarily anterior involvement. H: Postoperative AP view.

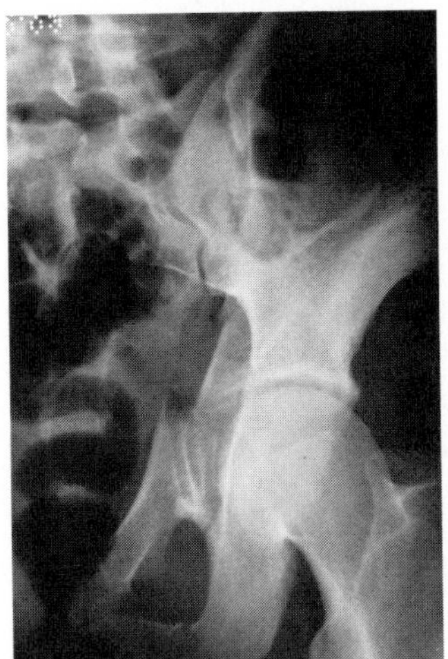

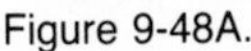

Figure 9-48A.

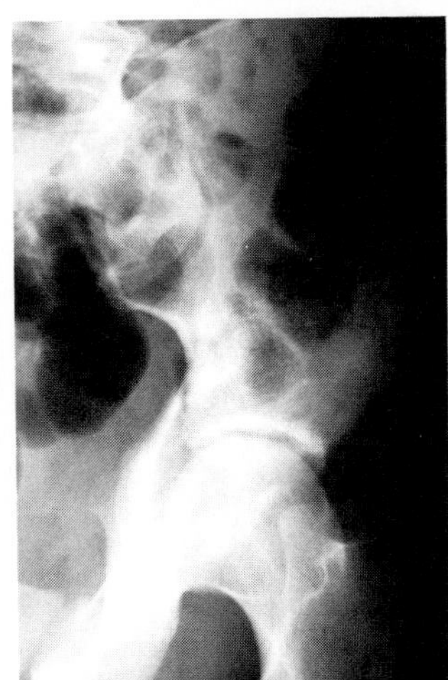

Figure 9-48B.

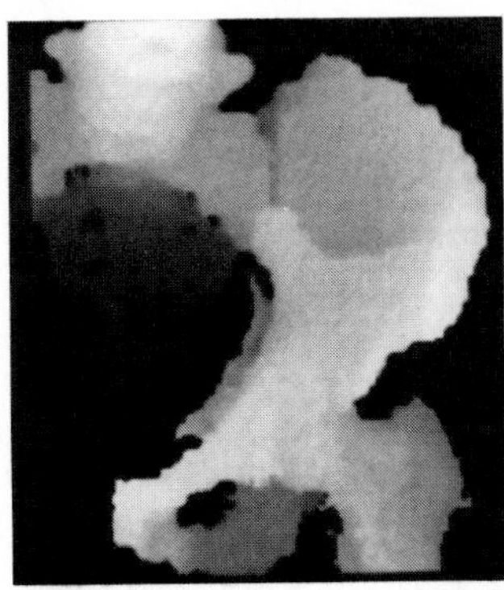

Figure 9-48C.

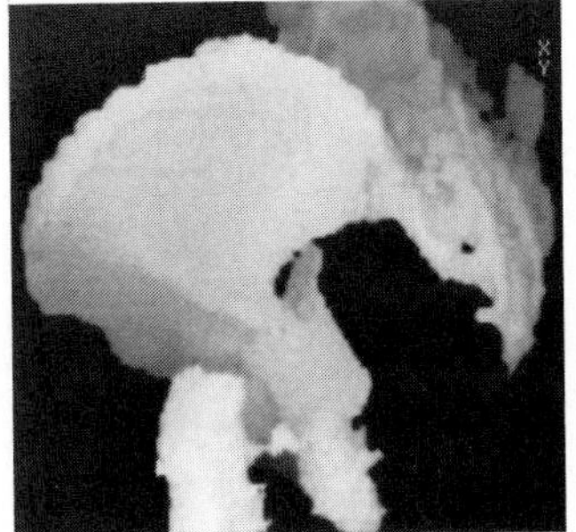

Figure 9-48D.

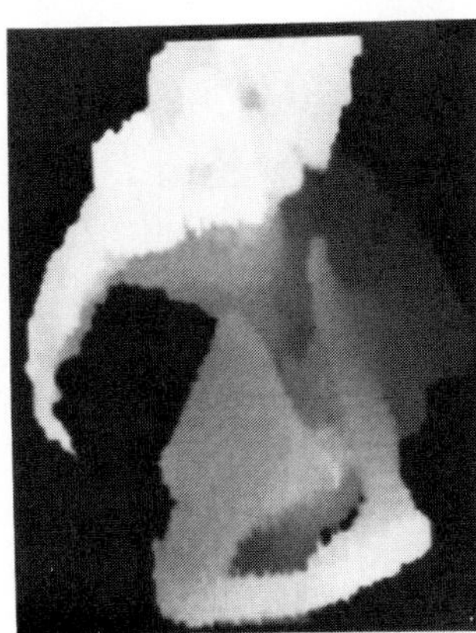

Figure 9-48E.

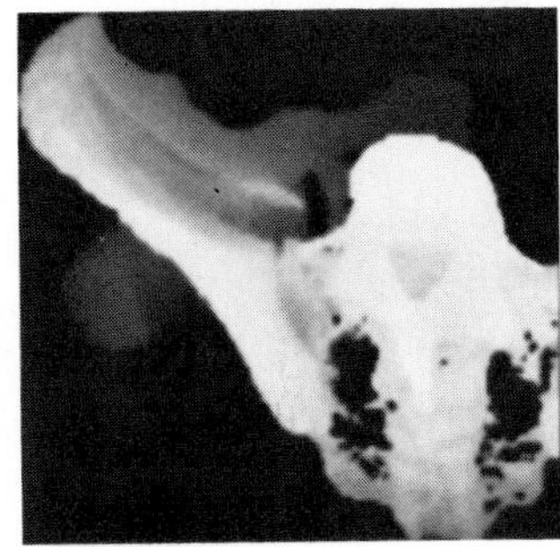

Figure 9-48F.

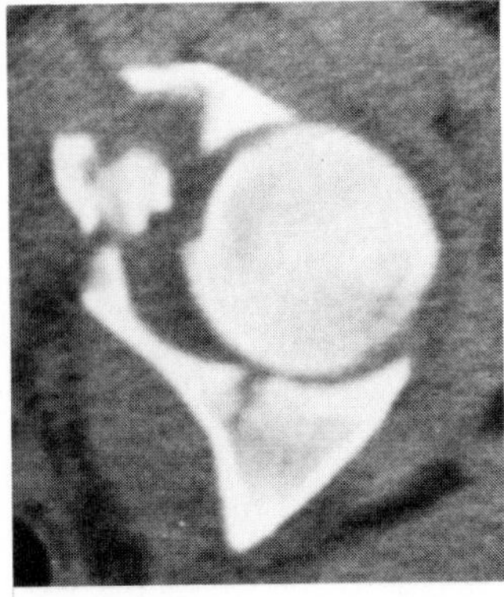

Figure 9-48G.

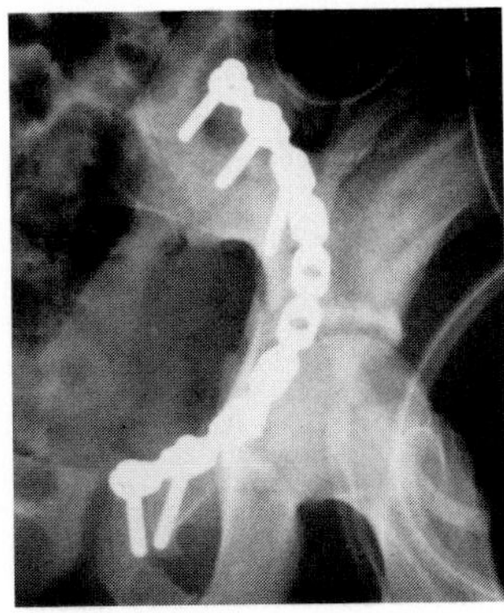

Figure 9-48H.

Figure 9-49. A highly comminuted and displaced both-column fracture with comminution of the ilium, a dislocation of the sacroiliac joint, and involvement of the superior ramus. The sacroiliac joint was immobilized through the ilioinguinal approach by a temporarily augmented displacement of the lateral iliac fracture, so that the screws could be inserted into the outside of the bone. A: Initial AP view. B: Initial inlet view. C: Obturator oblique view. D: Computed scan with iliac and sacroiliac involvement. E: Computed scan with intact posterior wall. F: Postoperative view.

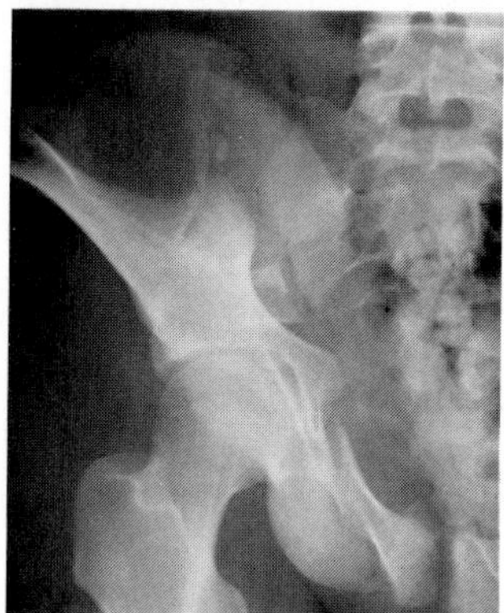

Figure 9-49A.

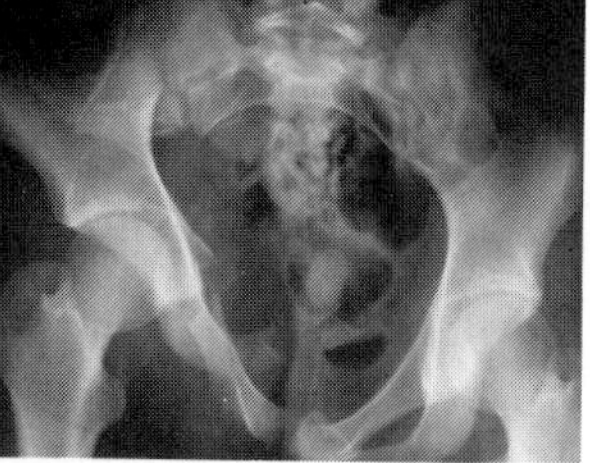

Figure 9-49B.

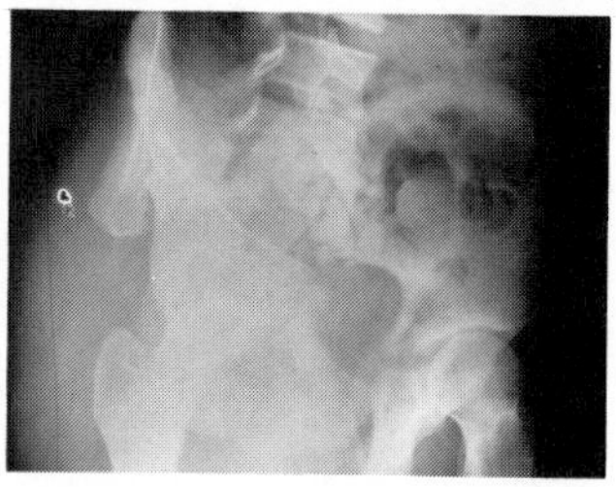

Figure 9-49C.

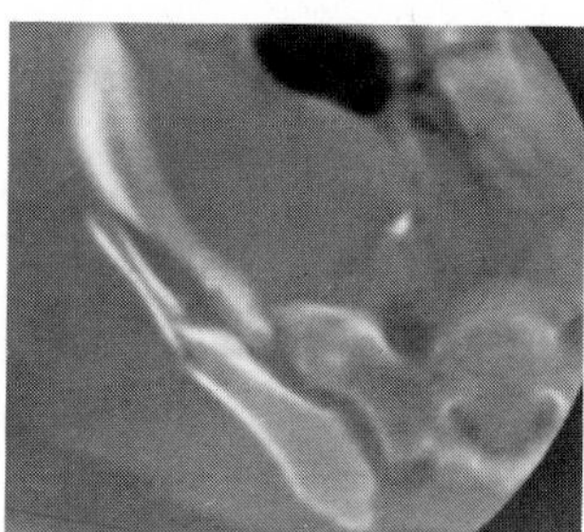

Figure 9-49D.

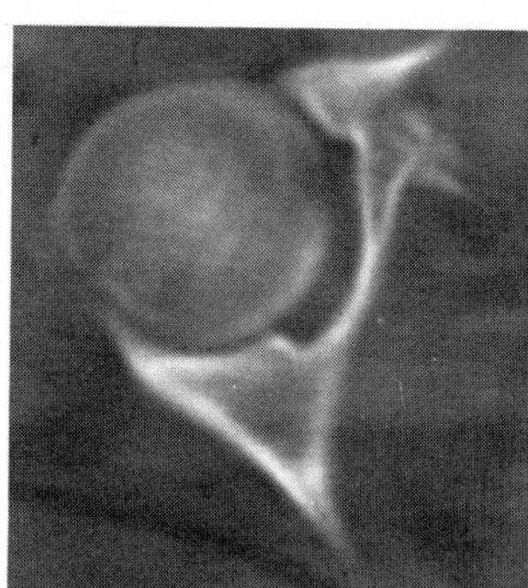

Figure 9-49E.

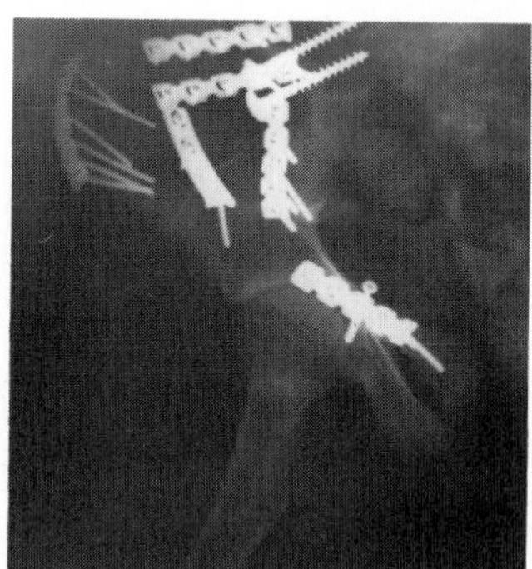

Figure 9-49F.

Figure 9-50. Schematic views of the stabilization of a both-column fracture with an extensile lateral approach. A: Primarily superior involvement of the anterior column is consistent with minimal extraarticular exposure of the anterior column and superior pubic ramus. B: With more extensive lateral comminution iliac plates are needed, along with an anterior column lag screw. C: For segmental involvement of the anterior column with a displacement of the crucial anterior wall portion, the anterior iliac fragment is displaced so that it hinges from the anterior inferior spine. A lag screw is inserted across the base of the acetabulum.

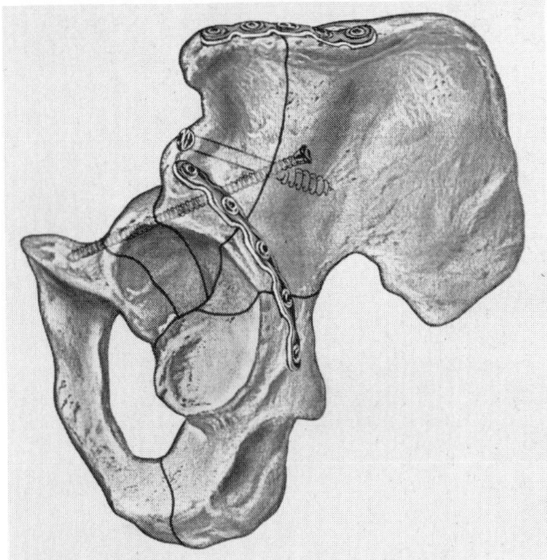

Figure 9-50A.

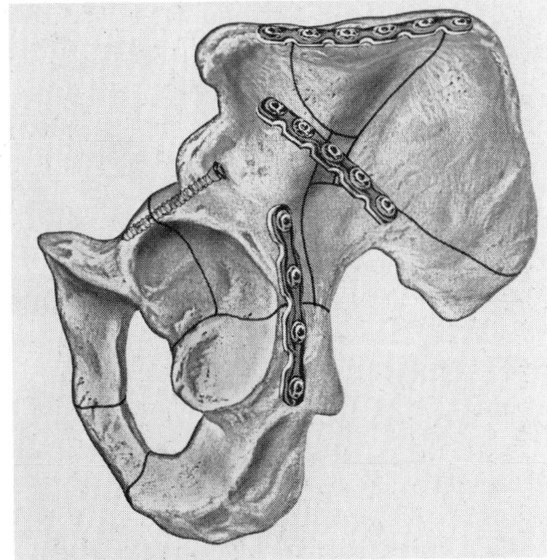

Figure 9-50B.

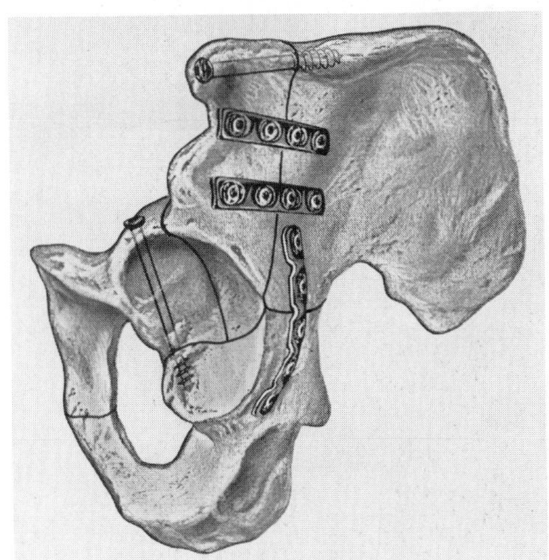

Figure 9-50C.

Figure 9-51. A both-column fracture with comminution of the anterior column. After careful review of the computed scans, the extraarticular nature of the anterior column involvement permits definition of the operative procedure. The extraarticular fragments are ignored, which greatly reduces the operative exposure, with concentration of the reduction on the highly displaced posterior column. A: Initial 3D scan, posterior view. B: Initial 3D scan, lateral view. C: Initial 3D scan, anterior-inferior view. D: Computed scan with minimal anterior column involvement of the articular surface. E: Postoperative AP view. F: Postoperative inlet view.

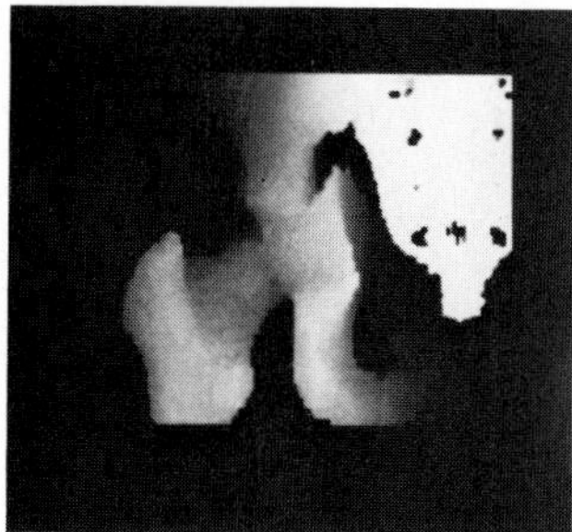

Figure 9-51A.

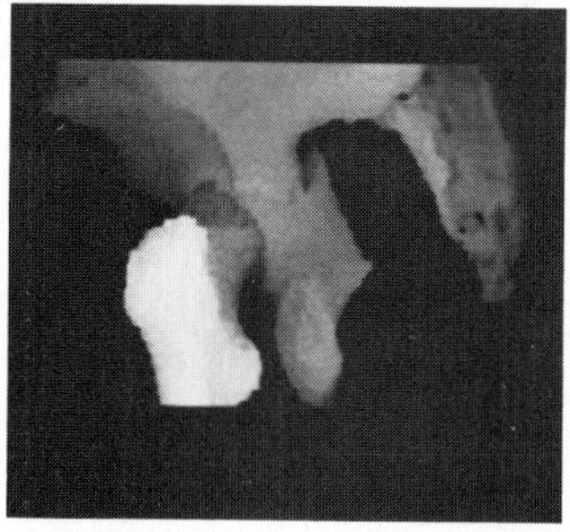

Figure 9-51B.

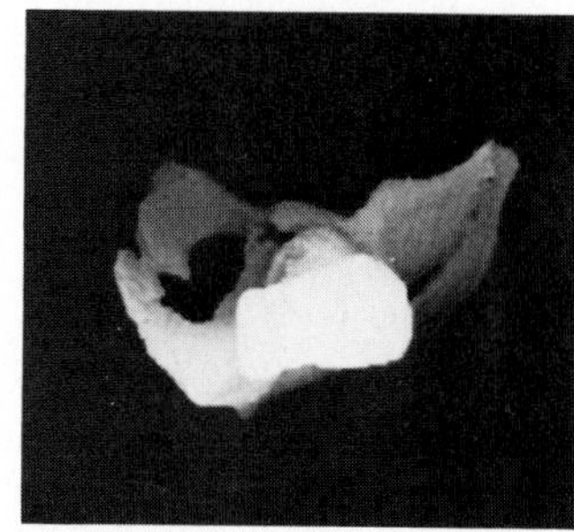

Figure 9-51C.

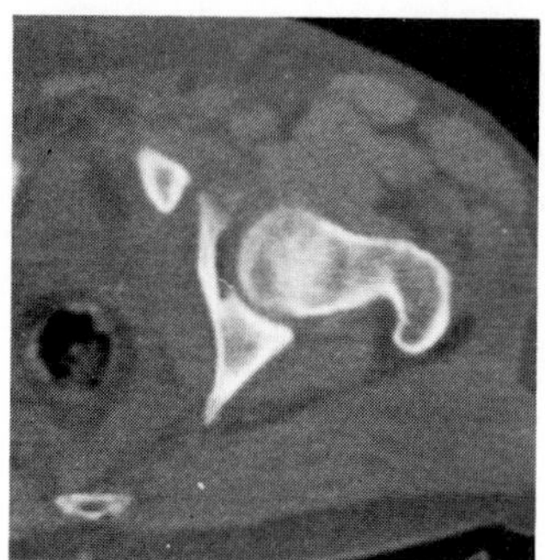

Figure 9-51D.

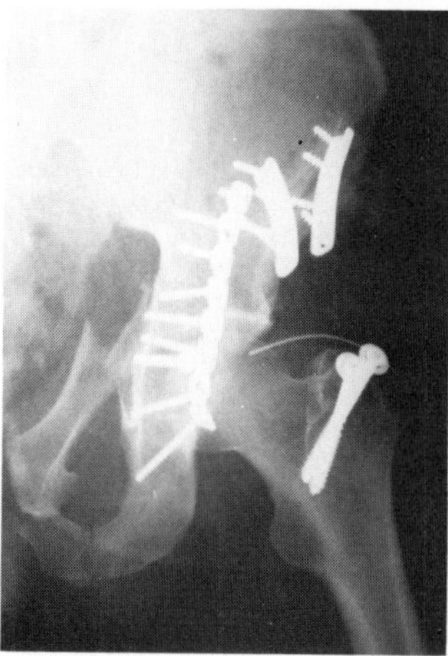

Figure 9-51E.

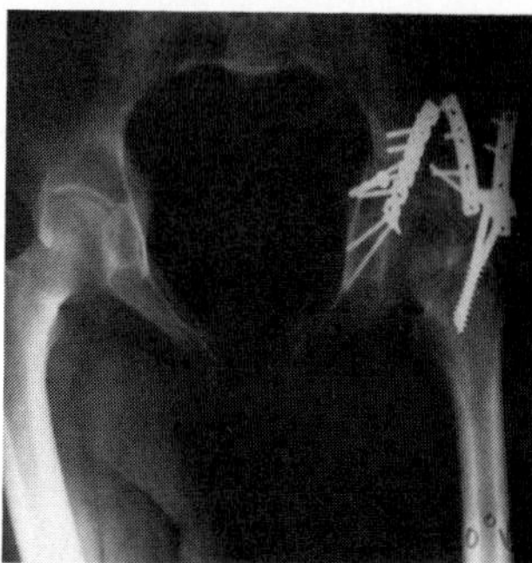

Figure 9-51F.

Figure 9-52. A highly comminuted both-column fracture with marked posterior column displacement and iliac comminution. A triradiate exposure permits an accurate anatomical reconstruction. A: Initial AP view. B: 3D scan, inner view. C: 3D scan, superior view. D: AP view, two months postoperative. E: Late obturator oblique view. F: Late iliac oblique view.

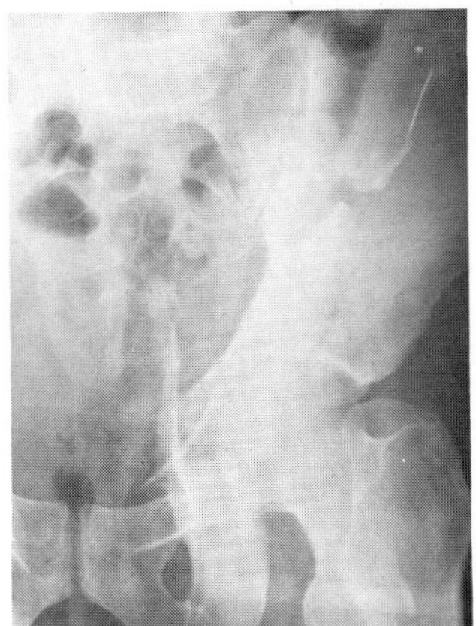

Figure 9-52A.

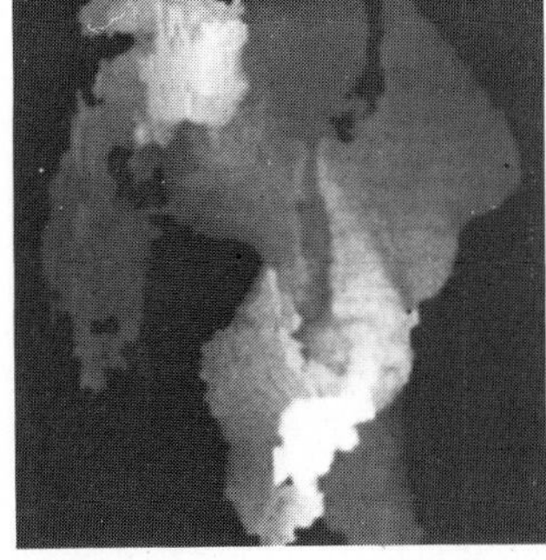

Figure 9-52B.

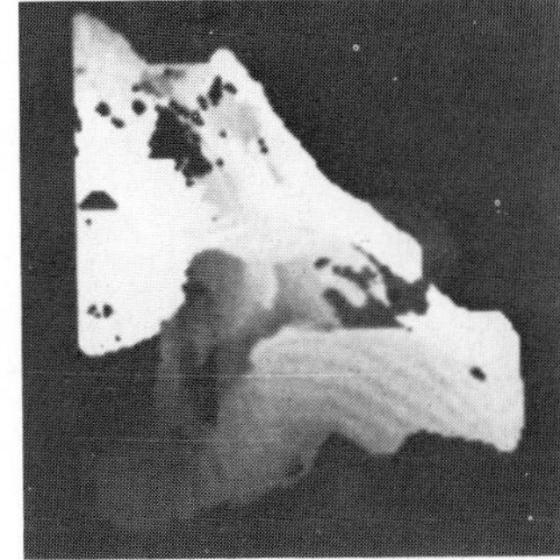

Figure 9-52C.

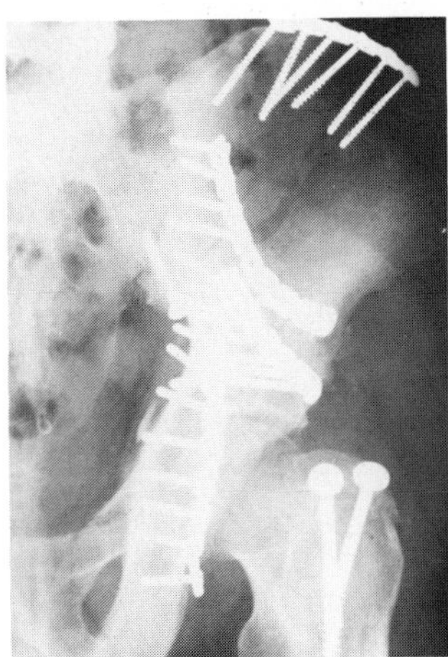

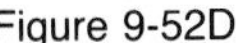

Figure 9-52D.

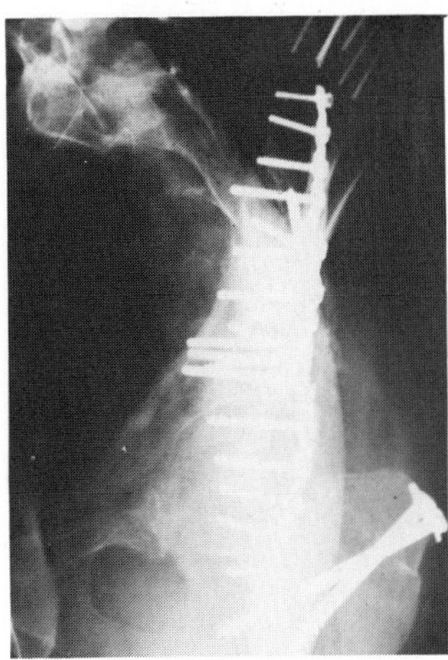

Figure 9-52E.

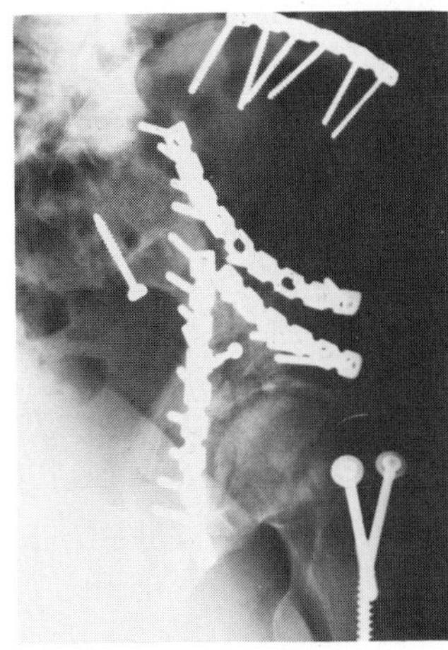

Figure 9-52F.

Figure 9-53. A highly comminuted both-column fracture with a segmental anterior column involvement. Through a triradiate approach, the anterior iliac crest fragment is hinged inwards on the rectus femoris to permit a reduction of the inferior half of the acetabulum. A 4.0mm cancellous lag screw secures the two lower fragments, then the reduction of the inferior half to the superior half of the innominate bone is completed and stabilized. A: Initial AP view. B: Inlet view. C: Obturator oblique view. D: 3D scan, anterior view. E: 3D scan, outer iliac oblique view. F: 3D scan, inner view. G: 3D scan, superior view, with marked protrusio. H: AP view, one year postoperative.

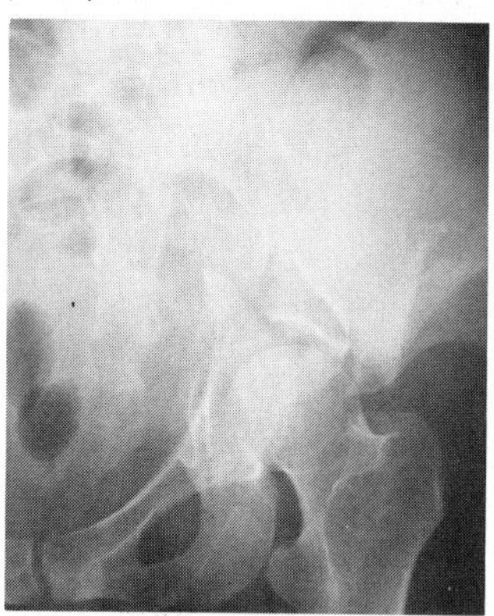

Figure 9-53A.

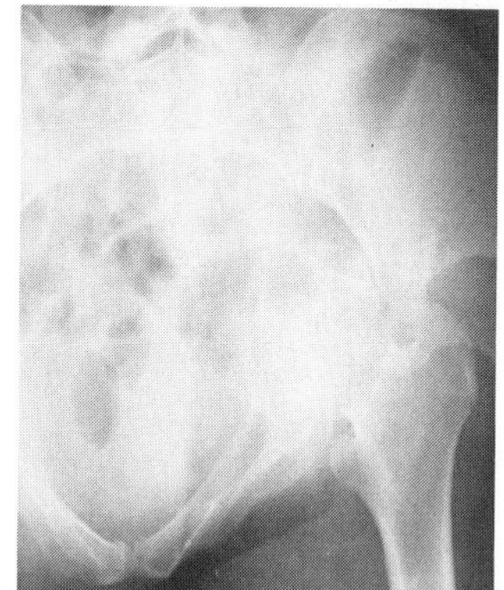

Figure 9-53B.

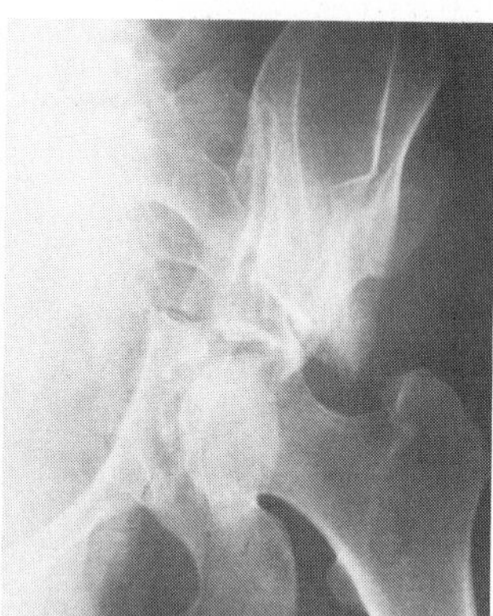

Figure 9-53C.

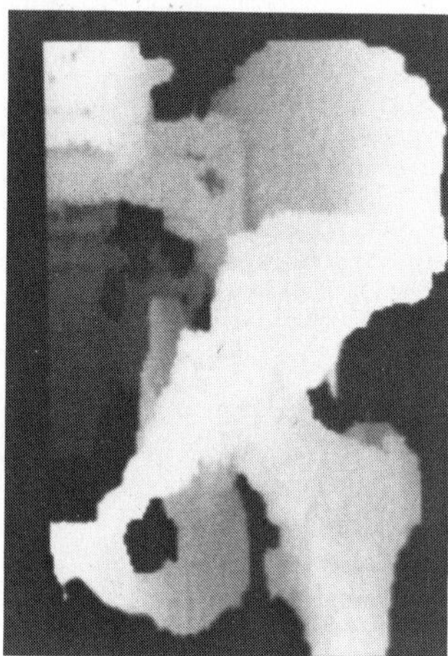

Figure 9-53D.

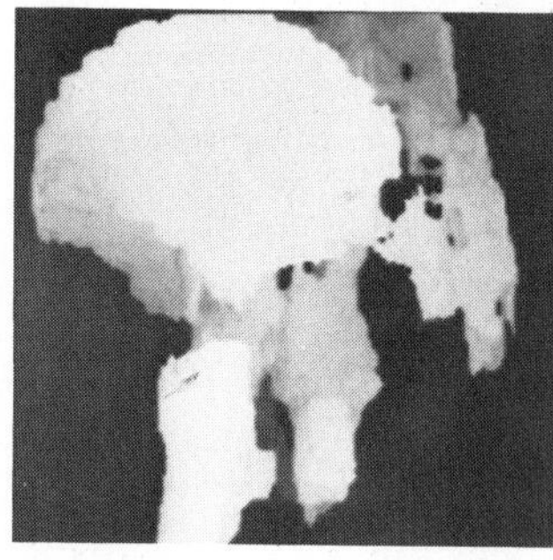

Figure 9-53E.

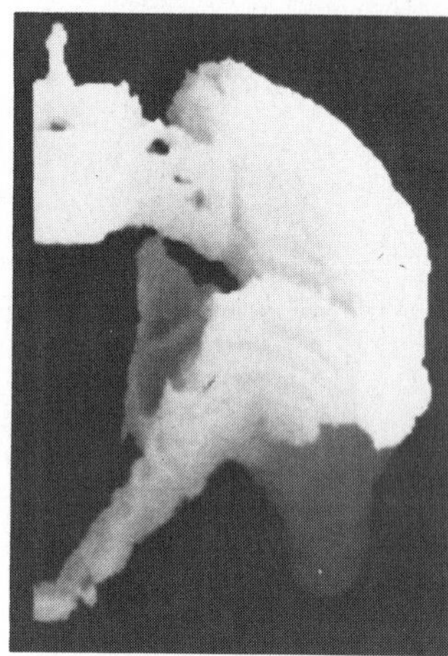

Figure 9-53F.

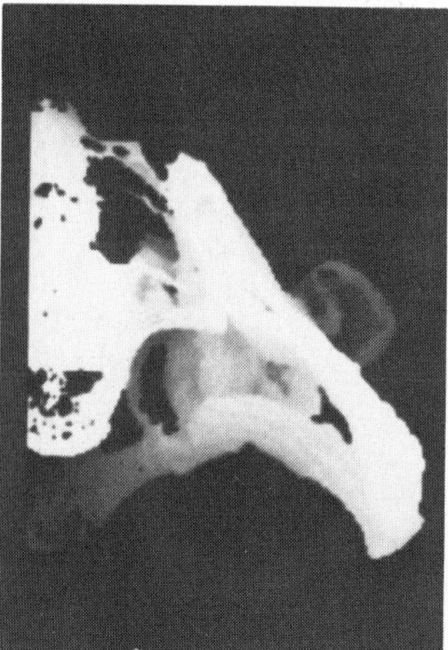

Figure 9-53G.

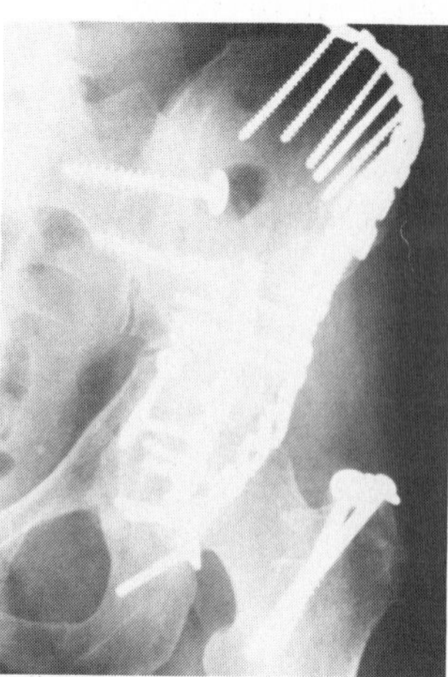

Figure 9-53H.

Figure 9-54. A highly displaced both-column fracture in an obese woman of 250 pounds illustrates an excellent reduction, particularly evident in the postoperative inlet view. A: Initial anterior 3D scan. B: Initial posterior 3D scan. C: 3D scan, superior view. D: 3D scan, inner view. E: Postoperative AP view at one year; a tension band wire supplemented the lag screw fixation of the greater trochanter. F: Late postoperative inlet view. G: Late iliac oblique view. H: Late obturator oblique view.

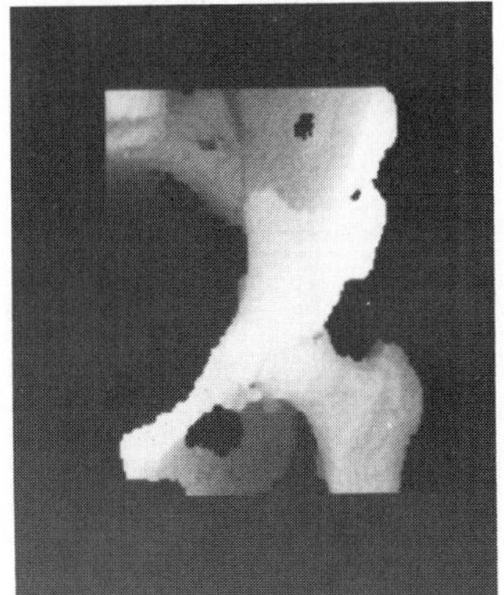

Figure 9-54A.

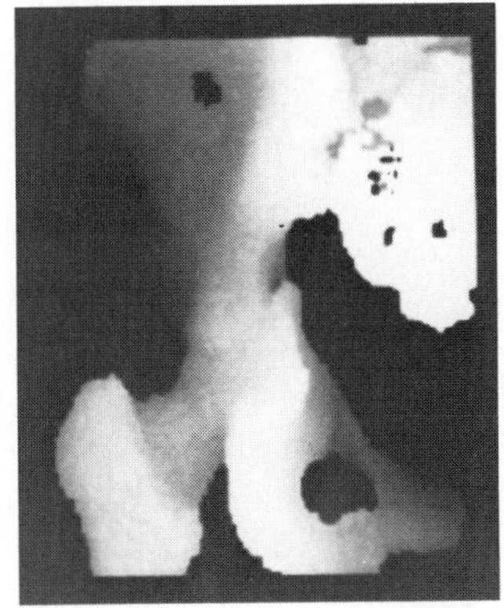

Figure 9-54B.

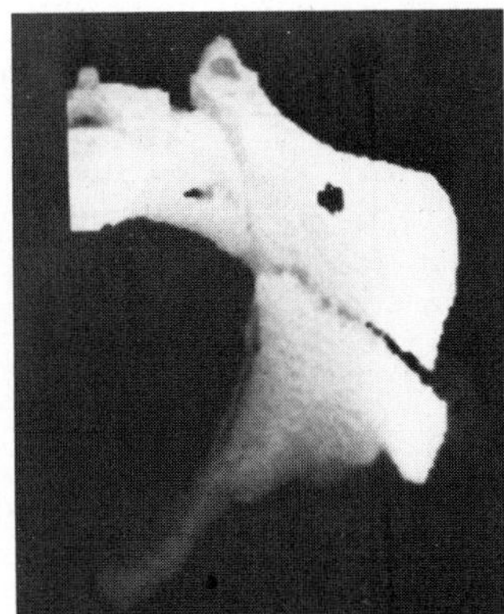

Figure 9-54C.

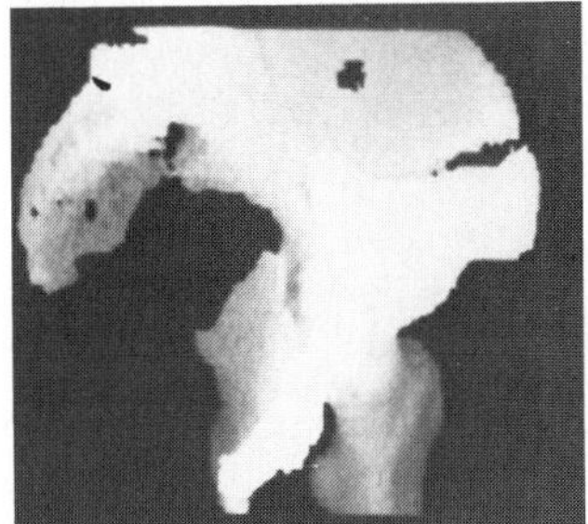

Figure 9-54D.

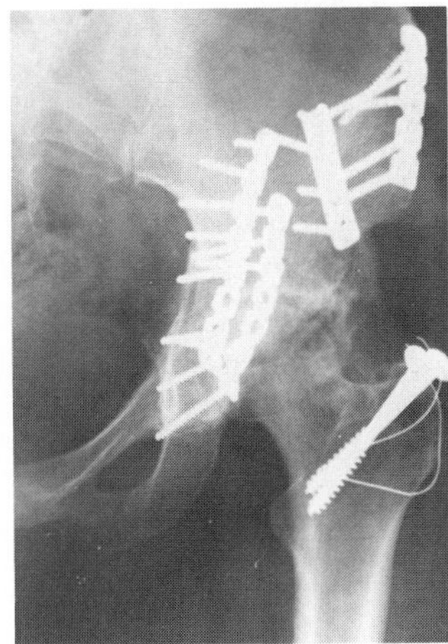

Figure 9-54E.

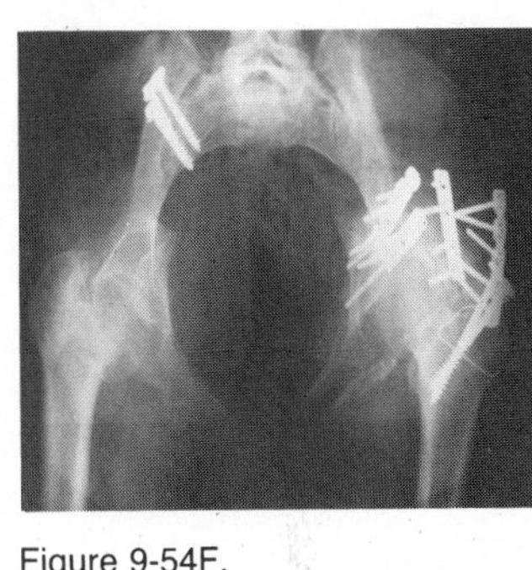

Figure 9-54F.

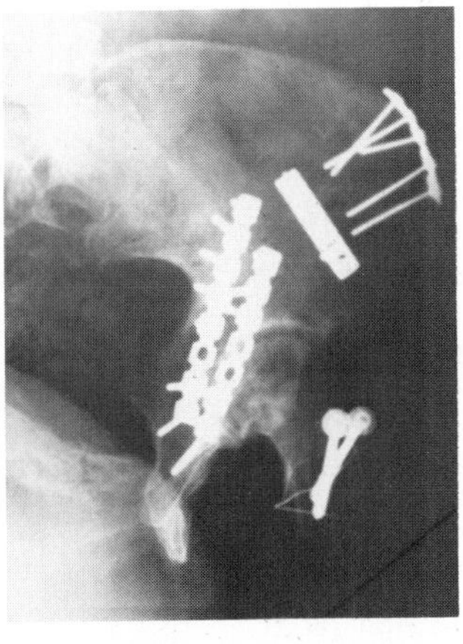

Figure 9-54G.

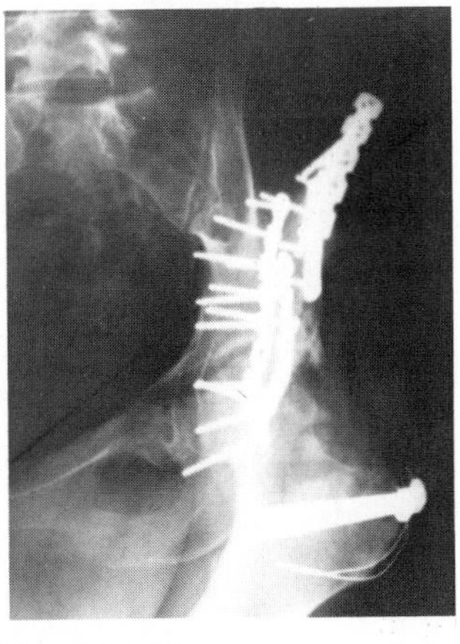

Figure 9-54H.

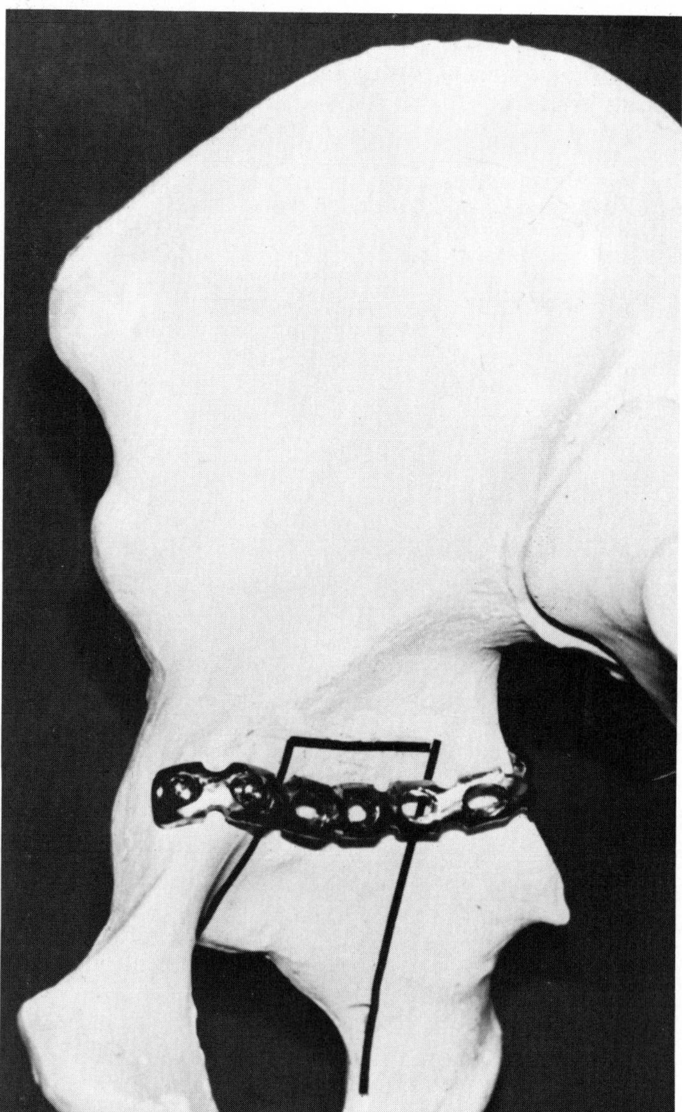

Figure 9-55. Stabilization of a large displaced fragment of quadrilateral surface is achieved with a 3.5mm reconstruction plate that is anchored from the anterior column to the posterior column. To expose this region, an extended lateral approach such as a triradiate incision is necessary.

# CHAPTER 10

# Techniques of External Fixation

In different clinics, various designs of pelvic frames are employed to stabilize a pelvic ring disruption. From a scrutiny of the mechanical attributes of the frames, the designs can be characterized as simple or complex.[1-5] The former design is used to immobilize a stable pelvic ring disruption or an unstable one when the application of supplementary internal fixation is planned. A complex frame is applied for the immobilization of an unstable pelvic ring disruption with a single site of posterior instability. While it can be used in conjunction with internal fixation to immobilize a bilateral posterior unstable injury, generally in such a case a simple frame is applied initially to the hemodynamically unstable patient and supplementary internal fixation is undertaken at a later date. In this chapter, guidelines for the selection of an appropriate frame are briefly reviewed. Techniques for the assembly of representative examples of simple and complex frames are presented.

## Preoperative Planning

At the time of presentation of the patient in the emergency room, the degree of hemodynamic instability, along with the identification of other potentially urgent surgical emergencies, provides guidelines for the acute application of the external pelvic frame. In the unstable clinical situation a single anteroposterior pelvic radiograph is reviewed in the emergency room; whenever possible, in the stable clinical situation supplementary pelvic inlet and outlet views and ideally a pelvic computed scan are scrutinized. By a combination of the clinical examination and the supplementary diagnostic studies, the appropriate type of frame is selected. While theoretically a simple frame can be converted to a complex design, in practice this modification is discouraged in view of the risk of wound infection when the second set of fixation pins is inserted into the anterior inferior spines. If the simple frame does not provide adequate stability, then supplementary immobilization is achieved by the application of an appropriate technique of internal fixation.

In the presence of an open pelvic disruption where a diversion colostomy is undertaken under the same general anesthetic as employed for external pelvic fixation, the general surgeons are advised to create the diversion colostomy in an upper abdominal quadrant to increase the space between the colostomy and the fixation pins.

## Application of a Simple Frame

The procedure is performed with the patient supine on the operating table. Ideally a pelvic deformity is corrected prior to the preparation of the cutaneous incisions necessary for insertion of the fixation pins. In clinical practice the pins provide a means to obtain the optimal mechanical advantage for the reduction. Also, the diastasis is optimally corrected with the patient in a lateral position. Realistically, the only correction of a deformity that can be achieved prior to the insertion of the fixation pins is a superior migration of a hemipelvis. In such a case, the procedure is undertaken on a fracture table to permit distraction of the relevant hemipelvis. Distraction can also be achieved by the use of a distal femoral or proximal tibial traction pin. Bilateral incisions are made along the anterior iliac crests for a length of 4cm to 5cm. The lateral femoral cutaneous nerve of the thigh is carefully protected. When a diastasis of the symphysis pubis exists, the incisions are made 2cm to 3cm medial to the iliac crests to avoid cutaneous tension after the pelvic ring has been reduced. The incision is extended to the subperiosteal plane. The periosteum is elevated on the inner or outer wall of the pelvis. Pilot holes are prepared with a 3.2mm drill bit and a 4.5mm tap. The holes are positioned 2.5 or 5cm apart with an orientation parallel to a line that extends from the anterior superior to the anterior inferior spine. Two 5mm half-pins of 180mm in length are inserted into the drill holes in either iliac crest (Figure 10-1). After irrigation of each wound, the fascia is repaired and the subcutaneous and cutaneous layers are loosely approximated. Dry dressings are applied to the pin sites.

To begin the assembly of a simple frame, a single universal ball joint is attached to each cluster of half-pins. Each ball joint is oriented with the wing nut positioned outside and caudad. A 100mm connecting rod is inserted into either ball joint so that it protrudes in an anterior direction with a modest medial displacement of its anterior end. Two articulation couplings are applied to the anterior ends of either connecting rod. Two other connecting rods of appropriate length are used to bridge from one hemipelvis to the other. The articulation couplings are loosely tightened. The patient is turned to a full lateral decubitus position so that the inferior half frame projects beyond the operating table. An appropriate closed reduction of the pelvis is undertaken by manual manipulation. The articulation couplings are loosened prior to the reduction. The 100mm connecting rods are grasped and manipulated to approximate the hemipelves and thereby obliterate a diastasis. Also, rotational manipulation of a displaced hemipelvis is undertaken. After the articulation couplings are tightened, the reduction is checked with intraoperative or postoperative radiographs, depending upon the urgency of other therapeutic measures (Figure 10-2).

For the typical frame, two connecting bars are used to bridge from one hemipelvis to the other so that either bar can be loosened without a loss of the reduction (Figures 10-3 and 10-4). Especially in an obese patient, inadvertently the frame may be assembled too close to the anterior abdominal wall. While this technical error is not evident in the operating room with the patient in the supine position, it is recognized once the patient sits in his bed so that his paunch impinges upon the frame. Also, the application of two connecting bars augments the rotational stability of the assembly. In a particularly lean and small individual who sustains a simple diastasis of less than 3cm, a somewhat simpler construction suffices (Figure 10-1E). A connecting rod of suitable length is loosely secured in either wing nut. A single articulation coupling joins the two connecting rods together at the midline. The diastasis is closed with the patient in a lateral decubitus position.

For the past three years a novel system has been employed to assemble a simple frame. The "Ultra-X" frame (Howmedica, Inc., Rutherford, New Jersey) possesses

Figure 10-1. Assembly of a simple pelvic frame. A: Insertion of the pins. B: Connecting adjacent pins with a ball joint. C: Insertion of 100mm rod into the ball joint. D: The complete frame. E: Modified frame for a small lean individual.

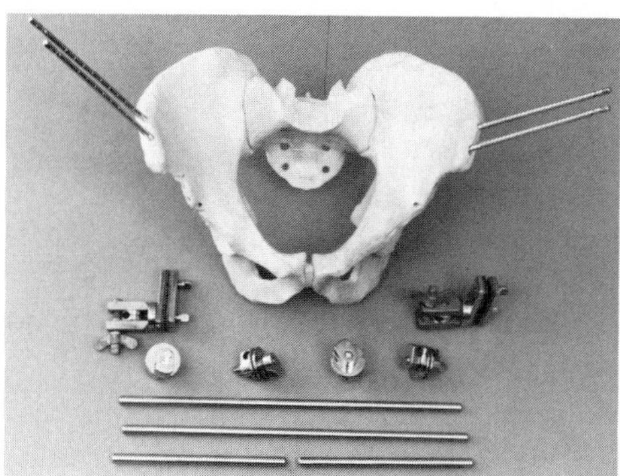

Figure 10-1A.

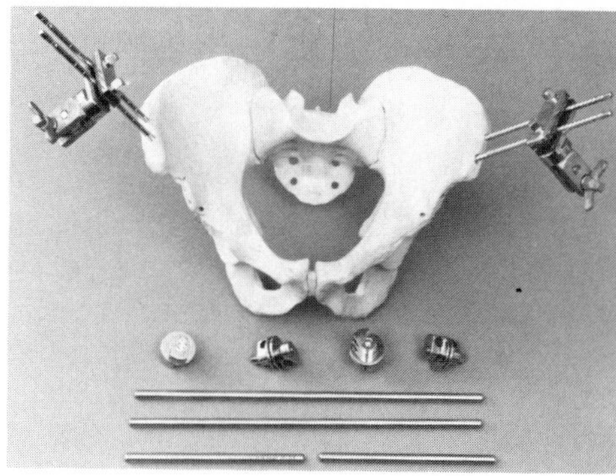

Figure 10-1B.

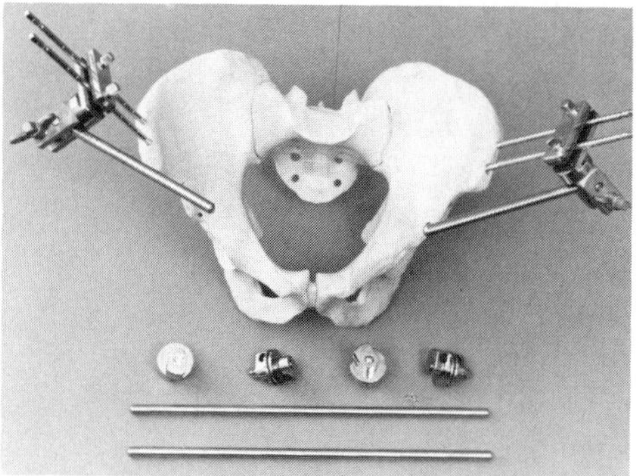

Figure 10-1C.

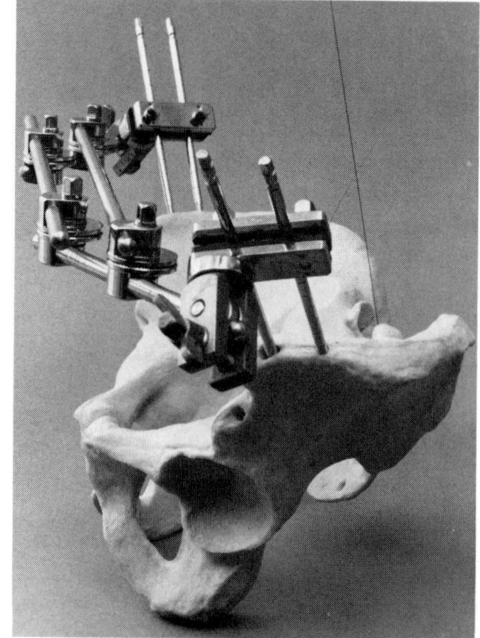

Figure 10-1D.

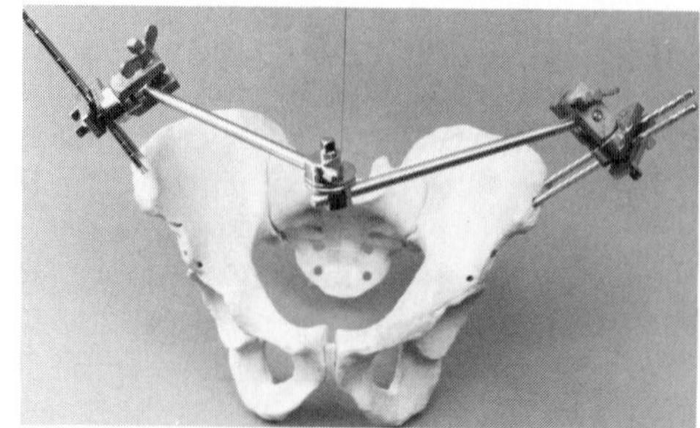

Figure 10-1E.

Figure 10-2. Radiographs and computed scans with typical cases for the use of a simple pelvic frame. A: Anteroposterior view with left ramus fractures and subluxation of the right sacroiliac joint. B: Computed scan of (A) through sacroiliac joints. C: Postoperative view with a simple frame.

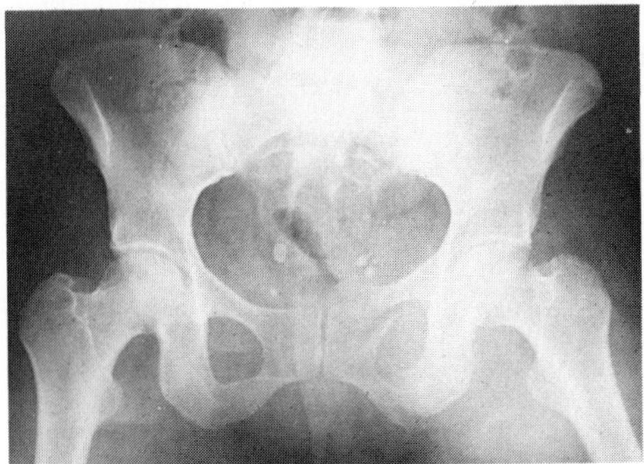

Figure 10-2A.

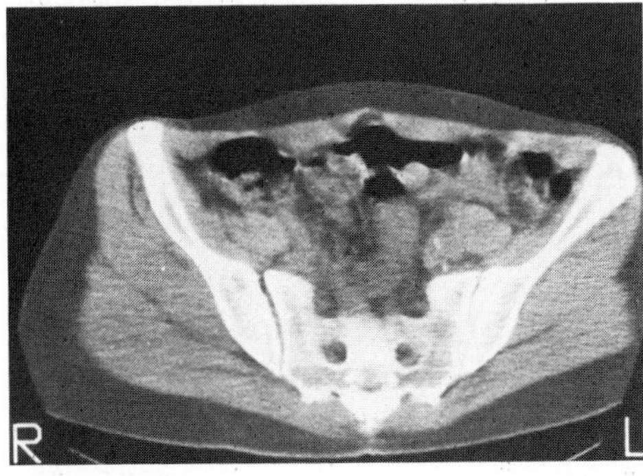


Figure 10-2B.

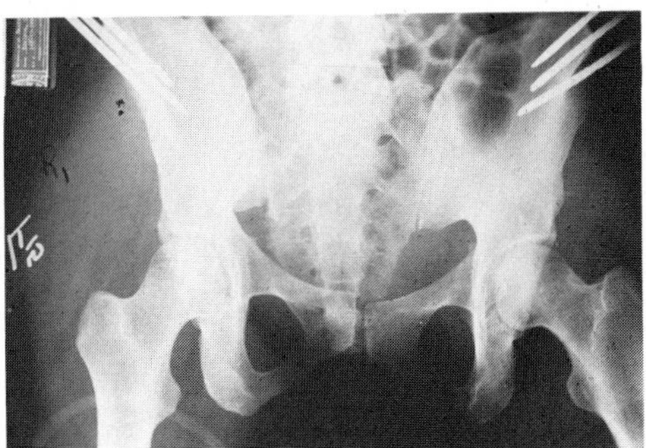

Figure 10-2C.

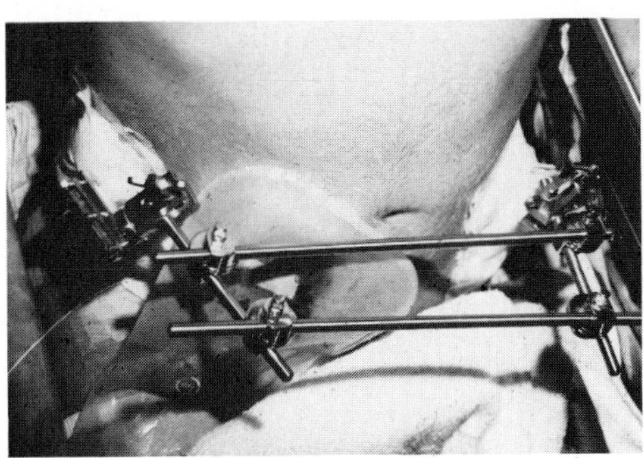

Figure 10-3. A typical simple frame erected with the provision for management of a diversion colostomy. This open pelvic fracture was provoked by a motorcycle accident.

Figure 10-4. Another simple frame design suitable for this lean young woman who sustained a pelvic disruption in a mining accident.

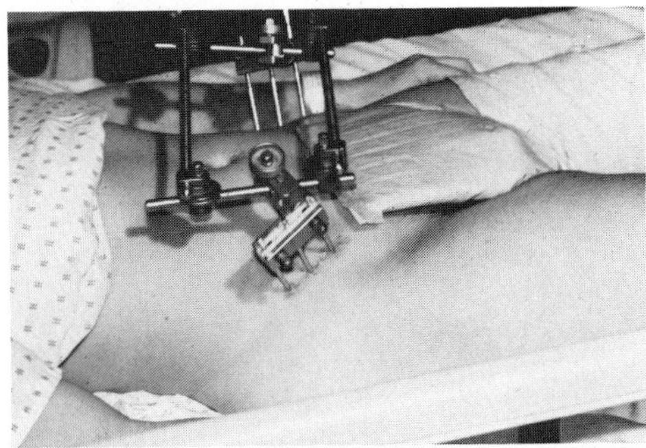

Figure 10-4A. Recumbent view.

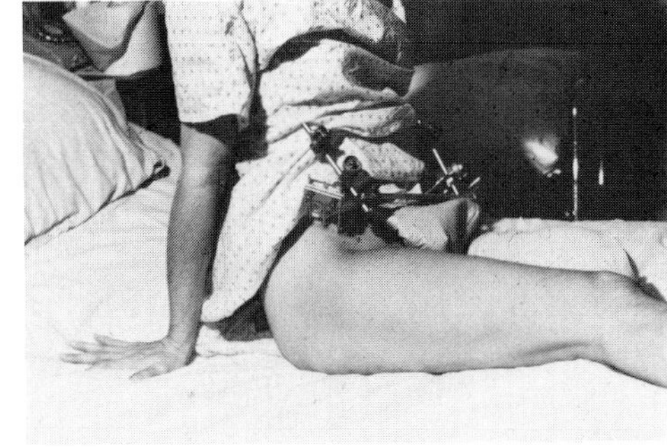

Figure 10-4B. Seated view.

three clamps (Figure 10-5) fabricated from a light-weight radiolucent graphite composite material. The clamps permit the insertion of obliquely oriented pins to augment the rigidity of the fixation and facilitate their insertion into the irregularly shaped pelvis (Figure 10-6). The radiolucent bars are available in three composite materials that possess various moduli. The most rigid bar possesses a stiffness equivalent to that of a stainless steel bar of comparable diameter. The two other bars possess rigidities that are 50% and 25% respectively of that of stainless steel. The alteration in the rigidity of a frame during the period of application may facilitate the rate of healing of the pelvis.

To assemble a simple frame from the Ultra-X System (Figure 10-7), a 3.2mm drill hole is inserted in the anterior superior spine with the use of an appropriate drill guide and drill sleeve. The drill hole is oriented parallel to a line that extends from the anterior superior to the anterior inferior spines. A 5mm half-pin of 180mm in length is inserted into the pilot hole by the use of a hand brace. A double pin clamp is applied to the pin. A drill sleeve is inserted into the second ball in the clamp. The drill sleeve is directed towards the superior gluteal ridge with an obliquity of about 25° with respect to the first 5mm half-pin. After the preparation of the second 3.2mm drill hole, the second 5mm half-pin is inserted through the clamp into the superior gluteal ridge. After irrigation and closure of the two incisions, dry dressings are applied to the pin sites. A 100mm connecting rod is inserted into the double pin clamps. Two rod-to-pin clamps are applied to either connecting rod. Two connecting rods of suitable length are used to bridge the hemipelves. With the patient in a lateral position, a closed reduction is undertaken and the clamps are tightened (Figure 10-8).

## Assembly of a Triangular Frame

In common with other pelvic frames, the procedure is performed with the patient on the operating table in a supine position. Bilateral curvilinear incisions are prepared along the anterior iliac crests for a distance of 8cm to 10cm (Figure 10-9). The lateral femoral cutaneous nerve of the thigh is carefully protected (Figure 10-10). When a diastasis of the symphysis pubis is present, each incision is made 2cm to 3cm medial to the iliac crest. Upon the extension of each incision to the subperiosteal plane, the periosteum is elevated on the inner and outer walls of the pelvis. The origins of the sartorius and the direct head of rectus femoris are incised from the anterior superior and anterior inferior iliac spines respectively. Initially, two 3.2mm pilot holes are prepared in the anterior inferior iliac spine with an interval of 2.5cm. Progressing from distal to proximal, the 5mm half-pins of 180mm in length are inserted for the full length of

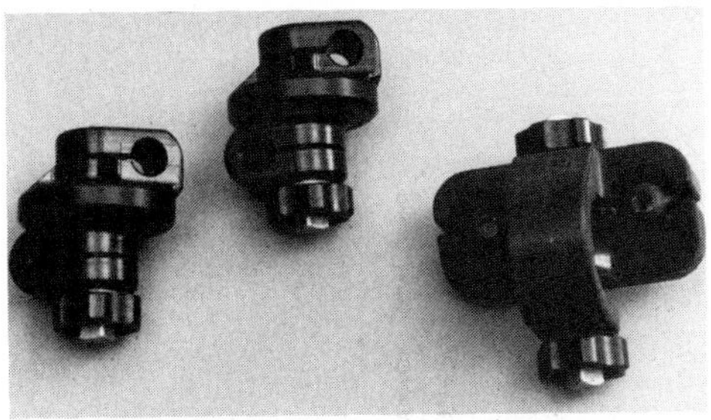

Figure 10-5. The Ultra-X radiolucent, lightweight, composite clamps. Left to right: 8mm/5mm rod-to-pin clamp; 8mm/8mm rod-to-rod clamp; double pin-to-rod clamp.

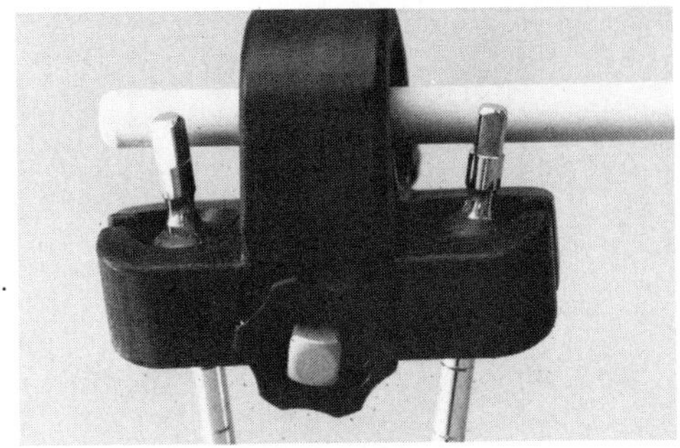

Figure 10-6. Close-up of double pin-to-rod clamp with obliquely oriented pins.

Figure 10-7. Simple pelvic frame assembled from Ultra-X components.

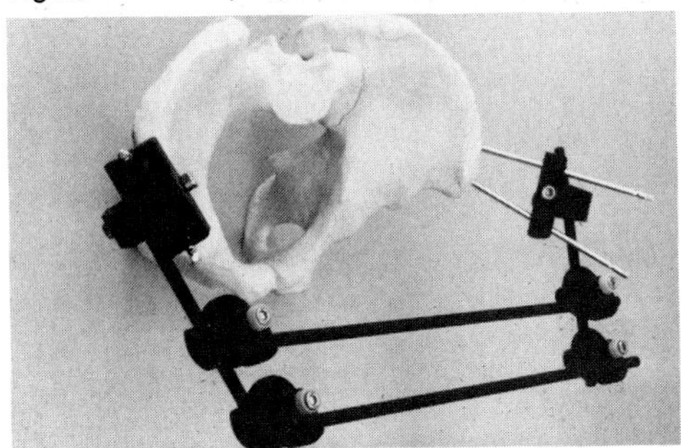

Figure 10-7A. Top view.

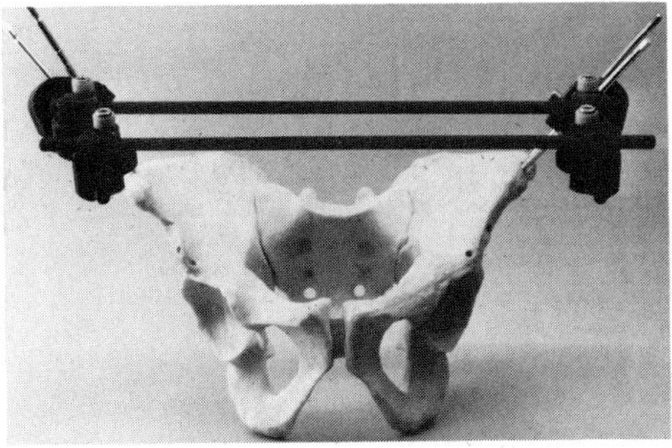

Figure 10-7B. Front view.

Figure 10-8. The use of a simple Ultra-X frame with posterior internal fixation for an unstable sacroiliac disruption with ramus fractures.

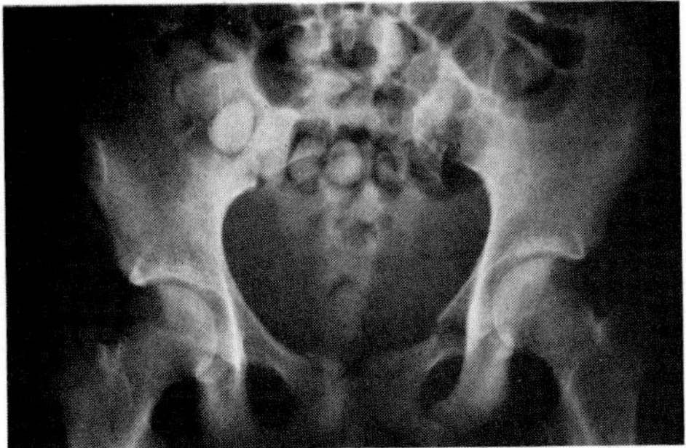

Figure 10-8A. Preoperative view.

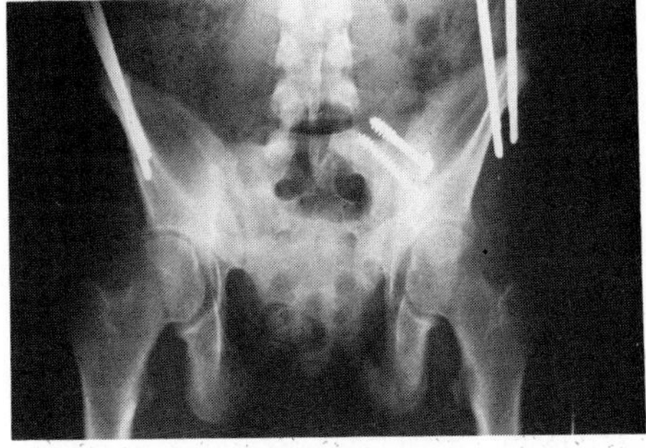

Figure 10-8B. Postoperative view.

the thread by the use of the hand brace. Two additional pins with a spacing of 2.5cm are inserted into appropriate drill holes in the anterior superior iliac crest. The angle between the two pin clusters is 40° to 50° (Figure 10-11). Upon irrigation and closure of the wounds, dry dressings are applied to the pin sites.

To assemble a Pittsburgh Triangular Frame (Figures 10-12 through 10-17), a double universal ball joint is attached to each cluster of half-pins. The outside wing

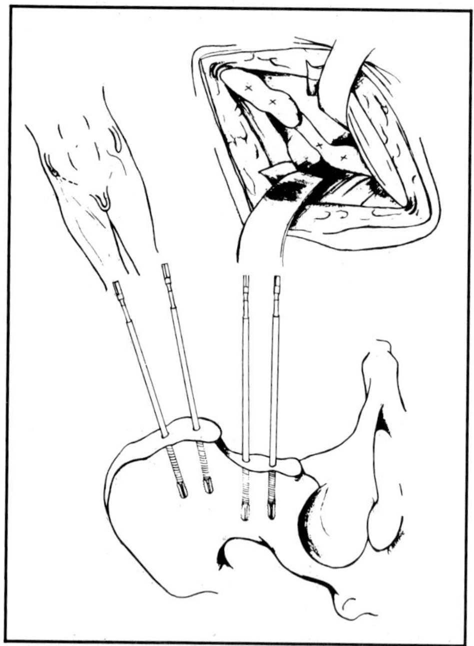

Figure 10-9. Insertion of the pins for a Pittsburgh Triangular Frame. Upper left: cutaneous incision. Upper right: exposure of bone to identify sites for pins. Lower: insertion of pins.

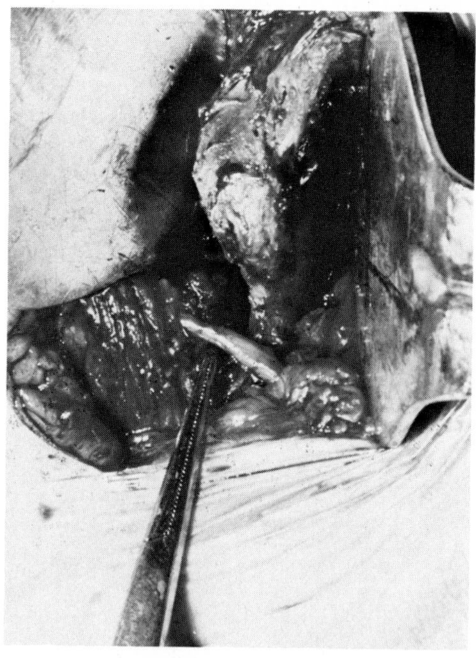

Figure 10-10. Lateral femoral cutaneous nerve of the thigh between the anterior superior and inferior spines.

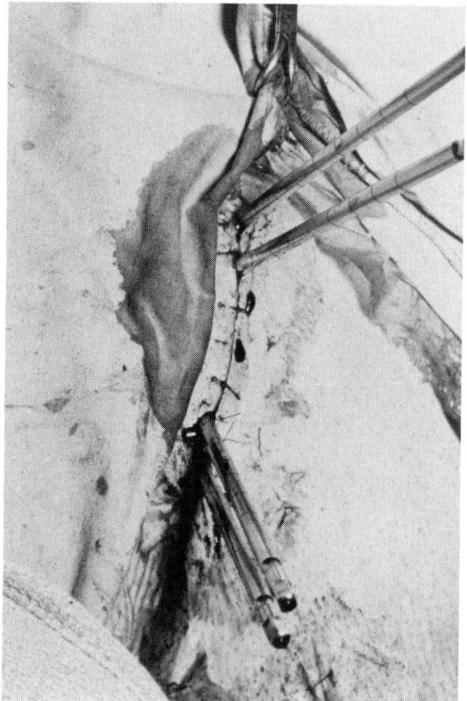

Figure 10-11. Protruding pin clusters with 40° to 50° obliquity.

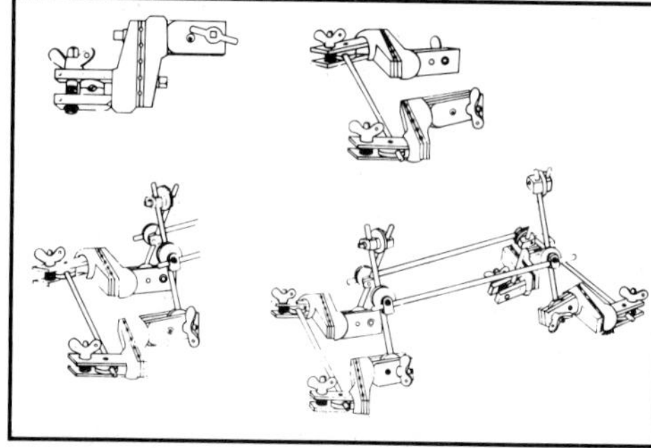

Figure 10-12. Assembly of a triangular frame. Upper left: double ball joint. Upper right: 100mm rod bridging adjacent double ball joints. Lower left: erection of a unilateral triangle. Lower right: complete frame.

Figures 10-13 to 10-16. Stages in the erection of a triangular frame.

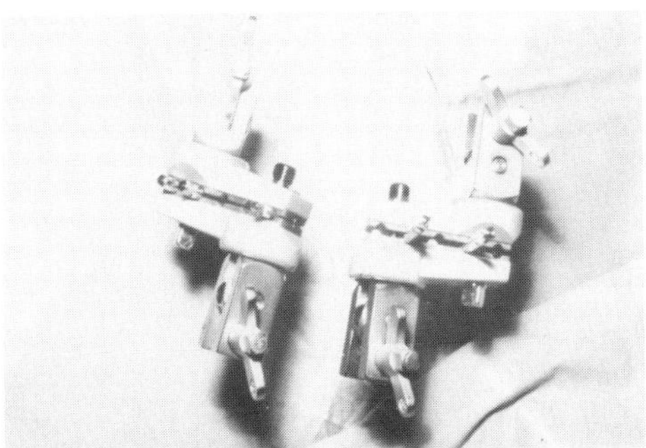

Figure 10-13. Double ball joints applied to adjacent pin clusters.

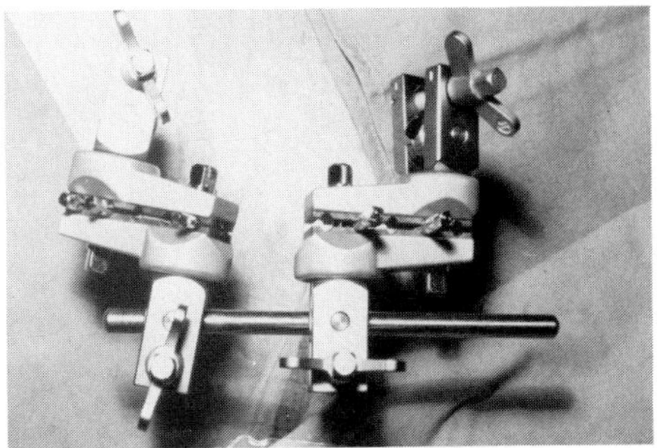

Figure 10-14. A 100mm connecting rod bridges the adjacent double ball joints.

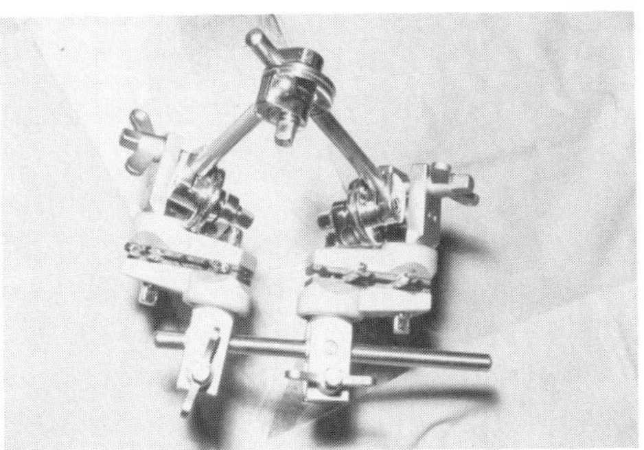

Figure 10-15. A triangular assembly on one hemipelvis.

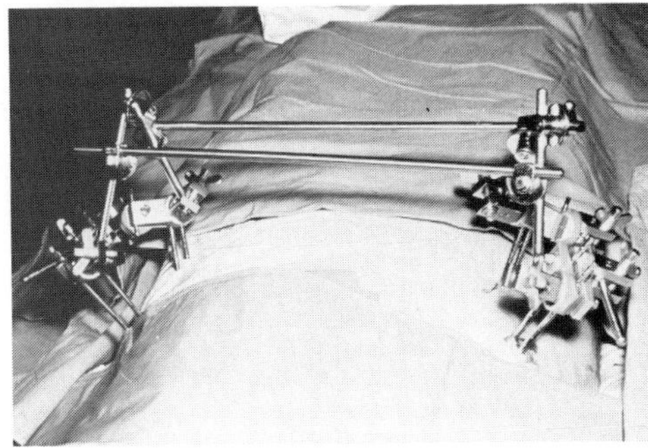

Figure 10-16. The complete frame.

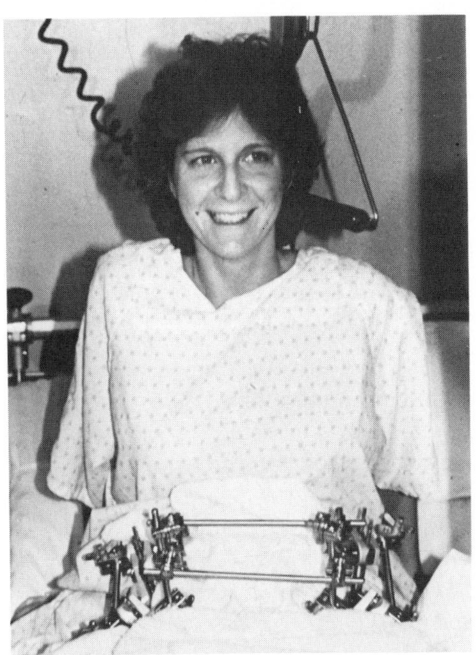

Figure 10-17. An erect patient with a triangular frame.

Figure 10-18. An unstable lateral compression injury managed with a triangular frame. A: Preoperative anteroposterior view. B: Postoperative view with the frame.

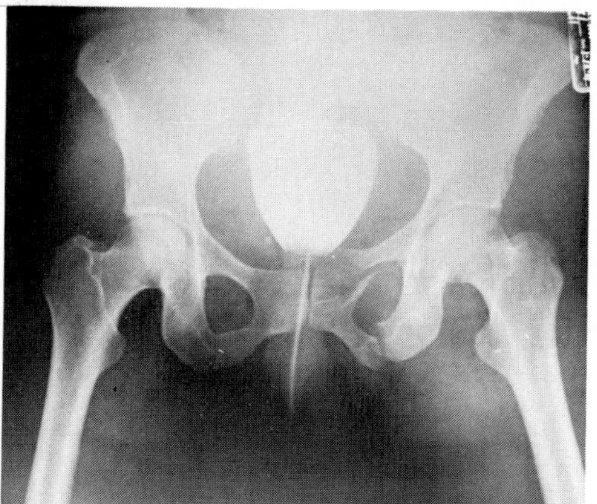

Figure 10-18A.

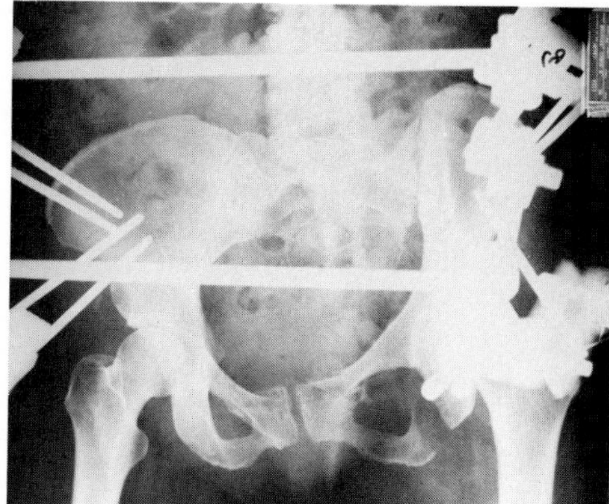

Figure 10-18B.

nuts are placed cephalad to avoid contact with the thigh during flexion of the hip. A 100mm connecting rod is inserted into the ball joints to bridge the ipsilateral pin clusters. Two 150mm connecting rods are inserted into the inner ball joints so that they complete a triangle. An articulation coupling is applied to each upright. The two uprights are connected at the apex of the triangle by a third articulation coupling. The superior articulation couplings and the ball joints are tightened with the T-wrench. Next the triangular uprights on each hemipelvis are bridged with two connecting rods of suitable length. The patient is turned to a lateral decubitus position. A closed reduction of the pelvis is undertaken by manual manipulation and the clamps are fully tightened. The rotational stability of the pelvis is greatly augmented by the separate horizontal connecting rods and by the use of two sets of half-pins per hemipelvis. The accuracy of the closed reduction is checked with intraoperative or postoperative radiographs (Figure 10-18).

## Hybrid Ultra-X Frames

With the new Ultra-X System, two types of modified frame constructions have been employed. The first design employs obliquely oriented pins inserted through a double pin clamp into the anterior superior and anterior inferior spines of either hemipelvis (Figure 10-19). These sites of insertion provide the optimal bone stock to immobilize the pelvis. A connecting rod of 150mm in length is inserted into either double pin clamp. A rod-to-rod connector is applied to either end of each connecting rod. Two horizontal bars of appropriate length are used

Figure 10-19. Modified Ultra-X frame for increased stability. A: Insertion of pins into anterior superior and anterior inferior spines. B: Assembled frame. C: Comparable frame on a patient who has a diversion colostomy and a urinary diversion for an open pelvic fracture with a complete urethral tear.

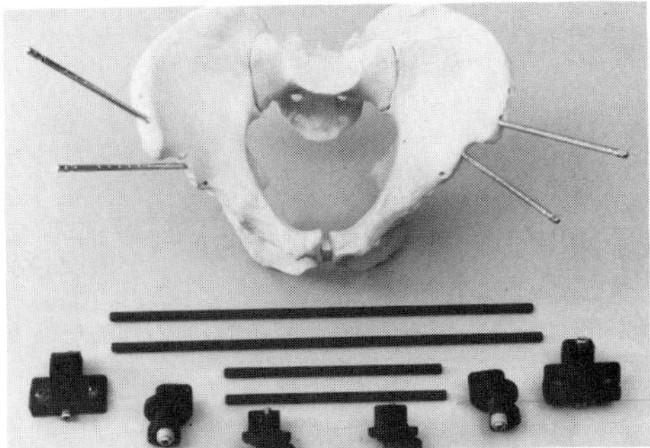

Figure 10-19A.

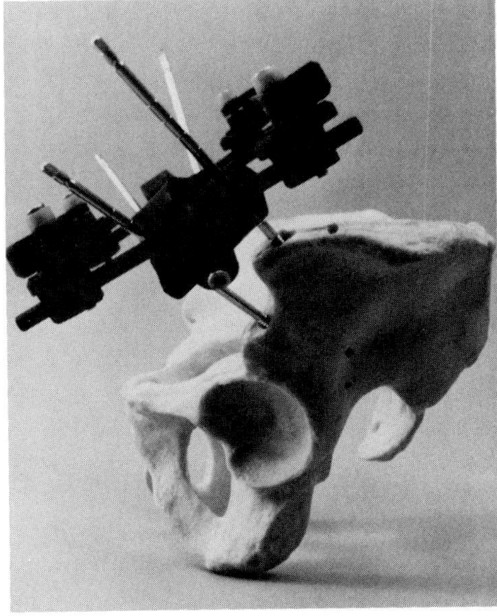

Figure 10-19B.

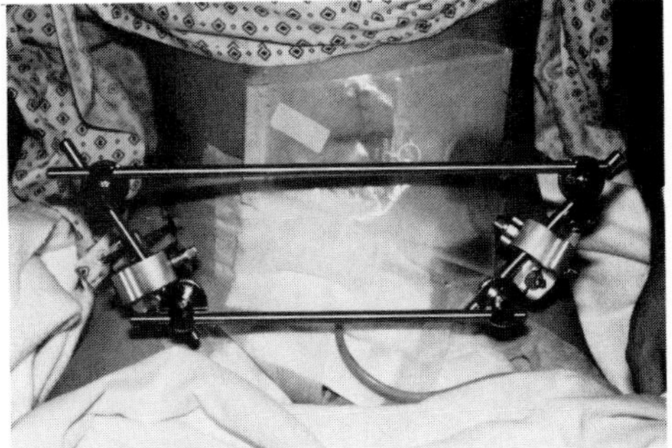

Figure 10-19C.

to bridge between the hemipelves. With this construction the increased separation of the two horizontal bars provides a way to augment the stability of the frame. This design is more stable than a simple rectangular frame but less stable than the triangular configuration.

Where a more stable configuration of the Ultra-X is desired, a third pin is inserted into either superior gluteal ridge. A pin to rod clamp is applied to the third pin. The triangular construction is erected by the hemipelvis. Two connecting bars are used to bridge between the hemipelves.

## References

1. Rubash HE, Mears DC: External fixation of the pelvis, in: AAOS Instructional Course Lectures. St. Louis, Mosby, 32:329, 1983.
2. Mears DC, Rubash HE: External and internal fixation of the pelvic ring, in AAOS Instructional Course Lectures. St. Louis, Mosby, 33:144, 1984.
3. Tile M: Fractures of the Pelvis and Acetabulum. Baltimore, Williams and Wilkins, 1984, p 121.
4. Slatis P: External fixation of the pelvic fractures, in Johnston RM (ed): Advances in External Fixation. Chicago, Year Book Medical Publishers, 1980, p 77.
5. Mears DC: External Skeletal Fixation. Baltimore, Williams and Wilkins, 1983, p 339.

# CHAPTER 11

# Postoperative Care

While the precise regimen for the postoperative care of a patient who has sustained a pelvic or acetabular fracture varies considerably depending upon the specific nature of the injury and the presence of a wide variety of associated injuries to the appendicular skeleton or spine, nevertheless, certain general principles provide helpful guidelines. The fundamental goal is to mobilize the patient as rapidly as possible without excessive likelihood for loss of the reduction.

## External Fixation of the Pelvis

Following the application of a simple or complex frame, certain routine measures are needed to minimize the likelihood of pin tract infection or premature loosening of the frame. The pin sites are left exposed provided that they remain dry. Cotton swabs soaked in hydrogen peroxide are used to clean the pin sites on a daily basis. If a pin site drains a small amount of serous fluid, a dry cotton dressing is applied. If a pin site becomes reddened with localized soft tissue swelling, a small release procedure is undertaken with a scalpel after the infiltration of a local anesthetic agent. A principal predilection for a pin tract infection around the pelvis is the presence of marked obesity. In such an instance, at the time of application of the external frame the cutaneous wounds are loosely approximated or packed in an open fashion with saline-soaked dressings. Until the frame is removed the open wounds are redressed on a twice daily basis. If a pin site develops frank purulent drainage, the frame is loosened from that pin to ascertain whether the pin remains anchored in the bone. If the pin is loose it is removed and the adjacent wound is debrided. Generally with the limited size of the anterior iliac crest, a loose infected pin cannot be replaced without an excessive predilection for pin tract infection of the new pin, with its close proximity to the infected one.

All of the available external frames are subject to spontaneous loosening of the clamps. The patient is provided with a wrench so that he or his family can tighten all of the nuts on a weekly interval until the frame is removed.

When external fixation is supplemented with appropriate internal fixation, at that time the external frame is temporarily removed; otherwise a suitable manipulation of the bone is hampered by the presence of the frame. The most typical supplementary procedure is an open reduction and internal fixation of the sacroiliac joint by the application of lag screws. The patient is positioned in a semiprone fashion so that the protruding external fixation pins on the inferior hemipelvis protrude beyond one edge of the table. Alternatively, a fracture table with a gap between the upper and lower portions can be employed so that the pins protrude in the intervening gap. After the supplementary internal fixation has been completed, the original external frame is reassembled. When a provisional external frame is replaced with definitive internal fixation, generally an attempt is made to design appropriate surgical incisions that do not cross the pin sites. In an uncommon instance when the incision transgresses a pin site, the open reduction and internal fixation is undertaken within a few days after the application of external fixation so that the risk of a wound infection is minimized.

For an isolated pelvic fracture or when other injuries permit, generally on the day after the application of external pelvic fixation, the patient is encouraged to undertake a bed to chair transfer. Frequently, multiple assistants are needed to perform the first transfer. Nevertheless, the upright posture of the patient facilitates both his pulmonary toilet and morale. At the very least he is encouraged to sit upright in his bed. The degree to which he can assume a fully upright posture depends upon his size and the position of the frame. Certain obese patients experience excessive impingement of the outer abdominal wall on the frame when they flex their hips beyond 60° to 80°. In a routine case of external pelvic fixation without supplementary internal fixation, bed to chair transfers are strongly encouraged to permit a patient to be discharged rapidly from the hospital to his home. Generally, gait training is deferred until the removal of the external frame. An external pelvic device does not afford rigid stability of the pelvis. If the injury is a diastasis with preservation of the sacroiliac ligaments, in a reliable patient a touchdown gait can be undertaken. Nevertheless, in many if not most cases, the magnitude of instability of the traumatized pelvis and the degree of stability of the reconstructed pelvis after the application of external fixation are unknown. A rapid postoperative initiation of gait training, therefore, provides a limited asset and a major potential liability if a satisfactory pelvic reduction is lost. Once the patient is comfortable with the bed to chair regime and can manage transfers independently or with the assistance of one person, he is discharged to his home. He is permitted to undertake showers on a daily basis.

When the posterior pelvic disruption is a fracture of the sacrum or posterior ilium, the frame is removed about six weeks after application. If, however, the injury represents an unstable dislocation of a sacroiliac joint, a longer period of immobilization of eight to ten weeks is employed. At that time the patient is readmitted to the hospital and the frame is removed after the administration of a short-acting general anesthetic agent. Upon the removal of the horizontal bars that connect the opposing hemipelves, the residual portions of the frame are grasped and manipulated to document the degree of pelvic stability. In those unusual instances when persistent instability is evident, the frame is reassembled. With the predilection for a delayed union or nonunion, conversion to internal fixation of the anterior and posterior disruptions is carefully considered. In the routine case once the frame has been dismantled and the pins have been removed, the pin sites are irrigated with betadine solution and dry dressings are applied. When the injury is a simple diastasis, the patient is encouraged to undertake a partial weightbearing gait with the use of crutches and a progression to full weight bearing during the subsequent month. In the presence of a more comminuted pelvic disruption, a period of progression from partial to full weight bearing continues for eight weeks. Twelve to sixteen weeks after the pelvic reconstruction, supplementary pelvic radiographs are obtained. Provided that a stable union is evident, a resumption of full activities is encouraged.

## Internal Fixation of the Pelvis

The application of internal fixation to both the anterior and posterior lesions or of posterior internal fixation to augment anterior external fixation restores a substantial degree of pelvic stability. Generally, when these techniques are employed the postoperative course with bed to chair transfers is supplemented with a touchdown gait. About six weeks later the patient progresses to a partial weightbearing gait, with progression to full weight bearing over the next six to eight weeks. The principal thrust of the postoperative regimen of physical therapy is progressive resistance exercises of the relevant muscle groups around the pelvis and lower extremities.

Following a pelvic reconstruction, removal of the internal fixation devices is rarely indicated. Symptomatic fixation devices usually are encountered on the anterior iliac crest or the rami. The former case is more notable in men where a belt can rub on a prominent plate or a screw. In a lean woman who undergoes plate fixation of the rami and symphysis, discomfort can present as dyspareunia.

## Internal Fixation of the Acetabulum

At the conclusion of the surgical reconstruction when the patient is transferred to his bed, his relevant lower extremity is placed in a continuous passive motion machine. Initially an arc of 30° to 50° is employed with a frequency of about one cycle per minute. The arc of motion is advanced as rapidly as tolerated by the patient, usually by twice daily adjustments. On the first postoperative day the patient is encouraged to sit in his bed; on the second postoperative day he is assisted with bed to chair transfers. At that time he attends physical therapy for active range of motion exercises of the hip, including flexion and extension, adduction and abduction, and rotation. He is provided with a skate board to encourage the adduction and abduction. Gait training is initiated as touchdown with about 25 pounds of force applied to the injured lower extremity. Progressive resistance exercises for the trunk and lower extremity are undertaken. The most important muscle group appears to be the abductors of the hip, although the quadriceps are crucial along with other groups. Generally, once the patient can perform independent transfers, 90° of active hip flexion, and walking with the use of two crutches, he is discharged to his home. He continues outpatient physical therapy for the subsequent period of six weeks with active motion exercises of the hip and progressive resistant exercises. Between two and four weeks after the surgical reconstruction in the absence of other injuries, he is encouraged to undertake swimming and riding a stationary bicycle. Six weeks after surgery, postoperative radiographs are obtained to document satisfactory alignment and early healing of the bone. Generally, a more vigorous progressive resistance exercise regime, undertaken in a Nautilus facility, is initiated on a thrice weekly basis, which continues for at least one year. Unless such a vigorous exercise program is undertaken for a prolonged period after acetabular and pelvic reconstruction, generally persistent symptomatic muscle weakness such as a gluteus medius lurch is evident. At the six-week period a partial weightbearing gait with about 50 to 80 pounds of weight bearing is encouraged. The degree of weight bearing is assessed by the use of a bathroom scale. A progression to full weight bearing ensues during the next four to six weeks. Further radiographic documentation of the acetabulum and hip joint is obtained at 12, 24 and 52 weeks after the injury. Full union of the bone should be evident at 12 weeks, while the possible formation of ectopic bone is judged on the succeeding radiographs. Other potential radiographic findings of interest include the features of avascular necrosis of the femoral head or traumatic arthritis of the hip.

## Pelvic and Acetabular Reconstruction

As a general rule all of the pelvic reconstructions share the need for vigorous progressive resistance exercises for a period of not less than one year following the injury. Such a regimen provides the greatest likelihood for a full functional recovery generally evident about a year after the surgery. When a sciatic nerve palsy or lumbosacral root injury accompanies the initial traumatic insult, appropriate functional bracing of the lower extremity is indicated. Typically a foot drop deformity is managed by use of an ankle-foot orthosis. The degree of recovery of the nerve injury is documented clinically and at the six-week period by multiple radiographic studies in the more severe cases. For the vast majority of pelvic and acetabular reconstructions, no consideration for removal of the internal fixation devices is given unless they are symptomatic. Following a transtrochanteric approach for an acetabular reconstruction in an aesthenic individual, stabilization of the greater trochanter by the use of lag screws can be followed by a complaint of local pain upon rolling over in bed. In such a case the trochanteric lag screws are easily removed.

No routine prophylactic treatment for thromboembolic problems has been undertaken. In addition to the potential for postoperative hemorrhagic complications, the use of heparin or oral anticoagulants is associated with a retardation of bone formation and fracture healing. While this limitation of anticoagulation discourages their use on a routine basis, they are employed in a patient who possesses a predilection for thromboembolic problems, such as massive obesity.

Following an acetabular reconstruction of a complex fracture where an extensile surgical exposure has been undertaken and when the surgical procedure has been delayed possibly because of concomitant traumatic problems, consideration of prophylactic treatment to retard ectopic bone formation is given. Of the available agents, the diphosphonates such as disodium etidronate do not appear to provide a beneficial action. Despite a few encouraging preliminary reports, the role of indomethacin also remains unclear at the present time. Undoubtedly, irradiation therapy is the most effective therapeutic agent to inhibit the formation of ectopic bone. A suitable therapeutic regime employs relatively small doses of 100 to 200 rads administered on alternate days from the time of the surgical procedure until a total of 1000 to 2000 rads have been given. Nevertheless, with its potential to inhibit the healing of bone and to provoke teratogenicity, it has not been employed for routine cases. When ectopic bone is excised after acetabular reconstruction in males greater than 40 years of age, the use of lower dose irradiation therapy has been associated with minimal recurrent ectopic bone formation.

# CHAPTER 12

# Late Problems

## Introduction

Perhaps more than any other type of traumatic disruption, a pelvic or acetabular fracture is apt to culminate in one of a variety of formidable late problems. Both as a result of conservative management and after operative intervention, late problems create the need for consideration of surgical reconstruction of the pelvis.[1-3] Such procedures remain in the forefront of surgery undertaken by a few clinical centers. With their extraordinary variety, complexity, and limited frequency, no useful statistical analysis of past experience is generally available. Nevertheless—with the authors' management of more than 150 cases of pelvic or acetabular disruption for late presentation, and 75 cases of nonunion, malunion, and infected nonunion, as well as other late cases presenting with symptomatic ectopic bone formation, traumatic arthritis, avascular necrosis of the femoral head, or allied neurological impairment—this chapter is meant to provide a clinical rationale for management of late problems based on the limited experience to date.

Despite the complexity of the procedures, highly encouraging results have been obtained, which are presented in the next chapter. The surgical complexities, which dwarf even those encountered with an acute associated fracture, necessitate careful preoperative planning referable to the indications for surgery, the optimal exposure, and techniques of reduction and stabilization. As a general principle, a symptomatic nonunion associated with a complaint of pain or pelvic instability possesses the best prognosis for a successful surgical correction.[4] Surgical reconstruction of a pelvic malunion yields somewhat varying results. The overall pelvic asymmetry can be greatly improved, while apparent limb length discrepancy can be corrected to a moderately satisfactory degree. Correction of sitting imbalance probably remains the most challenging objective. Correction of a painful stiff hip with or without an associated malunion or nonunion of the acetabulum has been greatly simplified by the recent innovation of cementless total hip replacement with acetabular components provisionally anchored by screw fixation.[5] An infected nonunion of the pelvis still possesses a greater potential mortality than any other type of late pelvic problem. The management of other late problems, including nerve impairment, ectopic bone formation, and allied hernias, also yield varying results.

## Late Presentation

Late presentation following a major pelvic or acetabular disruption is particularly likely to occur in the multiple trauma victim who sustains numerous other life-threatening problems, particularly a severe intracranial injury. To the present time, there is a general lack of awareness that acute stabilization of the pelvis can facilitate the overall recovery of the patient. Many trauma victims undergo acute management in an outlying hospital where the appropriate resources for pelvic and acetabular reconstruction are not available. With concomitant hemodynamic, pulmonary, or neurological instability the pelvic or acetabular reconstruction generally is deferred until the patient is transferred to a regional trauma center. Other patients are managed acutely with a conservative regime such as skeletal traction. An unsatisfactory reduction or a late loss of reduction of the fracture may not be recognized until a few weeks have ensued. Still other patients undergo an inadequate closed reduction with external fixation, or occasionally an open reduction with internal fixation, so that a subsequent surgical revision of the disruption merits serious consideration. While an almost unlimited variety of pelvic problems allied to late presentation are encountered clinically, some representative examples are given.

## Late Presentation of a Pelvic Disruption

Within a few days to a few weeks after the application of bed rest, a pelvic sling, or skeletal traction for the immobilization of a pelvic ring disruption, significant deformity may be documented by clinical scrutiny and radiological assessment. The most commonly encountered deformity is a persistent dislocation of a sacroiliac joint with widening of greater than 1cm or posterior migration of the ilium. Less frequently, marked superior migration of the ilium to provoke an apparent limb length discrepancy and difficulties with sitting secondary to asymmetry of the positions of the ischial tuberosities are encountered. Rotational deformity of the pelvis can present with a wide diastasis or overriding of the rami. In the presence of multiple ramus fragments, a displaced ramus fragment may project anteriorly as a tender subcutaneous prominence, or it may project inwardly to provoke dysfunction of the bladder or, in a woman, dyspareunia.

With a late presentation of a diastasis of the symphysis pubis and a displaced posterior iliac fracture, virtually an anatomical reduction can be achieved in a reproducible fashion even months or a few years after the time of the injury. When the posterior iliac fracture accompanies multiple ramus fractures, generally such a late presentation is adequately managed with an open reduction and internal fixation of the posterior ilium (Figure 12-1). Unless the rami are displaced by more than a few millimeters, generally they unite uneventfully. When a diastasis of the symphysis is accompanied by a dislocation of a sacroiliac joint with minimal rotational deviation of the involved hemipelvis, reapproximation of the anterior and posterior separations can be undertaken with relative ease even years after the initial injury. Unless both of the sites are stabilized, and even where only one site is symptomatic, persistent pain and instability are almost inevitable (Figure 12-2). When a symptomatic rotational deviation (Figure 12-3) or superior migration of a hemipelvis (Figure 12-4) follows the initial conservative management or an inadequate closed reduction and application of external pelvic fixation, effective correction of the rotational deviation or superior migration is difficult or impossible. Nevertheless, the late surgical reconstruction permits the reconstitution of a stable pelvic ring by reapproximation of the symphysis and the displaced sacroiliac joint, with alleviation of pain and mobility at the unstable sites. Persistent complaints of sitting imbalance, apparent limb length discrepancy, or occasionally a cosmetic problem in a lean patient are likely to follow the surgically induced malunion. If such a rotational deviation or posterior displacement of a hemipelvis

Figure 12-1: A late presentation of a posterior iliac fracture violating the left sacroiliac joint accompanied by multiple ramus fractures in a woman of 42 years. Patient presented two months after the time of injury, when multiple pins were employed to immobilize a femoral neck fracture.

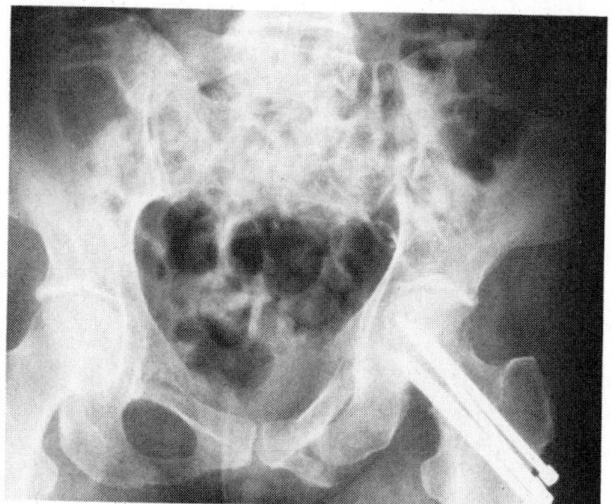

Figure 12-1A: Presenting AP view.

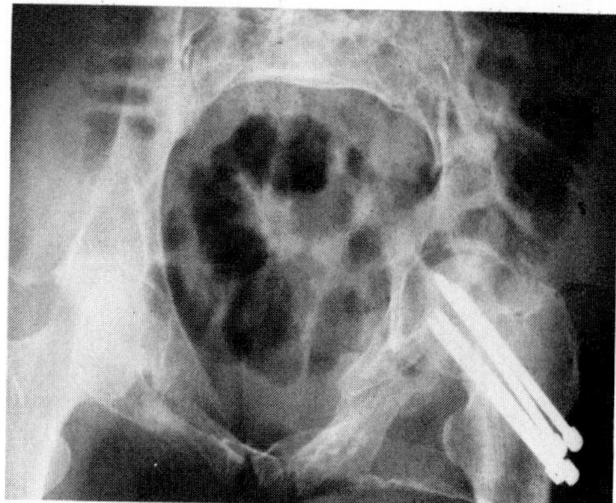

Figure 12-1B: Presenting inlet view.

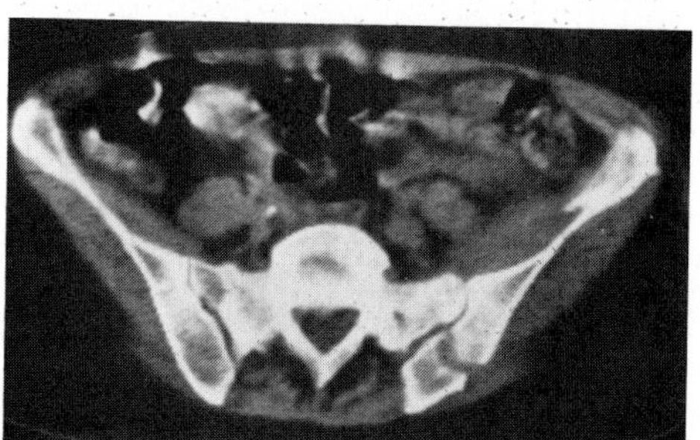

Figure 12-1C: Computed scan with posterior iliac fracture.

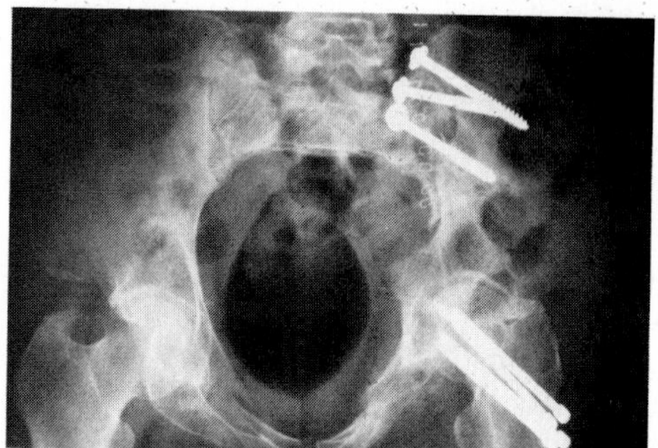

Figure 12-1D: Inlet view after internal fixation of the iliac fracture.

creates a prominence of the posterior superior spine at the time of the surgical reconstruction, even if the rotational or posterior displacement cannot be corrected the prominent posterior ilium is osteotomized to remove the potentially tender protuberance. As part of the surgical closure, the superior portion of the origin of the gluteus maximus is secured over the osteotomized surface of the bone to provide effective padding and cosmesis.

The most difficult late presentation is a markedly displaced sacral fracture with an associated anterior injury (Figure 12-5). By the use of the Double Cobra plate, reapproximation of the sacrum is readily achieved (Figure 12-6). A concomitant rotational deviation, however, has been difficult to realign anatomically. A surgical release of the contracted ipsilateral sacrospinous and sacrotuberous ligaments from the ischium facilitates the rotational correction with a corresponding temporary compromise to pelvic stability.

Figure 12-2: This Marine of 22 years fell from 100 feet when his parachute failed at low altitude. His unstable right hemipelvis was managed with a simple external frame. Upon removal of the frame, he complained of persistent pain at the symphysis, for which delayed internal fixation was undertaken. Afterwards he complained of sacroiliac pain on activity. Subsequently, a fusion of the sacroiliac joint was needed. With the poor initial reduction, the need for subsequent open reduction internal fixation of the anterior and posterior sites could have been anticipated and managed in a combined procedure. Internal fixation of the symphysis was performed at six months, and internal fixation of the sacroiliac joint at one year.

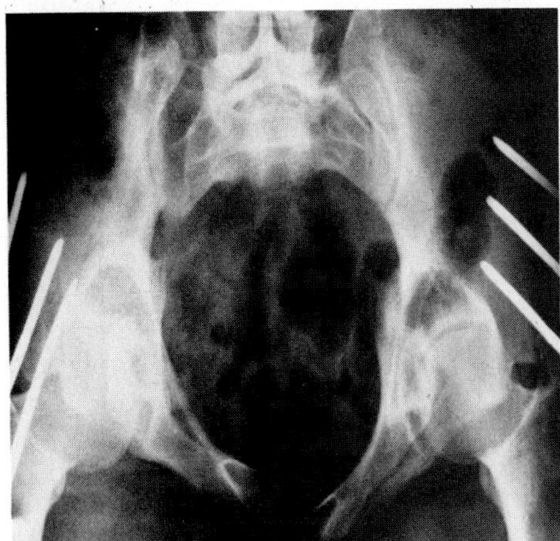

Figure 12-2A: Inlet view after external fixation.

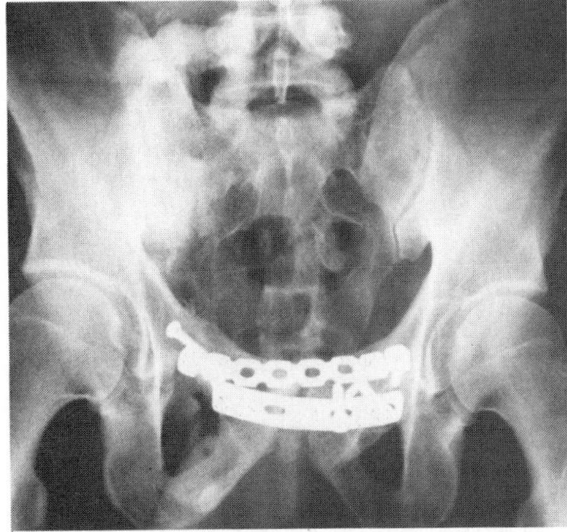

Figure 12-2B: AP view at six months.

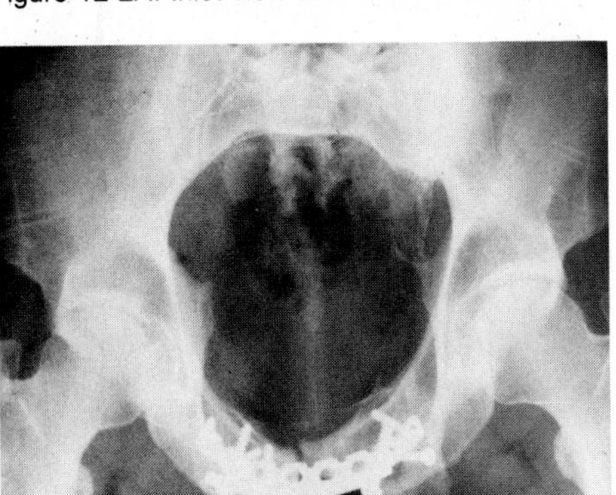

Figure 12-2C: Inlet view at six months.

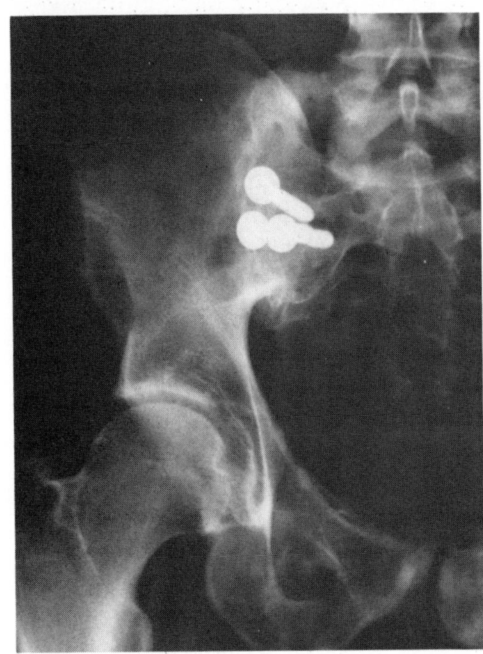

Figure 12-2D: AP view at one year.

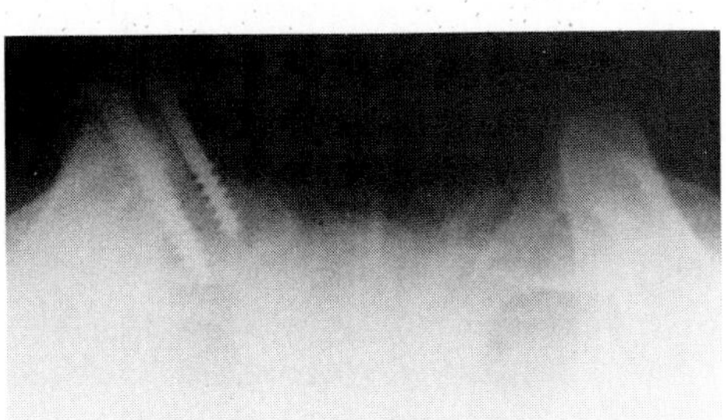

Figure 12-2E: Fergusson view at one year.

Figure 12-3: This female coal miner of 27 years was involved in a mining incident to provoke an open right sacroiliac dislocation with a diastasis and left ramus fracture. Initial management included application of a simple external frame and debridement of the sacroiliac joint. She also required a left above-knee amputation for a severe crush injury to the thigh. About eight weeks later, internal fixation of the sacroiliac joint was undertaken without realization of an anatomical reduction. One year later, she had persistent pain at the sacroiliac joint and symphysis. Ultimately, three years after her injury when the pain persisted, fusion of the sacroiliac joint and symphysis was undertaken. While the last procedure provided alleviation of discomfort of the sacroiliac joint and symphysis, correction of the persistent displacement of the right hemipelvis was not achieved. Her limb length discrepancy was corrected by modification of her left above-knee prosthesis.

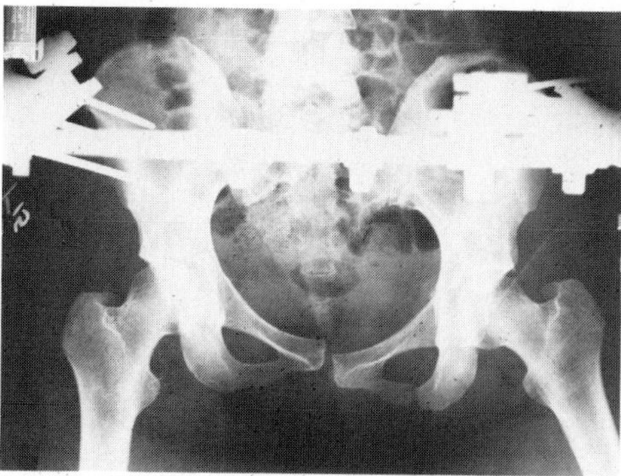

Figure 12-3A: AP view after external pelvic fixation.

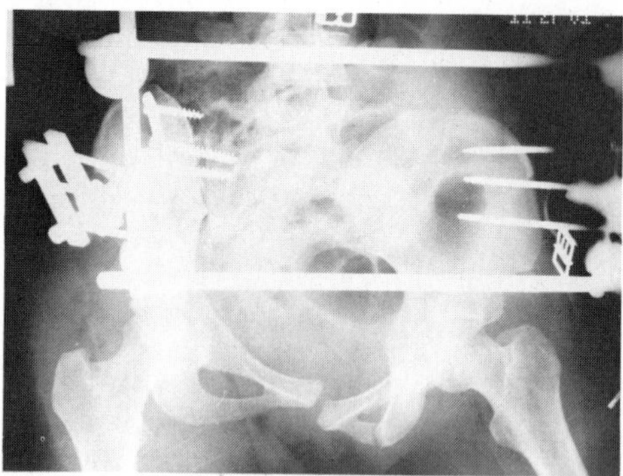

Figure 12-3B: Obturator oblique view after lag screw fixation of SI joint.

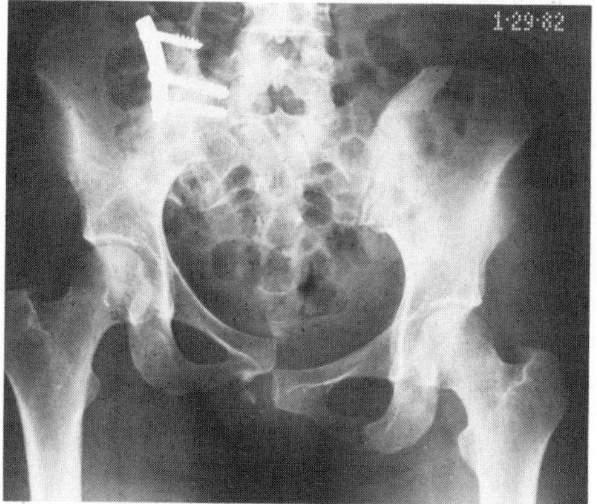


Figure 12-3C: AP view taken one year afterwards.

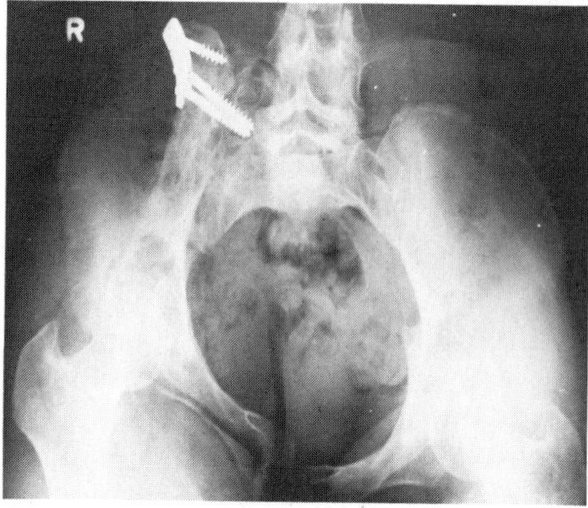


Figure 12-3D: Inlet view taken one year afterwards.

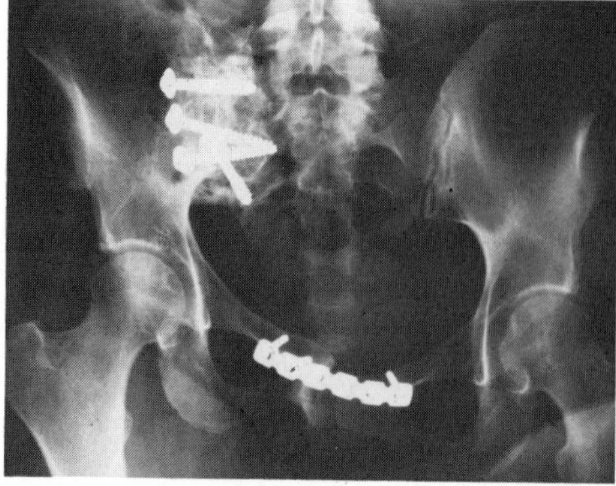

Figure 12-3E: AP view three years after injury.

Figure 12-4: This 13-year-old girl sustained a vertical shear injury to the right hemipelvis in a vehicular accident. Following her acute resuscitation, she was managed for five weeks with simple bed rest. At that time, sequential radiographs showed marked superior migration of the right hemipelvis. Open reduction and internal fixation of the posterior fracture dislocation was accompanied by external fixation to achieve a partial correction of the vertical displacement and a painless stable pelvis.

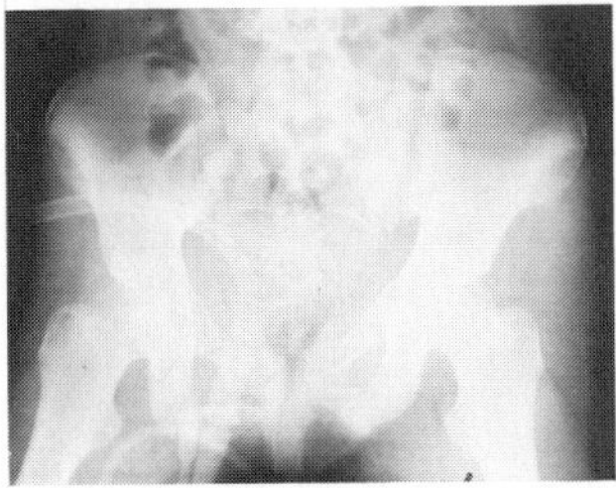

Figure 12-4A: Initial AP view.

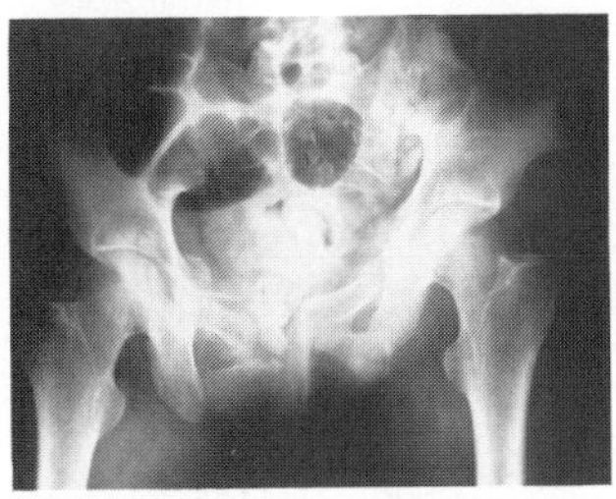

Figure 12-4B: Five weeks later.

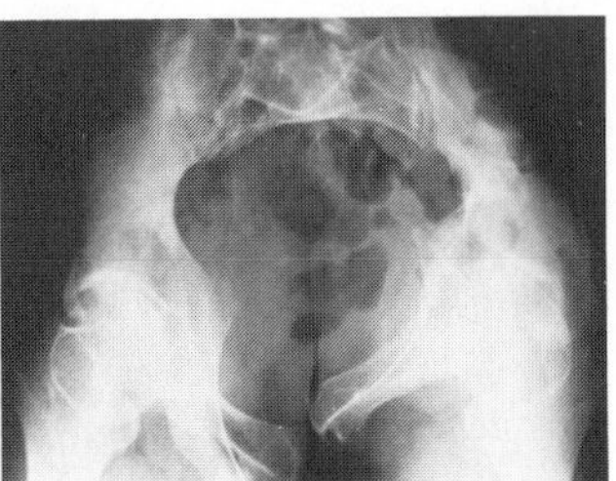

Figure 12-4C: Five weeks later.

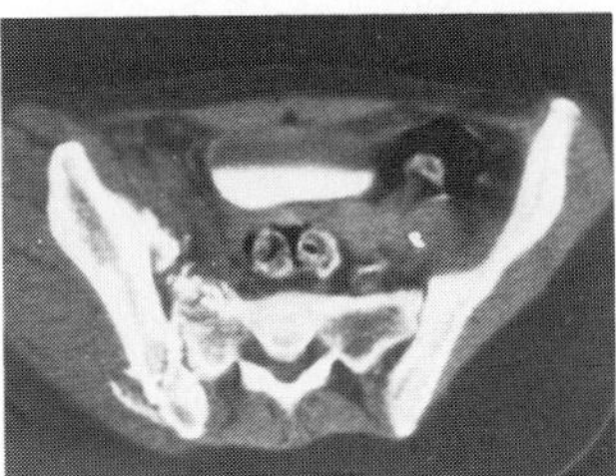

Figure 12-4D: Computed scan through SI joint.

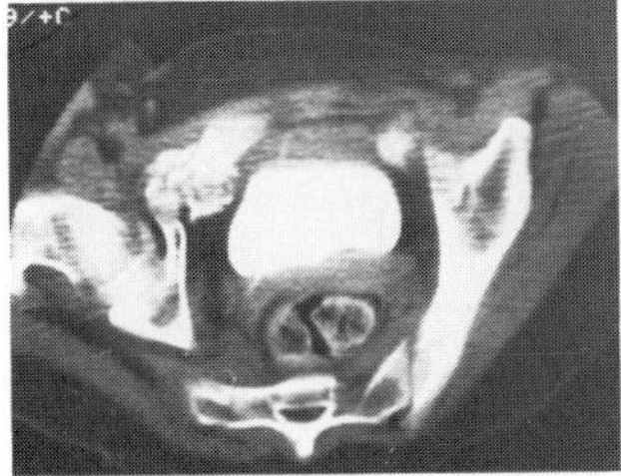

Figure 12-4E: Computer scan through right hip.

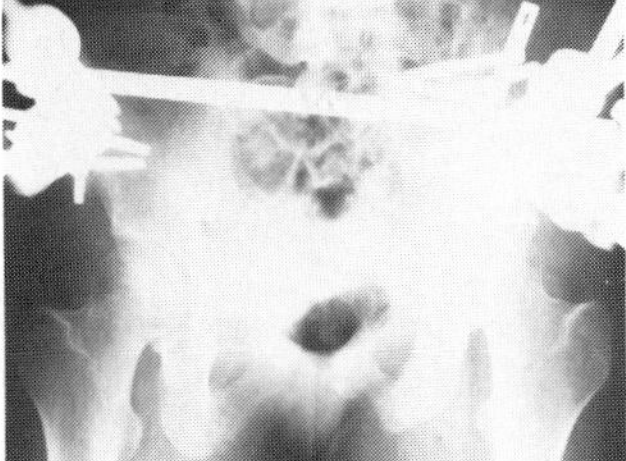

Figure 12-4F: Initial postoperative AP view.

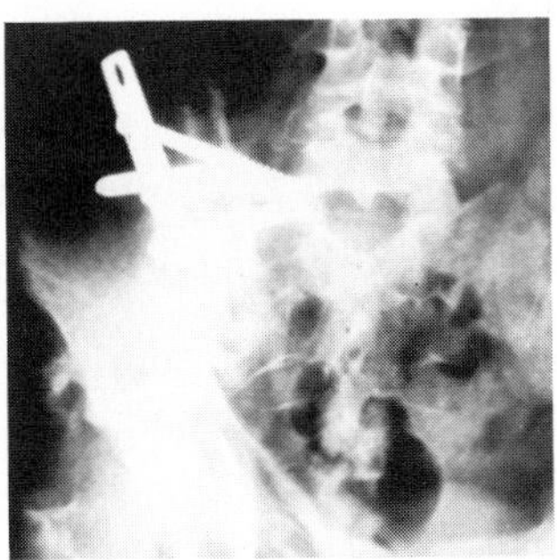

Figure 12-4G: One year post-operative AP view.

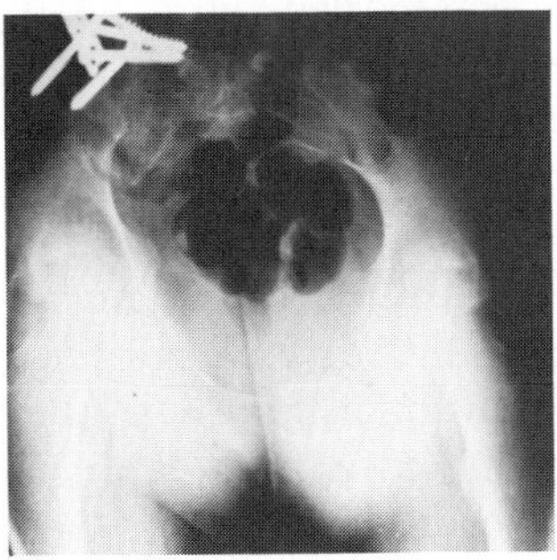

Figure 12-4H: One year post-operative inlet view.

As a general rule for rotational realignment of a deformed pelvis, the anterior reduction is undertaken prior to the posterior exposure. With the curvature of the rami, the quality of the open reduction is more easily ascertained. In the presence of superior migration of a hemipelvis, however, the initial exposure is made posteriorly so that the femoral distractor or comparable bone holding forceps can be employed to correct the deformity.

Figure 12-5: AP views of a woman of 24 years who was managed for an unstable left-sided sacral fracture with external fixation. In the absence of a preoperative inlet view or CT scan, a poor reduction was accepted. When the frame was removed, displacement ensued with a complaint of severe pain at the sacroiliac joint and mild discomfort at the symphysis. Subsequently, a complex reconstruction of the sacrum at the site of the sacral foramina with a potential for a neurological complication was necessary.

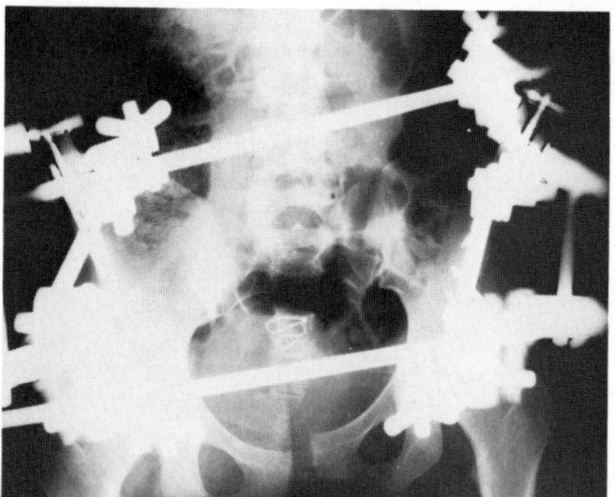

Figure 12-5A: AP view with external fixation.

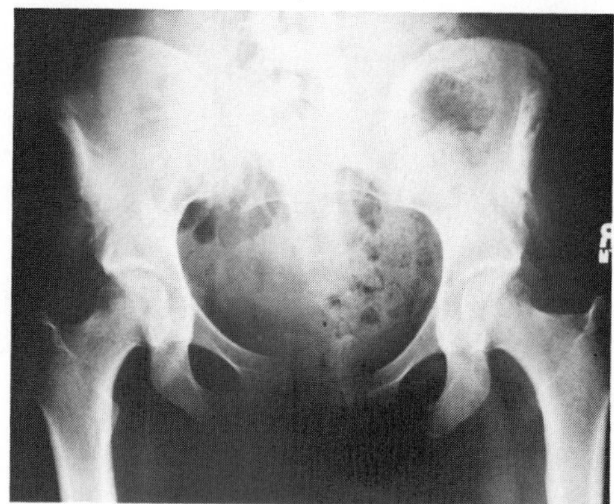

Figure 12-5B: AP view after removal of the frame with enhanced displacement.

## Late Presentation of Acetabular Disruptions

As Letournel has emphasized,[1] the presentation of an acetabular fracture more than three weeks after the time of the injury greatly compromises the accuracy attainable with an open reduction. Also, during the ensuing period, even in the presence of skeletal traction, further abrasive damage to the femoral head and the adjacent acetabulum frequently occurs. The pelvic fragments become osteoporotic during a period when granulation tissue tends to envelop them in their displaced positions. As the forces needed to achieve an anatomical reduction inevitably mount, so the softer bone fragments compromise the structural integrity of the anchorage sites available for the application of bone holding forceps. Nevertheless, surgical reconstruction may be indicated to prevent a high likelihood of a late dislocation or to lessen the risk of traumatic arthritis, which would otherwise be overwhelming. Even when a subsequent reconstructive procedure such as a total hip joint replacement is anticipated, the late pelvic and acetabular reconstruction can immeasurably simplify the subsequent arthroplastic procedure and greatly improve the anticipated longevity of the latter. While many examples where acetabular reconstruction appears to be indicated will be cited, there are a few cases where such surgery is contraindicated. In the presence of marked osteoporosis and comminution, the surgery possesses a poor chance for an effective result (Figure 12-7). In contrast, certain displaced transverse fractures or posterior column disruptions with minimal

Figure 12-6: A Nigerian female of 29 years presented one month after a vehicular accident for which she had been managed for a pelvic fracture with immediate external fixation and for her right femoral shaft fracture with an intramedullary rod fixation. The triangular frame was secured to the bone with 3mm pins. A postreduction inlet view and a computed scan were not obtained. Probably limited apposition of the sacral fracture was achieved. At the time of transfer of the patient, the pelvic ring showed a marked displacement of the sacral fracture. At the time of open reduction and internal fixation of the sacrum with the application of a Double Cobra plate, excellent apposition of the sacrum was obtained, although a correction of the rotational deviation was not possible. Nevertheless, a highly satisfactory cosmetic and symptomatic result was documented.

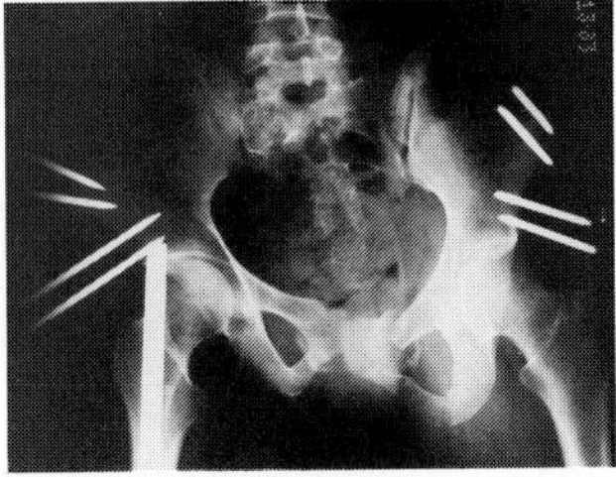

Figure 12-6A: AP view one month after external fixation.

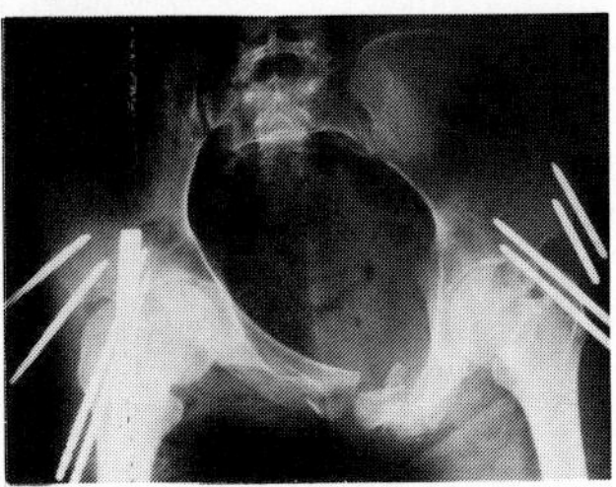

Figure 12-6B: Inlet view one month after external fixation.

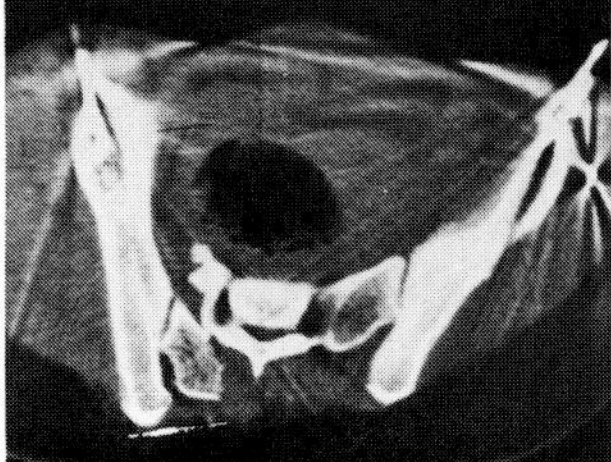

Figure 12-6C: Computed scans through upper part of the displaced sacral fracture.

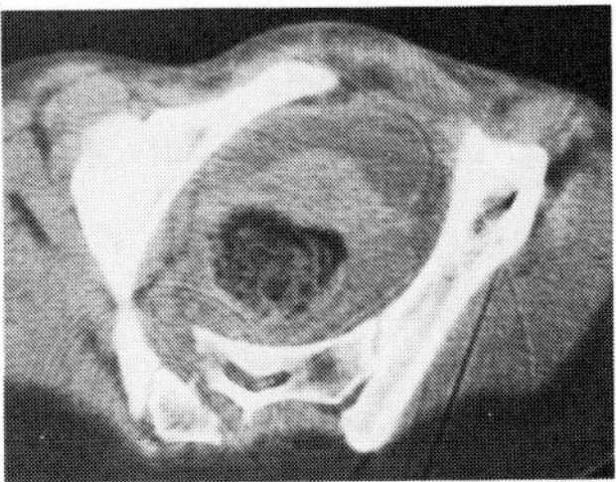

Figure 12-6D: Computed scan through lower part of the displaced sacral fracture.

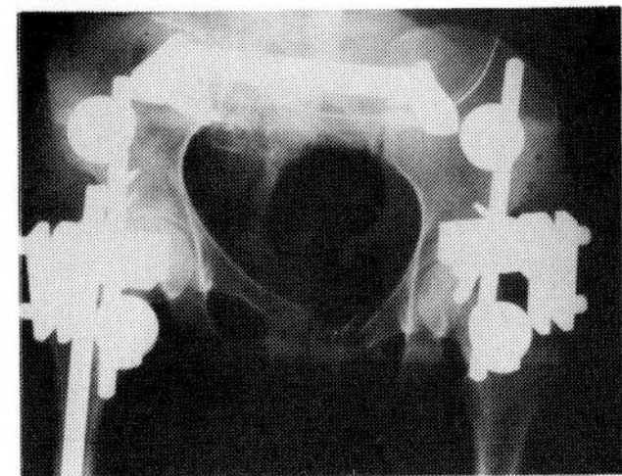

Figure 12-6E: Postoperative AP view with a Double Cobra plate.

comminution can be undertaken with little more difficulty than a comparable acute injury.

One other indication for nonsurgical management is the late presentation of a highly comminuted both-column fracture with secondary congruence of the acetabular fragments around the femoral head (Figure 12-8). On the one hand, the nonoperative result may be a good one. Furthermore, this fracture pattern rarely is subject to an accurate reduction at the time of a late surgical reconstruction (Figure 12-9). While the latter example possessed a Harris Hip Rating of 92, the residual pelvic deformity nevertheless indicates that little correction of the displaced fracture fragments was achieved by the surgical procedure. Probably the result would have been as good or better if nonoperative management had been undertaken. In the example evident in Figure 12-10, a similarly displaced both-column fracture managed by skeletal traction provided a satisfactory painless mobile hip for ten years, after which late degenerative changes with pain and stiffness

Figure 12-7: This woman of 66 years with marked senile osteoporosis presented with a highly comminuted transverse fracture with dislocation of the ipsilateral sacroiliac joint. An open reduction and internal fixation was undertaken. Shortly after surgery, the fixation failed with a loss of the reduction. One year later, she presented with a painful nonunion-malunion of the hemipelvis and avascular necrosis of the femoral head. A further anticipated reconstruction is immensely complicated by the severe osteoporosis. A-D: Computed 3D scans of the pelvis. E & F: Postoperative radiographs taken one year after surgical reconstruction.

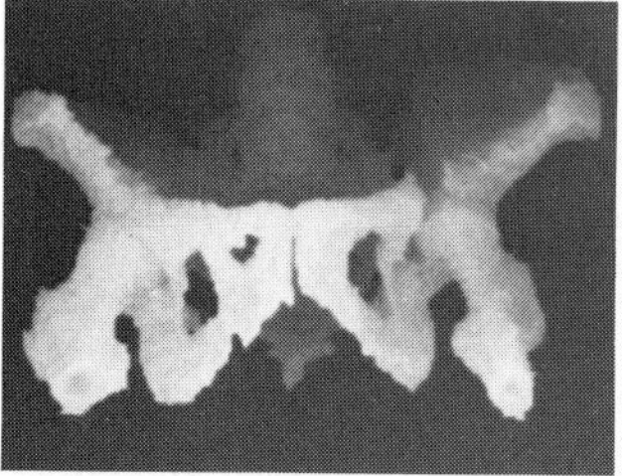

Figure 12-7A: AP view

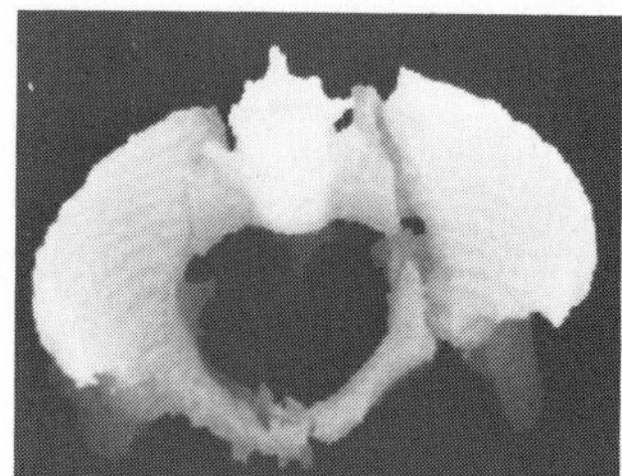

Figure 12-7B: Inlet view

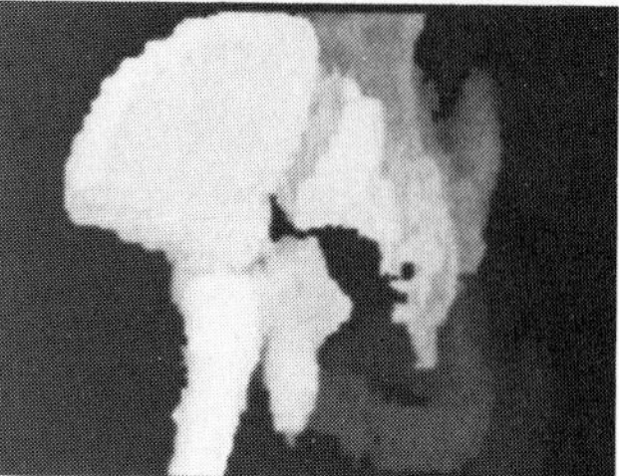

Figure 12-7C: Iliac oblique view

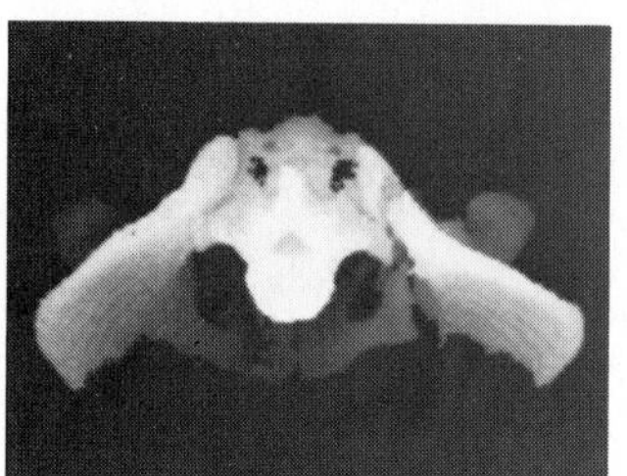

Figure 12-7D: Top view

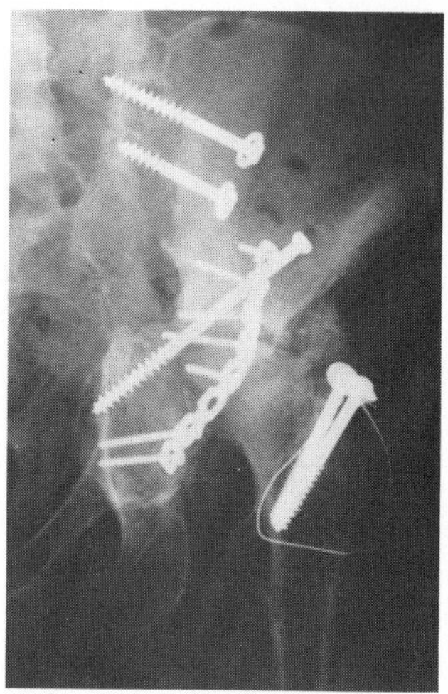

Figure 12-7E: AP view.

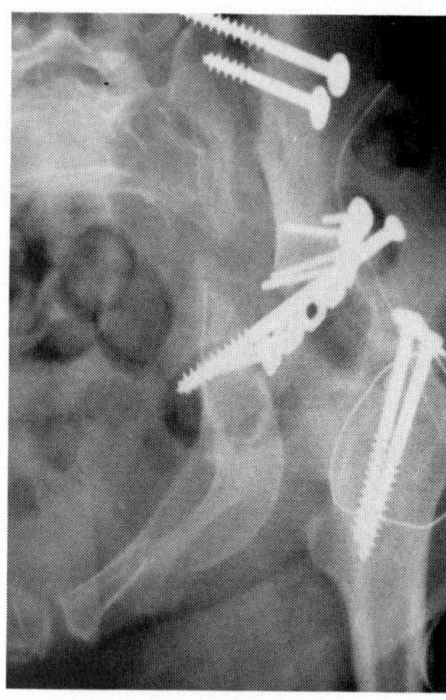

Figure 12-7F: Inlet view.

initiated consideration of total hip replacement with anticipated technical difficulties.

Late presentation of a posterior wall disruption with persistent subluxation or dislocation of the femoral head is an absolute indication for surgical reconstruction. While many of these cases may be destined to progress to a total hip joint replacement, the late surgical reconstruction of an acetabulum compromised by a deficient or ununited posterior wall is extraordinarily difficult (Figure 12-11). During the exposure, particular care is needed to avoid devascularization of the posterior wall fragment. The capsular origin to the fragment is obscured by scar formation so that the fragment is readily devitalized. Once the fragment is completely displaced, the exposed femoral head can be subluxed to facilitate the removal of the fracture callus. The femoral head and posterior wall region are carefully examined for evidence of a fracture or impaction of the former and marginal

Figure 12-8: This man of 45 years presented six weeks after a vehicular accident provoked a highly comminuted both-column fracture, which was managed with skeletal traction. While the radiographs indicate substantial persistent displacement, secondary congruence provides a more favorable prognosis. These radiographs were taken one year later when a painless mobile hip was documented.

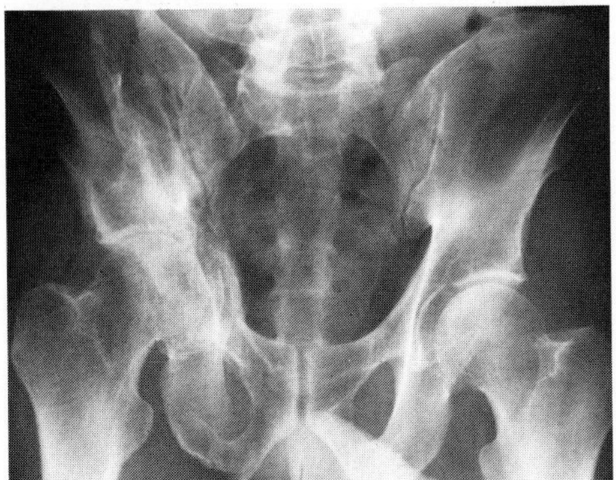

Figure 12-8A: AP view of the pelvis.

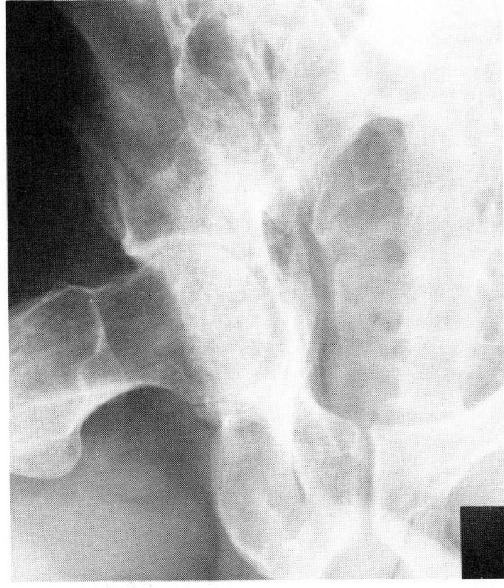

Figure 12-8B: Lateral radiograph of hip.

impaction of the latter. Such an area is carefully elevated around the femoral head, while the hip is positioned with 30° of abduction and flexion. Bone graft is packed into the deficiency in the impacted region between the inner and outer tables of the pelvis. With a large posterior wall fragment, lag fixation is afforded by the application of two or three 4.5mm cortical screws. The screws are inserted by retrograde drilling each gliding hole prior to the reduction of the fragment. For a late presentation where the wall fragment is small or somewhat osteoporotic, the use of a supplementary 3.5mm reconstruction plate to buttress the posterior column is strongly recommended.

With a late presentation of a posterior wall disruption, avascular necrosis of the femoral head with marked collapse (Figure 12-12) is likely to ensue. In such an instance, even though the posterior wall reconstruction is effectively undertaken, the femoral head can shrivel up to 50% of its normal size, whereupon it is subject to spontaneous dislocation. In other cases with a posterior wall fracture dislocation, an associated fracture of the femoral head is not recognized acutely. Unless a large fracture fragment sheared from the femoral head is reconstructed at the time of the acetabular repair, a late spontaneous dislocation is likely to occur (Figure 12-12). Once the late dislocation occurs, either endoprosthetic replacement of the femoral head or, in

Figure 12-9: Postoperative radiographs taken one year after delayed surgical reconstruction of a highly comminuted both-column fracture. This woman of 35 years possessed a very good clinical result but marked persistent central and posterior displacement of the acetabulum.

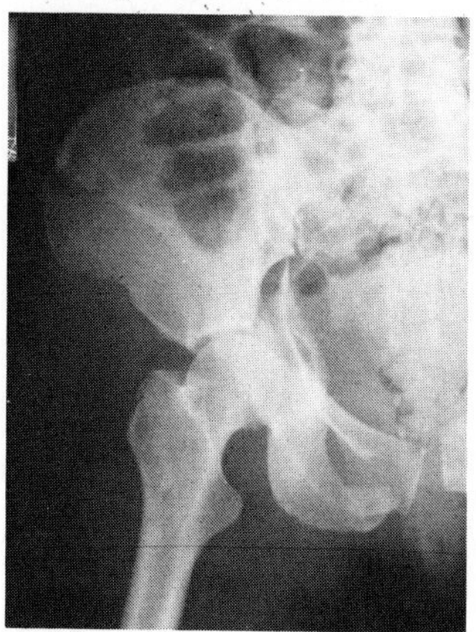

Figure 12-9A: Preoperative AP view.

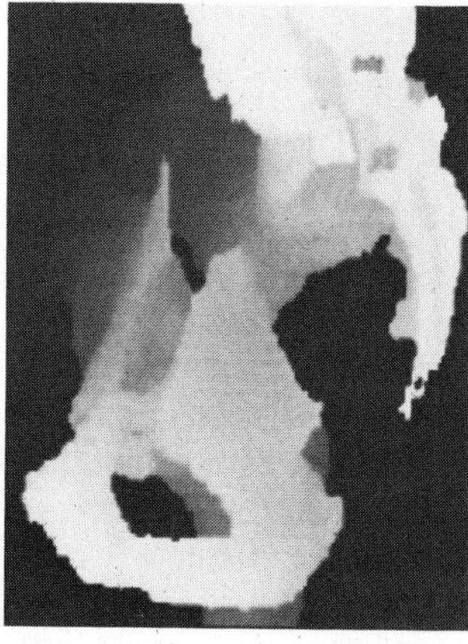

Figure 12-9B: Inner view in a 3D computed scan.

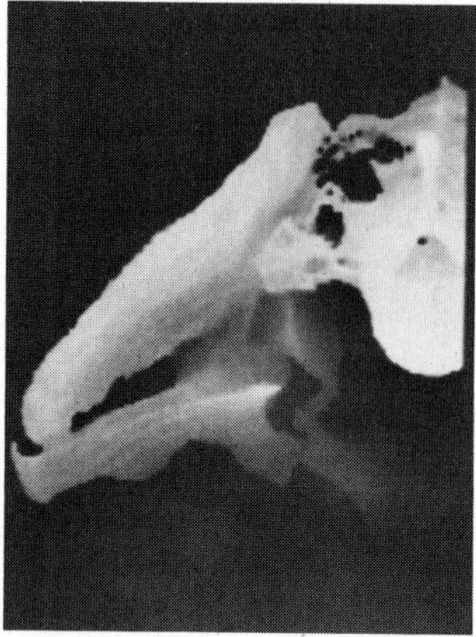

Figure 12-9C: Top view in a 3D computed scan.

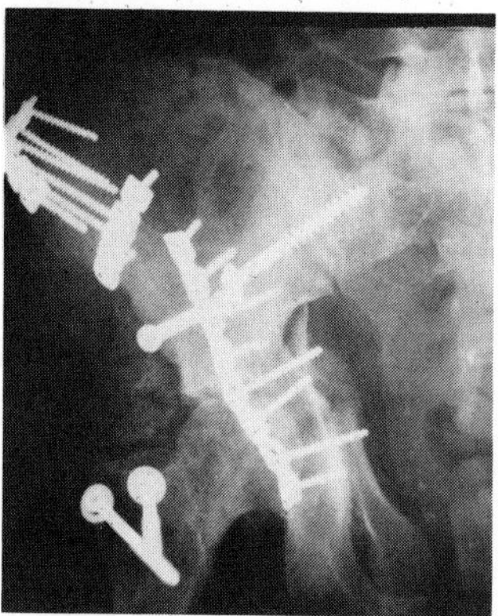

Figure 12-9D: AP view one year after surgery.

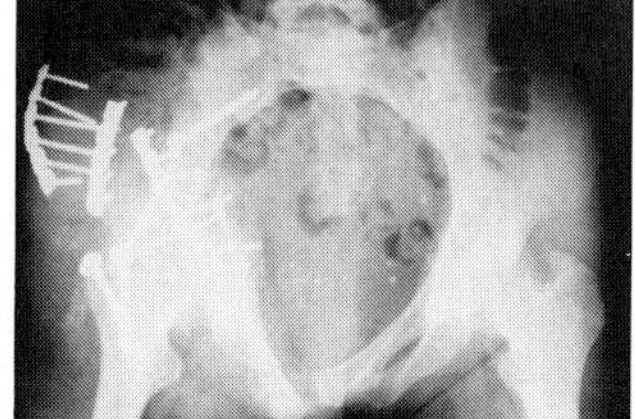

Figure 12-9E: Inlet view one year after surgery.

the presence of substantial acetabular disruption, a total hip joint replacement is indicated.

In the presence of a posterior column or a posterior column with a posterior wall disruption, a late presentation provides a more difficult reduction of the displaced portion of the column (Figure 12-13). If the posterior column is markedly displaced, then a surgical release of the sacrospinous and sacrotuberous ligaments is needed to facilitate an accurate reduction. Once the posterior column is restored, the posterior wall is reconstructed around the relocated femoral head.

With a displaced transverse fracture, a late presentation necessitates an extensile exposure of both the anterior and posterior aspects of the fracture so that the callus can be removed and an accurate reduction can be achieved (Figure 12-14). If the transverse fracture is

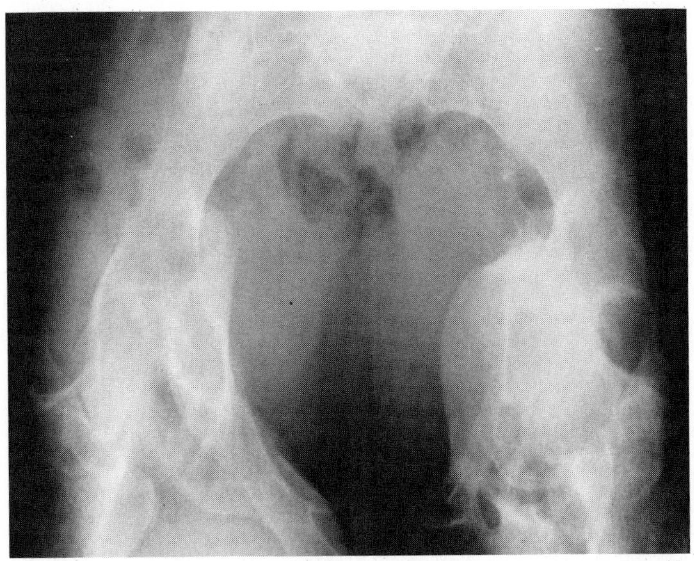

Figure 12-10: In this inlet view taken ten years after a both-column fracture initially managed with skeletal traction, marked protrusio is evident that was consistent with a satisfactory result for many years.

accompanied by a displacement of the ipsilateral sacroiliac joint, then an anterior approach to the sacroiliac joint is needed to debride the joint and undertake an anatomical reduction. Unless this maneuver precedes the acetabular reduction, restoration of a congruent acetabulum is impossible. The sacroiliac joint can be visualized over the top of the iliac crest or around the front of the ilium by release of the sartorius and rectus femoris. Frequently, the most difficult aspect of the open reduction is the rotational correction of the inferior fracture fragment. This maneuver is facilitated by the insertion of a femoral distraction pin or femoral head extractor into the ischial tuberosity and a release of the sacrospinous and sacrotuberous ligaments.

For the comminuted associated variants, such as a transverse with posterior wall, "T" type, or both-column fracture, an extensile exposure is needed to achieve a rigorous debridement of all of the fracture lines (Figures 12-15 to 12-17). As the callus is removed from the fractures, a persistent and ever increasing ooze is encountered with the potential for a substantial blood loss, much greater than a comparable acute fracture. A hypotensive anesthetic regime and the use of a "cell saver" lessens the need for transfusion. Despite a late presentation in many instances, an excellent functional and anatomical result can be achieved. A greater predilection for ectopic bone formation exists, although a surprisingly good functional recovery is possible if, about one year after the initial surgical procedure, upon its maturation, the ectopic bone is removed.

In certain instances, particularly with an inexperienced surgical team, an initial open reduction and internal fixation of an associated fracture is wholly unsuccessful

Figure 12-11: This man of 48 years presented one month after a vehicular accident when he had been examined in three other hospitals for his complaint of hip pain. His hip remained dislocated with a posterior wall fracture complicated by a fracture of the femoral head and marginal impaction. During surgical reconstruction, the area of acetabular impaction was carefully elevated and bone graft was applied to the corresponding defect. While the postoperative radiographs document an excellent reduction, the prognosis is poor with persistent damage to the femoral head.

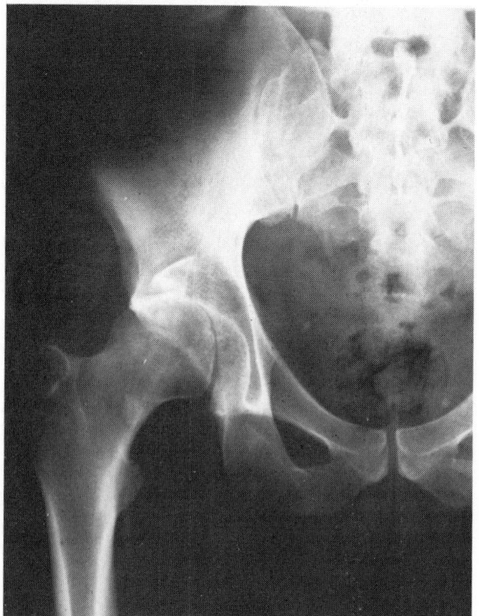

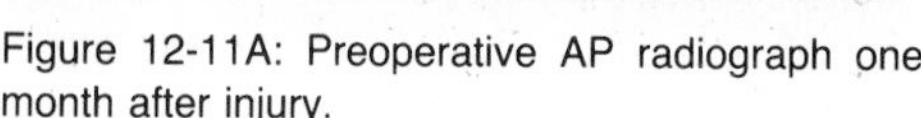

Figure 12-11A: Preoperative AP radiograph one month after injury.

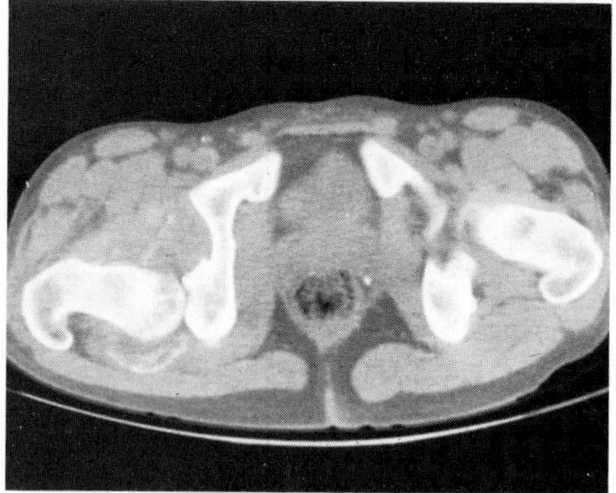

Figure 12-11B: Computed scan with posterior wall fragment, marginal impaction, and defect on anterior portion of the femoral head.

with inadequate visualization of the articular surface (Figure 12-18). In such a case, after transfer of the patient to a regional trauma center a consideration for a second operative approach may arise. Each case merits a meticulous scrutiny particularly of the magnitude of the persistent displacement, the age of the patient, and the presence of other medical problems. Particularly where the first procedure was limited to the iliac disruption and the residual periarticular portion of the hip joint was not exposed, a highly satisfactory reconstruction of the displaced columns can be achieved. If the first surgical wound is not suitable for the second reconstructive procedure, then a modified surgical exposure may be necessary. In this example initially a both-column fracture in a young woman of 23 years was managed at a local hospital by an iliofemoral exposure. Only the propagation of the anterior column fracture across the lateral ilium to the iliac crest was visualized and secured with a single pin. When the apex of the wound adjacent to the anterior superior spine underwent a superficial necrosis, the patient was transferred to our care. The partial sloughing of the anterior exposure precluded the use of a triradiate approach or an extended iliofemoral approach. A lengthy Kocher-Langenbeck

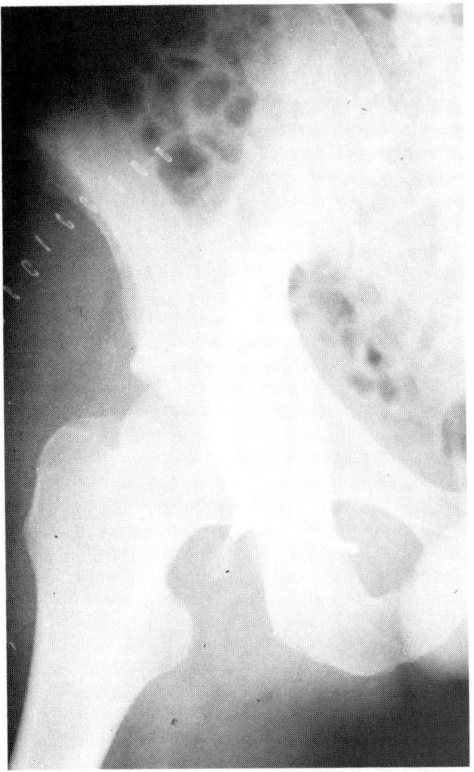

Figure 12-11C: Postoperative AP radiograph.

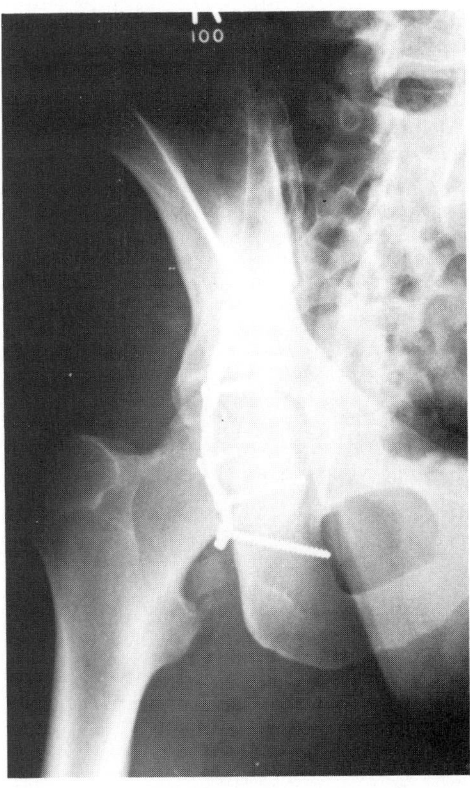


Figure 12-11D: Postoperative obturator oblique radiograph.

posterolateral exposure was therefore employed to visualize both the posterior and anterior columns. A highly satisfactory reduction was achieved. The patient did develop ectopic bone formation, which was excised one year afterwards with restoration of rotation and full flexion of the hip.

By scrutiny of the radiographs (Figure 12-19) taken a few months after an associated acetabular or pelvic fracture, the degree of the union of displaced fracture fragments and the quality of the articular surfaces of the femoral head and opposing acetabulum may not be subject to accurate characterization, even when supplementary computed scans, 3D scans, and tomographs are studied. Frequently, a computed scan shows an apparently mobile ununited fracture site when, at the time of surgery, a substantial degree of union is documented. A computed scan can be suggestive of a nonunion with apparent gaps between adjacent fracture fragments when a subsequent surgical exposure reveals the presence of stable bony bridges between the fragments. When a patient complains of persistent pelvic pain for many months after the time of his injury so that a surgical correction is indicated, the procedure is

Figure 12-12: This 360-pound man of 28 years was transferred to us about two months after his injury secondary to a vehicular accident with persistent instability of the femoral head. His transfer had been delayed by an open tibial fracture with secondary infection and a major pulmonary embolus requiring intravenous anticoagulation. In his initial operation, a solid fixation of the transverse fracture was achieved, although inadequate stabilization of the supplementary posterior wall fragment was realized. About one month later his hip dislocated spontaneously. At the time of reoperation, about two months after the first procedure, the anterior half of the femoral head was shriveled and the posterior wall fragment was markedly displaced. Conversion to a Harris-Galante total hip replacement was performed with lag fixation of the posterior wall.

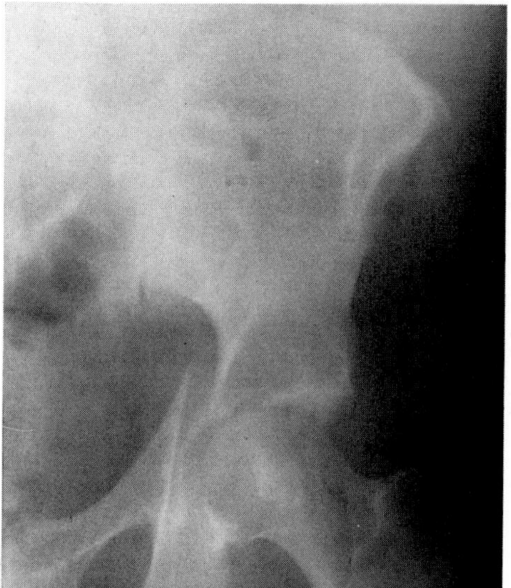

Figure 12-12A: Presenting AP radiograph.

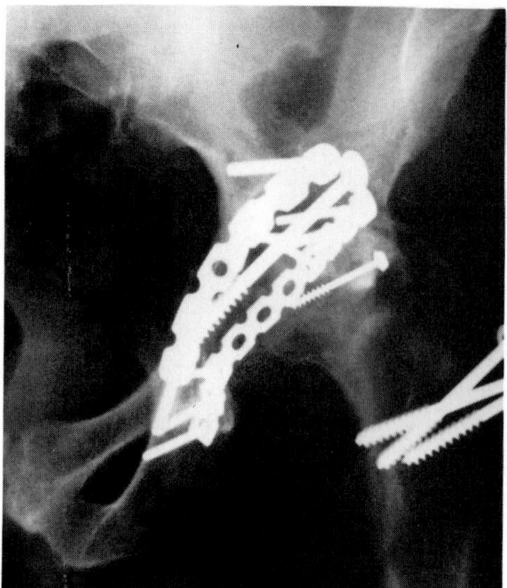

Figure 12-12B: Initial postoperative view.

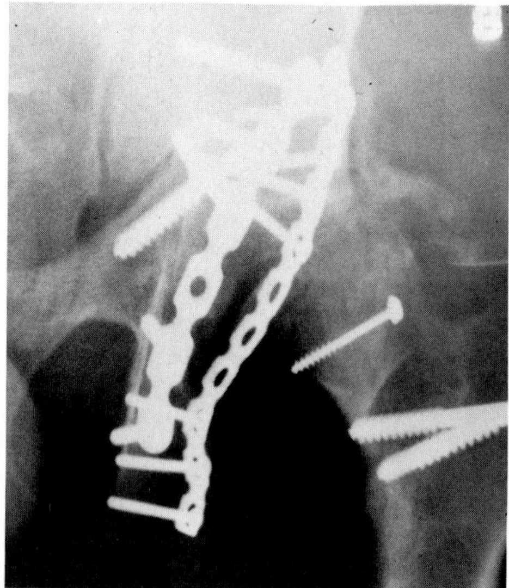

Figure 12-12C: Two months afterwards with recurrent posterior dislocation and displacement of posterior wall fragment.

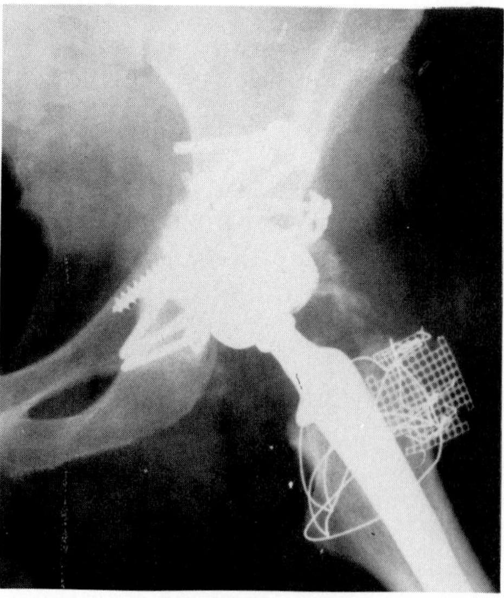

Figure 12-12D: Subsequent postoperative view after total hip replacement.

Figure 12-13: This white 15-year-old girl presented five weeks after a vehicular injury, when she was managed for a left acetabular fracture with skeletal traction. Her mother became concerned about the persistent fixed internal rotational deformity of her left lower extremity. Careful scrutiny of the AP view reveals a somewhat smaller left femoral head than the right. In the iliac oblique view the posterior column disruption is evident, although the posterior subluxation of the femoral head is relatively obscure. In the 3D computed scan, the posterior subluxation of the femoral head locked upon the residual wall was evident, along with the displaced posterior column and sacroiliac joint. In this instance, a large defect in the femoral head was evident.

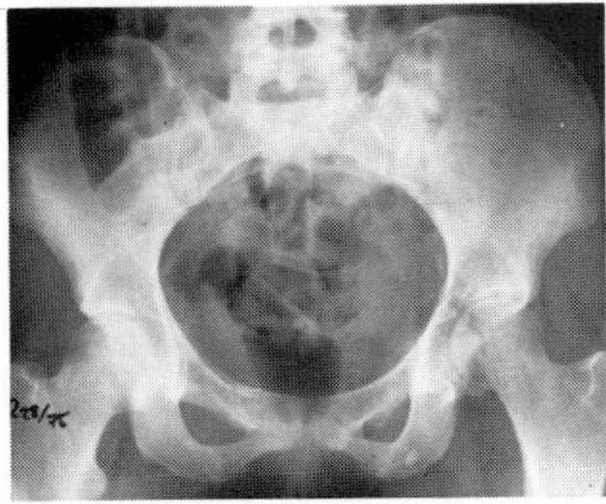

Figure 12-13A: Preoperative AP view.

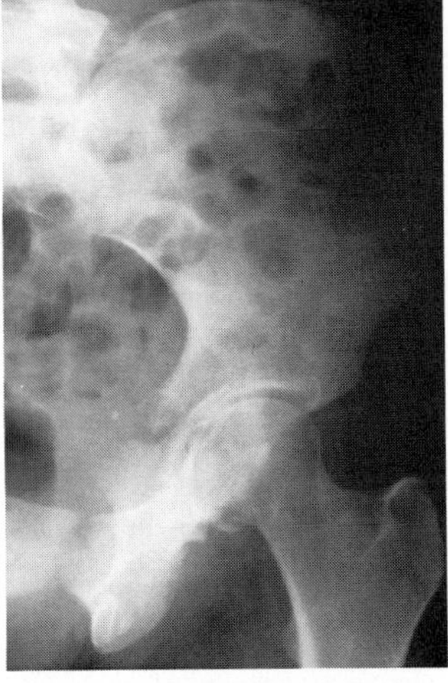

Figure 12-13B: Preoperative iliac oblique view.

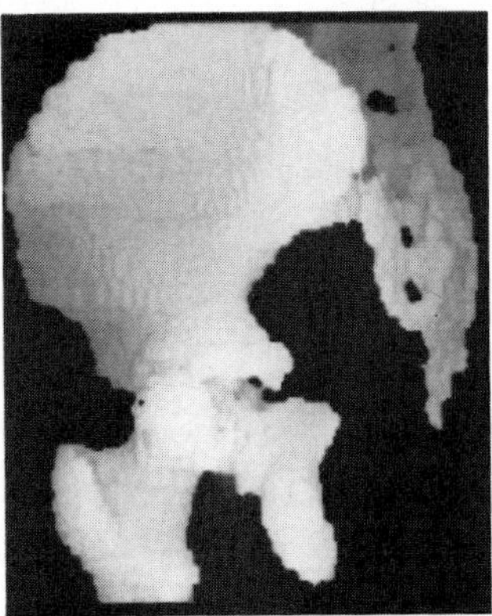

Figure 12-13C: 3D iliac oblique view, posterior column fracture.

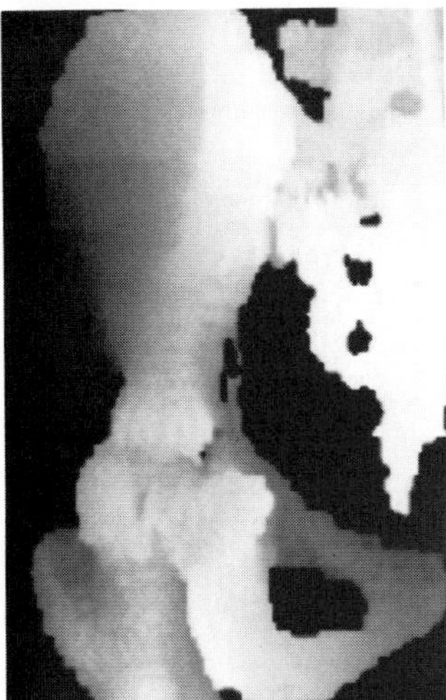

Figure 12-13D: 3D obturator oblique view, subluxed SI joint and femoral head locked on residual posterior wall.

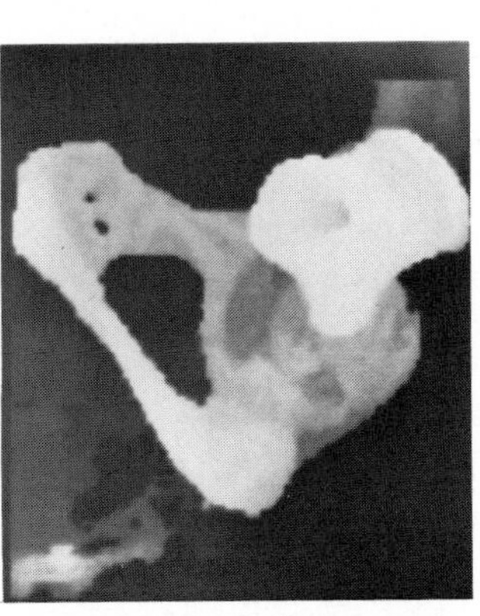

Figure 12-13E: 3D view, posterior displacement of femoral head.

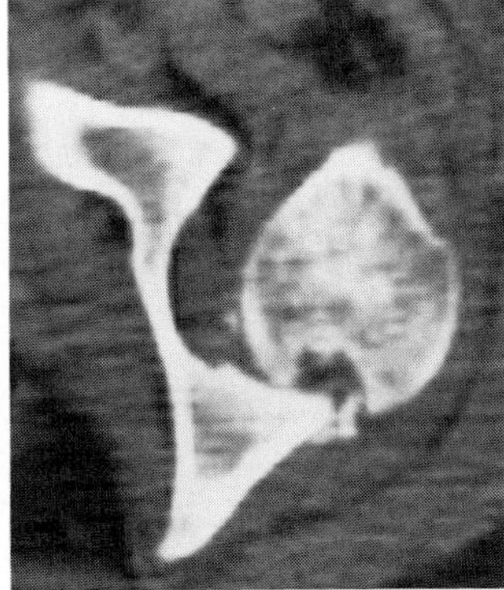

Figure 12-13F: Conventional computed scan, femoral head engaged upon posterior wall.

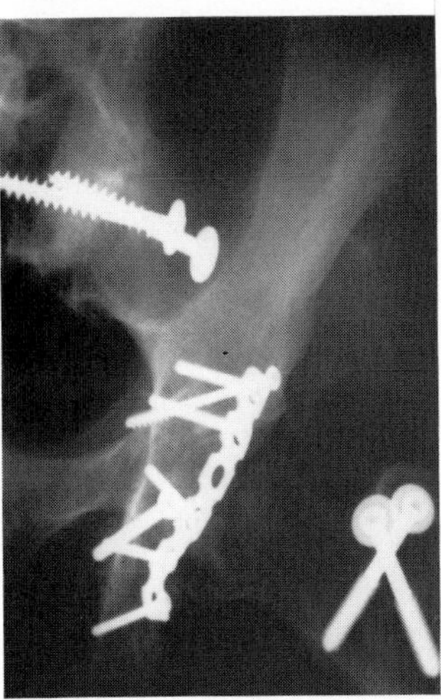

Figure 12-13G: Postoperative view.

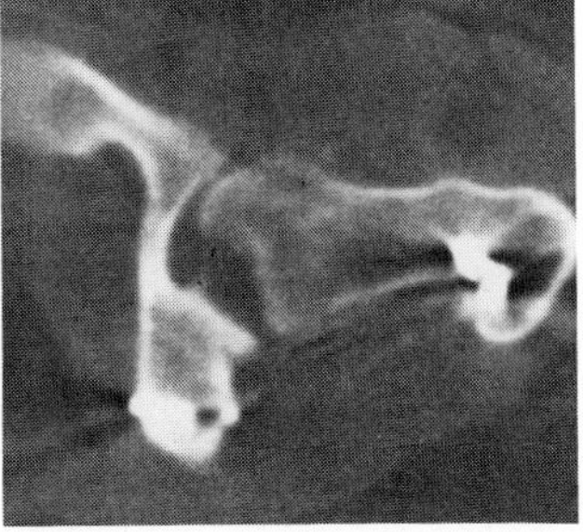

Figure 12-13H: Postoperative computed scan reveals located femoral head with large defect.

Figure 12-14: This white woman of 22 years was involved in a motorcycle accident when her cycle struck a car at high speed. She sustained a right transverse acetabular fracture with bilateral unstable sacroiliac joints and bilateral femoral shaft fractures. The open Grade III left femoral shaft fracture became infected so that an above-knee amputation was required. A persistent Serratia marcescens infection necessitating multiple debridements delayed transfer to our center for pelvic reconstruction until four months after injury. At that time the right femur was healed, but persistent displacement of the pelvis remained. Reconstruction of the acetabulum and sacroiliac joints provided an excellent realignment of the pelvis. Subsequently, she progressed to avascular necrosis of the right femoral head so that an endoprosthetic replacement was required.

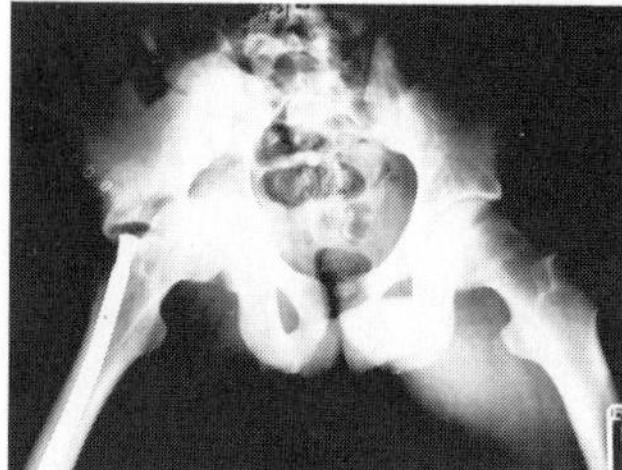

Figure 12-14A: AP view four months after injury.

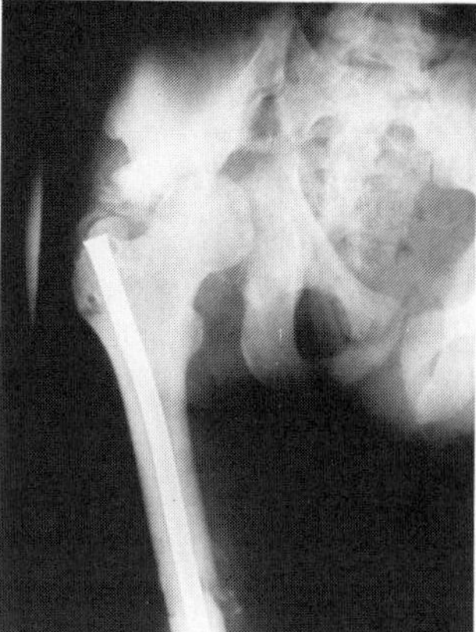

Figure 12-14B: Obturator oblique view four months after injury.

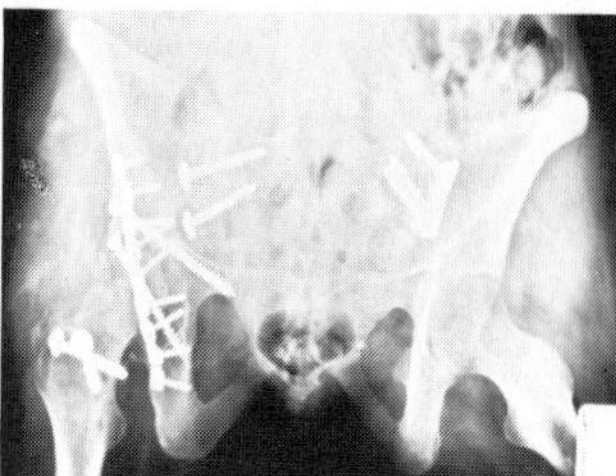

Figure 12-14C: Postoperative outlet view.

planned as an exploration of the apparent pseudoarthrosis with a possible application of autologous iliac bone graft to persistent clefts, or an open reduction and internal fixation to a mobile nonunion. For a symptomatic acetabular nonunion at the time of a late open reduction and stabilization, provisions are made for a possible cementless total hip joint replacement. While the primary goal is the restoration of an anatomical hip joint, in many instances the intraoperative visualization of severe abrasive damage or incongruity of the articular surfaces precludes any realistic likelihood for an effective surgical restoration. Even a careful preoperative scrutiny of a complete radiographic series and a computed scan is notoriously misleading as a guide to the quality of the articular surfaces. In younger adults, for a marginal case, admittedly, an anatomical reconstruction is preferred. But for an adult more than 60 years of age, in a comparable marginal case a cementless total hip replacement is undertaken. The recent introduction of an acetabular component anchored by multiple screws so that the metallic backing can be utilized as a hemispherical plate greatly simplifies the reconstruction (Figure 12-20).

## Late Presentation of a Complex Pelvic and Acetabular Disruption

Generally such a case presents as a patient who

Figure 12-15: This cardiovascular surgeon of 34 years presented six weeks after a vehicular accident that provoked a highly comminuted transverse fracture with a posterior wall fragment and posterior subluxation of her left hip. An anatomical reduction was followed by a full functional recovery and return to work within six months and skiing in 12 months.

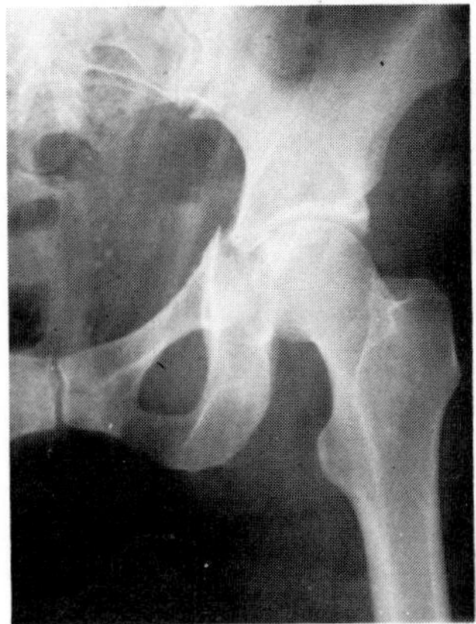

Figure 12-15A: Preoperative AP view.

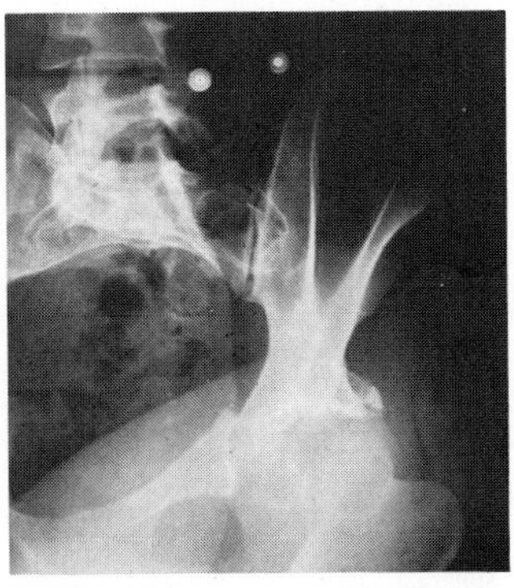

Figure 12-15B: Preoperative obturator oblique view.

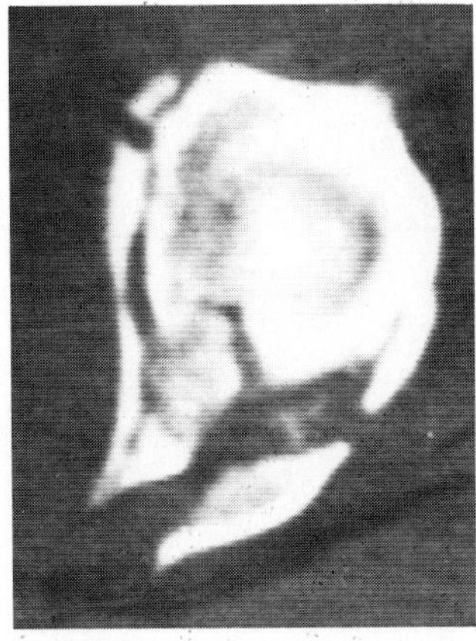

Figure 12-15C: Computed scan of dome.

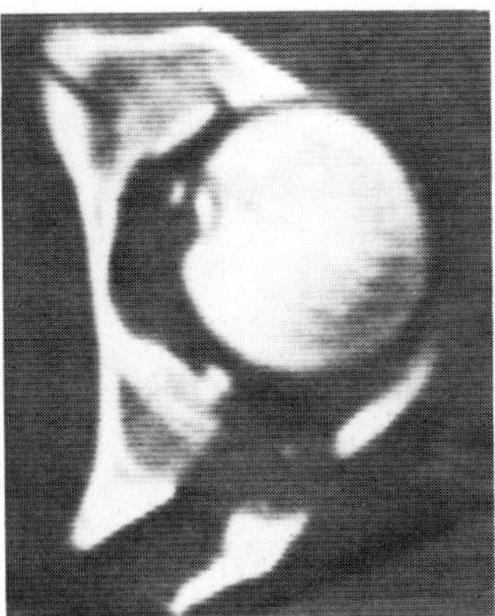

Figure 12-15D: Computed scan of central acetabulum.

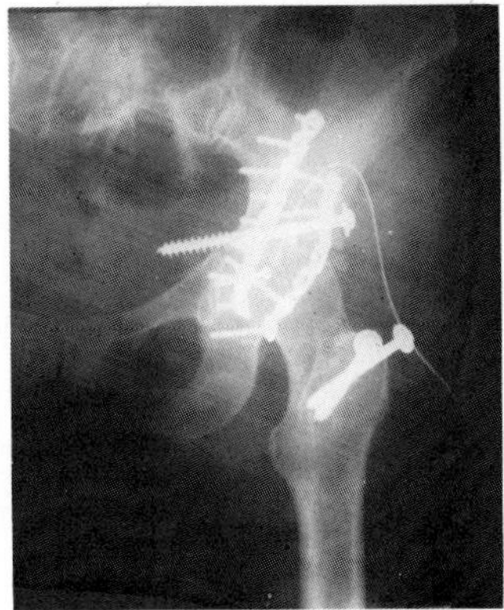

Figure 12-15E: Postoperative AP view. The poorly directed lag screw was removed prior to a subsequent pregnancy and vaginal delivery.

sustained an extraordinary multiple traumatic insult with a prolonged period of management in an intensive care unit and late referral to address an unstable pelvis and acetabular disruption. Usually the acetabular articular surfaces have deteriorated so that ultimately a total hip joint replacement will be indicated. Nevertheless, the deferred reconstruction of the pelvis can be undertaken with a later conversion to a total hip joint replacement if and when the latter procedure is indicated (Figure 12-21). Without the availability of a 3D computed scan, an accurate characterization of such a markedly displaced pelvic injury can be difficult or impossible. The associated iliac disruptions are difficult

Figure 12-16: This obese female with a both-column fracture was referred six weeks after her injury with an ipsilateral sacroiliac dislocation when skeletal traction, including the use of a greater trochanteric pin, failed to provide a satisfactory reduction. Two weeks after insertion the infected greater trochanteric pin was removed for debridement and serial dressing changes. A highly satisfactory, if imperfect, reduction was achieved that has provided a pain-free mobile hip for more than three years.

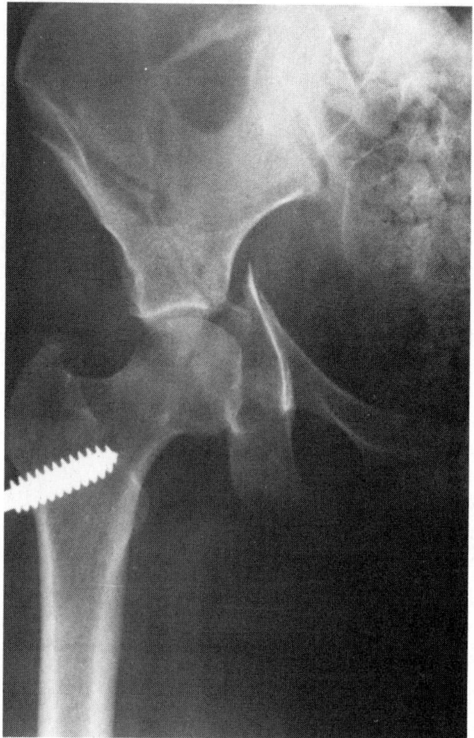

Figure 12-16A: Preoperative AP view.

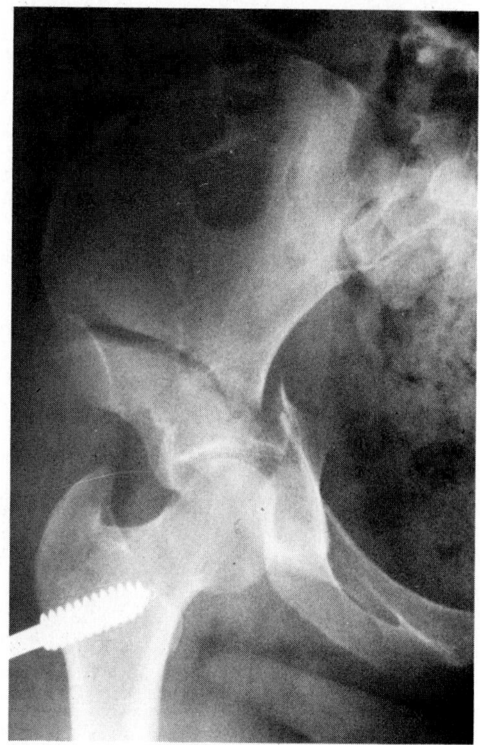

Figure 12-16B: Preoperative inlet view.

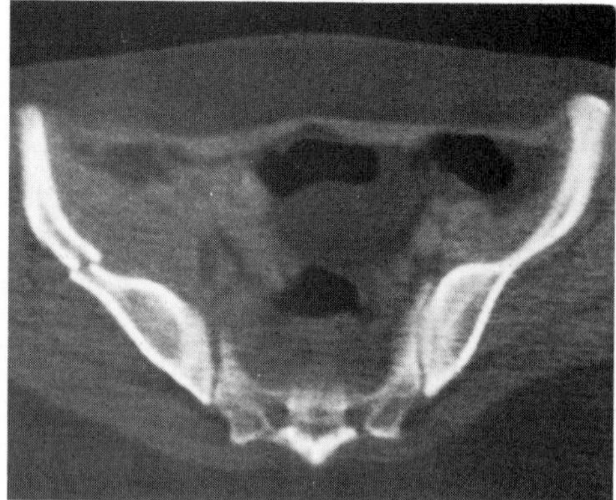

Figure 12-16C: Computed scan of subluxed sacroiliac joint.

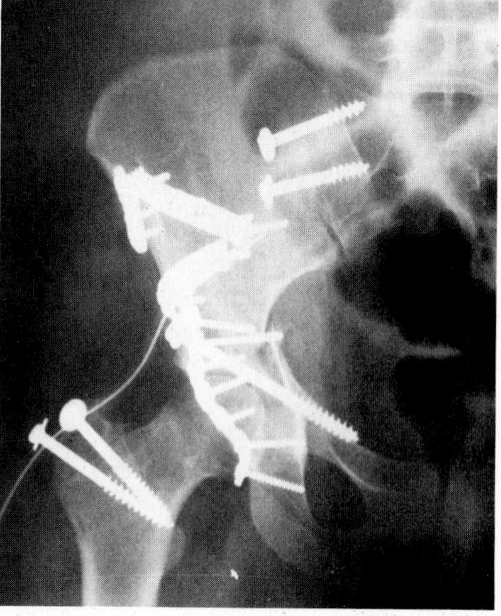

Figure 12-16D: Postoperative AP view.

Figure 12-17: This 43-year-old laborer was involved in an industrial accident with severe multiple traumatic insults including a ruptured thoracic aorta. He presented for pelvic reconstruction about seven weeks later for a both-column fracture with a segmental anterior column disruption. These radiographs were taken two years later when he had returned to work as a laborer walking more than two miles a day. The persistent displacement of the anterior column is typical of such a late reduction.

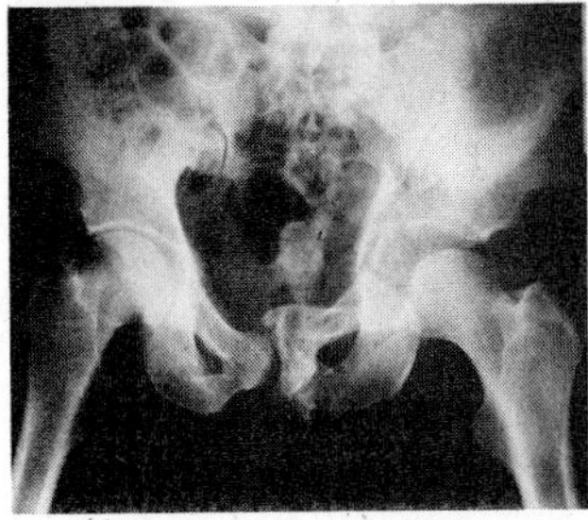

Figure 12-17A: Preoperative AP view.

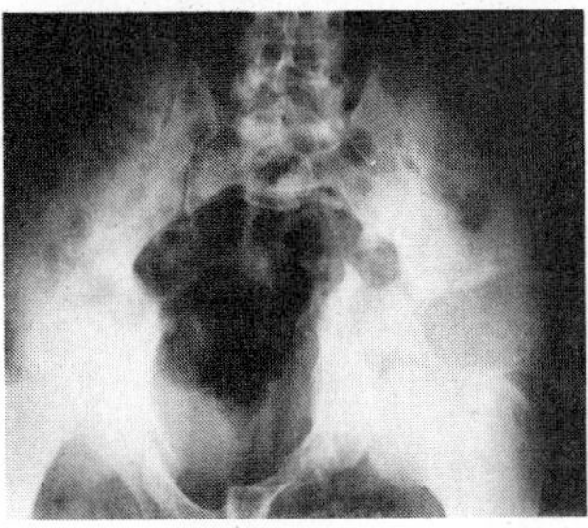

Figure 12-17B: Preoperative inlet view.

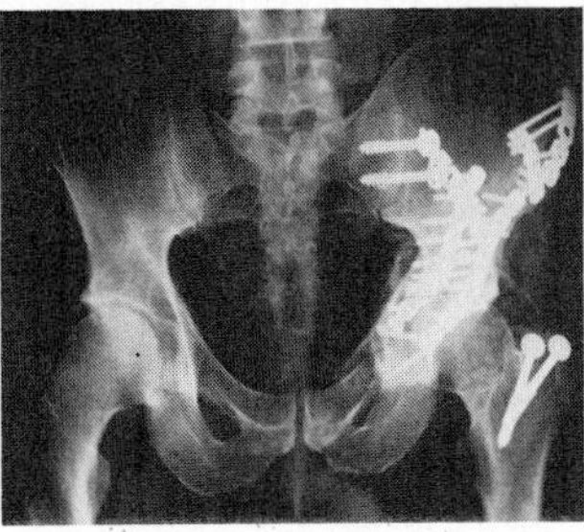

Figure 12-17C: Postoperative AP view.

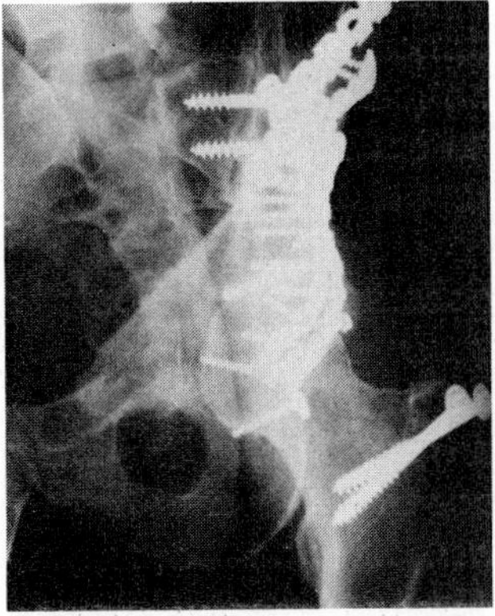

Figure 12-17D: Postoperative obturator oblique view.

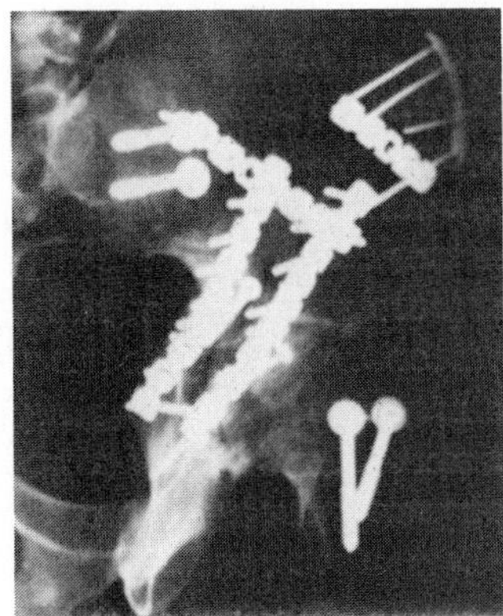

Figure 12-17E: Postoperative iliac oblique view.

to classify as unstable or partly united. Even a careful scrutiny of conventional series of pelvic radiographs and computed scans is notoriously misleading for the distinction of an unstable partly united ilium from a healed innominate bone with persistent clefts between bridges of healing bone. For such late reconstructions, as a general principle, when an acetabular fracture is accompanied by a sacroiliac joint, the ipsilateral sacroiliac disruption is subject to the initial open reduction and internal fixation (Figure 12-22). Subsequently the acetabulum is addressed, followed by the rami and a contralateral pelvic insult. Where an anatomical reconstruction of the hip is precluded by marked deterioration of the articular surfaces, a total hip joint replacement is undertaken. Previously, a Mueller ring was used as a hemispherical plate to permit a reconstruction of the acetabulum with the concomitant application of a cemented acetabular component (Figure 12-23). With the early promising results of the cementless

Figure 12-18: This white woman of 23 years was knocked from a bridge by a passing concrete mixer, to fall from a height of more than 50 feet, sustaining a both-column fracture and other injuries. Initially, through a limited iliofemoral approach two pins were inserted across the iliac fracture. When the wound sloughed, she was transferred to Pittsburgh where about eight weeks later an extended Kocher-Langenbeck approach was employed to correct the substantial persistent posterior displacement. About one year later, ectopic bone was removed to restore about 0-120° of flexion, 30° of internal rotation and abduction.

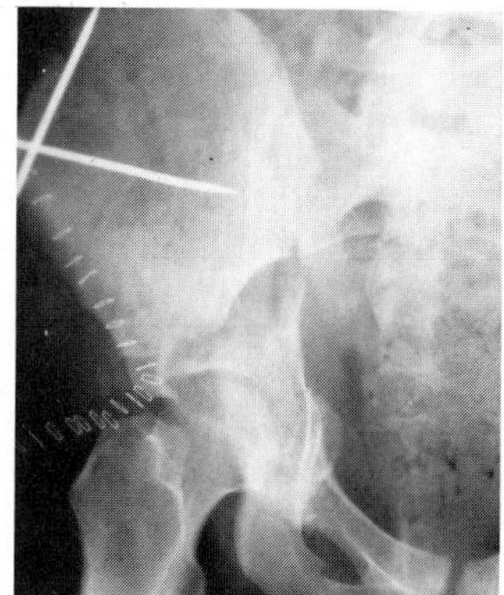

Figure 12-18A: AP view taken eight weeks after injury.

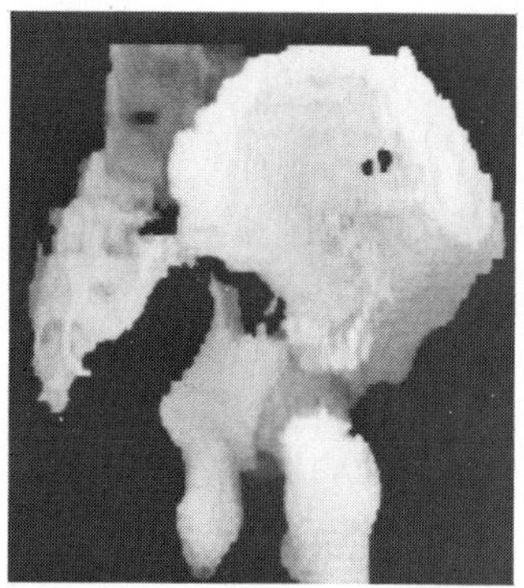

Figure 12-18B: Iliac oblique 3D scan taken at the time of 12-18A.

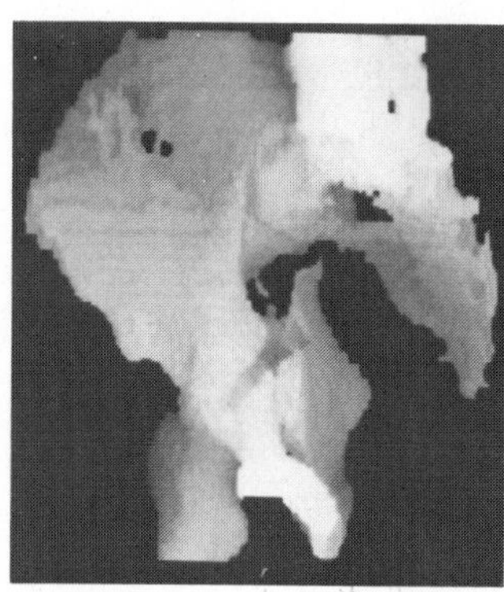

Figure 12-18C: Inner oblique 3D scan taken at the time of 12-18A.

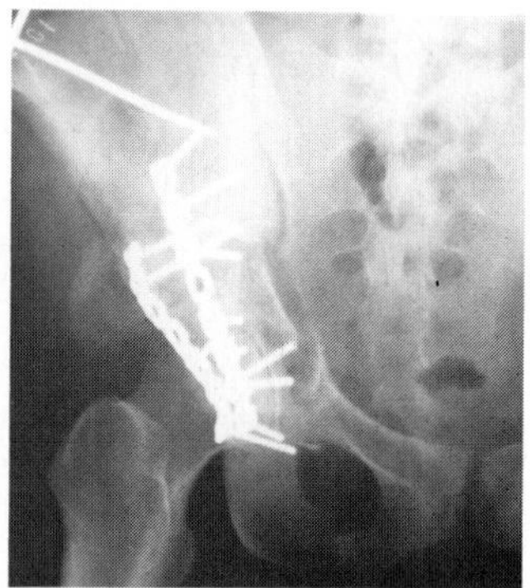

Figure 12-18D: AP view after the second surgical procedure.

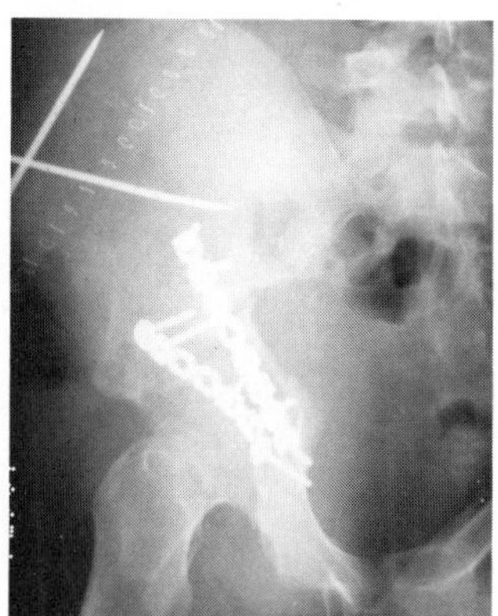

Figure 12-18E: Iliac oblique view after the second surgical procedure.

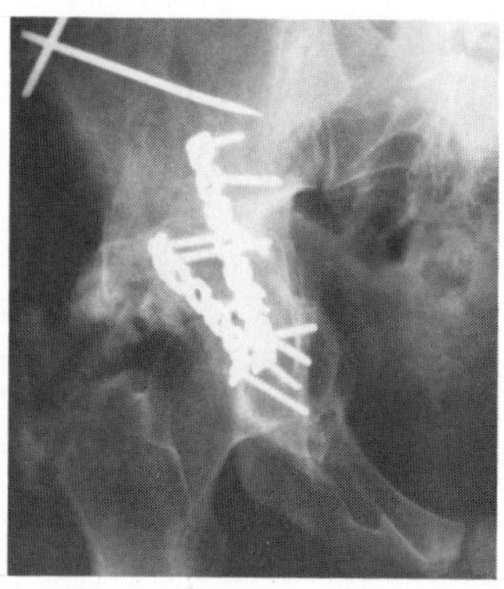

Figure 12-18F: One year afterwards, ectopic bone provoked limitation in flexion, abduction, and internal rotation.

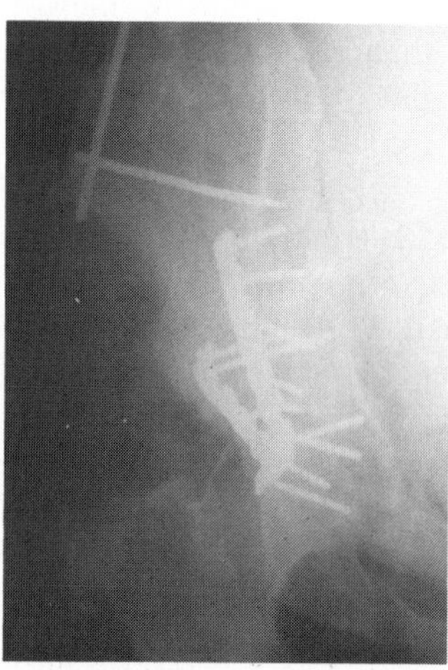

Figure 12-18G: AP view after excision of ectopic bone.

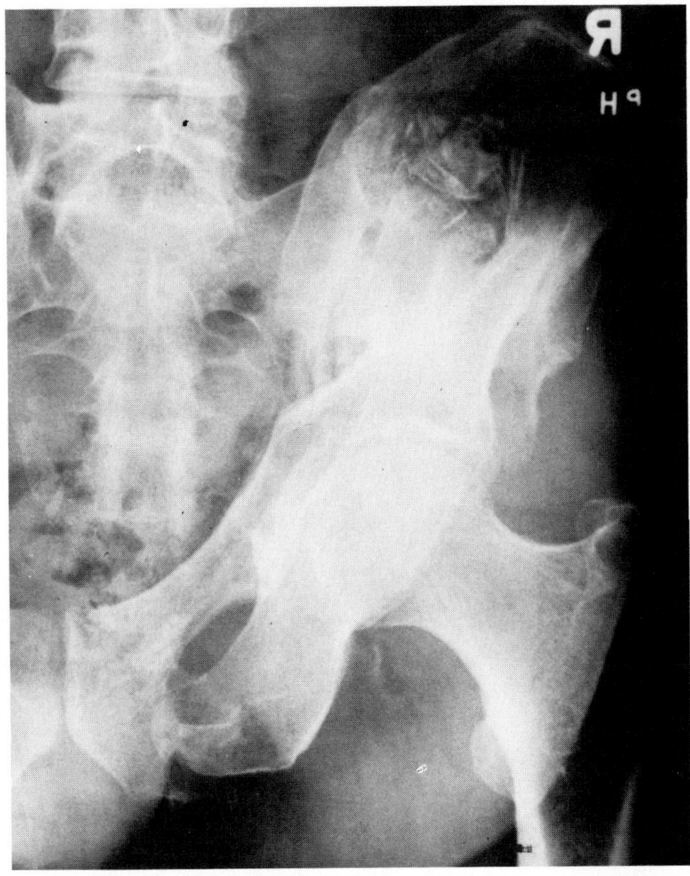


Figure 12-19: This white man of 50 years was struck by lightning while standing on top of a tall ladder. He sustained a highly comminuted both-column fracture, which was treated by skeletal traction. Six months later he continued to complain of persistent iliac pain for which an exploration was undertaken. The stable partial union was documented at that time when the defects were obliterated with autologous iliac crest bone graft. A scrutiny of multiple radiographic views and computed scans failed to provide an accurate characterization of the degree of osseous healing.

acetabular component anchored by resort to supplementary screws, the use of cement is limited to those instances of severe osteoporosis where effective screw fixation cannot be undertaken.

## Nonunion

While the distinction between a late presentation and a pelvic nonunion is a continuous gradation, for the purposes of this discussion a nonunion is defined as a fracture that persists more than six months after the time of the initial injury. At that time generally a marked soft tissue contracture accompanies the persistent deformity. Frequently, substantial osteoporosis associated with immobilization and disuse further complicates the surgical attempt to correct a persistent deformity. While the elimination of a large gap at the site of a nonunion/malunion has been highly successful as with late presentation, the correction of a concomitant rotational displacement has been disappointing.

Figure 12-20: This 28-year-old laborer on an oil rig sustained a fall from more than 100 feet to provoke a complex pelvic fracture with bilateral acetabular fractures and a dislocation of the right sacroiliac joint. His initial radiograph taken through a pneumatic pressure garment shows relatively minor pelvic displacement that markedly increased when he was maintained in skeletal traction for the next six weeks. He presented to our clinic about four months after his injury when he elected to defer surgical reconstruction. Two months later, when he experienced left hip pain, he represented for surgical reconstruction when a complete loss of articular cartilage in the hip joint was observed. A cementless Harris-Galante total hip joint replacement was undertaken and he returned to work two months later.

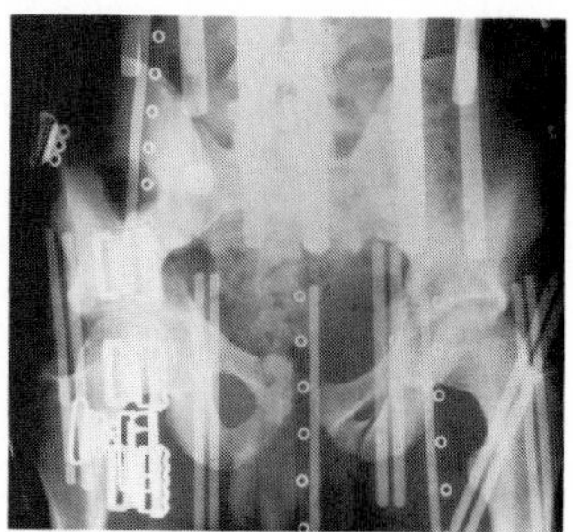

Figure 12-20A: Initial posttraumatic view in MAST suit.

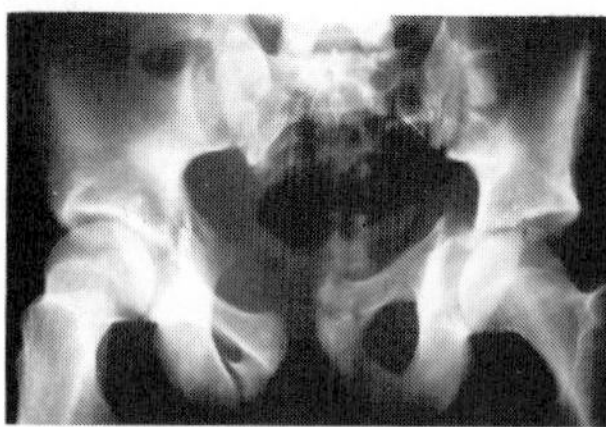

Figure 12-20B: Six weeks after injury in skeletal traction.

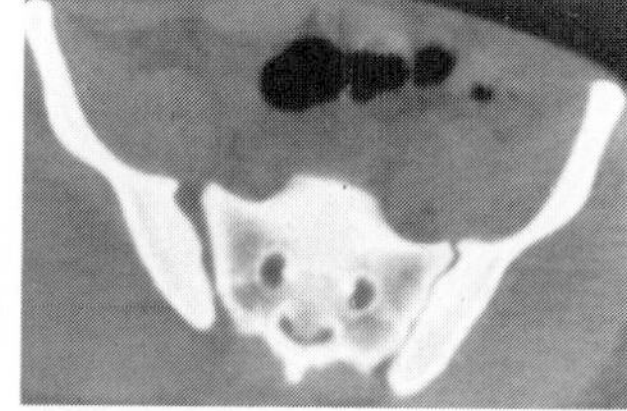

Figure 12-20C: Posttraumatic computed scan indicative of a dislocated SI joint.

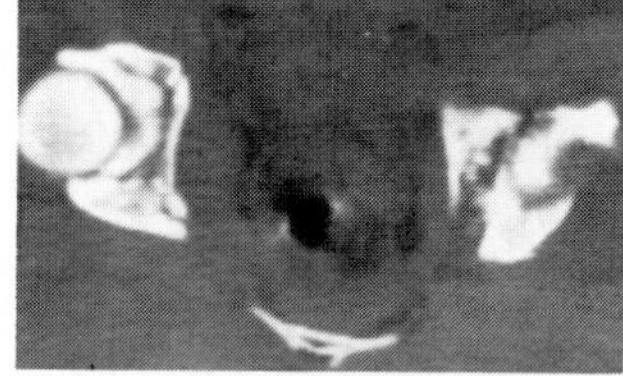

Figure 12-20D: Posttraumatic computed scan, comminuted bilateral acetabular domes.

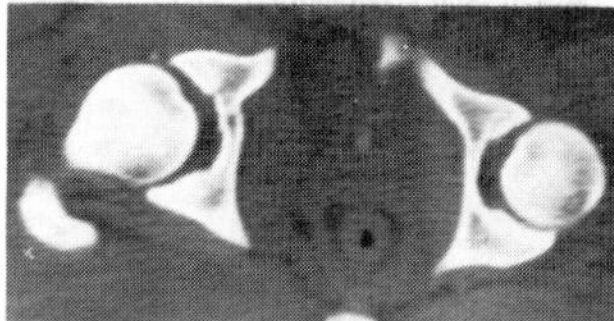

Figure 12-20E: Posttraumatic computed scan shows relatively intact quadrilateral surfaces.

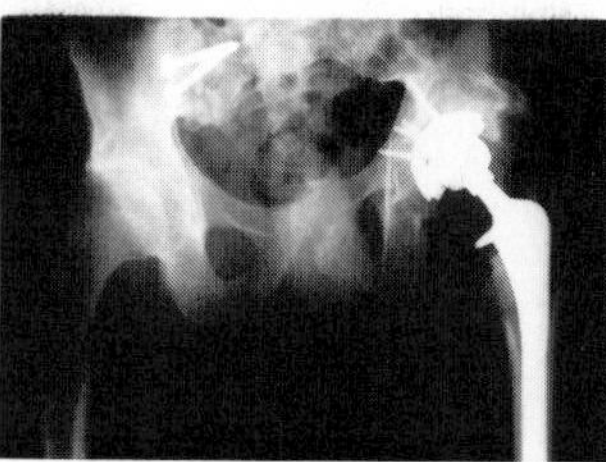

Figure 12-20F: Postoperative view after H-G THR and lag screw fixation of right SI joint.

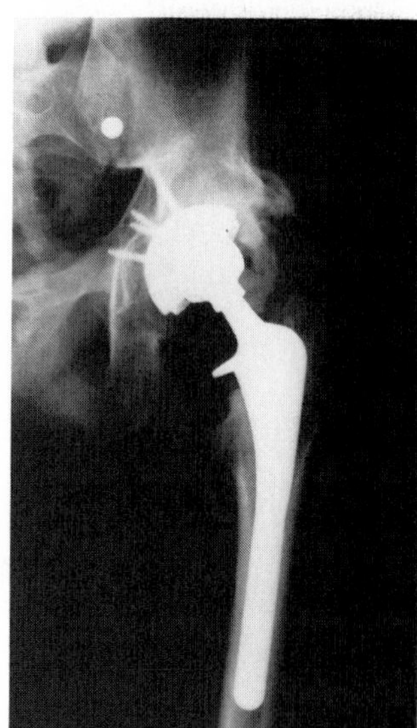

Figure 12-20G: Six months after total hip joint replacement.

Figure 12-21: This black man of 28 years was severely crushed in an industrial accident. He presented to us about 18 months later with severe bilateral pelvic pain and instability. In the subsequent reconstructive procedure, the bilateral iliac nonunions and the nonunion-malunion of the left both-column fracture were reconstructed. The patient did well for about one year, when he developed recurrent left hip pain. At that time, a total hip joint replacement with a Mueller ring was undertaken. Since then the patient has returned to gainful employment as a laborer.

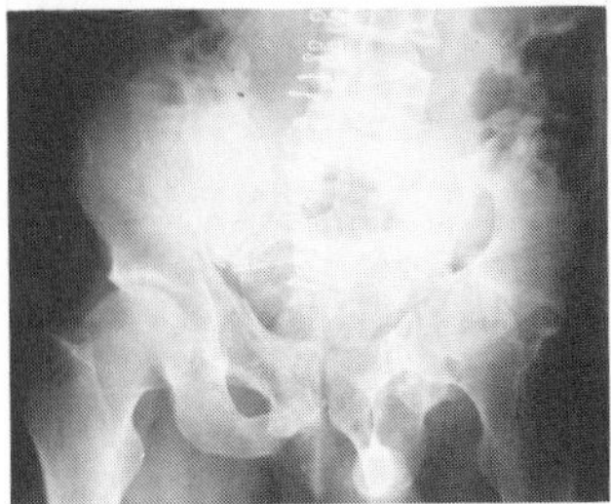

Figure 12-21A: Preoperative AP view.

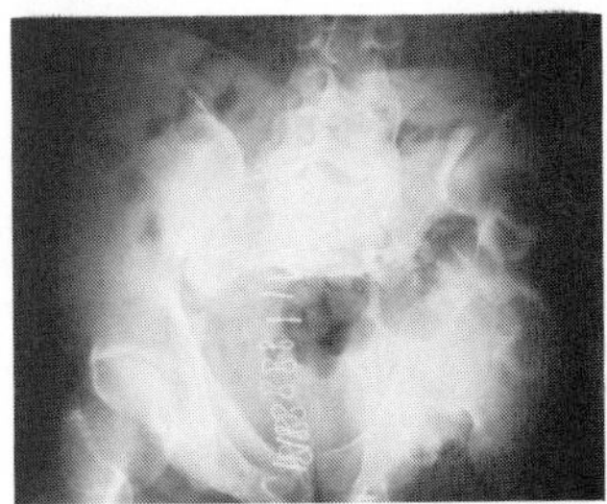

Figure 12-21B: Preoperative inlet view.

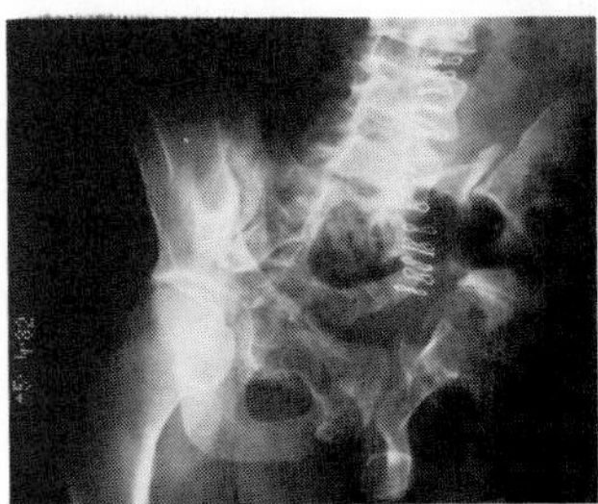

Figure 12-21C: Preoperative iliac oblique view.

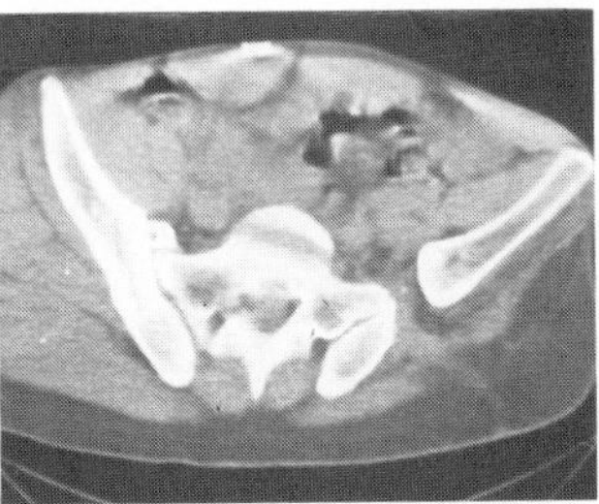

Figure 12-21D: Preoperative computed scan through the SI joints.

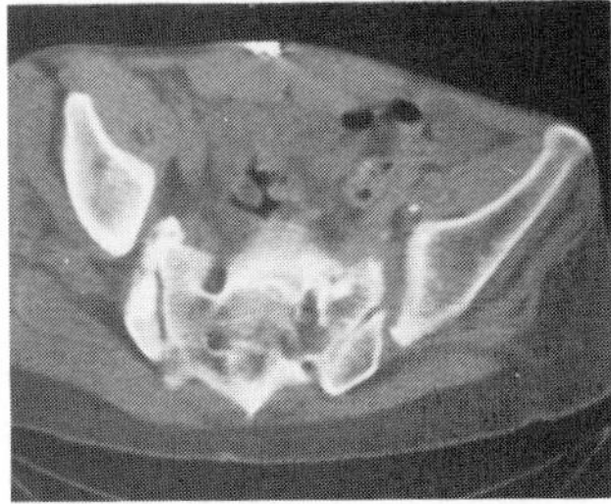

Figure 12-21E: Preoperative computed scan through the sacrum.

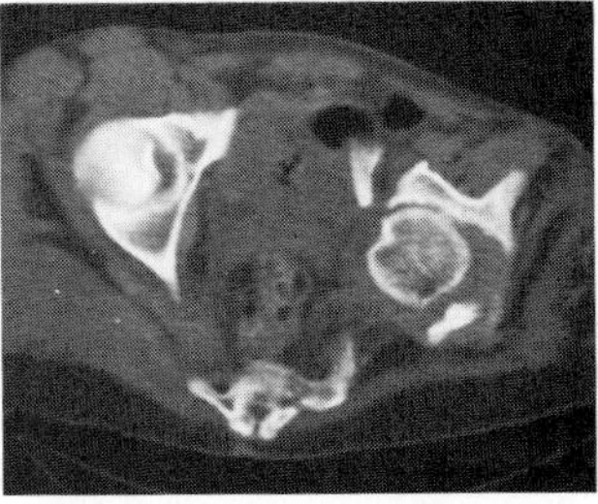

Figure 12-21F: Preoperative computed scan through the hip joints.

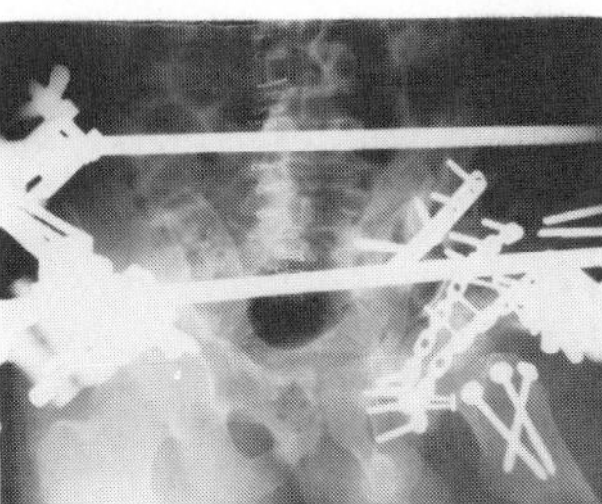

Figure 12-21G: Initial postoperative AP view with supplementary external frame.

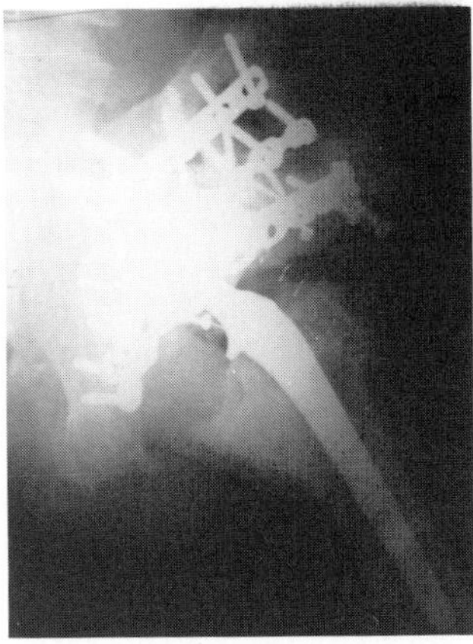

Figure 12-21H: After secondary total hip joint replacement.

Figure 12-22: This male of 45 years presented one year after a vehicular accident with a nonunion-malunion of his left sacroiliac joint, a mobile diastasis, and a transverse with posterior wall acetabular disruption. At the time of the surgical reconstruction, the femoral head was relatively spared and possessed considerable intact articular cartilage. While the procedure provided a restoration of pelvic stability, the need for a subsequent arthroplasty of the hip joint is anticipated.

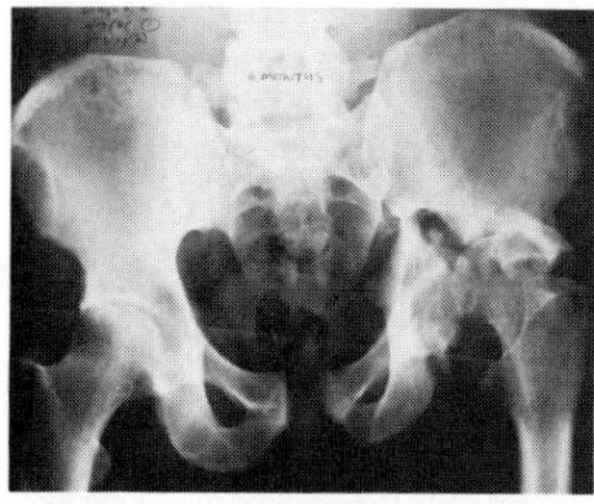

Figure 12-22A: Preoperative AP view.

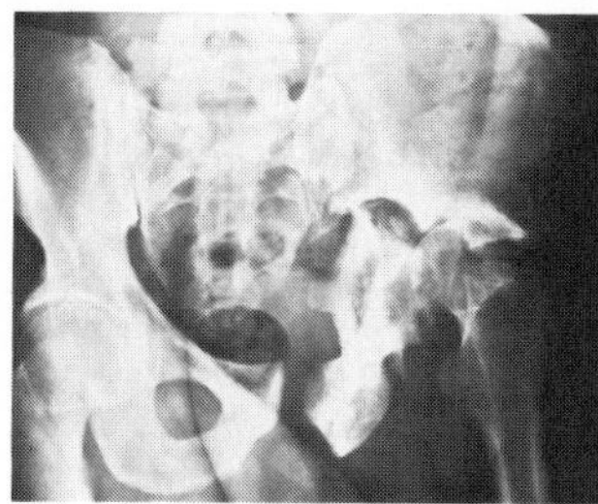

Figure 12-22B: Preoperative iliac oblique view.

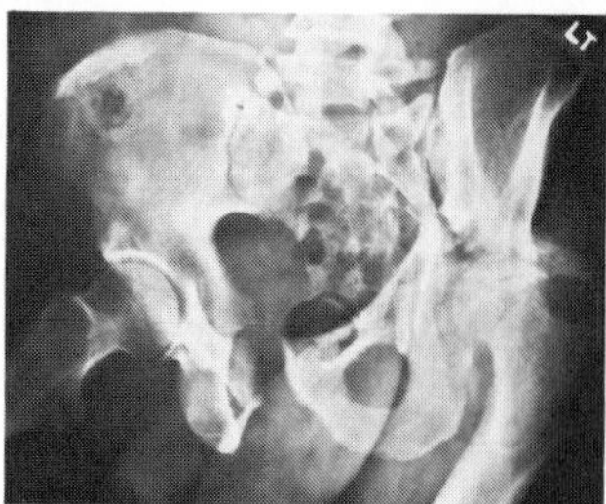

Figure 12-22C: Preoperative obturator oblique view.

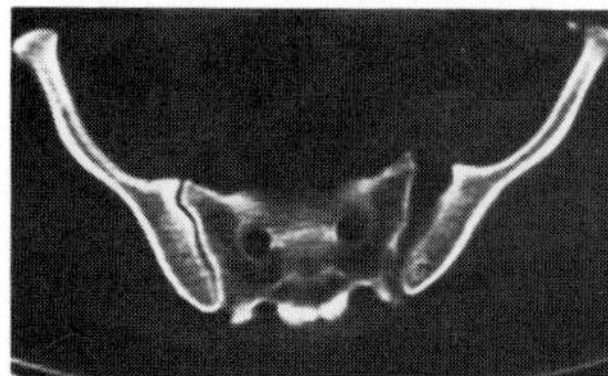

Figure 12-22D: Preoperative computed scan through dislocated SI joint.

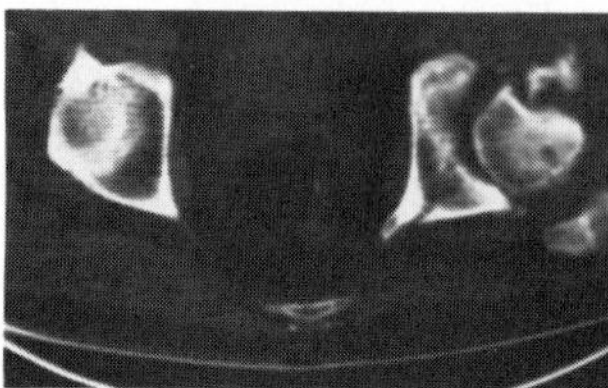

Figure 12-22E: Preoperative computed scan through hip joint.

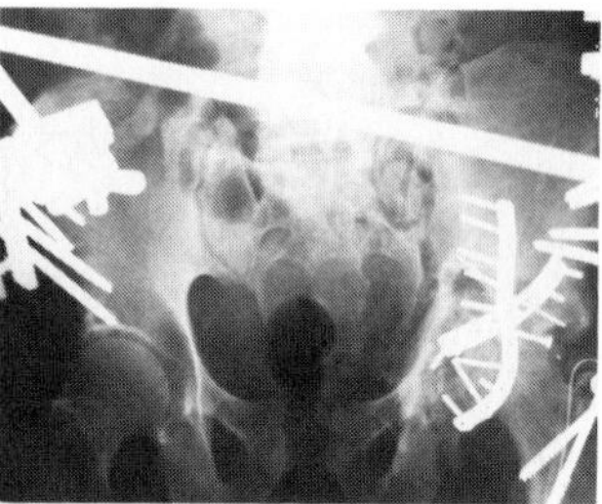

Figure 12-22F: Initial postoperative AP view.

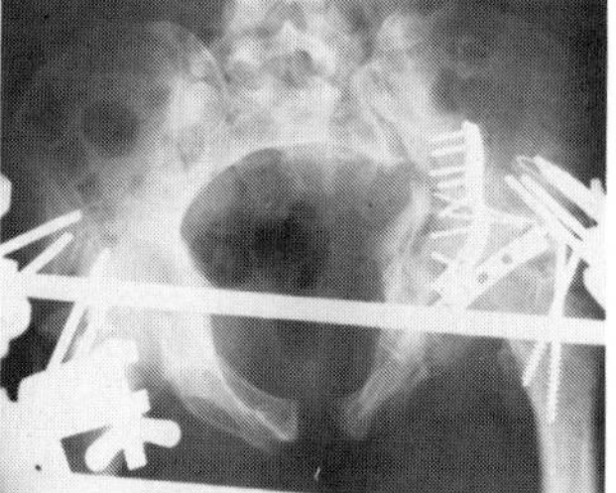

Figure 12-22G: Initial postoperative inlet view.

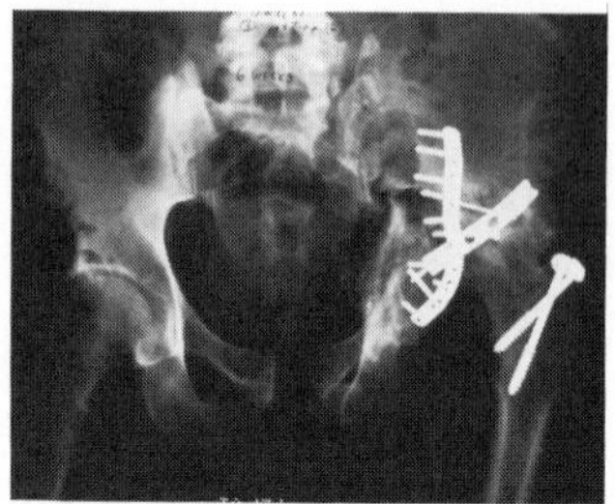

Figure 12-22H: Six weeks afterwards, when the external frame is removed.

## Pelvic Nonunion

Of the broad spectrum of symptomatic pelvic nonunions, probably the most frequently encountered pattern is a painful subluxed or dislocated sacroiliac joint accompanied by a diastasis of the symphysis pubis or multiple ramus fractures. Despite the presence of unstable anterior and posterior disruptions, most of the patients with a late presentation complain of posterior pain; only about 20% complain of a painful diastasis or nonunion of a ramus. Whether the painful sacroiliac joint is attributable to a nonunion or to traumatic

Figure 12-23: In a vehicular accident, this diabetic man of 58 years sustained a right sacroiliac dislocation, diastasis, and left transverse with posterior wall fracture, for which he was managed with external fixation and skeletal traction. One year later, at the time of presentation to our center, persistent mobile nonunions of all the disrupted sites remained with traumatic arthritis of the hip. Open reduction and internal fixation was undertaken with the use of a Mueller ring as a "hemispherical plate" along with a total hip joint replacement.

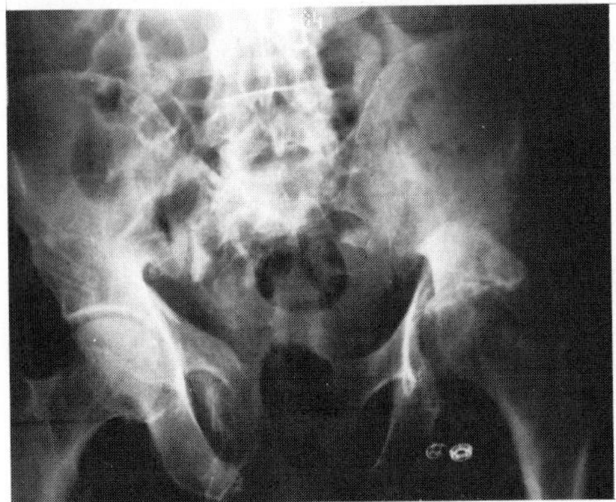

Figure 12-23A: Preoperative AP view.

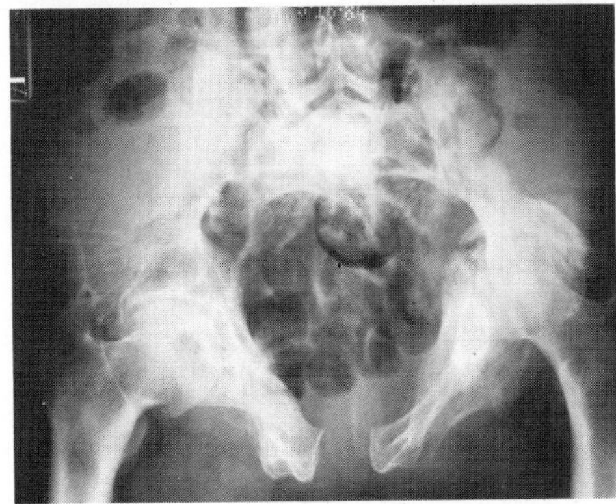

Figure 12-23B: Preoperative inlet view.

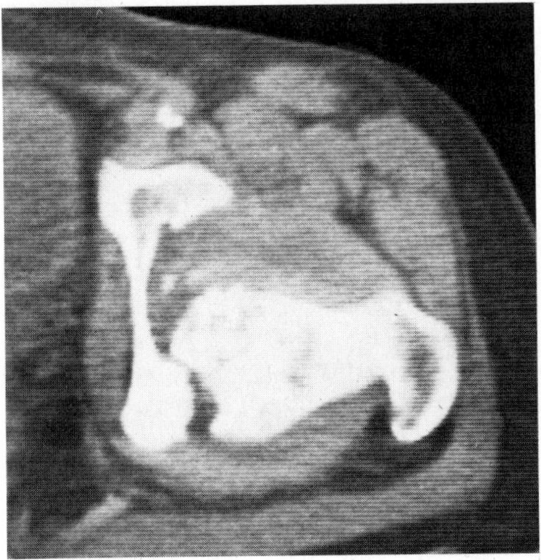

Figure 12-23C: Preoperative computed scan with posterior subluxation of the femoral head.

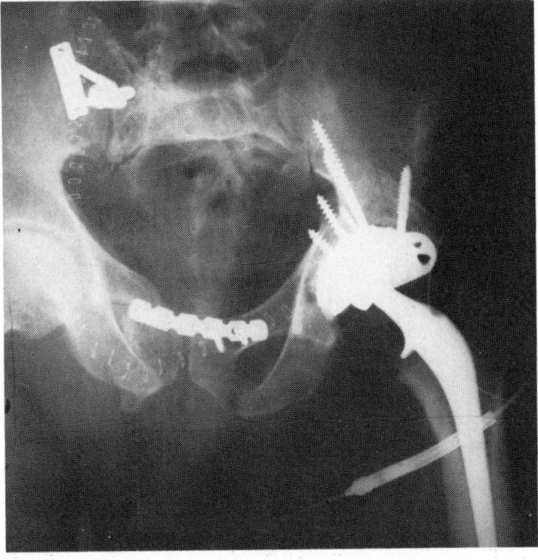

Figure 12-23D: Postoperative view.

arthritis is irrelevant from the therapeutic point of view. When the anterior lesion is a ramus fracture that has united or a minimally displaced symphysis, then a fusion of the symptomatic sacroiliac joint suffices (Figure 12-24). Where the anterior and posterior disruption through the sacroiliac joint is accompanied by a diastasis of the symphysis pubis, even though one site is asymptomatic, unless a fusion of both sites is undertaken the likelihood for a persistent painful failed fusion is substantial (Figure 12-25). Stabilization of both the symptomatic and asymptomatic sites, therefore, is indicated. Upon a debridement of the sacroiliac joint, conventional lag screw fixation is undertaken, along with plate fixation of the

Figure 12-24:This white woman of 19 years presented one year after a vehicular accident with a painful left sacroiliac joint. Her right rami fractures and symphysis were minimally displaced and asymptomatic. Six months after the fusion of her sacroiliac joint she became a cheerleader at her university.

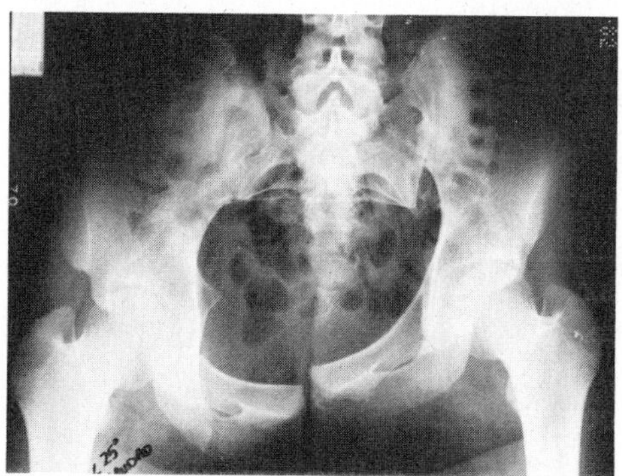

Figure 12-24A: Preoperative AP view.

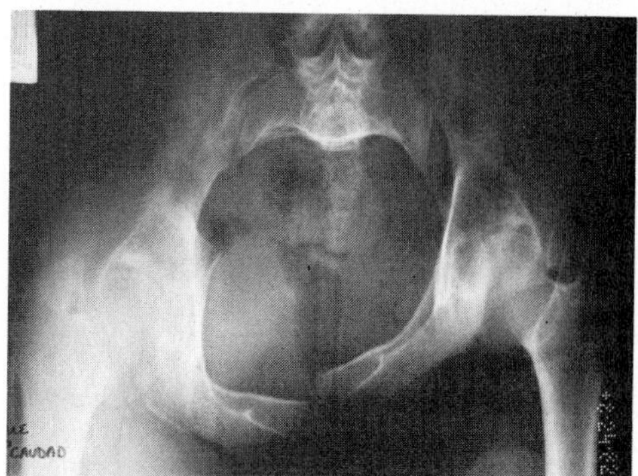

Figure 12-24B: Preoperative inlet view.

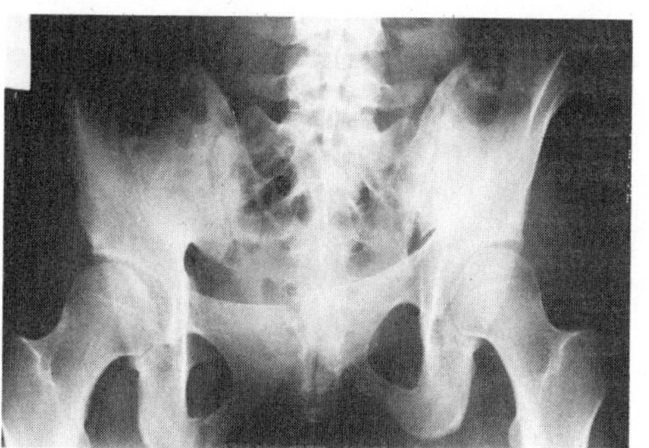

Figure 12-24C: Preoperative outlet view.

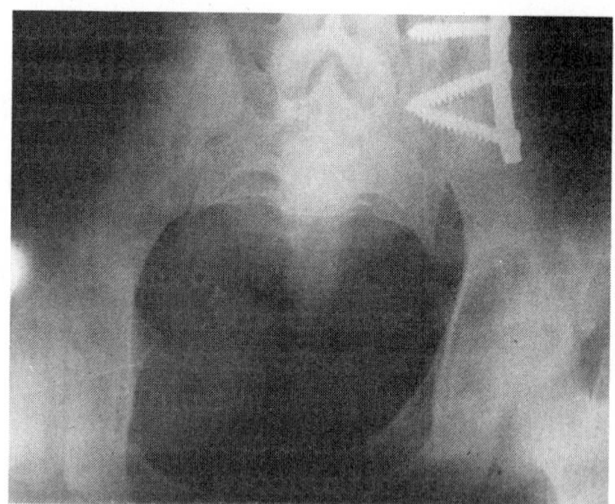

Figure 12-24D: Inlet view, one year postoperative.

Figure 12-25: This white man of 26 years presented one year after a left sacroiliac dislocation and diastasis with persistent sacroiliac pain. At that time a sacroiliac fusion was undertaken, which failed to provide relief of discomfort. Ultimately, a revision of the sacroiliac fixation combined with stabilization of the symphysis pubis was needed.

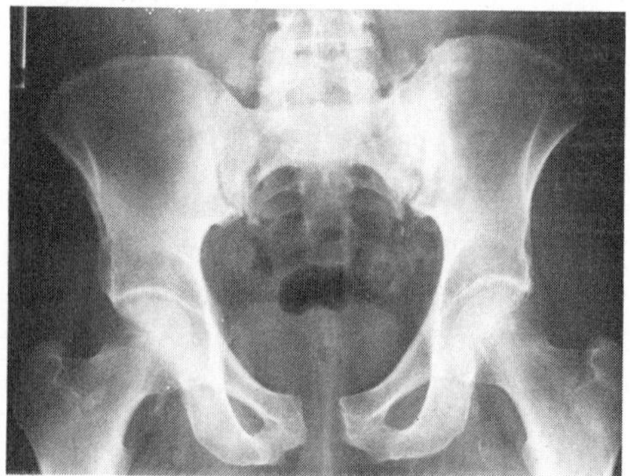

Figure 12-25A: Preoperative AP view.

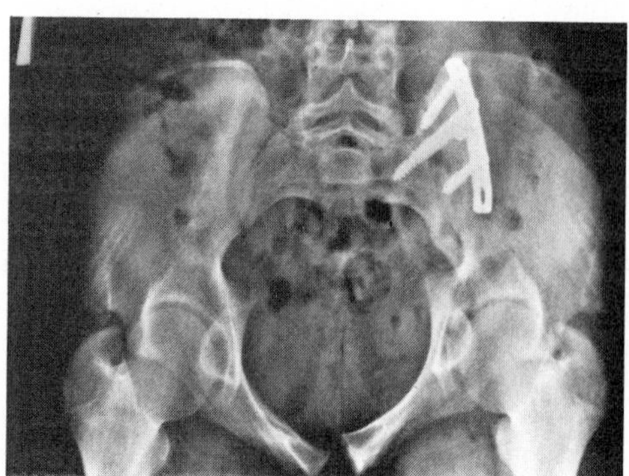

Figure 12-25B: Postoperative inlet view one year after failed SI joint fusion.

Figure 12-26: This 46-year-old accountant presented two years after a motorcycle accident with an unstable left hemipelvis and a wide diastasis. At the time of surgical reconstruction, the bladder was carefully moved from the diastasis prior to plate fixation.

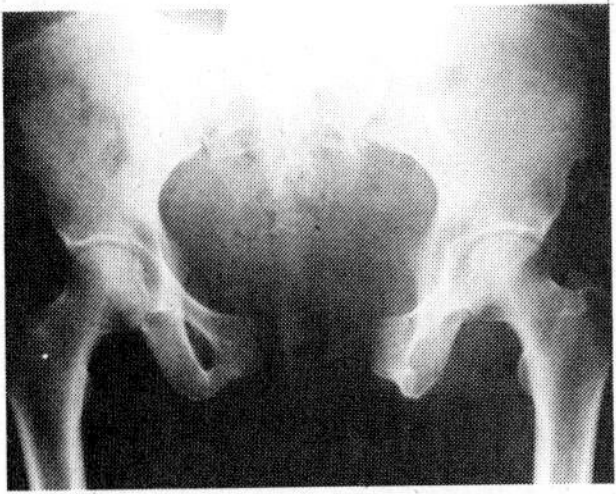
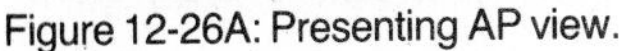

Figure 12-26A: Presenting AP view.

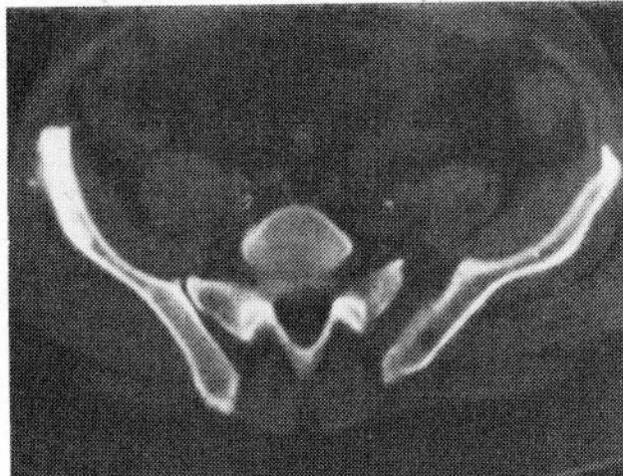

Figure 12-26B: Computed scan with dislocation of left SI joint.

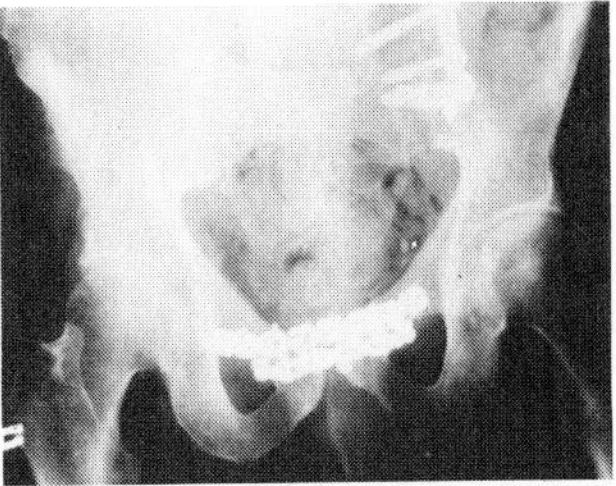

Figure 12-26C: Postoperative view one year afterwards.

symphysis. In the presence of a wide diastasis with a nonunion of the sacroiliac joint, frequently the urinary bladder is scarred between the opposing rami (Figure 12-26). The first surgical exposure is directed toward the symphysis so that the bladder can be carefully repositioned posterior to the rami. Unless the orthopaedic surgeon is knowledgeable in manipulation of the bladder, collaboration with a urologist is advisable. Prior to the procedure, a Foley catheter is inserted to facilitate identification of the urethra. While the opposing rami are approximated, a finger is used to palpate the position of the urethra and to ensure that it is not trapped within the symphysis. A six-hole 3.5mm reconstruction plate is applied to the superior surface of the superior pubic rami. In the presence of osteoporosis either a 4.5mm plate is used or, in more severe cases, a second plate is applied across the anterior surface of the symphysis. For the second stage, with the patient in a lateral to a semi-prone position, the sacroiliac joint is approached through the conventional posterior longitudinal incision. The joint is thoroughly debrided and lag screws are inserted through the lateral ilium into the ala of the sacrum and the first sacral body. With the potential for a persistent rotational malalignment of the unstable hemipelvis and compromised contact of the sacrum or the ilium, each drill bit is inserted cautiously through the ilium into the sacrum. As the drill bit courses across the sacroiliac joint, it is palpated by a finger inserted into the posterior aspect of the joint. This method permits a verification of the appropriate orientation of the drill hole with its entry into the sacrum.

In the presence of a nonunion of the sacroiliac joint and associated ipsilateral ramus disruptions, lag screw fixation of the superior pubic ramus accompanies a comparable lag screw fixation of the sacroiliac joint (Figure 12-27). The superior or iliac portion of an iliofemoral incision is suitable for such an exposure, whereupon the glutei, external oblique, and iliopsoas muscles are elevated from the outer and inner tables of the ilium respectively. The fixation of the superior pubic ramus is undertaken by the use of a cannulated screw. Once a suitable entry site is identified on the lateral ilium adjacent to the superior gluteal ridge, the guide wire for the screw is inserted under image intensification. A lengthy screw is inserted over the guide wire, and conventional lag screw fixation of the sacroiliac joint is undertaken. In the presence of bilateral sacroiliac nonunions and a diastasis, plate fixation of the symphysis is accompanied by use of the Double Cobra plate to immobilize both sacroiliac joints (Figure 12-28).

When a posterior iliac nonunion accompanies multiple ramus fractures, the former problem can be managed with lag screws inserted into the posterior iliac crest (Figure 12-1). This is one example of a type of sacroiliac disruption where a fusion of the sacroiliac joint is unnecessary. Theoretically, a sacral nonunion would not require immobilization of the sacroiliac joints (Figure 12-29). When the Double Cobra or comparable posterior plate is used, however, the sacroiliac joints are immobilized, although they are not formally fused. To date no problems associated with immobilization of both sacroiliac joints have been identified.

On four occasions the Double Cobra plate was used as the only method of surgical stabilization for a pelvic nonunion malunion. In three such cases a successful outcome ensued (Figure 12-29). In one other case (a woman of 35 years with painful mobile nonunions of a right-sided sacral fracture and contralateral ramus fractures), the application of a Double Cobra plate with a fusion of the posterior nonunion failed to provide relief of the pain and mobility of the anterior nonunion (Figure 12-30). In a second operation the superior pubic ramus was immobilized with a plate, which culminated in a stable, painfree outcome. Currently, rigorous immobilization of both the posterior and anterior nonunion sites is recommended.

Certain pelvic nonunions are associated with marked pelvic distortion and bone loss. For example, a woman of 32 years (Figure 12-31) underwent a resection of her right sacroiliac joint for a chondrosarcoma that culminated in an unstable pelvic nonunion with posterior pain. Three years after her initial resection and at the time of the pelvic reconstruction, the patient had no evidence of recurrent tumor. An exact replica of her pelvis was prepared by the use of a CAD/CAM technique based upon a computed scan of her pelvis (Contour Medical Systems, Inc., Mountain View, California). The model provided a way to obtain measurements of the

Figure 12-27: This nonunion of the left superior pubic ramus and left-sided sacral fracture presented 18 months after injury in a man of 41 years.

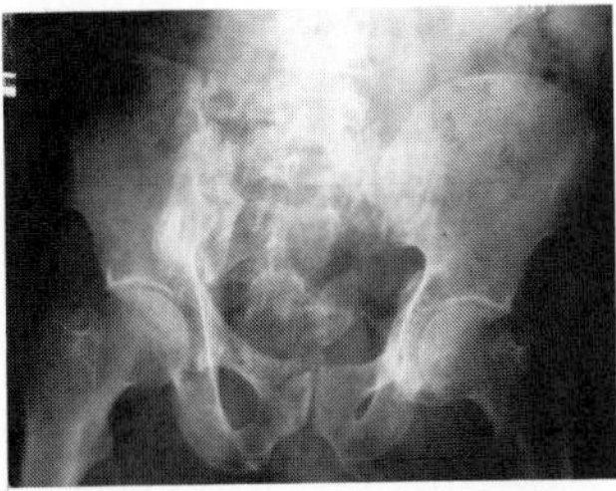

Figure 12-27A: Presenting AP radiograph.

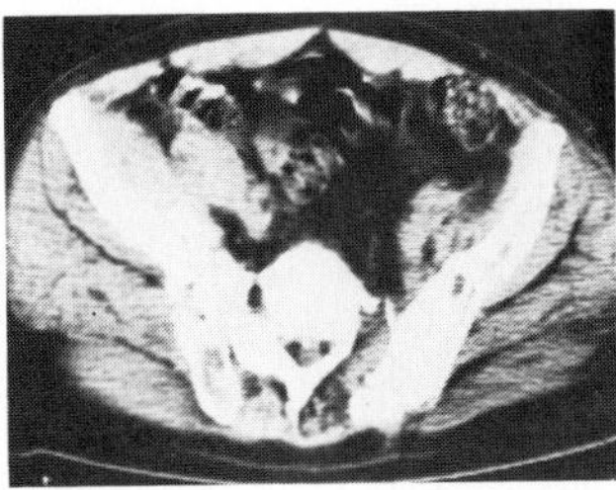

Figure 12-27B: Computed scan through sacral nonunion.

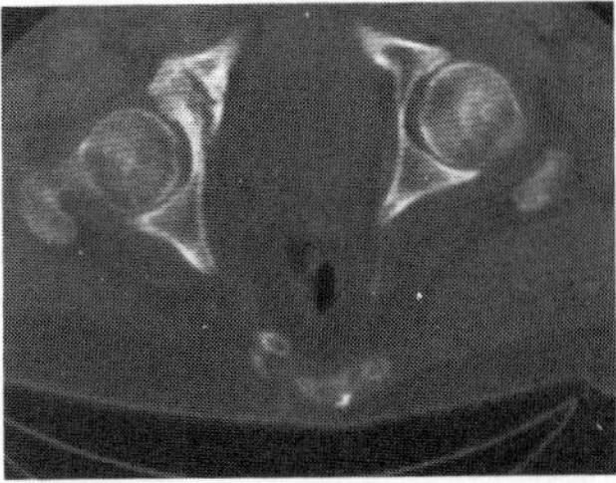

Figure 12-27C: Computed scan through nonunion of superior ramus.

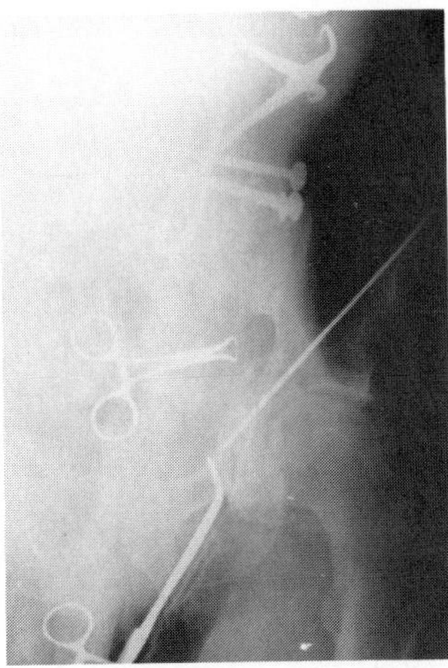

Figure 12-27D: Intraoperative view with Kirschner wire inserted across the nonunion of the ramus.

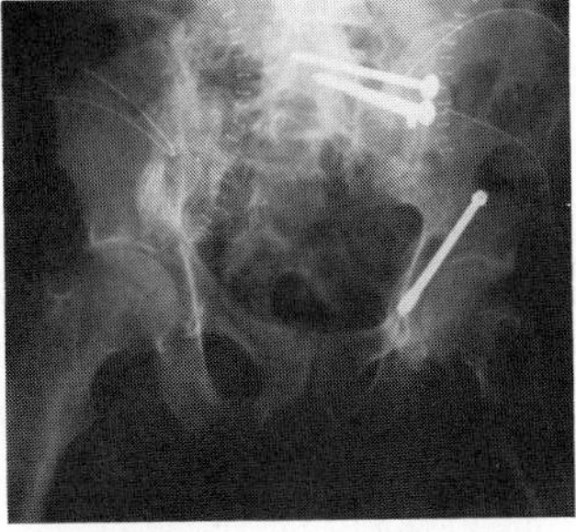

Figure 12-27E: Postoperative AP view after supplementary lag screw fixation of the sacral nonunion.

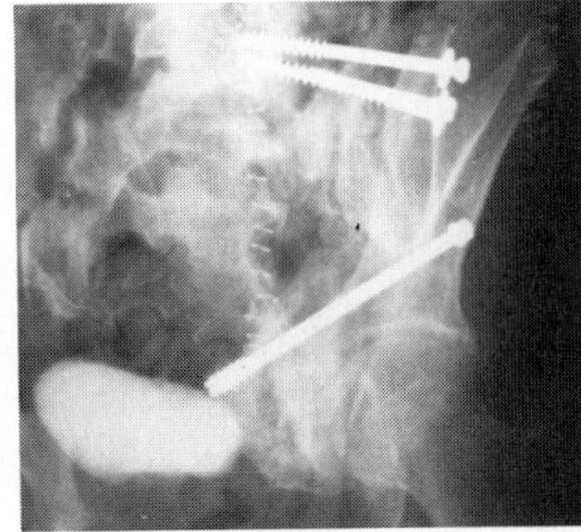

Figure 12-27F: Postoperative obturator oblique view.

available bone stock and to determine whether a conventional Double Cobra plate could be employed for posterior fixation along with a supplementary plate across the symphysis. Assessment of the model also was used to determine whether a supplementary free iliac crest vascularized bone graft was needed to augment the bone stock. Confirmation of the adequacy of the local bone stock was made upon scrutiny of the model, so that the need for a free contralateral vascularized iliac crest bone graft was obviated.

## Pelvic Malunion

A late pelvic ring deformity with or without concomitant nonunion provides a formidable reconstructive problem. While the elimination of a painful mobile nonunion can be undertaken in a moderately reproducible way, the correction of a rotational deviation of the pelvis remains a difficult surgical undertaking. One example, a nonunion-malunion involving both sacroiliac joints

Figure 12-28: This diabetic man of 52 years presented one year after a vehicular accident with a painful nonunion-malunion of bilateral sacroiliac joints and a wide diastasis.

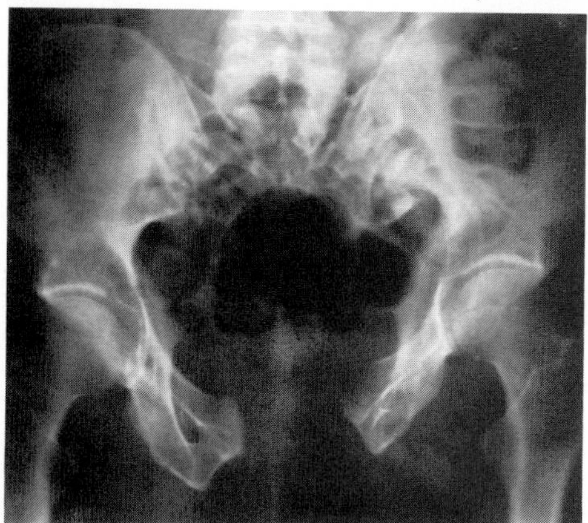

Figure 12-28A: Preoperative AP view.

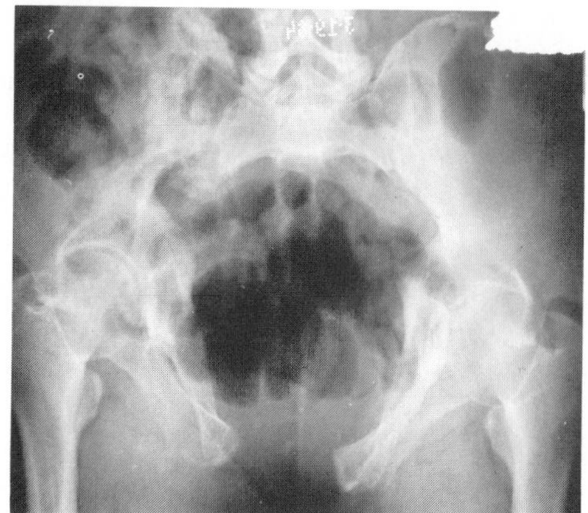

Figure 12-28B: Preoperative inlet view.

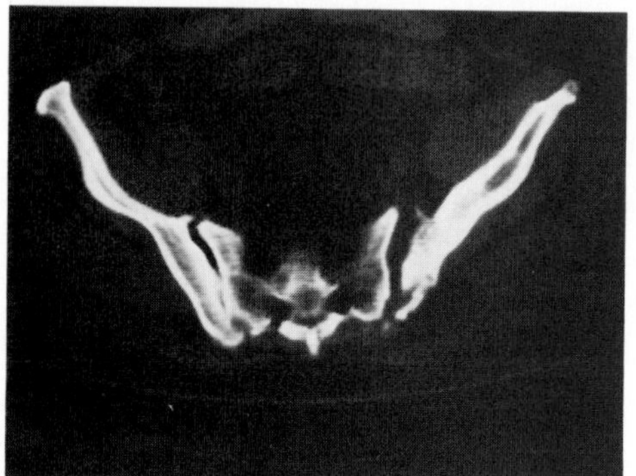

Figure 12-28C: Preoperative computed scan.

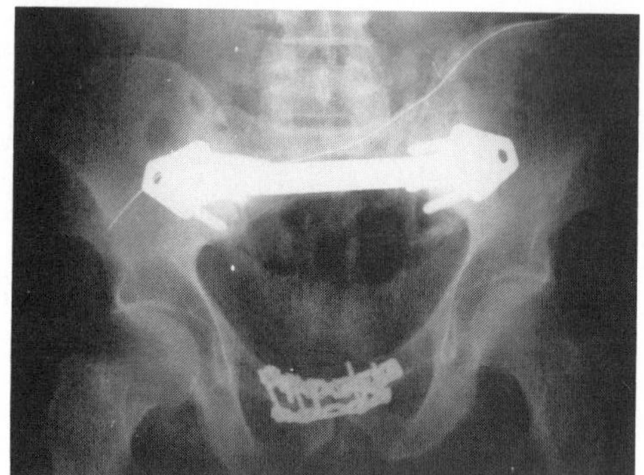

Figure 12-28D: Postoperative view.

(Figure 12-32), management of the left ilium and the symphysis was highly successful in terms of alleviation of discomfort at the several sites of involvement, although comparison of the preoperative and postoperative radiographs shows little evidence of significant cosmetic correction. Nevertheless, the patient was able to resume a heavy laboring job within nine months after the reconstructive procedure. Where there is a rotational asymmetry about the midline (Figure 12-33) highly satisfactory cosmetic correction can be achieved, although an anatomical realignment of the pelvic ring clearly is not realized. The first stage of the procedure is an exploration of the diastasis of the symphysis. The bladder is removed from its abnormal site, interposed between the adjacent rami. After the rami are reapproximated and stabilized with a plate, the sacroiliac joints are reduced and stabilized sequentially or by the use of a Double Cobra plate. Another highly successful correction was achieved in a woman of 26 years who

Figure 12-29: This white woman of 64 years presented one year after her accident with a painful sacral nonunion-malunion and ipsilateral rami disruptions. She achieved alleviation of her posterior discomfort by immobilization with a Double Cobra plate.

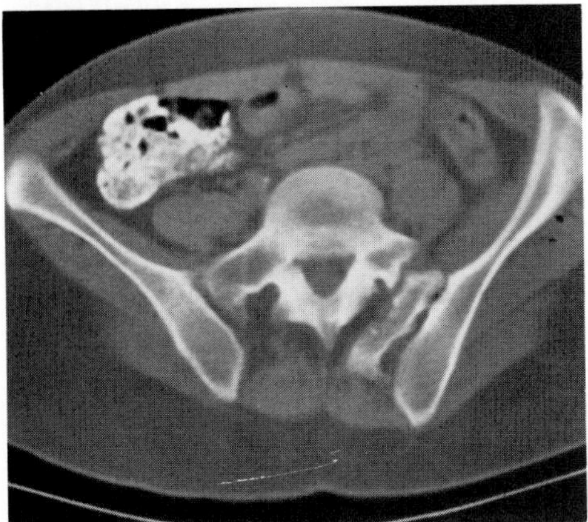

Figure 12-29A: Preoperative computed scan.

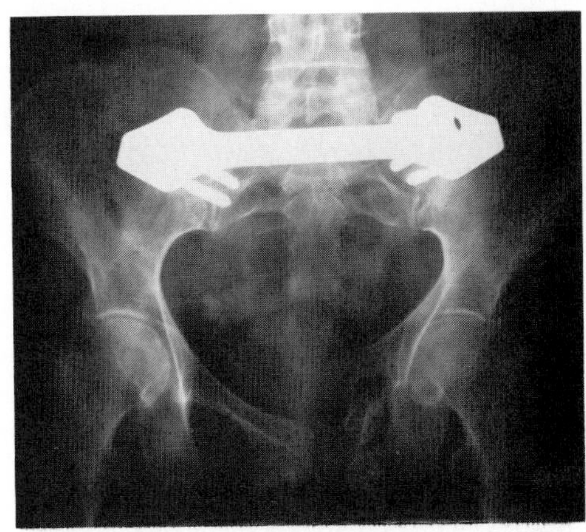

Figure 12-29B: Postoperative AP view.

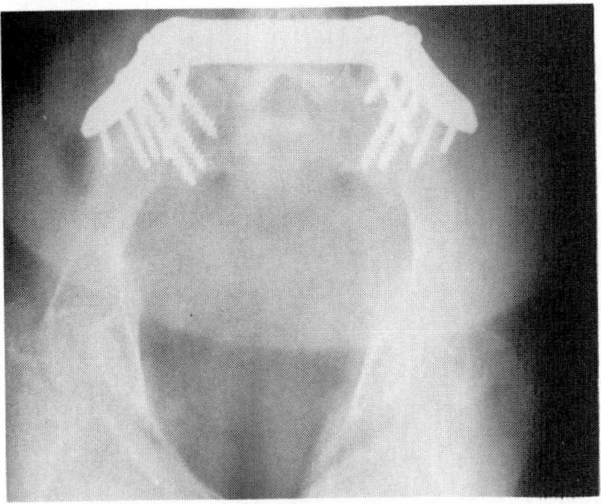

Figure 12-29C: Postoperative inlet view.

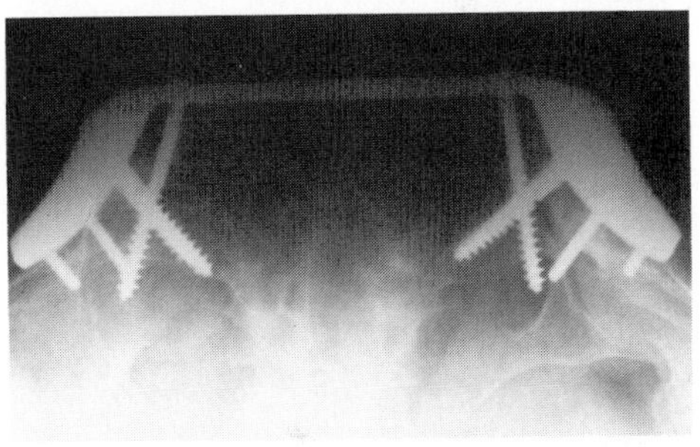

Figure 12-29D: Postoperative Fergusson view.

sustained a pelvic fracture complicated by a closed head injury (Figure 12-34). She remained unrousable for eight weeks when she was managed in bed in a fetal position. Her pelvic injuries included bilateral sacroiliac dislocations and an acetabular fracture. Her pelvis underwent a rotational deformity with approximately 90° of anteflexion with respect to the lumbar spine. The acetabular fracture progressed to a hip fusion with an abduction contracture of 45°. Two years later, the patient presented to us unable to stand with an upright posture. For derotation of the pelvis on the lumbar spine, the anesthetized patient was placed on an appropriate operating table in a kneeling position. The sacroiliac joints were osteotomized and the bottom of the table was extended to achieve the pelvic reduction. Stabilization was achieved by the use of a Double Cobra plate. One week later the hip fusion was converted to a total hip joint replacement. With these procedures the

Figure 12-30: This osteoporotic white woman of 35 years presented with a painful mobile right-sided sacral fracture and contralateral ramus disruption for which lag screw fixation of the sacrum and a Double Cobra plate were applied. One year later, she continued to complain of pain and motion at the rami fractures, for which a secondary reconstruction of the superior pubic ramus was successfully undertaken.

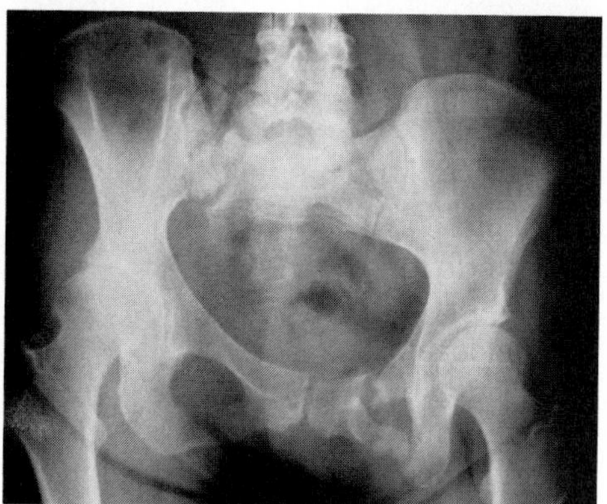

Figure 12-30A: Presenting AP view.

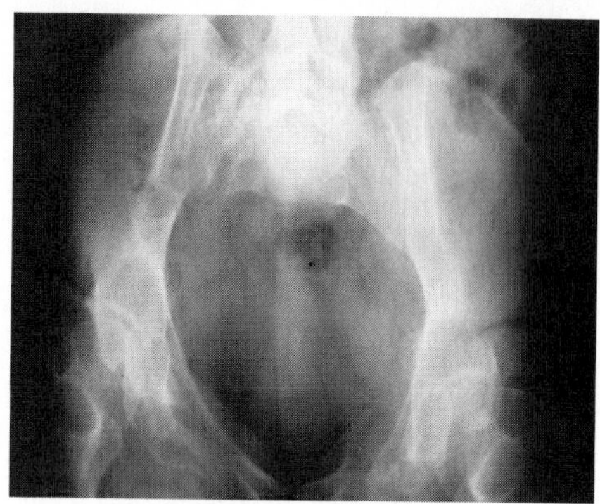

Figure 12-30B: Presenting inlet view.

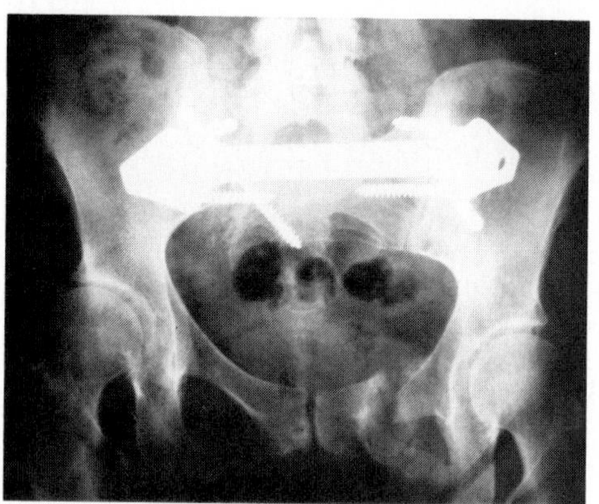

Figure 12-30C: Initial postoperative AP view.

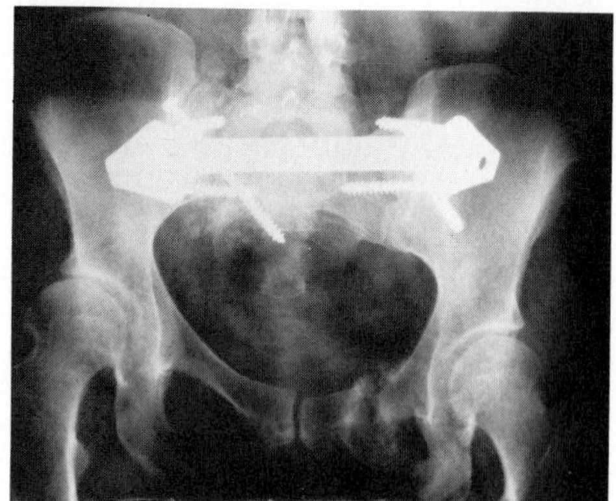

Figure 12-30D: AP view one year postoperative, with persistent painful mobile ramus.

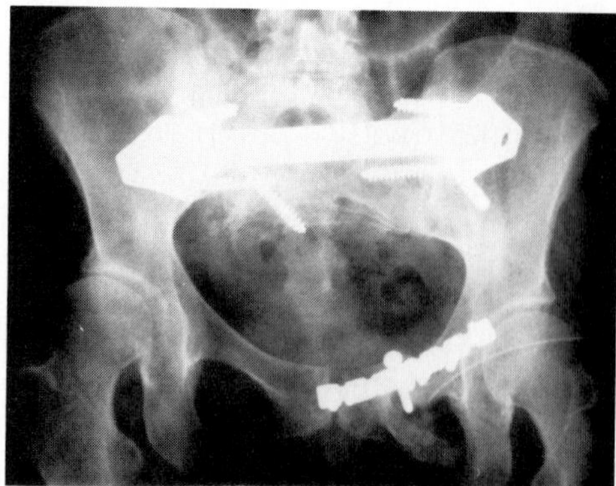

Figure 12-30E: Subsequent postoperative view after stabilization of left ramus.

Figure 12-31: This woman of 32 years underwent a resection of a chondrosarcoma of the right sacroiliac joint that culminated in a painful nonunion-malunion of the right hemipelvis, for which a subsequent reconstructive procedure was undertaken.

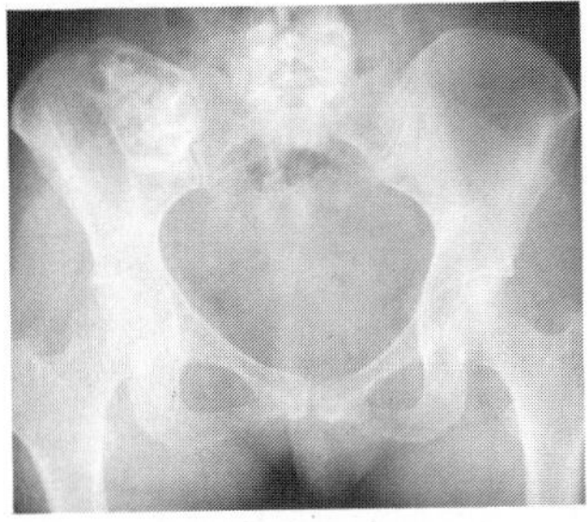

Figure 12-31A: Initial AP view with presence of tumor.

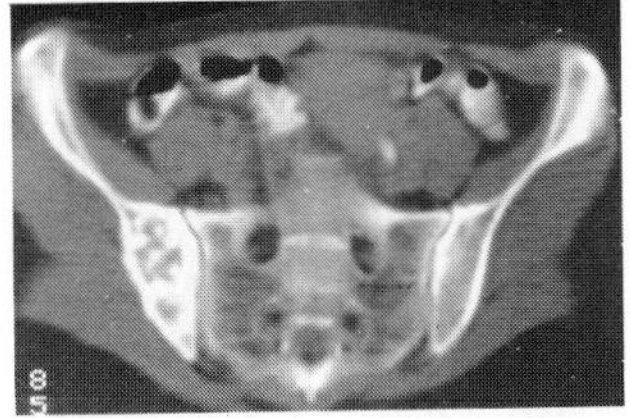

Figure 12-31B: Corresponding computed scan.

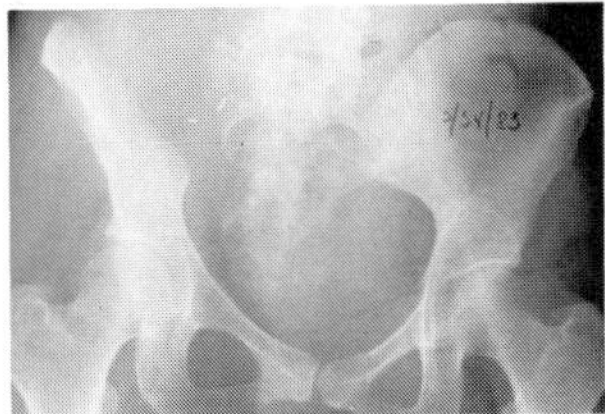

Figure 12-31C: Initial postoperative AP view.

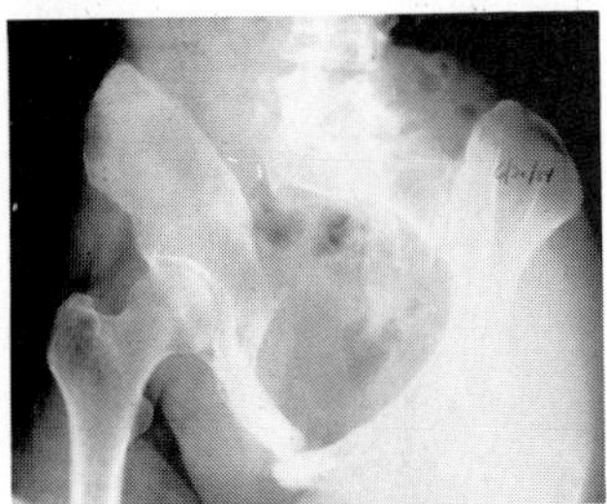

Figure 12-31D: Inlet view, 14 months postoperative.

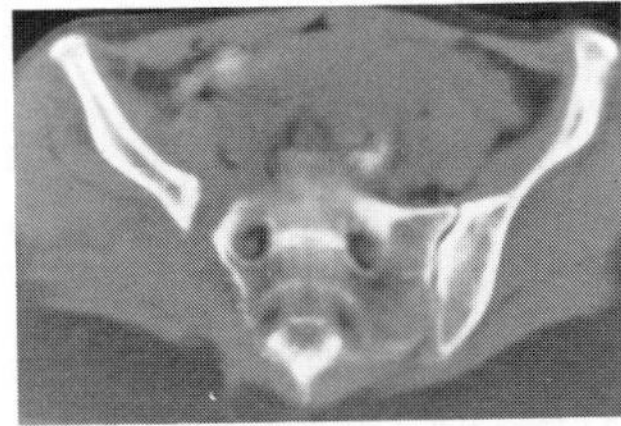

Figure 12-31E: Computed scan, 18 months after the surgical resection.

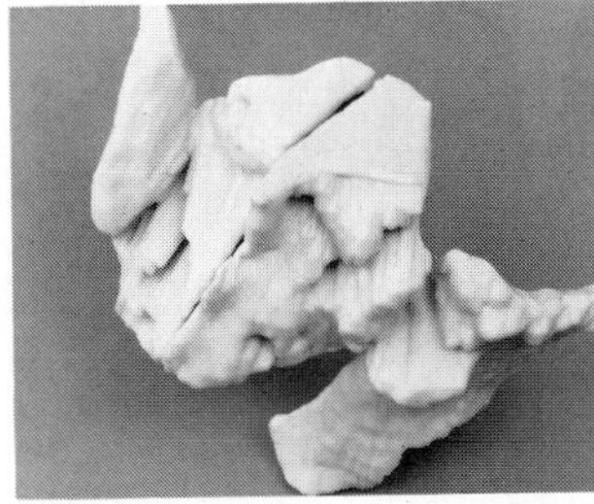

Figure 12-31F: CAD-CAM model of pelvis, posterior view.

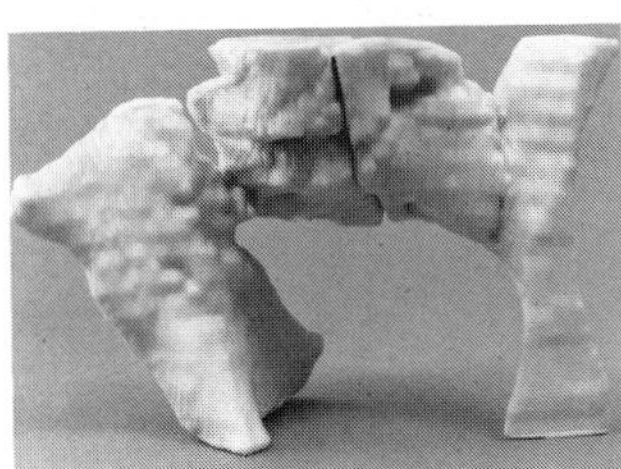

Figure 12-31G: CAD-CAM model of pelvis, anterior view.

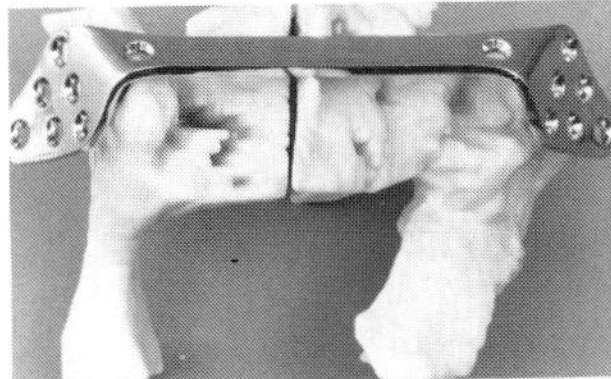

Figure 12-31H: Preoperative planning with Double Cobra plate.

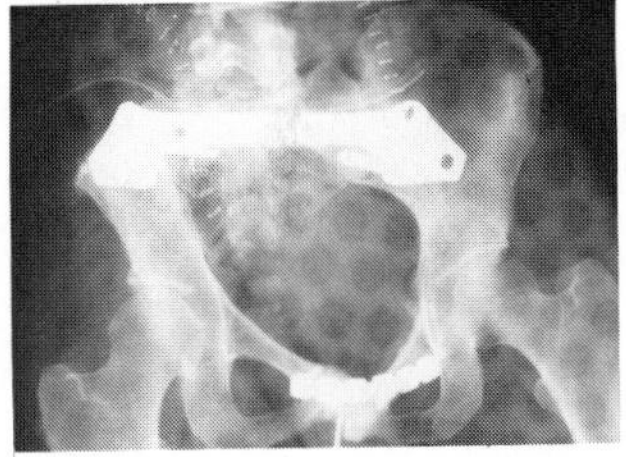

Figure 12-31I: Subsequent postoperative AP view.

patient reassumed an upright posture and the ability to undertake an independent gait.

The correction of sitting imbalance with apparent limb length discrepancy and rotational deformity is probably the most difficult pelvic correction. Either the affected side of the pelvis can be realigned or, in certain instances, a simpler correction can be achieved by osteotomy of the unaffected side of the pelvis. When a distal displacement of the affected high riding hemipelvis is planned, an intraoperative neurological evaluation with sensory evoked potentials is recommended so that a traction injury to the lumbosacral plexus or sciatic nerve can be avoided. With the enormous force of distraction required to anatomically realign the pelvis, a partial

Figure 12-32: This nonunion-malunion of the symphysis, left ilium and bilateral sacroiliac joints in a 36-year-old laborer was surgically reconstructed with excellent alleviation of discomfort, but poor correction of the persistent deformity.

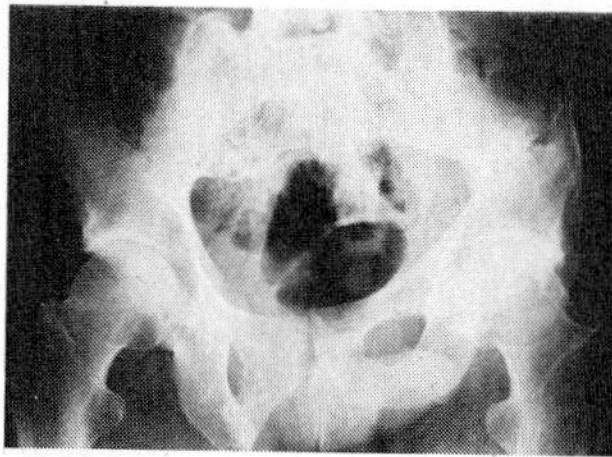

Figure 12-32A: Presenting AP view, two years after vehicular accident.

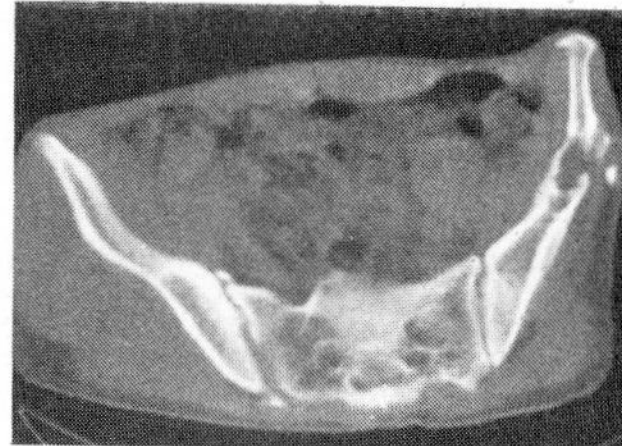

Figure 12-32B: Presenting computed scan of posterior pelvis.

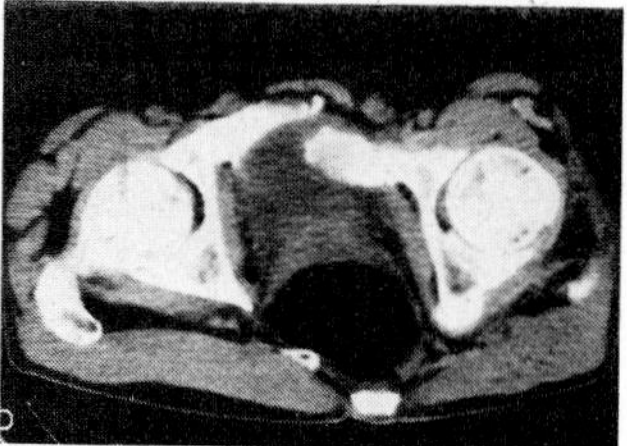

Figure 12-32C: Presenting computed scan of rami and hip joints.

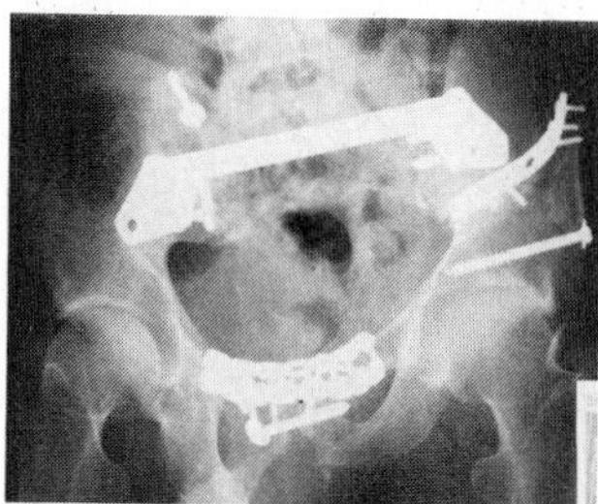

Figure 12-32D: Initial postoperative view.

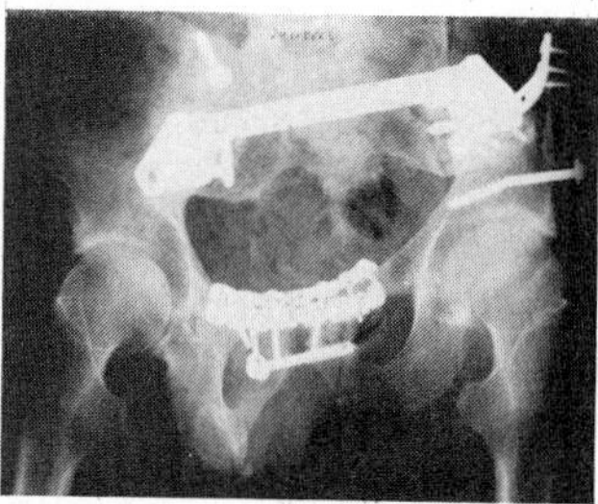

Figure 12-32E: Six months later, painfree result was evident. Note fractured iliac screw.

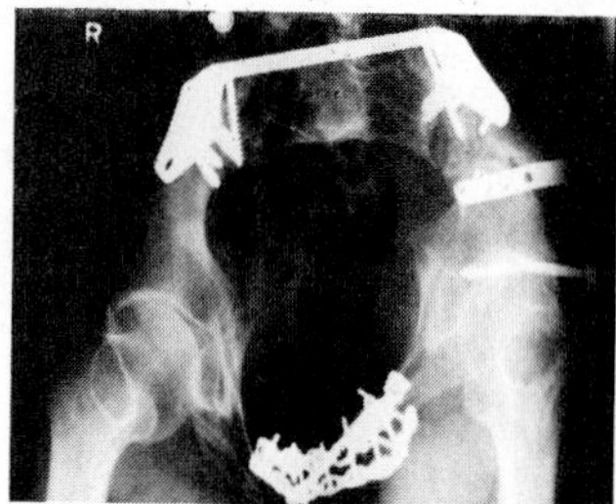


Figure 12-32F: Inlet view six months after surgery.

correction may be the best that realistically can be attained. During an attempt to achieve longitudinal distraction the pelvis may undergo concomitant rotational deviation. Unless a careful scrutiny of the pelvis is undertaken, the undesirable rotational displacement is unrecognized. An example of an unsuccessful attempt to correct a superior migration of the right hemipelvis is shown (Figure 12-35). During the procedure, longitudinal distraction applied by resort to a femoral distractor provoked rotational deviation that was not recognized until the postoperative radiograph was examined.

When the nonunion-malunion transgresses the sacrum, especially the sacral foramina, or even a sacroiliac joint with an associated superior migration of a hemipelvis, a correction of the discrepancy of the superior acetabulum and ischial tuberosity is most simply corrected by an osteotomy of the ilium (Figure 12-36). In this example a 55-year-old woman, who nine months earlier sustained a vehicular accident, complained of persistent sacral pain with an apparent limb length discrepancy of 4cm. Through a curved incision around the iliac crest, cancellous lag screws were inserted into the sacral ala and first sacral body to immobilize the

Figure 12-33: This woman of 24 years presented three years after a vehicular accident with a painful pelvic nonunion-malunion and marked pelvic obliquity. For her initial injury—a diastasis, left-sided ramus fracture, left sacroiliac dislocation, and right sided sacral fracture—she was managed with bed rest. When marked external rotational deformities of both ilia ensued, a pelvic sling was applied, which provoked overriding of the rami and marked pelvic obliquity. The subsequent surgical reconstruction provided a satisfactory cosmetic correction and relief of posterior pelvic pain, although persistent rotational deformity is evident by radiographic assessment. (Figures A and B reproduced with permission of Williams and Wilkins.)

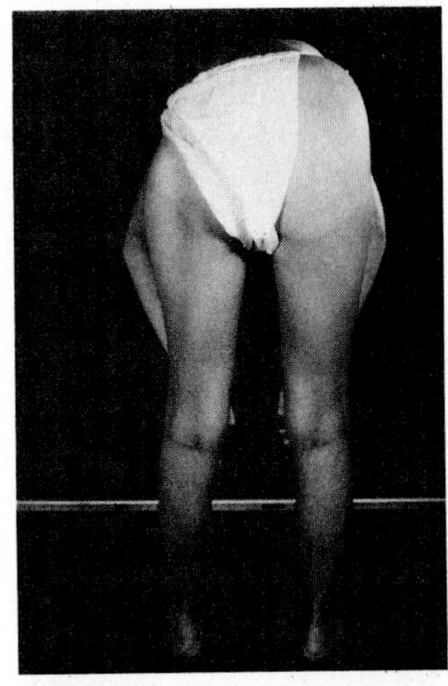

Figure 12-33A: Preoperative photograph documents pelvic obliquity.

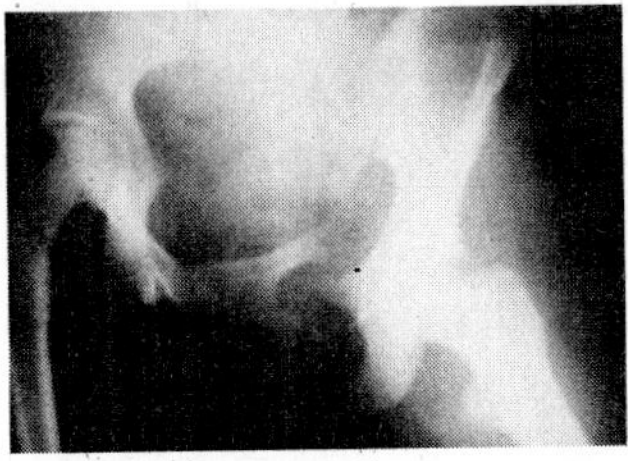

Figure 12-33B: Initial posttraumatic radiograph.

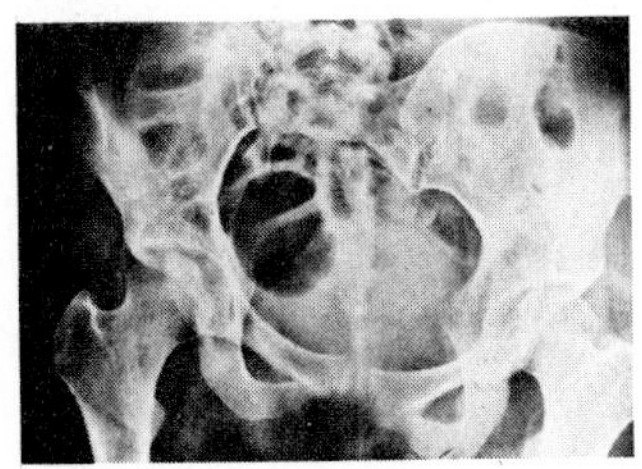

Figure 12-33C: Two weeks after injury, external rotational deformities of both ilia are evident.

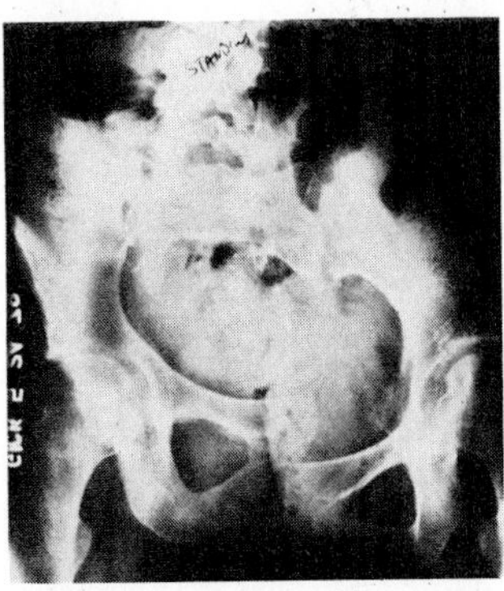

Figure 12-33D: Presenting radiograph with overriding rami and pelvic obliquity.

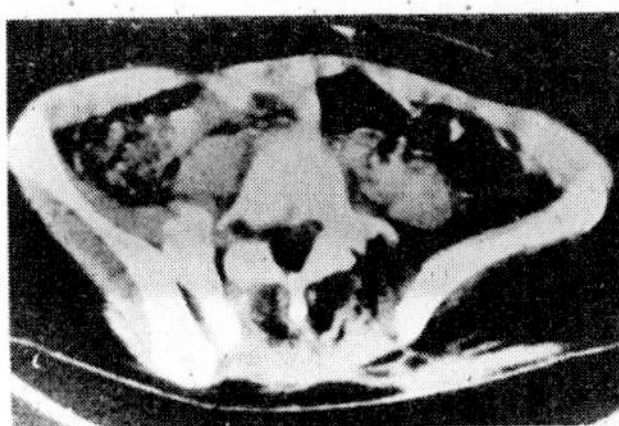

Figure 12-33E: Presenting computed scan.

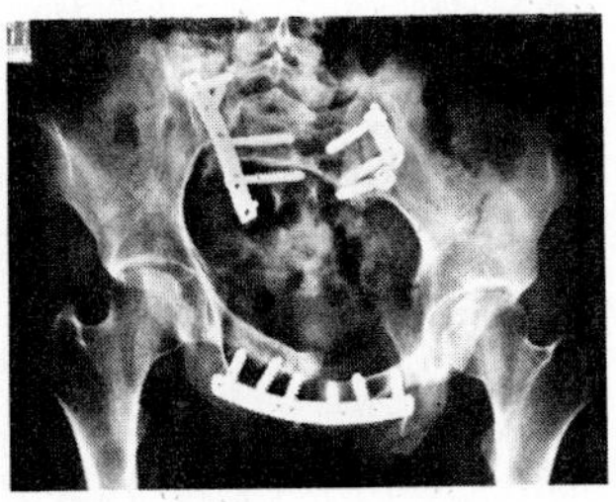

Figure 12-33F: Postoperative AP view.

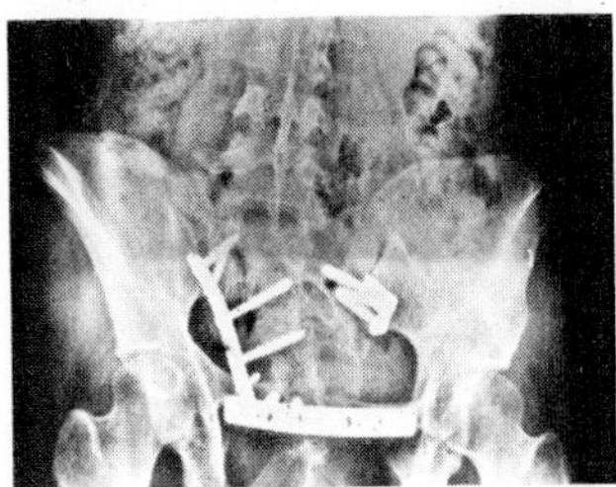

Figure 12-33G: Postoperative outlet view.

Figure 12-34: This woman of 26 years sustained a pelvic fracture complicated by a closed head injury for which she was managed with bed rest. Two years later she presented to us when marked displacement of the sacral fracture was accompanied by a spontaneous hip fusion secondary to the acetabular fracture. Her pelvis was anteflexed 90° with respect to the lumbosacral spine. A two-stage reconstruction consisted of derotation of the pelvis on the sacrum and a total hip joint replacement.

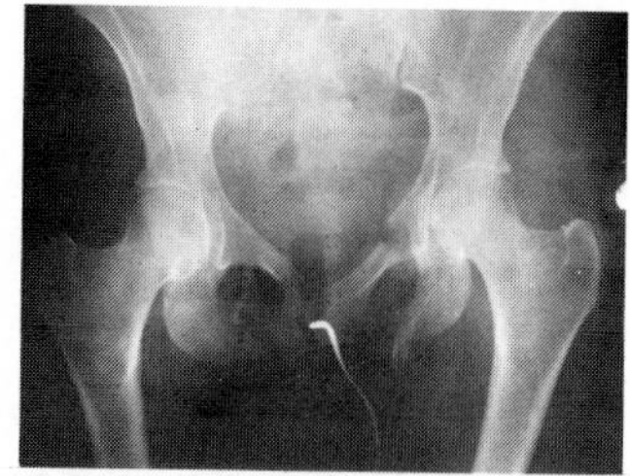

Figure 12-34A: Initial anteroposterior radiograph with relatively little pelvic or acetabular displacement.

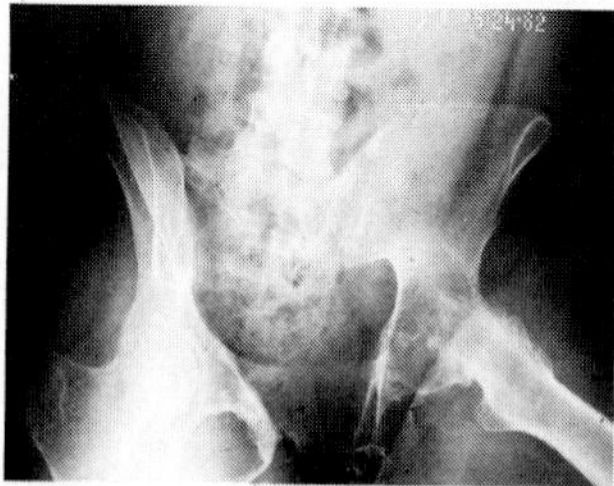

Figure 12-34B: Presenting AP view two years afterwards.

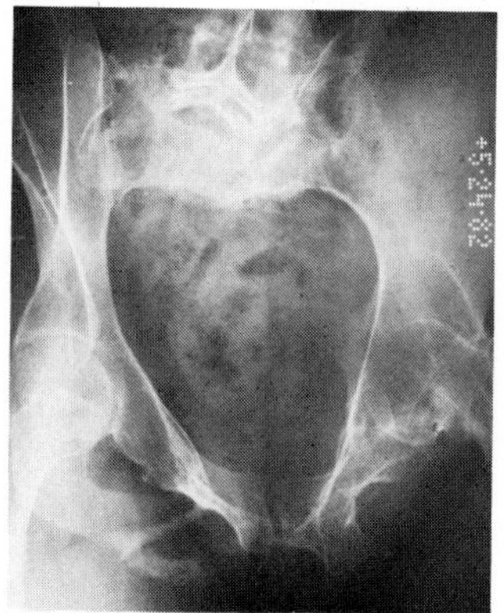

Figure 12-34C: Presenting inlet view two years afterwards.

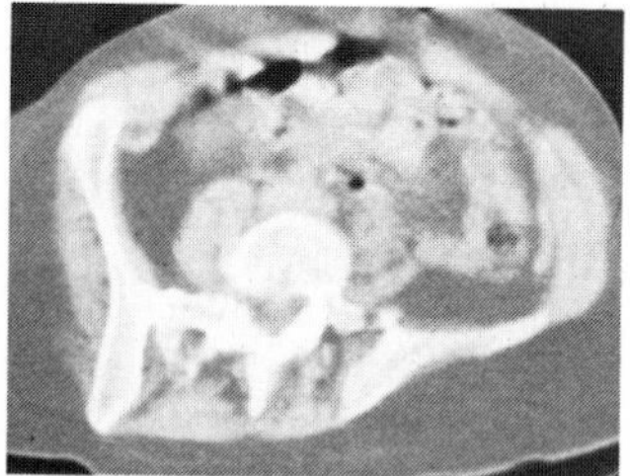

Figure 12-34D: Computed scan through malunion-nonunion of the SI joints.

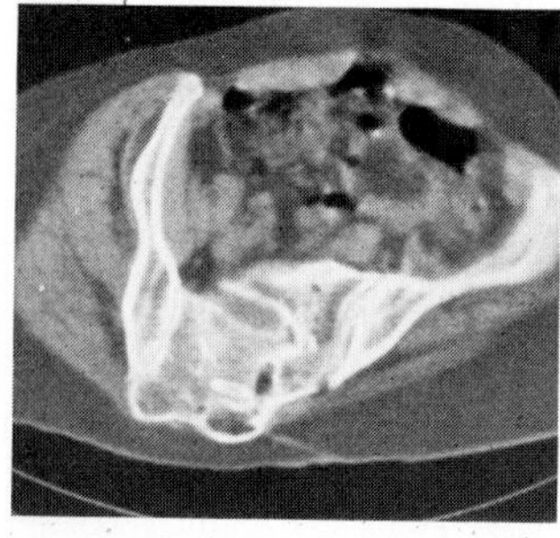

Figure 12-34E: Computed scan through malunion-nonunion of the sacrum.

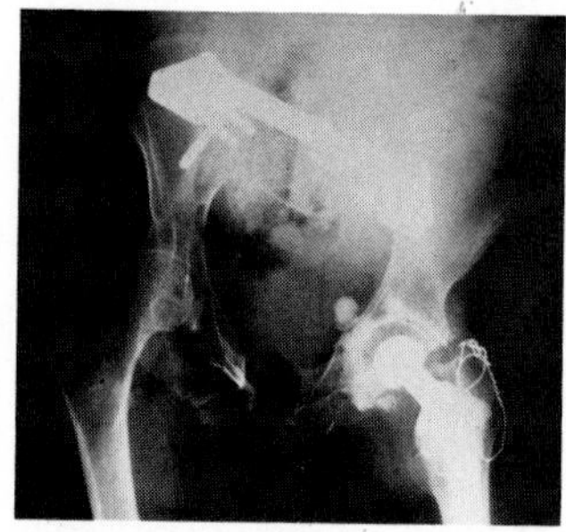

Figure 12-34F: Postoperative AP view.

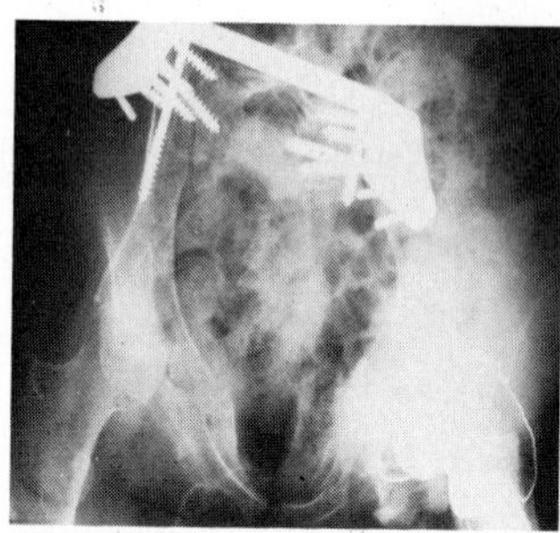

Figure 12-34G: Postoperative inlet view.

partial union of the sacrum. Then, an osteotomy was created from the anterior margin of the greater sciatic notch to the anterior inferior spine. The femoral distractor was applied from the posterior column to the posterior ilium for distraction of the acetabulum in a distal and anterior direction. After 3cm of correction had been obtained, a rectangular segment of lateral ilium centered on the superior gluteal ridge was harvested with a power oscillating blade and applied to the osteotomy site. The stabilization was completed with

Figure 12-35: This 17-year-old boy sustained a four-part rami fracture and diastasis with a fracture dislocation of the right sacroiliac joint. While his initial radiograph was relatively undisplaced, substantial superior migration of the right hemipelvis ensued eight weeks after the application of skeletal traction, when independent ambulation was resumed. While the subsequent surgical procedure provided relief of right-sided sacroiliac pain, it failed to correct the discrepancy in the height of the ischial tuberosities with an associated complaint of sitting imbalance. In E and F, postoperative radiographs document persistent pelvic deformity.

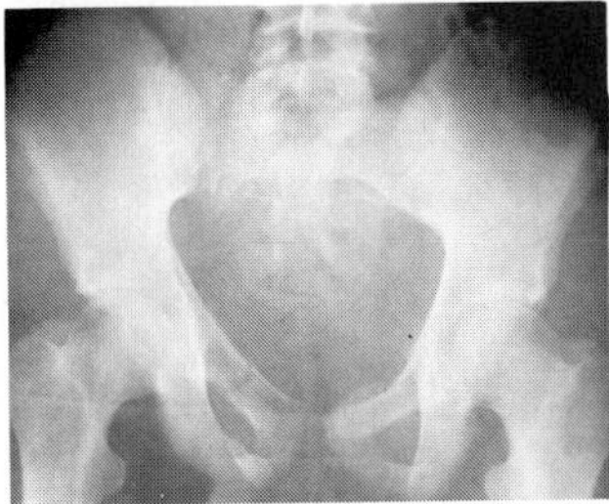

Figure 12-35A: Initial posttraumatic AP view.

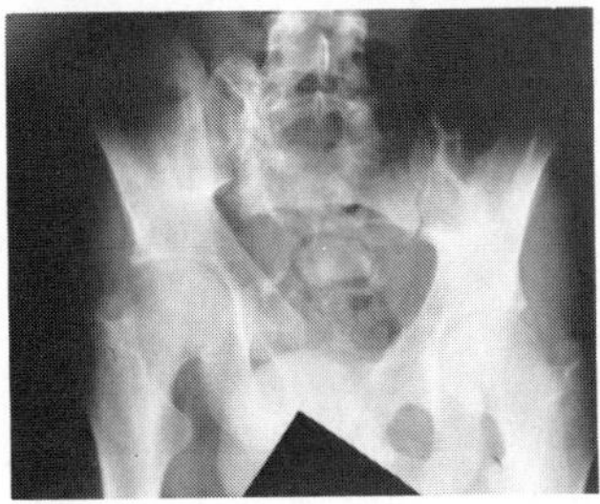

Figure 12-35B: Two months after injury, subsequent AP view documents superior migration of right hemipelvis.

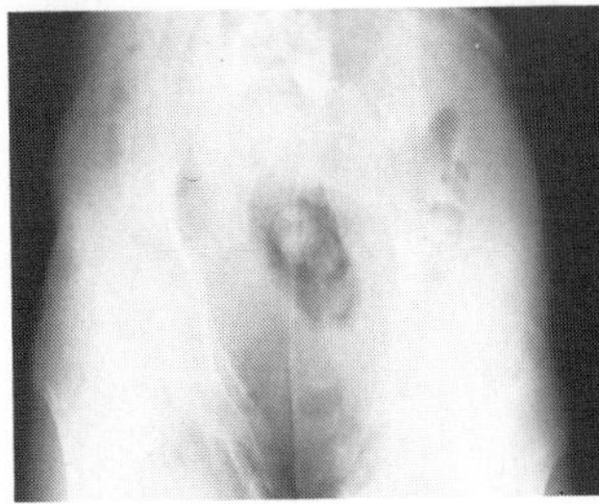

Figure 12-35C: Two months after injury, inlet view.

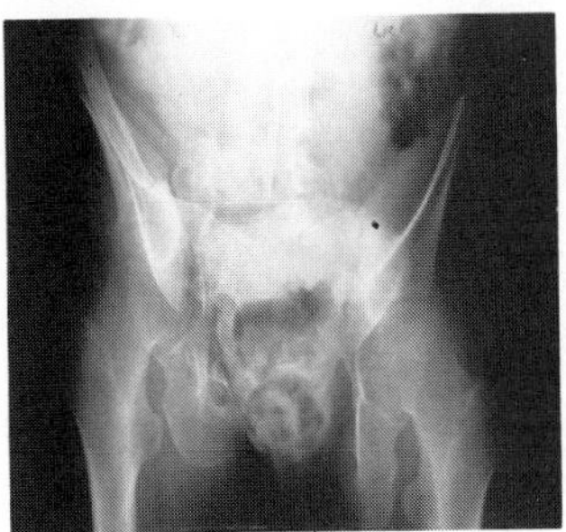

Figure 12-35D: Two months after injury, outlet view.

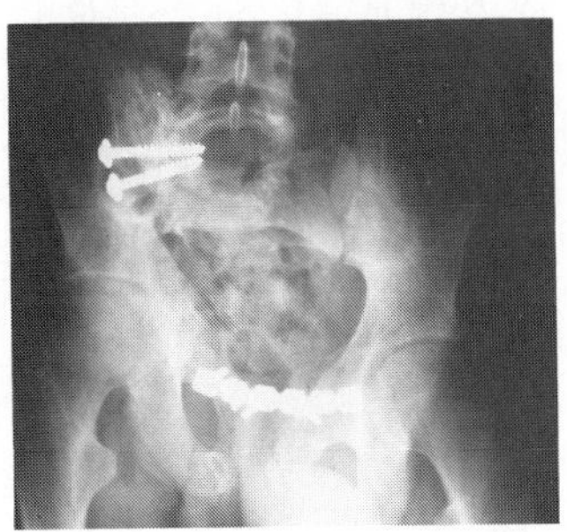

Figure 12-35E: Inlet view with malrotation of the right hemipelvis.

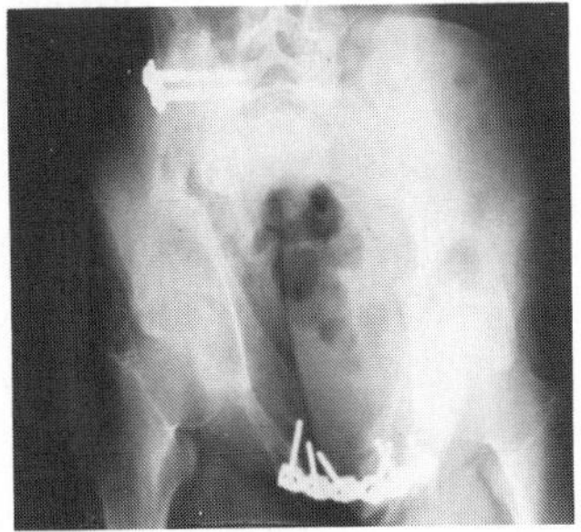

Figure 12-35F: Outlet view with discrepancy in the position of the acetabuli.

3.5mm reconstruction plates applied to the anterior and posterior ends of the osteotomy. In the postoperative radiograph, a near-anatomical correction of the position of the right acetabulum is evident.

## Acetabular Nonunions

A patient with a nonunion of the acetabulum can present a year or more after the time of his acute traumatic insult with a complaint of pain, deformity, stiffness, or instability. Rarely his hip joint shows adequate preservation of the femoral head and the articular surface of the acetabulum, so that an intact hip joint can be reconstructed. The most extensive experience with this problem has been documented by Letournel,[1] who records many favorable results with a prolonged period of hip function after the late reconstruction. Also, the late reconstruction may provide a limited period of adequate function of the intact hip and the optimal restoration of the bone for the ultimate

Figure 12-36: This woman of 55 years presented nine months after a vehicular accident with a painful nonunion of a sacral fracture and superior migration of the right hemipelvis. Surgical reconstruction included lag screw fixation of the sacrum with a lengthening osteotomy of the right ilium for the correction of a 4cm apparent limb length discrepancy.

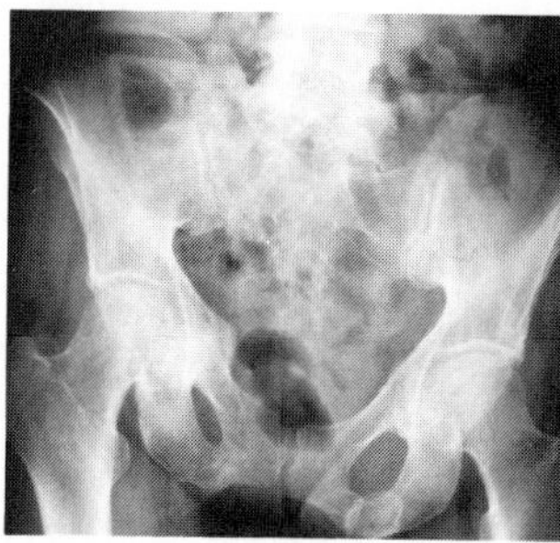

Figure 12-36A: Presenting AP view.

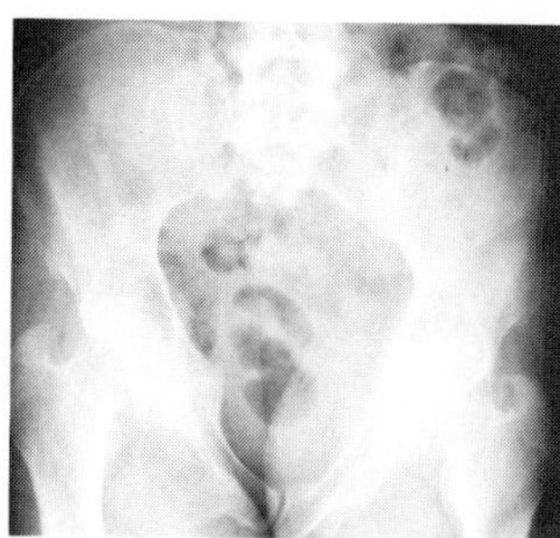

Figure 12-36B: Presenting inlet view.

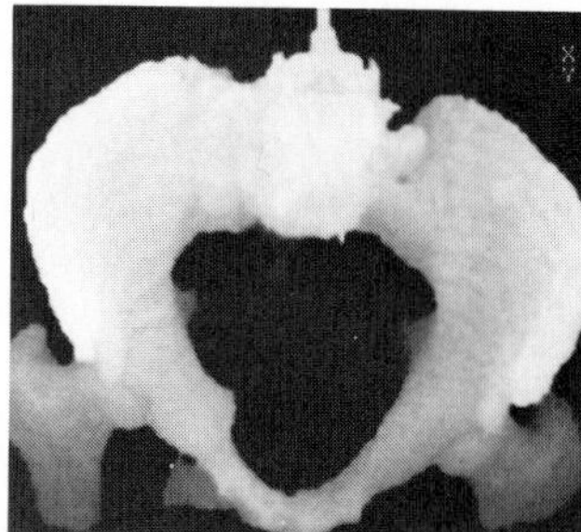

Figure 12-36C: Presenting 3D computed inlet view.

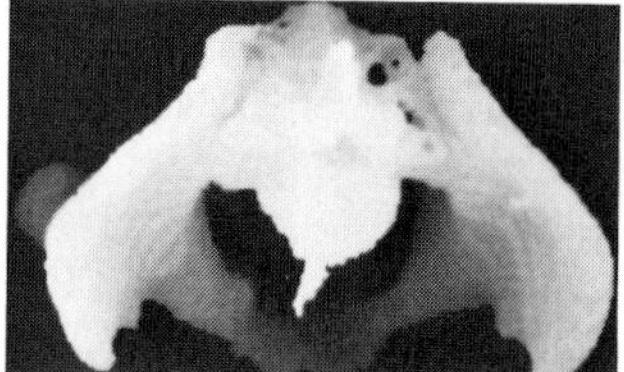

Figure 12-36D: 3D computed superior view.

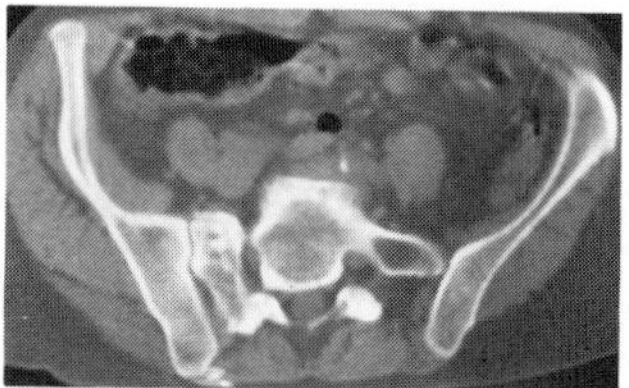

Figure 12-36E: Computed scan with sacral nonunion.

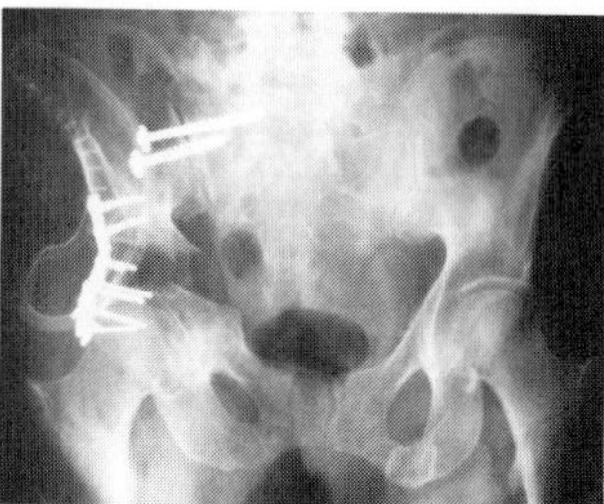

Figure 12-36F: Postoperative view.

Figure 12-37: This woman of 38 years presented one year after a "T" posterior wall acetabular fracture with severe hip pain and stiffness. Severe abrasive damage precludes anatomical reconstruction so that total hip joint replacement is indicated.

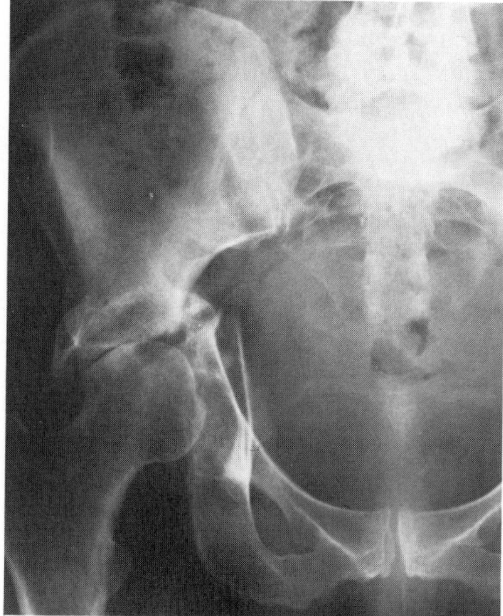

Figure 12-37A: AP view.

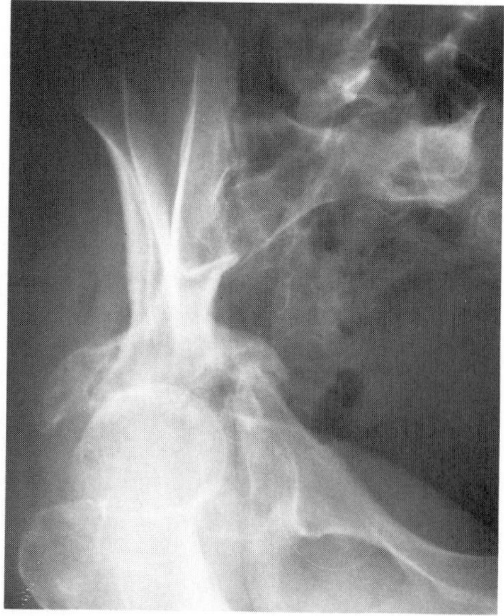

Figure 12-37B: Obturator oblique view.

Figure 12-38: This man of 34 years presented one year after a both-column fracture with persistent pain and instability. An open reduction and internal fixation with partial correction of the deformity achieved a highly effective result so that he has resumed employment as a law enforcement officer, with a normal gait with more than 120° of flexion.

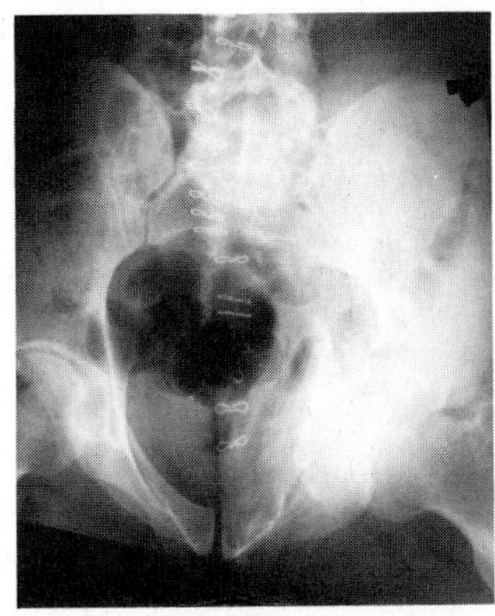

Figure 12-38A: Presenting inlet view.

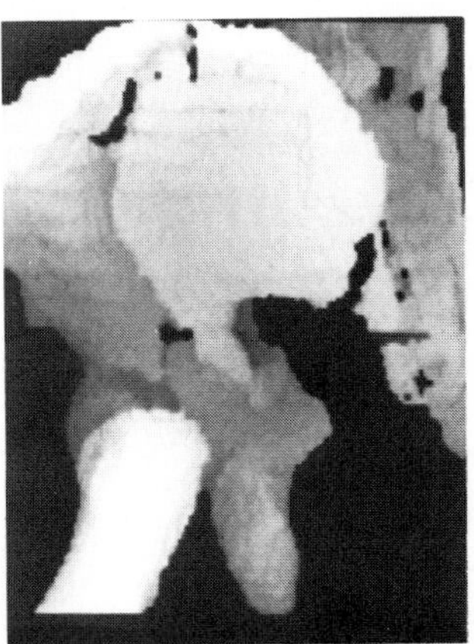

Figure 12-38B: 3D scan of both-column fracture as iliac oblique view.

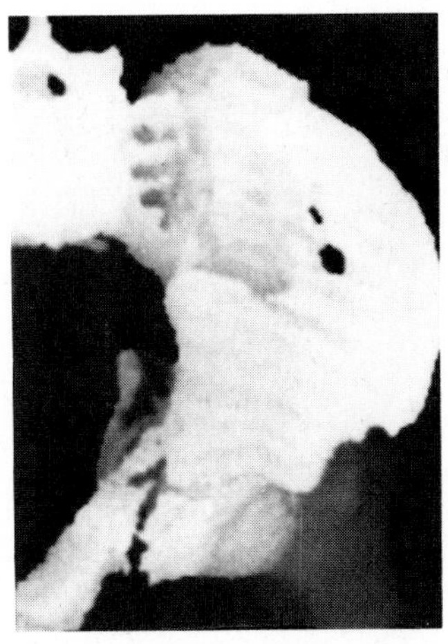

Figure 12-38C: 3D scan of both-column fracture as superior view.

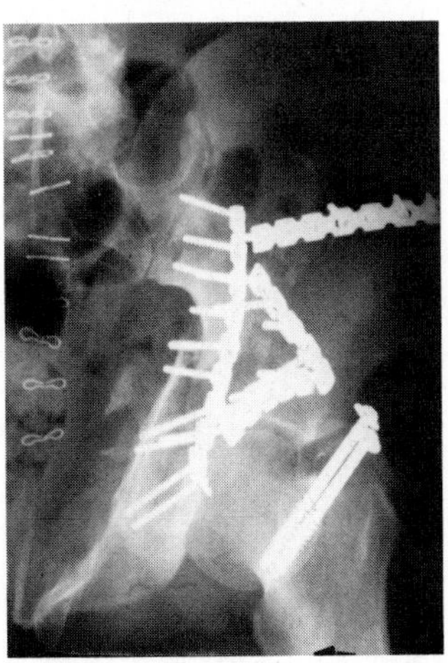

Figure 12-38D: One year postoperative result.

total hip joint replacement. Most of the cases that present a year or more after the time of injury with a symptomatic nonunion of the acetabulum possess overwhelming degenerative changes, so that a total hip joint replacement is required as part of the pelvic reconstruction (Figure 12-37). Probably the best candidate for a late reconstruction of an acetabular nonunion with a likelihood for the restoration of an intact hip is a displaced transverse fracture or occasionally a posterior wall or column fracture (Figure 12-38). Most of the displaced associated fracture variants possess such incongruity that the femoral head is eroded in one or more sites and possesses an inadequate articular surface. When the hip joint is reconstructed, the general principles discussed under late presentation are followed.

Many of the patients who present about one year after the time of their initial injury with persistent pain possess radiographs and a computed scan indicative of a partial

Figure 12-39: This white man of 45 years presented one year after a limited acetabular reconstruction culminated in a painful hip. Scrutiny of preoperative radiographs and a computed scan failed to ascertain whether there was a persistent nonunion or solely traumatic arthritis. At the time of surgery, a united acetabulum with persistent clefts was encountered so that a cementless total hip replacement was undertaken.

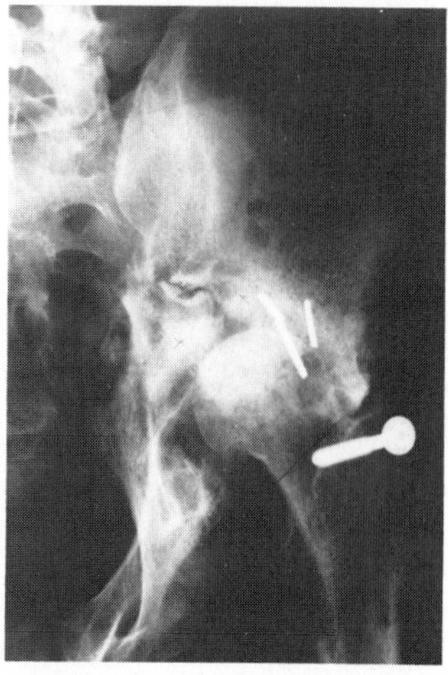

Figure 12-39A: Presenting AP radiograph.

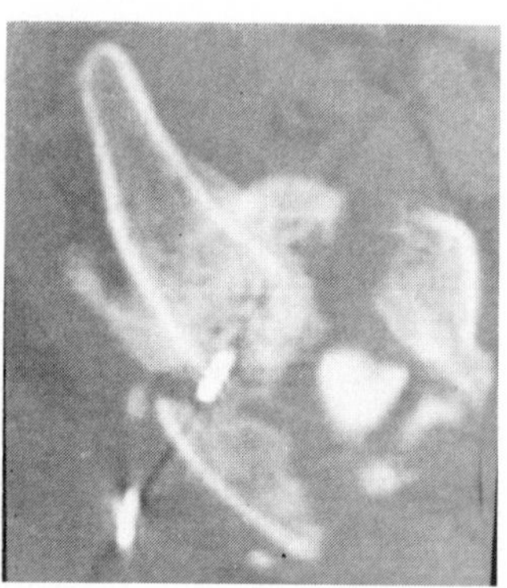

Figure 12-39B: Computed scan through dome.

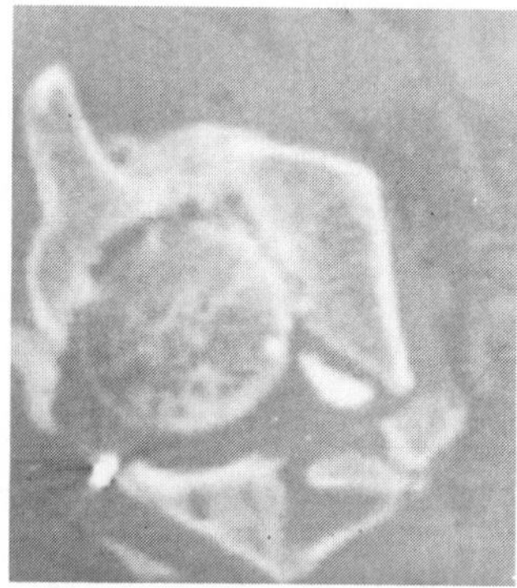

Figure 12-39C: Computed scan through hip joint.

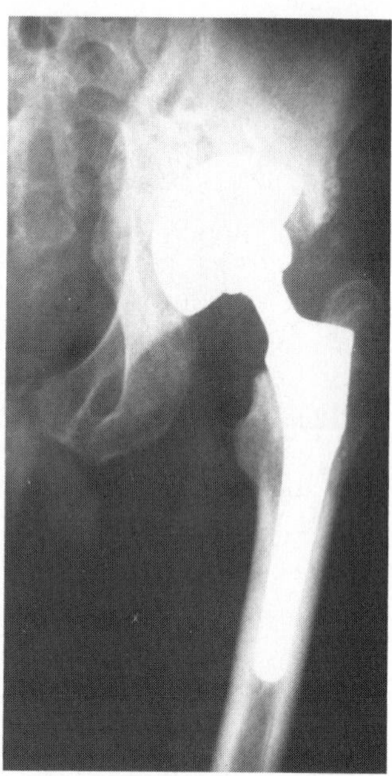

Figure 12-39D: Postoperative view.

union (Figure 12-39). In this example, a man of 45 years who presented after a limited acetabular reconstruction, a thorough scrutiny of the radiographs failed to provide a distinct confirmation of whether a reconstruction of the ununited acetabulum was possible or whether severe deterioration of the hip necessitated a total hip joint replacement. At the time of surgery, union of the acetabulum was documented with severe articular changes of the acetabulum and opposing femoral head, so that a cementless total hip joint replacement was indicated. With the substantial acetabular displacement, a 62mm PCA acetabular component (Howmedica, Inc., Rutherford, New Jersey) was employed to achieve a stable fit.

For the diverse acetabular problems including nonunions, malunions, and protrusio where supplementary bone graft is needed, an acetabular component with screw fixation such as the Harris-Galante model (Zimmer, Inc., Warsaw, Indiana) is strongly preferred. Prior to their availability, a Mueller ring was employed as a "hemispherical plate" for anchorage of the various acetabular fragments with or without the use of supplementary bone graft. With this device, however, supplementary methylmethacrylate cement was needed to anchor the acetabular component of a conventional total hip joint replacement into the ring. With the availability of a metallic acetabular backing anchored by supplementary screws, the need for bone cement is obviated. For an acetabular nonunion with protrusio and supplementary posterior displacement, usually the femoral head is the preferred source of bone graft for restoration of the acetabular component in an anatomical position[6,7] (Figure 12-40). In this example of a both-column nonunion with secondary traumatic arthritis, the femoral head permitted a correction of the acetabular displacement in a woman of 35 years who is the mother of nine children and a welder in a shipyard. She returned to work about four months after the total hip joint replacement. As the magnitude of protrusio increases, the role of the femoral head for augmentation of the acetabular bone rapidly mounts (Figure 12-41). In the presence of a persistent mobile nonunion and protrusio, reapproximation of the columns and the use of the femoral head for bone graft accompanies the fixation and total hip replacement (Figure 12-42).

Another source of an acetabular nonunion is a pathological fracture, such as this example in a woman of 61 years with multiple myeloma (Figure 12-43). The patient was managed for a right acetabular lesion with chemotherapy and radiation therapy. One year later she presented with a nonunion of the acetabulum in a "T" configuration complicated by severe avascular necrosis of the femoral head. A Mueller ring provided a way to stabilize the acetabular nonunion and to attach a conventional acetabular component with bone cement. During the insertion of a Mueller ring or an acetabular component anchored by screw fixation, special care is needed to avoid a vascular injury of the external iliac vessels by an errant drill bit or screw that penetrates the inner table of the pelvis. In a complex pelvic reconstruction, the innominate bone is likely to be displaced so that the position and proximity of the external iliac vessels to the remaining acetabular roof

Figure 12-40: One year after an industrial accident provoked a both-column acetabular disruption that initially was managed with longitudinal and greater trochanteric traction, this 35-year-old female welder presented with a painful acetabular nonunion and traumatic arthritis of the hip. For the cementless H-G total hip joint replacement, the femoral head was employed as bone graft behind the acetabular component.

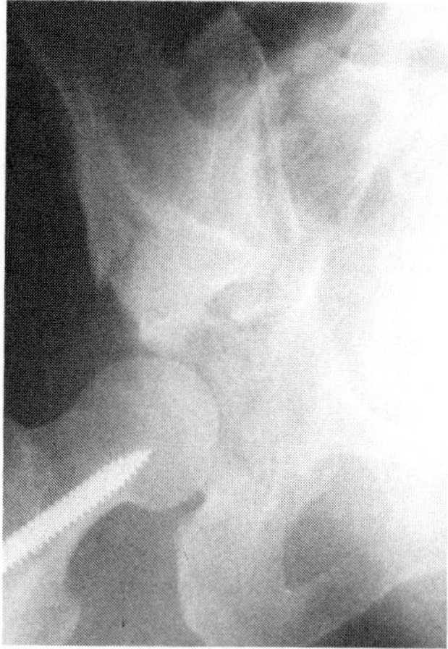

Figure 12-40A: Early posttraumatic radiograph with skeletal traction.

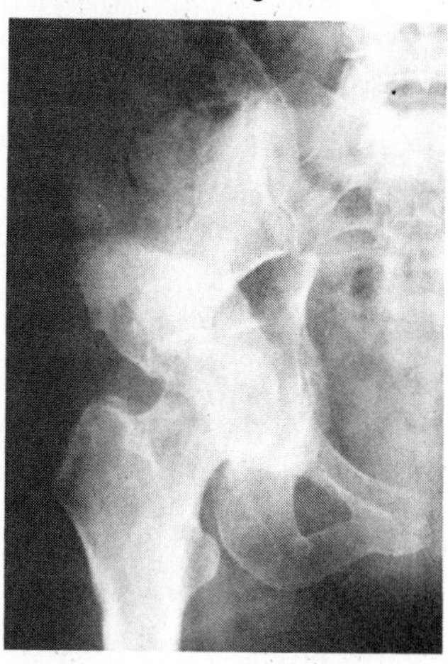

Figure 12-40B: Presenting AP view with marked displacement of posterior column.

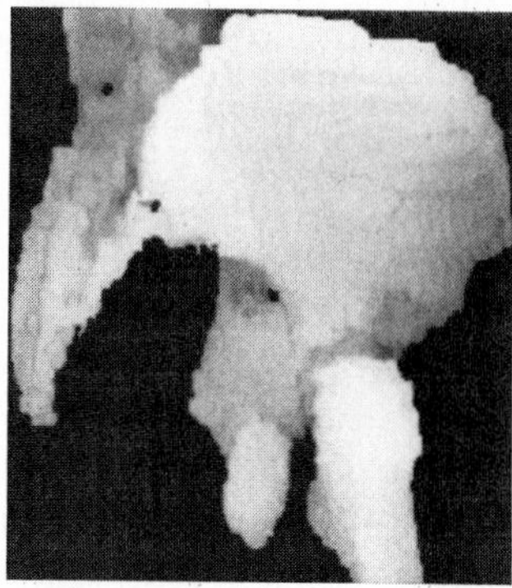

Figure 12-40C: 3D computed iliac oblique view.

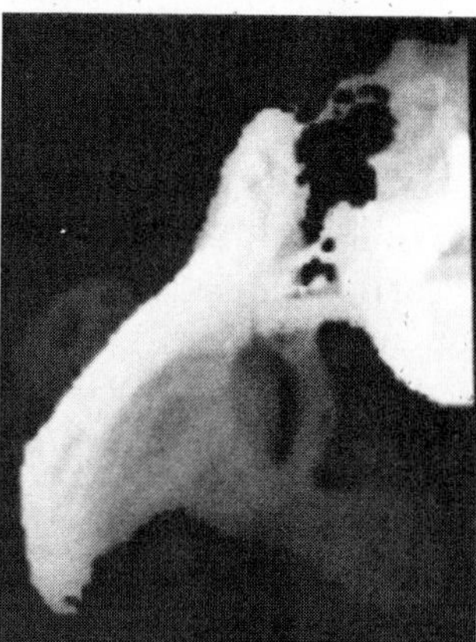

Figure 12-40D: 3D computed superior view.

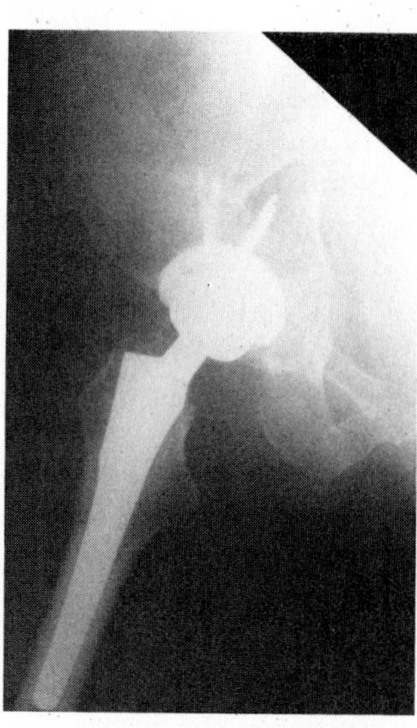

Figure 12-40E: Postoperative view.

are not appreciated. Usually the vessels are scarred to the adjacent acetabular roof and anterior column so that they do not retract as readily as in a typical virgin total hip joint replacement. If a drill bit exits through the typically osteoporotic inner table, possibly coated with callus, a distinct end point is not encountered so that excessive penetration is not evident. In the presence of a nonunion of the anterior column, where screws are employed to immobilize the nonunion as well as to anchor

Figure 12-41: In this example of severe protrusio secondary to a displaced transverse fracture with traumatic arthritis, the application of the femoral head for bone graft to augment the acetabulum is crucial.

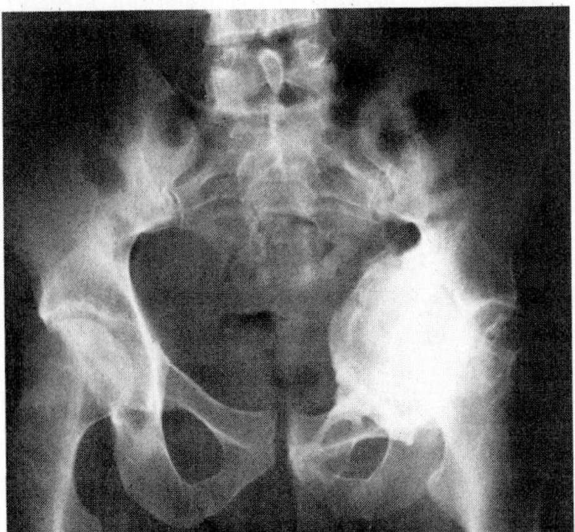

Figure 12-41A: AP view.

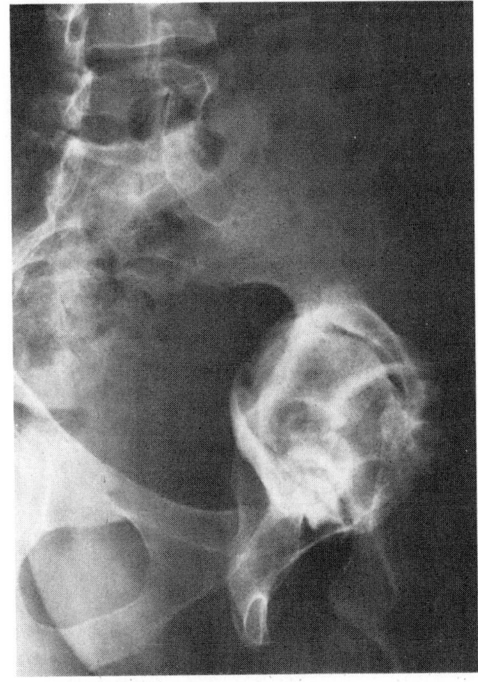

Figure 12-41B: Iliac oblique view.

the acetabular component, the use of supplementary image intensification is helpful to document the appropriate orientation and penetration of the drill bit and screws.

A nonunion of a posterior wall fracture with or without an associated posterior column disruption is a relatively common sequel to an initially unsuccessful surgical reconstruction. The problem arises when the posterior wall fragment is inadequately secured with lag screws. If the wall fragment is reduced prior to the preparation of the gliding holes, an errant direction of the holes and subsequently of the screws creates a predilection for premature loss of fixation (Figure 12-44) or penetration of the hip joint by a screw (Figure 12-45). Such a maldirected screw may explain catastrophic deterioration of the hip, which previously has been attributable to avascular necrosis of the femoral head. Where the fixation of the wall fragment fails prematurely, the fragment displaces secondary to posterior subluxation of the femoral head. Frequently, even years later at the time of a total hip joint replacement, a fibrous nonunion of the posterior wall fragment can be anticipated. With the instability and malalignment, fixation of a conventional acetabular component by the use of bone cement becomes exceedingly difficult. The posterior wall needs to be stabilized with screws or a buttress plate. Again, for

Figure 12-42: This white woman of 26 years sustained a "T" fracture, for which lag screw fixation and the application of iliac crest bone graft was undertaken acutely. When she progressed to a painful acetabular nonunion-malunion with severe avascular necrosis of the femoral head, she was transferred to our center, where a pelvic reconstruction with a cementless H-G total hip joint replacement was undertaken. Prior to the insertion of the acetabular component, fibrous nonunions of the anterior and posterior columns were curetted and obliterated with bone graft harvested from the femoral head. An H-G total hip replacement was undertaken.

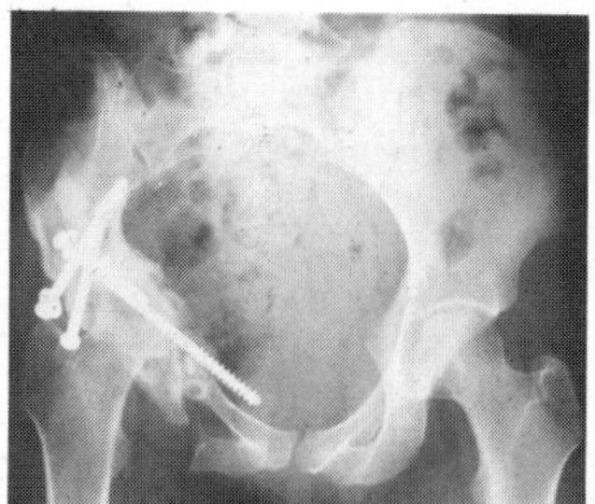

Figure 12-42A: Preoperative AP view.

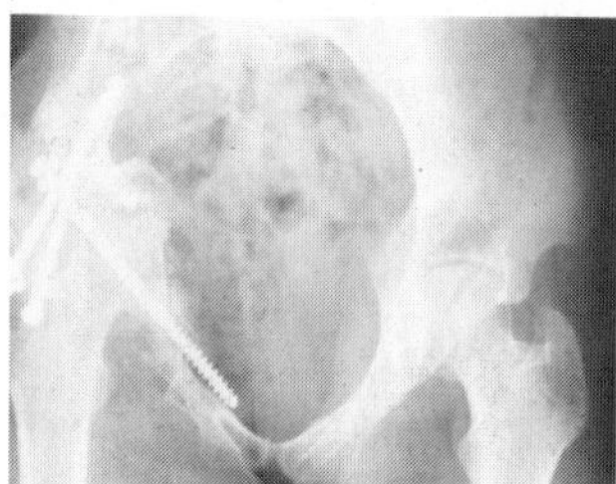

Figure 12-42B: Preoperative inlet view.

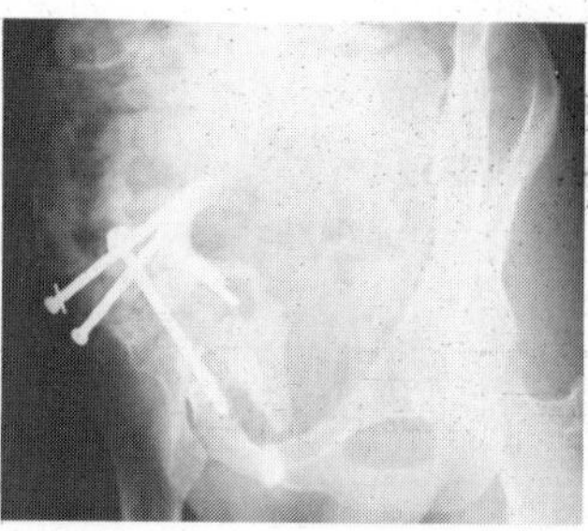

Figure 12-42C: Preoperative iliac oblique view indicative of extensive harvesting of iliac crest at the time of initial surgery and the marked protrusio.

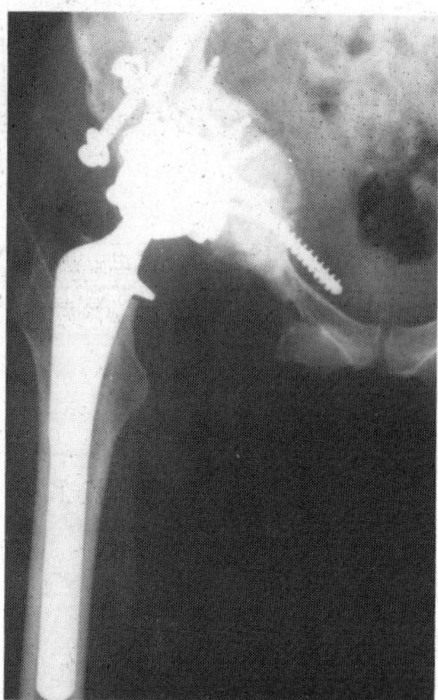

Figure 12-42D: Postoperative AP view.

Figure 12-43: This woman of 61 years presented with a "T" acetabular nonunion secondary to multiple myeloma with radiation therapy and allied avascular necrosis of the femoral head.

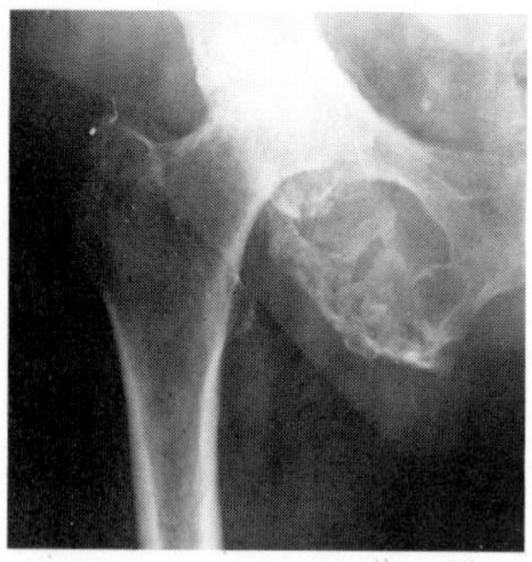

Figure 12-43A: Preoperative radiograph.

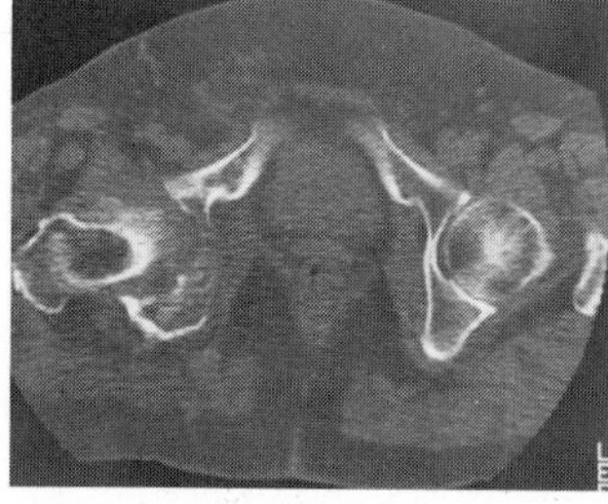

Figure 12-43B: Preoperative computed scan.

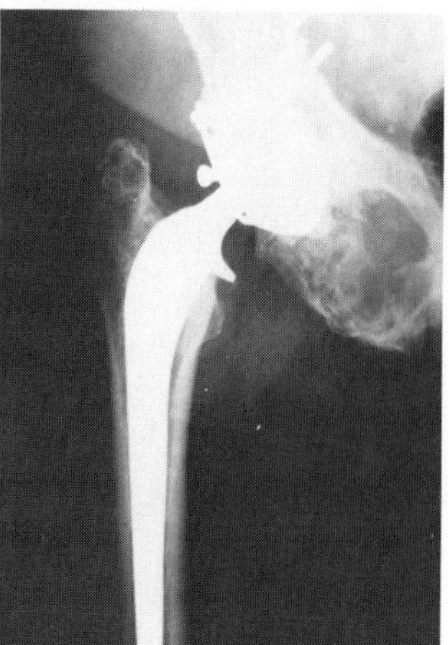

Figure 12-43C: Postoperative radiograph one year after surgical reconstruction.

Figure 12-44: This obese male of 260 pounds sustained bilateral acetabular fractures with a minimally displaced left transverse pattern and a contralateral posterior column and wall disruption. For the right hip, two lag screws were employed to secure the posterior wall, while the posterior column was not reduced. Subsequently, the screws disengaged from the posterior wall with recurrent subluxation of the hip joint. At the time of presentation one year later, and the then-available total hip joint replacements, a difficult stabilization of the acetabular component ensued. With adequate initial surgical reconstruction, this problem would have been avoidable.

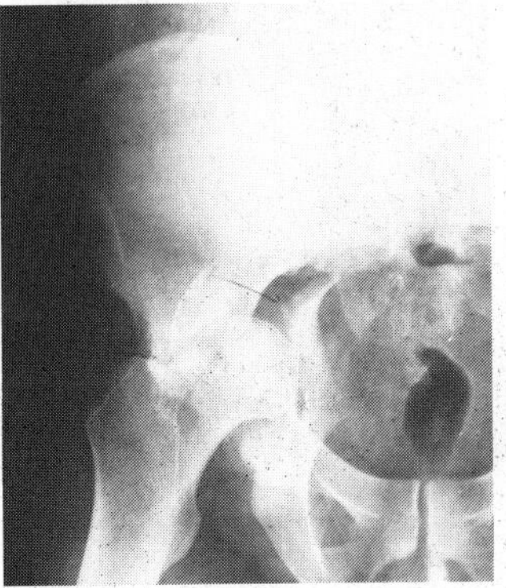

Figure 12-44A: Initial posttraumatic view.

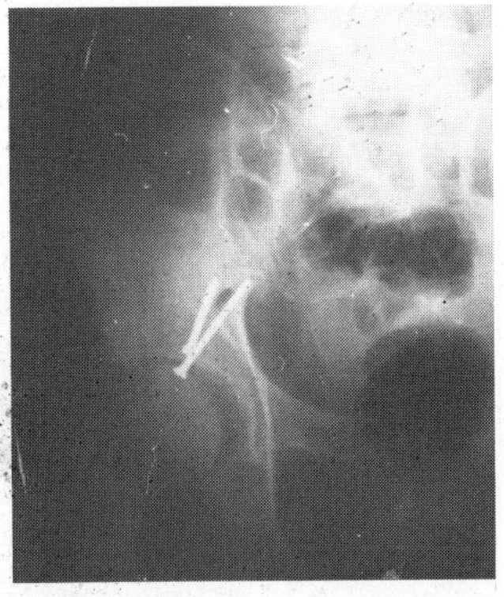

Figure 12-44B: After limited internal fixation.

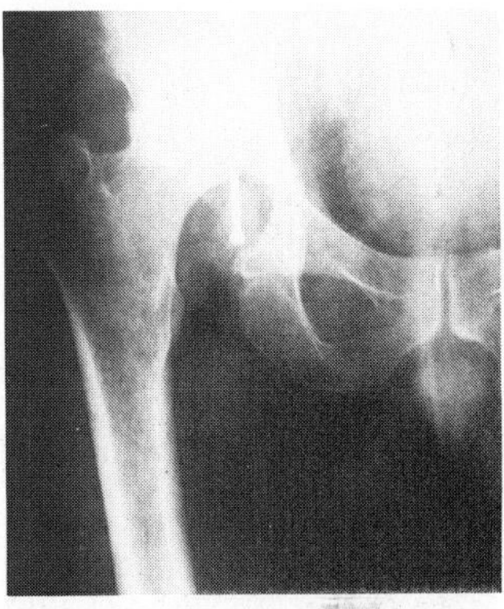

Figure 12-44C: Two months later, the fixation had failed and recurrent subluxation of the femoral head was evident.

this problem, the H-G total hip replacement represents a major technical improvement.

Another late acetabular problem, a nonunion-malunion of a posterior wall fracture with traumatic arthritis of the hip joint and a nonunion of a midshaft femoral fracture (Figure 12-45), is amenable to immobilization of both nonunions with a special total hip joint replacement. The acetabulum is reconstructed by resort to lag screws while a long-stem femoral component permits immobilization of the femoral nonunion. An excellent late functional result was documented in this woman of 68.

When an acetabular nonunion-malunion accompanied by profound osteoporosis necessitates a total hip joint replacement, the provision for adequate fixation of the acetabular component becomes a formidable undertaking or a technical impossibility (Figure 12-46). In this instance, a woman of 66 years with severe postmenopausal osteoporosis presented over a year after a vehicular accident with a nonunion-malunion of a highly comminuted both-column fracture. At the time of surgery, anchorage of the acetabular component by conventional cement technique in the displaced, comminuted osteoporotic remnants of the acetabulum was impossible. Screw fixation for the anchorage of a cementless acetabular component in the osteoporotic bone was wholly ineffective. After the application of a large amount of autologous bone graft to the acetabulum, a cemented bipolar device was inserted for the total hip

Figure 12-45: This woman of 68 years presented one year after a left posterior wall disruption with a midshaft femoral fracture. She had persistent dislocation of the hip joint with a screw violating the joint and a nonunion of the femur. A total hip joint reconstruction employing a Mueller ring and a long stem prosthesis corrected both problems.

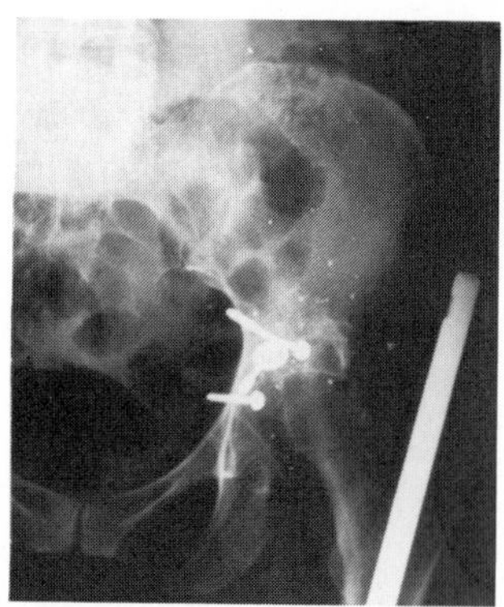

Figure 12-45A: Presenting view.

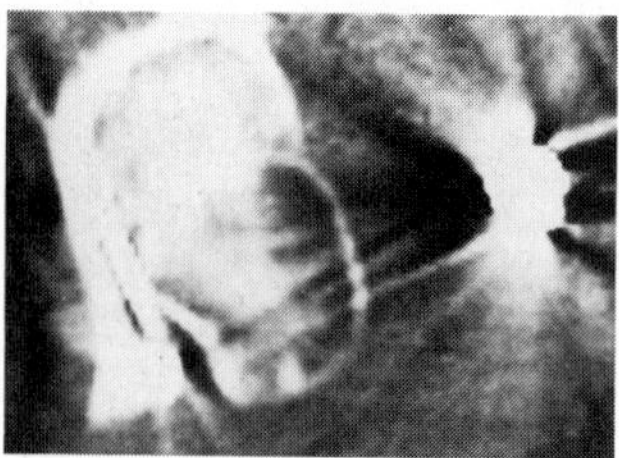

Figure 12-45B: Computed scan with a screw in the hip joint.

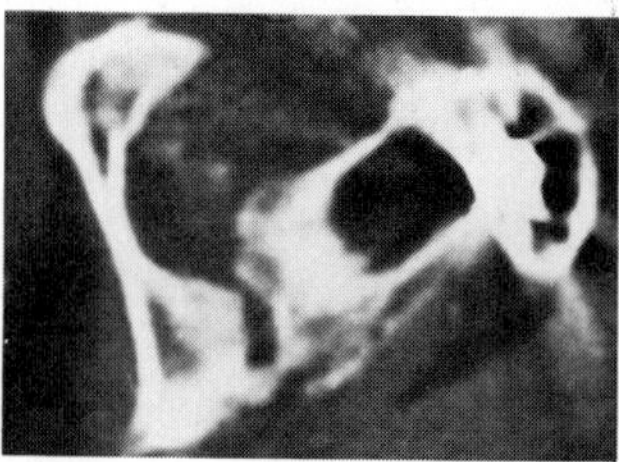

Figure 12-45C: Computed scan shows persistent dislocation of the femoral head.

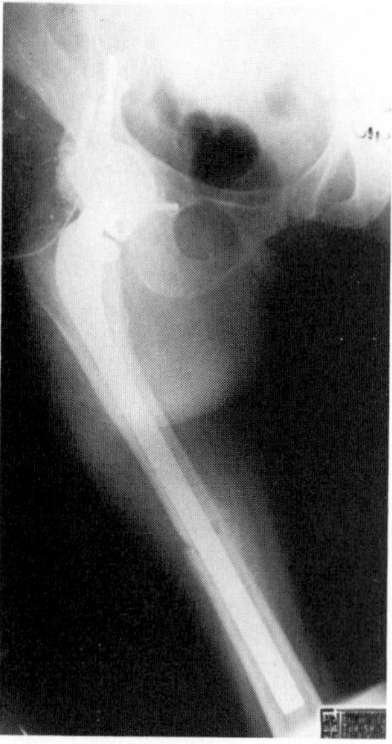

Figure 12-45D: Postoperative view.

replacement. This solution has provided an effective result for 18 months after surgery in this woman of about 98 pounds. Even if the bipolar device slowly migrates into the bone graft and becomes painful, a conversion to a conventional cemented acetabular component is feasible once the acetabulum has united.

An acetabular malunion of the inferior half of the acetabulum or of the posterior column can be associated with sitting imbalance (Figure 12-47). Here both the discomfort secondary to sitting imbalance as well as the incongruity of the acetabulum with a predilection for traumatic arthritis of the hip can be corrected by a rotational displacement of the ramus fragment. In this example, inadequate correction of the acetabulum was achieved.

Figure 12-46: This osteoporotic woman of 66 years presented one month after she sustained a highly comminuted both-column fracture for which internal fixation provided inadequate fixation of the soft bone fragments. One year later a cemented PCA bipolar total hip joint replacement was undertaken with the application of bone graft to the persistent nonunion of the osteoporotic acetabulum.

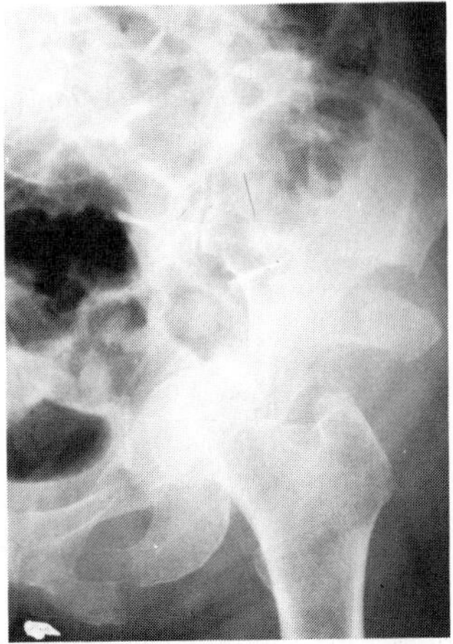

Figure 12-46A: Presenting AP view.

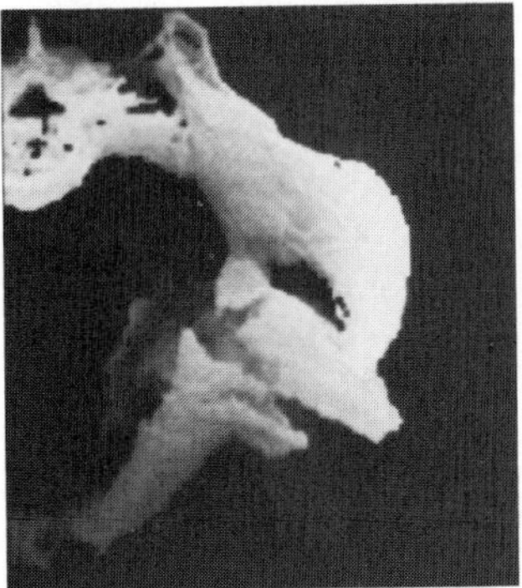

Figure 12-46B: Presenting 3D computed superior view.

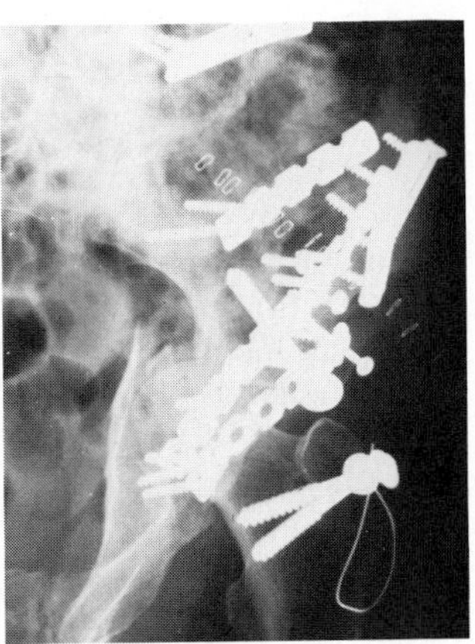

Figure 12-46C: One year afterwards.

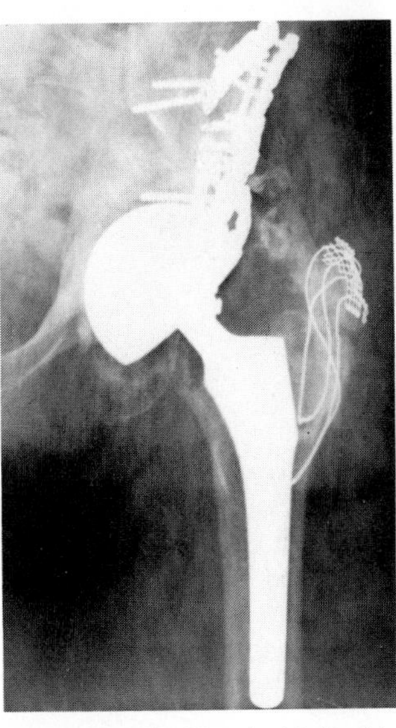

Figure 12-46D: After the bipolar hip replacement.

Figure 12-47: A malunion of a transverse acetabular fracture with marked rotation of the inferior acetabulum and sitting imbalance.

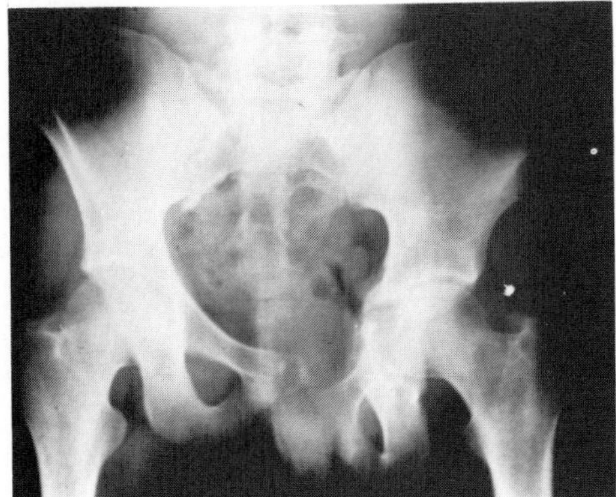

Figure 12-47A: Preoperative view.

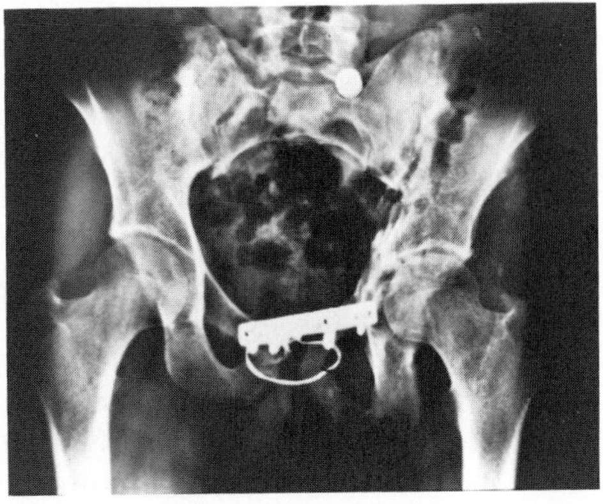

Figure 12-47B: Postoperative view.

Figure 12-48: This woman of 61 years was struck by a car while walking across a street, sustaining a ruptured thoracic aorta and numerous appendicular fractures along with a left-sided pelvic and acetabular disruption. Her pelvic injury was managed with skeletal traction. One year later she presented with a mobile nonunion of the sacroiliac joint and a "T" posterior wall acetabular nonunion-malunion, for which pelvic reconstruction and a total hip joint replacement were undertaken.

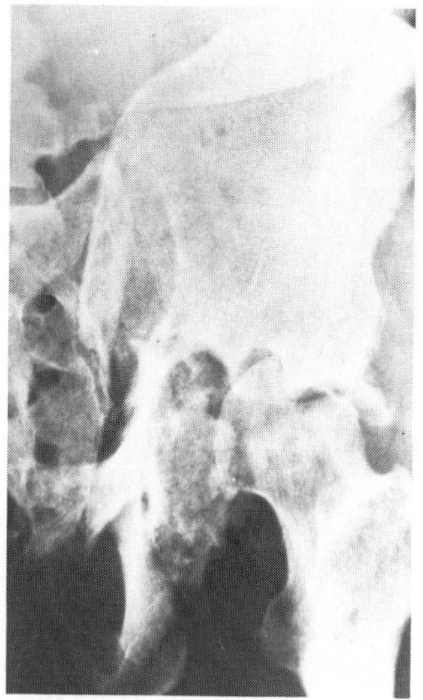
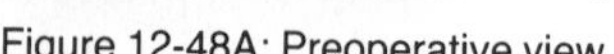

Figure 12-48A: Preoperative view.

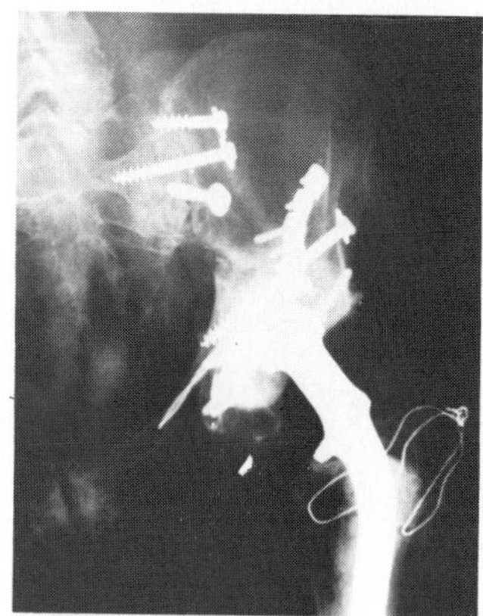

Figure 12-48B: Postoperative AP view.

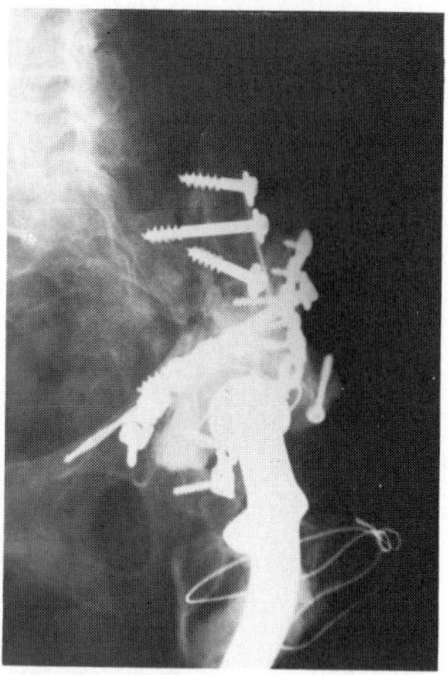

Figure 12-48C: Postoperative obturator oblique view.

## Nonunion-Malunion of Complex Pelvic and Acetabular Fractures

With the extraordinary force needed to provoke a complex pelvic fracture and the likelihood for major associated life-threatening problems, it is not surprising that many patients present with late clinical problems secondary to their pelvic disruption. The problems may arise as a result of the initial unstable clinical state of the patient or from a lack of awareness among the surgical team that reconstructive surgery is feasible. Hopefully, in the future, many of these cases will be managed with early reconstruction of the pelvis and acetabulum so that the late problems are avoided.

Many of these problems are associated with extensive displacement of virtually the entire pelvic ring so that a precise characterization of the deformity is virtually impossible. Especially in young adults, whenever the hip joint appears to be potentially viable the acetabular and pelvic nonunion is reconstructed, even though a later total hip joint replacement may become necessary. The reconstruction starts with the acetabular nonunion-malunion and progresses to the adjacent ilium. Where the ipsilateral sacroiliac joint is involved, anterior debridement and anatomical location of that site is needed before a concentric acetabular reduction can be undertaken. For the more severe cases, bilateral osteotomies through the fibrocartilaginous malunion-nonunion sites are necessary. Initially, combinations of external and internal fixation were employed (Figures 12-21 and 12-22). The provision for external fixation limited the exposure and somewhat simplified the surgical technique; nevertheless, the external fixation pins provided a potential for pin tract infection with a possible extension to the acetabulum. External fixation also provided a transient and less rigid method of stabilization than a comparable technique of internal fixation in a situation where a prolonged period of healing was anticipated. More recently solely internal fixation has been utilized for the immobilization of a late pelvic reconstruction. Once the pelvis has been restored to a stable anatomical configuration, if traumatic arthritis of the hip ensues, a relatively uncomplicated total hip joint replacement can be undertaken in a conventional way.

In the presence of a transverse or "T" acetabular fracture with a nonunion/malunion of the sacroiliac joint (Figure 12-48), a triradiate approach permits exposure of all of the sites of disruption. Initially, an anterior approach to the sacroiliac joint is undertaken for debridement and immobilization of the joint by the use of lag screws. This step restores the anatomical alignment of the superior half of the acetabulum. Then the transverse and vertical elements of the acetabular nonunion are debrided, reduced, and immobilized with lag screws so that the total hip joint acetabular component can be inserted into a stable base. With the potential for substantial residual malalignment even after the open reduction, particular care is required to orient the acetabular component properly and, thereby, avoid the potential for a late recurrent dislocation of the hip. When the acetabular nonunion-malunion is accompanied by an unstable diastasis of the symphysis and an unstable nonunion-malunion of the contralateral pelvis such as the sacroiliac joint (Figure 12-23), then all of the disrupted sites require immobilization to recreate an intact pelvic ring. Otherwise, persistent late pain and instability at one or more of the nonunion sites is almost inevitable.

For the most difficult bilateral cases, a staged surgical reconstruction is preferred (Figure 12-49). In this example a helicopter pilot fell from a height of about 200 feet when his craft sustained an engine failure. He presented to us about two years later with superior migration of the left hemipelvis as a nonunion-malunion accompanied by a "T" fracture nonunion-malunion of the contralateral pelvis. He had a marked sitting imbalance with a discrepancy in the ischial tuberosities of 8cm and bilateral pelvic pain. In the first surgical procedure, the left hemipelvis was stabilized and an attempt was made to reconstruct the "T" fracture. While this procedure provided alleviation of the left pelvic pain, it did not correct the sitting imbalance and right-sided pelvic and hip pain. About one year later a cementless total hip joint was undertaken. At this stage the right ischial tuberosity was osteotomized and repositioned as a posterior wall and column for the acetabular component. The procedure provided an effective correction of the sitting imbalance and a pain-free hip.

In a nonunion-malunion involving an entire hemipelvis, a T-type incision has been particularly helpful (Figure 12-50). A posterior curved extension of an ilioinguinal incision continues around the iliac crest to the posterior superior spine. The T extension of the incision continues from the iliac crest, superficial to the superior gluteal ridge across the greater trochanter. The extended ilioinguinal approach provides adequate exposure for reconstruction of the anterior column, as well as the sacroiliac joint. The longitudinal limb of the incision is employed for a restoration of the acetabulum, as well as the total hip joint replacement. With extraordinary malalignment of the various parts of the pelvis, including the acetabulum, proper alignment of the metallic backing is particularly difficult. In this case where a Bateman prosthesis had been inserted into the nonunion-malunion of the pelvis and acetabulum, the device provoked erosion of the entire roof of the acetabulum. A new roof was created from fragments of autologous iliac crest bone graft, which were secured by screws inserted through the acetabular metal backing along with supplementary lag screws. This patient also possessed a symptomatic inguinal hernia secondary to the bony deficiency in the superior pubic ramus. The hernia was corrected as part of the surgical closure.

## Late Infections

Infections can provide clinical problems either as a result of therapeutic intervention or as a sequel of an open fracture. While many of the problems are potentially avoidable, all of them require prompt recognition and definitive management.

### Pin Tract Infection

Both external skeletal fixation pins and traction pins can progress to a pin tract infection. External fixation pins are prone to infection if the skin is tented around the pin or if the bone is thermally necrosed at the time of insertion. Such problems are minimized by preparation of the cutaneous incision superficial to the ultimate

Figure 12-49: This helicopter pilot of 61 years fell 200 feet, provoking a vertical shear injury of the left hemipelvis and a "T" fracture of the right acetabulum for which conservative treatment was employed. Two years later, the bilateral unstable painful hemipelves were managed with open reductions and stabilization by resort to internal and external fixation. One year later, a cementless right total hip joint replacement with correction of persistent sitting imbalance was performed.

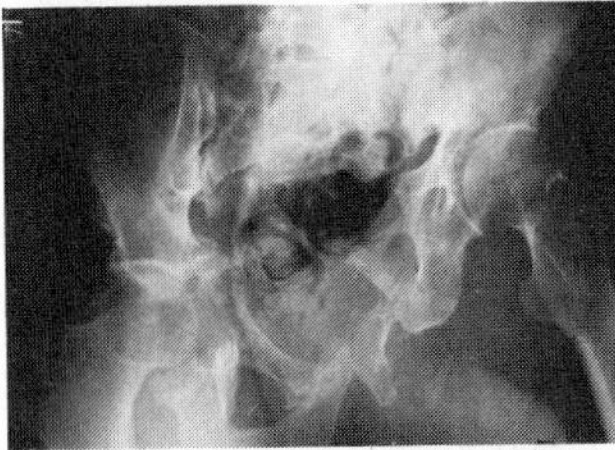

Figure 12-49A: Presenting AP view.

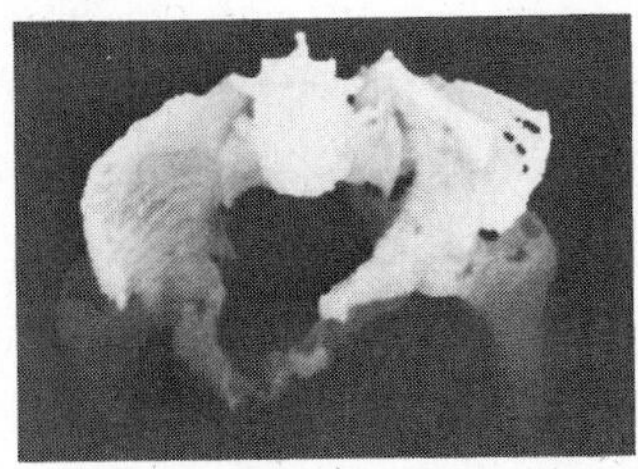

Figure 12-49B: Presenting 3D computed inlet view.

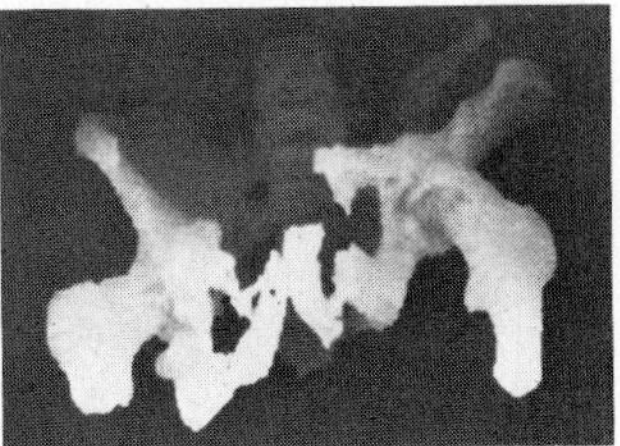

Figure 12-49C: Presenting 3D computed outlet view.

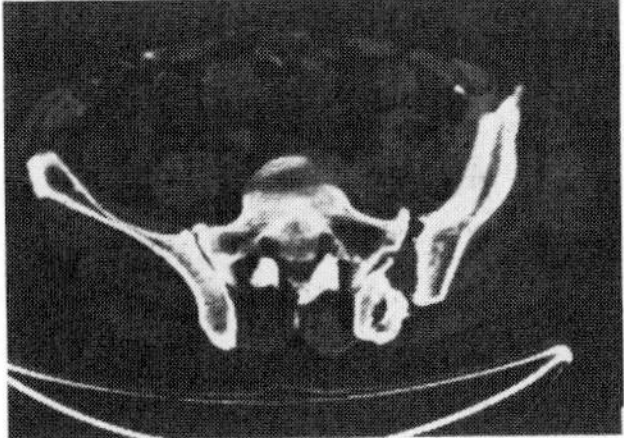

Figure 12-49D: Computed scan of disrupted SI joint.

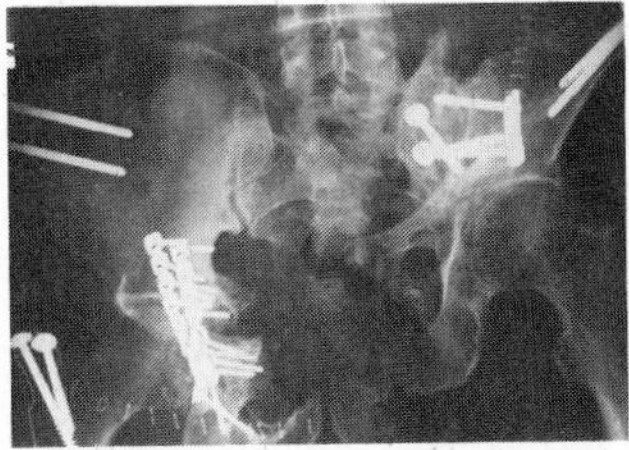

Figure 12-49E: Initial postoperative radiograph.

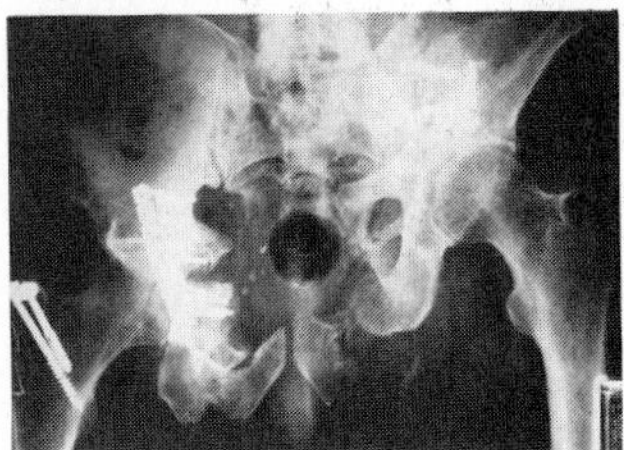

Figure 12-49F: One year later with a painful right hip and sitting imbalance.

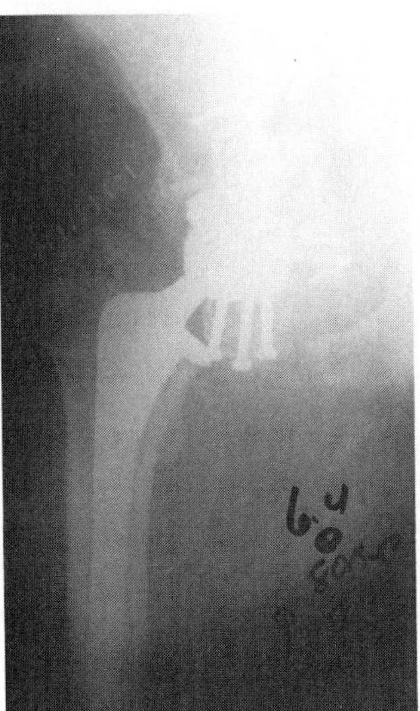

Figure 12-49G: Postoperative view of H-G total hip replacement.

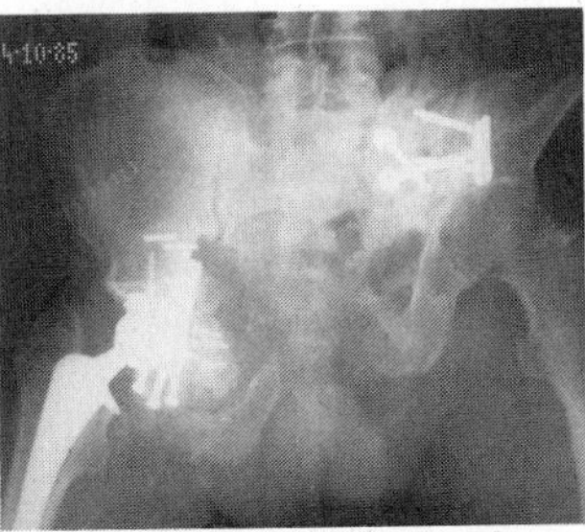

Figure 12-49H: AP view taken six months later.

Figure 12-50: This man of 40 years presented six years after sustaining a right-sided pelvic disruption with a sacroiliac dislocation, a transverse acetabular fracture, and a diastasis. Following conservative management when hip pain ensued, a Bateman prosthesis was inserted. Persistent pain and instability of the right hemipelvis was followed by migration of the Bateman prosthesis. The secondary reconstruction included lag screw fixation of the sacroiliac joint, the application of plate fixation with a large iliac crest bone graft to the symphysis, and acetabular reconstruction with multiple screws and an H-G total hip joint replacement.

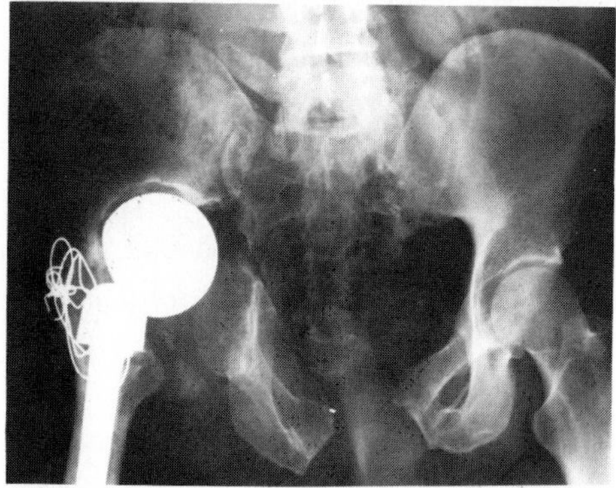

Figure 12-50A: Presenting AP view with Bateman prosthesis.

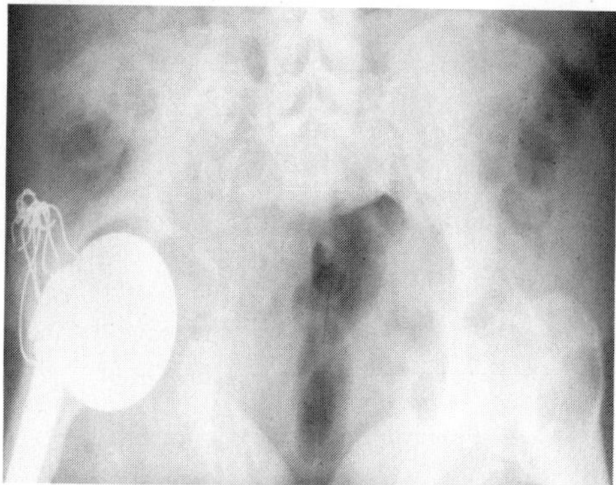

Figure 12-50B: Inlet view.

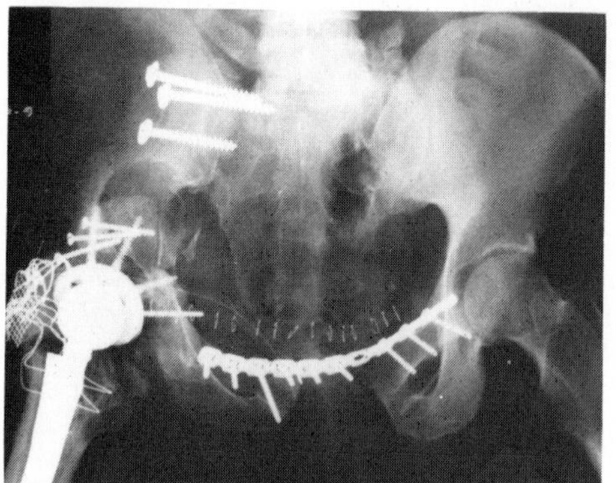

Figure 12-50C: Postoperative AP view of pelvis.

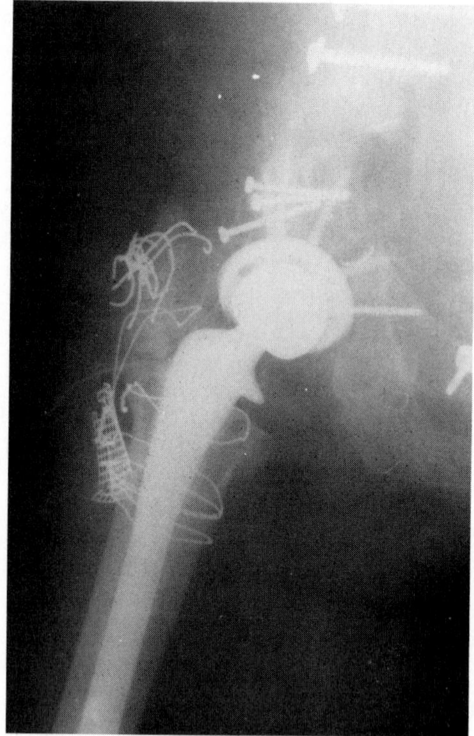

Figure 12-50D: Postoperative view of hip.

position of the bone after a closed pelvic reduction has been undertaken. Predrilling with a sharp bit and insertion of the pin with a hand brace minimize the thermal damage to bone. In a markedly obese individual a particularly loose closure is undertaken or the wound is packed completely open until the pins are removed. Once a pin shows evidence of purulent drainage, it is removed and the pin tract is debrided. Generally with the limited bone stock available in the pelvis, such a pin is not replaced. If the stability of the external fixation is thereby markedly compromised, consideration is given to supplementation or conversion to suitable internal fixation. If a pin site shows evidence of purulent drainage at the time of definitive removal of the frame, the pin site is debrided with a curette.

With the application of skeletal traction, particularly by resort to a greater trochanteric pin, infection of the intertrochanteric bone is relatively common and a potentially catastrophic problem (Figure 12-16). A pin inserted in such cancellous bone is particularly liable to spontaneous loosening and infection. Once that site becomes infected, it creates a predilection for a postoperative wound infection if an open reduction and stabilization of an acetabular fracture is undertaken by a lateral exposure. In some cases, admittedly, an ilioinguinal or an iliofemoral approach can be employed to minimize the risk of cross-contamination of the surgical incision from the pin site. With the limited likelihood for lateral traction applied by resort to a greater trochanteric pin with or without supplementary longitudinal traction, to provide an accurate reduction of a centrally displaced acetabular fracture this technique is strongly discouraged. Once a greater trochanteric pin site has become infected, a thorough debridement of the site with appropriate antibiotic therapy is indicated. Generally, a deferral of definitive surgical intervention for the acetabular fracture for two to four weeks greatly complicates the subsequent open reduction and increases the likelihood for postoperative ectopic bone formation.

## Postoperative Wound Infections

With the excellent blood supply of the skin, subcutaneous tissues, and muscle superficial to the pelvis, postoperative wound infections of the pelvis and acetabulum appear to be relatively uncommon. The resistance of the soft tissues to infection, however, can be markedly compromised by a major contusion or abrasive injury, which accompanies many of the fractures. Whenever possible the surgical exposure is modified to circumvent the contused or abraided skin. During the exposure if necrotic subcutaneous fat or greater trochanteric bursa is encountered with a lateral compression type of acetabular or pelvic fracture, the necrotic material is debrided. The potential interval between the superficial muscles and the skin is carefully preserved as a myocutaneous flap for optimal maintenance of the cutaneous blood supply. In the presence of a comminuted pelvic or acetabular fracture, a muscular origin or insertion in each major bone fragment is carefully preserved. If a major fragment is totally devascularized and postoperative infection occurs, the fragment necroses with a fulminant infection and requires surgical removal. During the early postoperative period if the wound shows evidence of serous drainage, the patient is maintained at bed rest until the drainage subsides. If the wound shows progressive reddening and initiation of purulent drainage, a surgical exploration and debridement is performed promptly. During the debridement a culture is taken and appropriate intravenous antibiotics are initiated. If totally devitalized bone is encountered it is removed. The wound is loosely closed and suitable intravenous antibiotics are administered. Of our own clinical experience with four infected acetabular fractures and no late infection after a pelvic reconstruction, three cases resolved with debridement and antibiotic therapy. One other case culminated in a hip fusion. The last fracture was a comminuted both-column insult with iliac extension where the extensive surgical approach included a stripping of most of the iliac crest. The devitalized bone became infected so that resection of the ilium and posterior column was necessary. Ultimately, when the infection had resolved a hip fusion was performed by the use of a Cobra plate.

Another possibility is the presentation of an infected nonunion of the greater trochanter following a closure of an acetabular fracture that includes internal fixation of the greater trochanter. In one instance, a young adult male managed for a both-column fracture with an anatomical reduction and stabilization of the acetabulum progressed to a symptomatic bursitis of the greater trochanter. Three months after the acetabular repair the greater trochanteric screws were removed. At this time an infected nonunion of the greater trochanter ensued when the patient was transferred to our care. Following a thorough debridement the four viable greater trochanteric bone fragments were secured with lag screw fixation and a supplementary tension band wire. A stable union followed without evidence of drainage for the next two years.

## Infected Nonunion of the Pelvis

In our experience with two infected nonunions of the pelvis, both formidable problems followed an open fracture with an extensive anterior wound. In one case (Figure 12-51), a coal miner of 55 years who was involved in a collapse of a mine shaft presented to us about nine months after his injury with a wholly exposed bladder and an unstable hemipelvis. While external pelvic fixation

Figure 12-51: This coal miner of 55 years sustained a mining injury with an open pelvic fracture and exposed bladder. An initial attempt at wire fixation of the symphysis failed so that a painful unstable nonunion-malunion of the pelvis ensued. About nine months later, at presentation external fixation was applied. The patient succumbed two days later to septicemia.

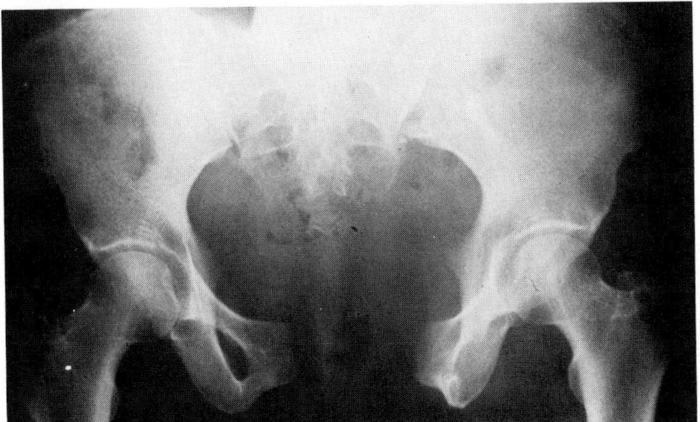

Figure 12-51A: Initial AP view.

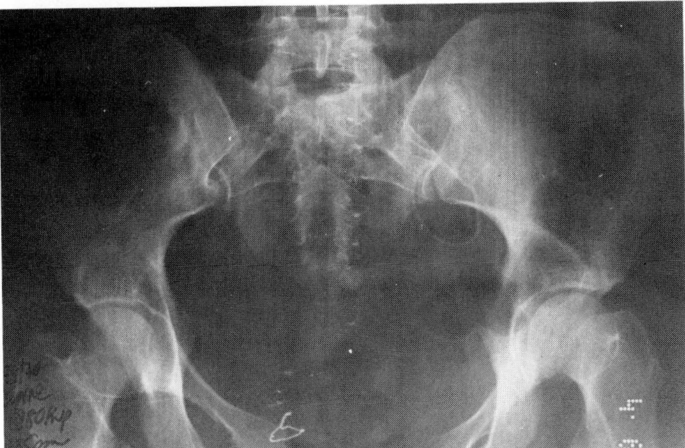

Figure 12-51B: Nine months afterwards, at presentation.

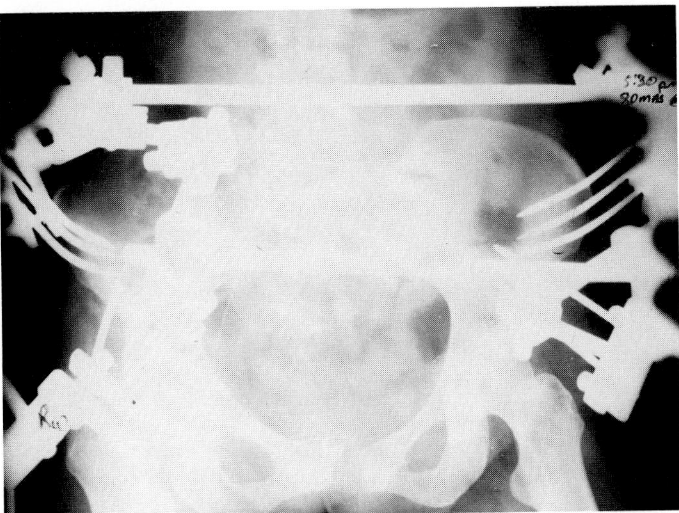

Figure 12-51C: After pelvic external fixation.

Figure 12-52: Photographs, schematic diagrams, and radiographs present a woman of 20 years who sustained an open pelvic ring fracture when her jeep overturned, pinning her beneath it. (Reproduced with permission of Williams and Wilkins).

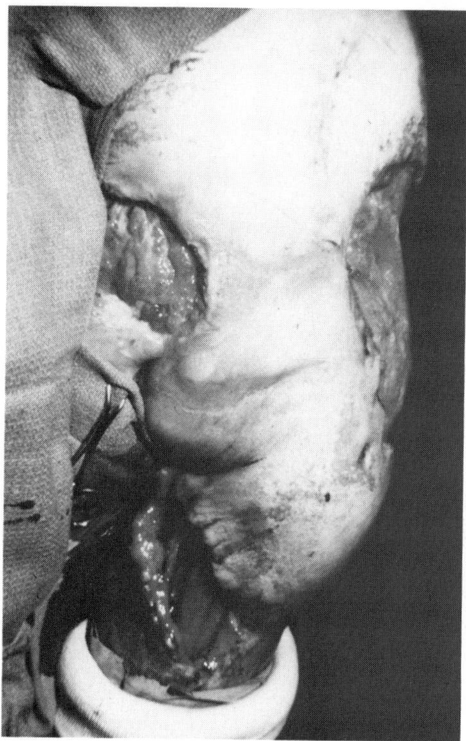

Figure 12-52A: One year after injury at the time of presentation.

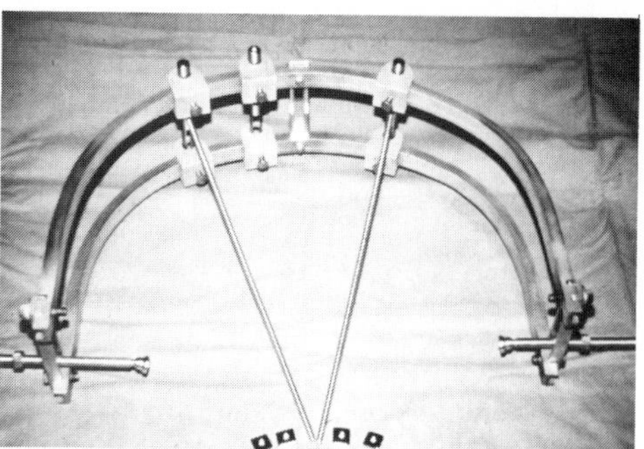

Figure 12-52B: Appearance of the special frame and instruments designed for management.

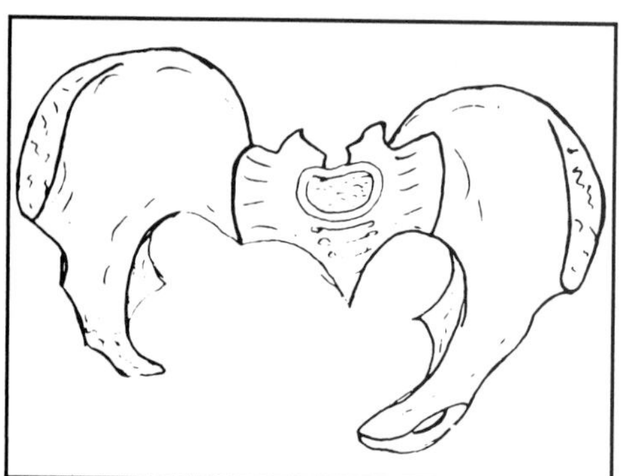

Figure 12-52C: Pelvic inlet diagram prior to osteotomy through the malunion-nonunion of the right SI joint.

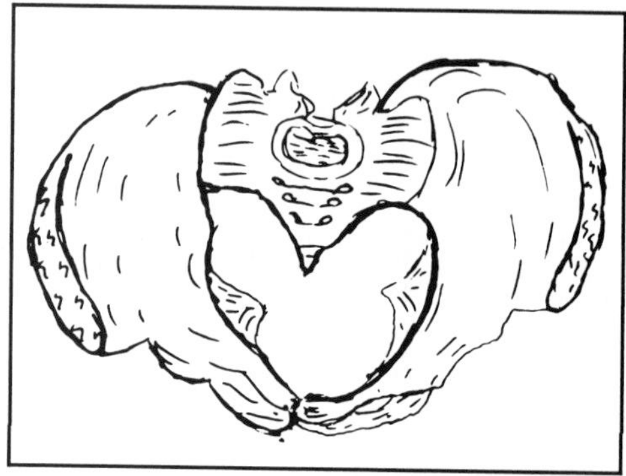

Figure 12-52D: Pelvic inlet diagram after osteotomy.

was applied along with a debridement, the patient died of an overwhelming pseudomonas septicemia including pulmonary involvement, two days after his presentation to us. The other patient, a young woman of 20 years (Figures 12-52 and 12-53), presented one year after a vehicular accident when she sustained a wide abduction

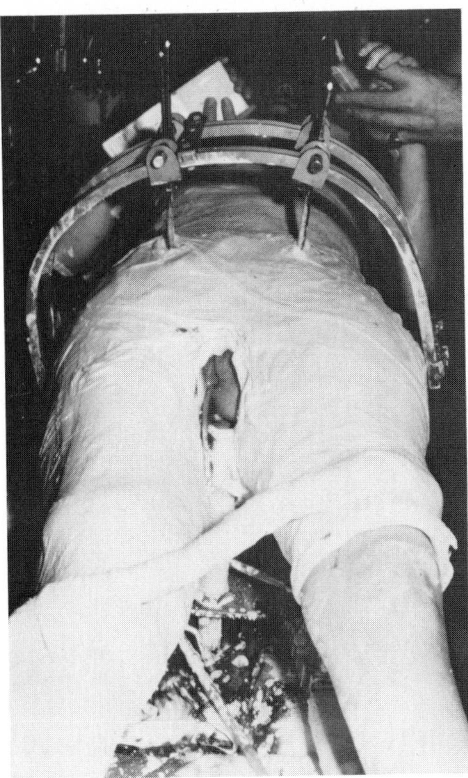

Figure 12-52E: After the application of external fixation and hip spica.

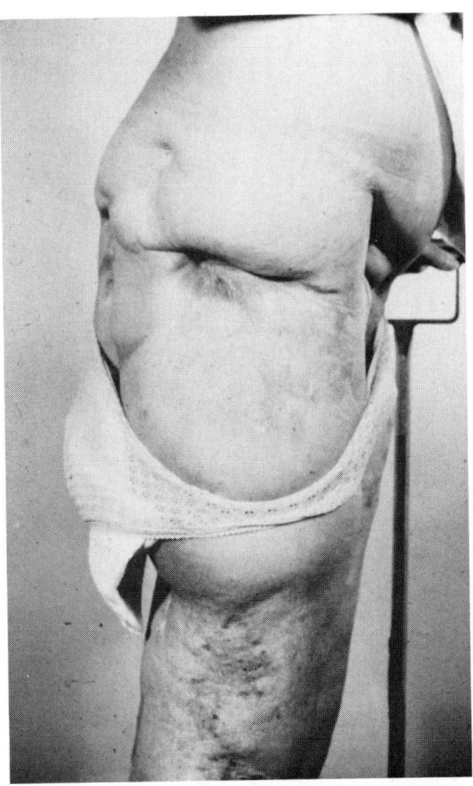

Figure 12-52F: Four months later, after closure of the wounds.

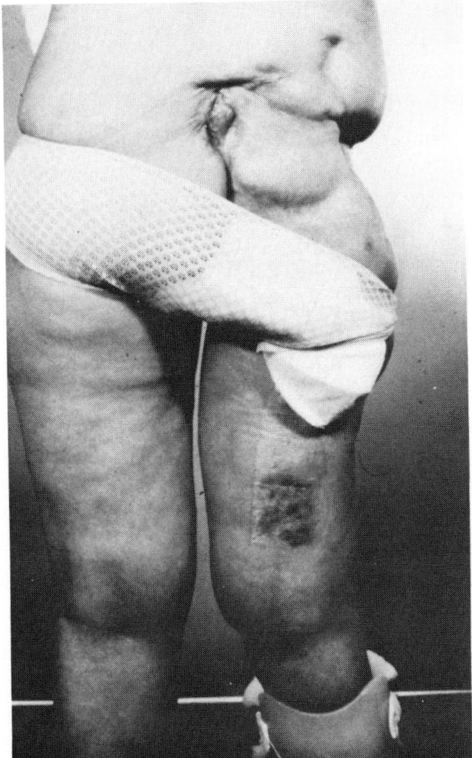

Figure 12-52G: Four months later, after closure of the wounds.

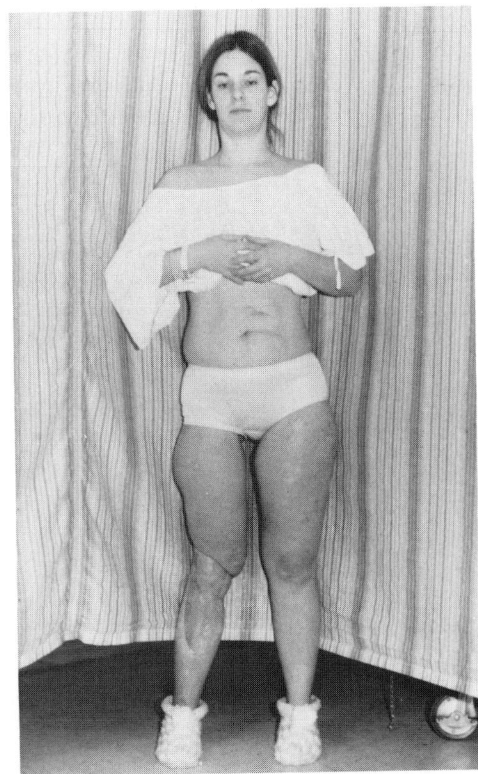

Figure 12-52H: Two years later, after plastic revision.

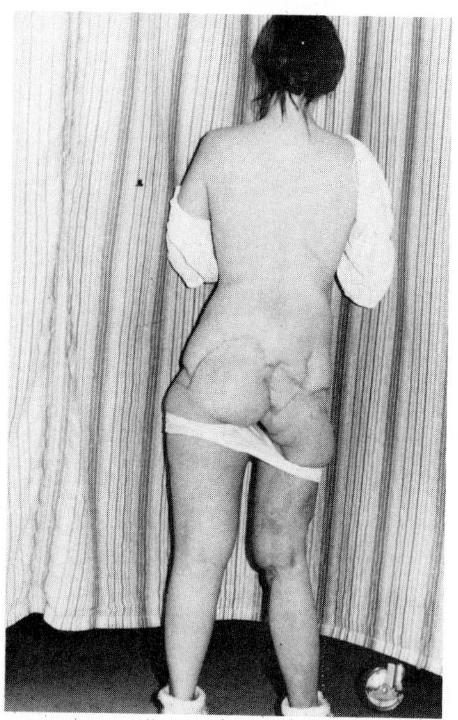

Figure 12-52I: Two years later, after plastic revision.

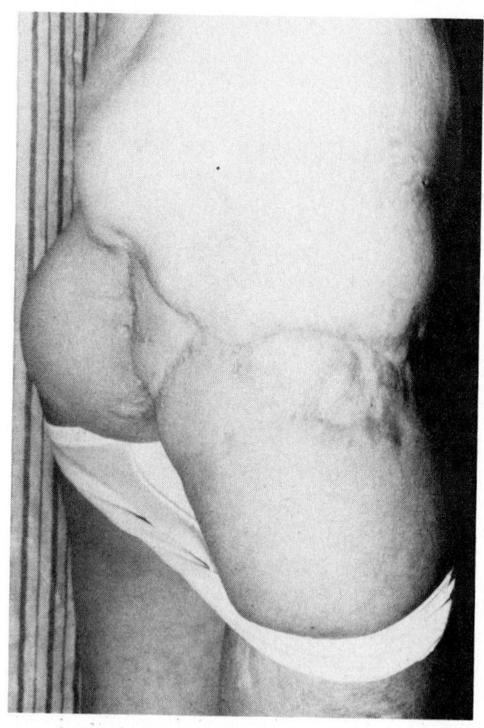

Figure 12-52J: Two years later, after plastic revision.

insult with an open pelvic ring disruption and an ipsilateral acetabular fracture. Initially she was managed with skeletal traction and bed rest, but progressed to an infected nonunion. Probably the massive wound infections encountered in both of these cases were associated with feculent contaminiation and the absence of a diversion colostomy. On the day of presentation she sustained a cardiac arrest from hypokalemia secondary to electrolyte loss through the massive open wounds. A few days after her successful resuscitation, external pelvic fixation and debridement were undertaken and a diversion colostomy was prepared. During the next month multiple debridements were performed and split thickness skin grafts were applied. Then a closing-wedge osteotomy of the widened sacroiliac joint was undertaken to recreate a pelvic ring with bony continuity. Six weeks afterwards the external frame was removed. Four months after presentation to us, gait training was initiated. About one year later, plastic reconstructive surgery was performed to irradicate a large avulsive loss and associated disfigurement of the buttock. Approximately five years later, following completion of her college education, she underwent a successful Cesarean section to deliver a normal boy. For these late open infected problems, external fixation is generally preferred to minimize the devascularization of the bone. Unusually large fixation pins with an outside diameter of 6mm may be needed to obtain fixation in the osteoporotic bone. Along with a diversion colostomy and appropriate antibiotic therapy, intravenous hyperalimentation merits consideration to facilitate the healing of bone and allied soft tissues.

## Ectopic Bone Formation

Following pelvic surgery a variable degree of ectopic bone formation is a common sequel. In certain instances bone forms at the sites where external fixation pins were inserted (Figure 12-54). To date, associated symptomatic problems have not been documented. When a lateral or posterolateral exposure of an acetabular fracture is undertaken by resort to a Kocher-Langenbeck incision, or especially with a transtrochanteric lateral approach or a comparable extensile iliofemoral approach, ectopic bone formation occurs in up to 70% of the cases. In most instances the ectopic bone is of a small amount and constitutes merely a radiological finding (Figure 12-55). In other cases, however, extensive ectopic bone formation provokes stiffness of the hip or a continuous deep seated pain (Figure 12-56). In our experience the greatest predilection for extensive ectopic bone is documented after a large individual presents with a highly comminuted acetabular fracture and undergoes a surgical reconstruction by resort to an extensile lateral approach, particularly more than two weeks after the time of the injury. In the high risk cases, prophylactic application of disodium etidronate or indomethacin has been undertaken without obvious lessening of the tendency for ectopic bone formation. While prophylactic irradiation in doses as low as 500 to 1000 rads has been considered, this method has been employed solely for those cases where ectopic bone was excised about one year after an acetabular reconstruction. While it is the one available technique that appears to provide a distinct lessening for the tendency to ectopic bone formation, it is precluded from routine application by its potentially adverse side effects, including teratogenicity and delayed healing of bone and adjacent soft tissues.

When ectopic bone formation culminates in a complaint of marked stiffness of the hip, especially with associated discomfort apparently unrelated to traumatic arthritis, consideration for removal of the bone is undertaken. Maturation of the heterotopic bone is assessed by the use of serial radiographs and a technetium bone scan. Generally, the surgical removal is undertaken about one year after the initial trauma, when the predilection for recurrent ectopic bone formation is minimized (Figure 12-57). Prior to the surgery a computed scan of the hip

Figure 12-53: Anteroposterior radiographs of the same patient.

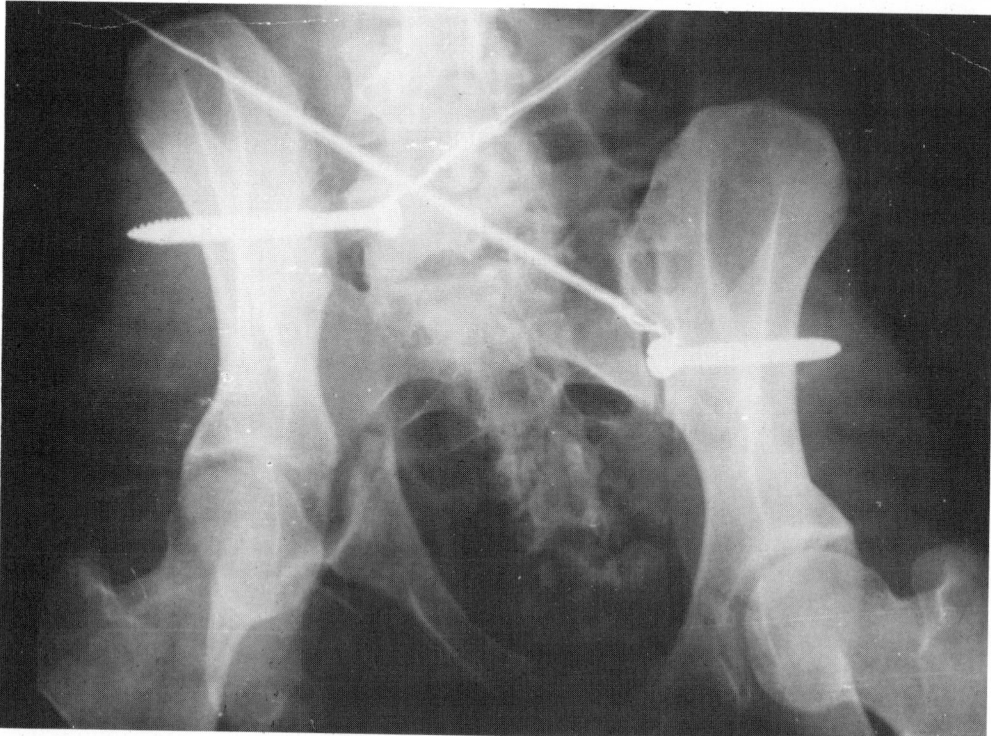

Figure 12-53A: After an unsuccessful attempt to employ skeletal traction wire. (Reproduced with permission of Williams and Wilkins).

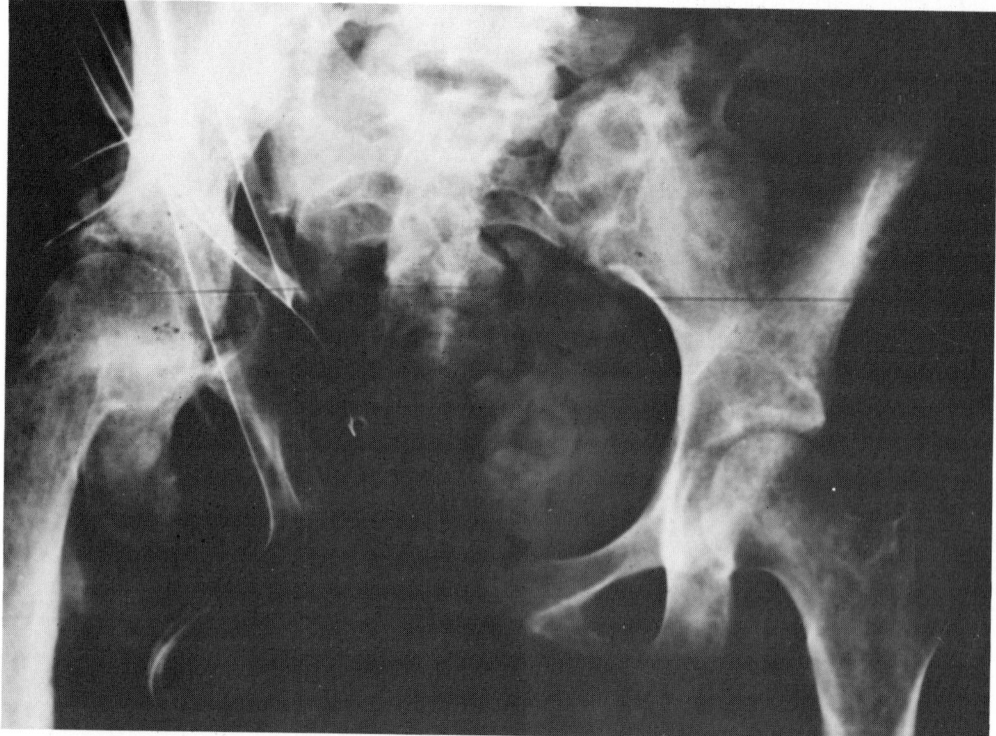

Figure 12-53B: One year later, at the time of presentation.

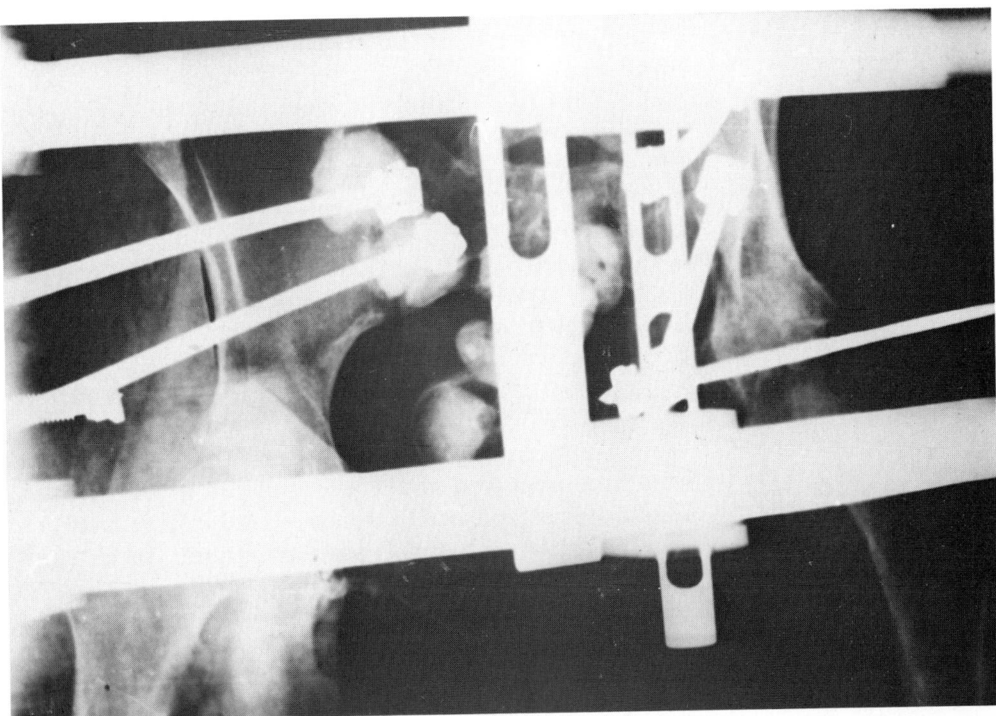

Figure 12-53C: View with pelvic frame.

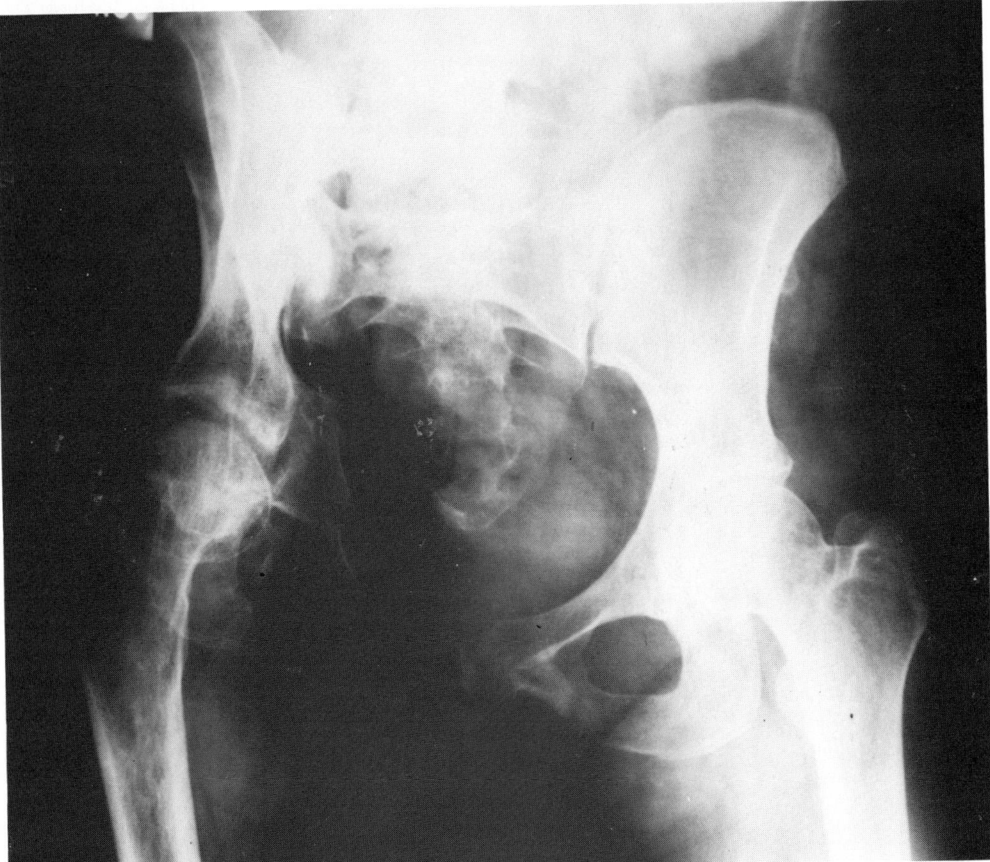

Figure 12-53D: Four months later, when the pelvis is united.

is undertaken to determine the location and extent of the ectopic bone. In the presence of extensive ectopic bone around the hip joint, which obliterates the radiographic details of the articular surfaces, the computed scan provides a crucial characterization of the magnitude of degenerative change. At the time of surgery, the capsular blood supply to the femoral head is carefully preserved. Generally, the superior capsule is incised longitudinally for removal of the ectopic bone. Usually a layer of capsule separates the femoral head and adjacent acetabulum from the ectopic bone. This deeper capsular layer is carefully preserved. Frequently, a large lip of ectopic bone accumulates around the acetabular rim and adjacent to the greater trochanter. When the initial exposure includes a release of the origins of the indirect and direct heads of the rectus femoris, usually the ectopic bone extends from the capsular region to the anterior inferior spine. During the surgical procedure the hip joint is manipulated to confirm the restoration of satisfactory mobility. If a particular limitation of motion is detected, a search for residual ectopic bone usually provides a suitable explanation so that further appropriate resection can be performed. Once the ectopic bone has been thoroughly removed, an intraoperative radiograph is taken to confirm the adequacy of the surgery. In the early postoperative period a continuous passive motion machine is employed to facilitate a rapid return of hip motion.

In men more than 40 years of age and postmenopausal women where extensive ectopic bone is removed, postoperative irradiation in low doses has been given (Figure 12-58). Typically, the regime provides 1000 rads administered incrementally as 200 rads given on alternate days starting the day after the surgery. With or without the irradiation, excision of proliferative ectopic bone has been notable for a considerable improvement in motion of the hip where congruent articular surfaces are present. The procedure is particularly effective to correct a fixed flexion contracture, a limitation of flexion to less than 100°, or marked limitation of abduction or internal rotation (Figure 12-59).

In those caes of ectopic bone accompanied by moderate or severe traumatic arthritis, provisions for concomitant total hip joint replacement are made. After the ectopic bone has been thoroughly removed, the articular surfaces are inspected. If they appear to be relatively intact, then the wound is closed. If a substantial loss of congruity and erosion of the articular surfaces or avascular necrosis of the femoral head are evident, then a total hip joint replacement is performed (Figure 12-60). Nevertheless, the potential for severe recurrent ectopic bone formation exists, which can culminate in a fused hip (Figure 12-61).

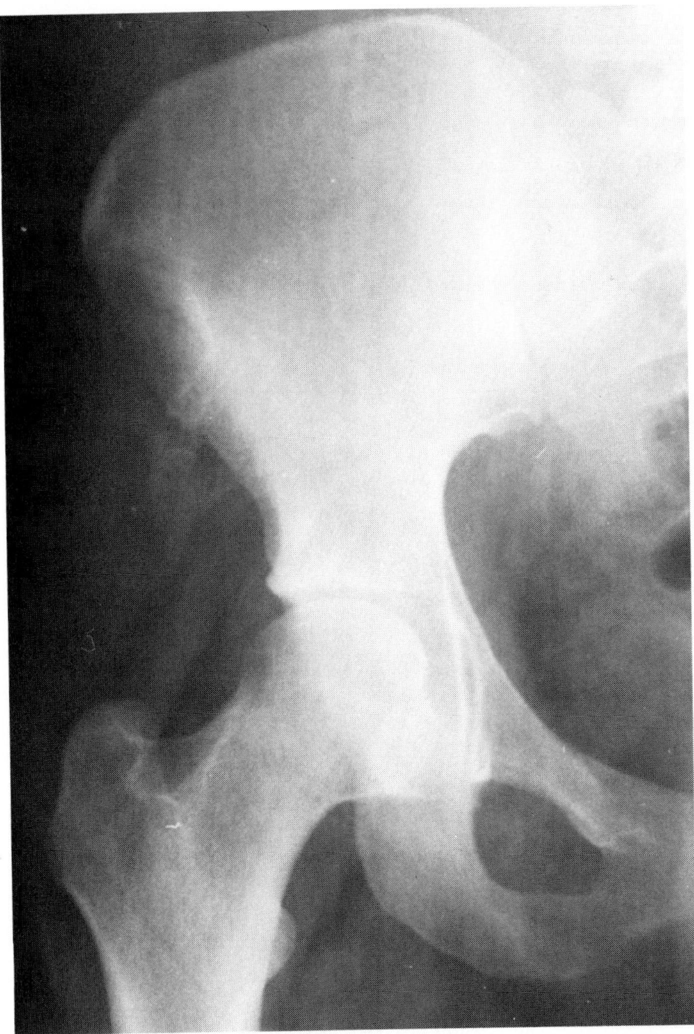

Figure 12-54: One year after removal of a Pittsburgh triangular frame, ectopic bone formation is evident at the site of the two pins inserted into the anterior inferior spine.

## Nerve Injury

A persistent neurological problem secondary to traumatically induced or, rarely, iatrogenically provoked injuries to the lumbosacral plexus or sciatic nerve is a relatively common cause of disability following a pelvic or acetabular disruption.[2] The incidence of nerve injury secondary to pelvic trauma including temporary neurological deficit is about 10% to 15%. Certain fracture patterns are particularly susceptible to associated neurological injury. Bilateral unstable vertical shear injuries head the list, with an incidence of up to 46%.[8] Pelvic disruptions associated with a dislocation of a hemipelvis, a sacral fracture, or a posterior fracture-dislocation of the hip are notoriously susceptible to allied nerve injury.[9,10] Most disruptions of the sacroiliac joint produce an L-5 lesion, while sacral fractures initiate an

Figure 12-55: Limited postoperative ectopic bone formation after a triradiate approach, seen one year after surgery.

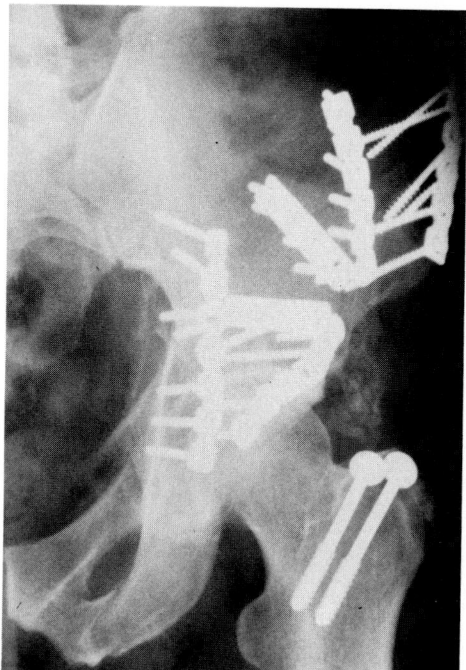

Figure 12-55A: AP view.

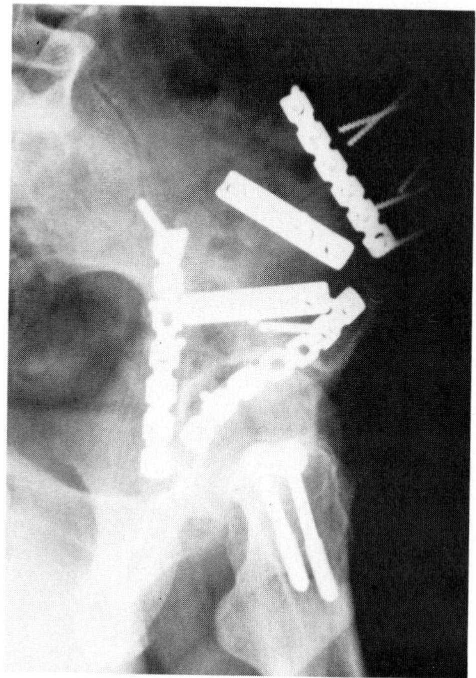

Figure 12-55B: Iliac oblique view

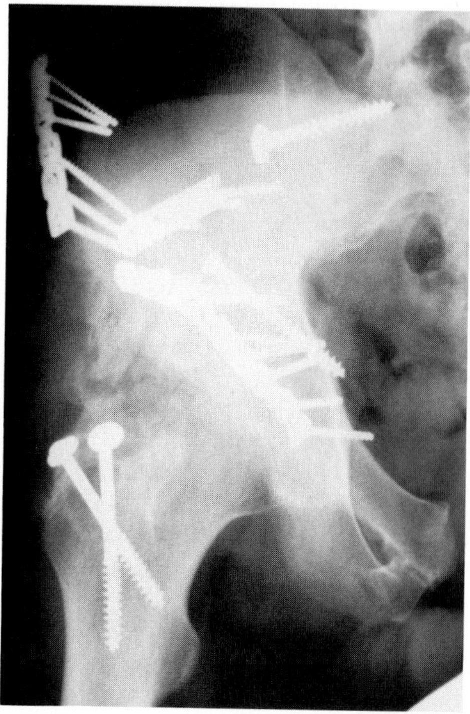

Figure 12-56: Severe postoperative ectopic bone formation one year after a triradiate approach for a both-column fracture.

Figure 12-57: One year after an initial reconstruction of a both-column fracture, this woman of 26 years underwent excision of mature ectopic bone with an excellent restoration of hip motion.

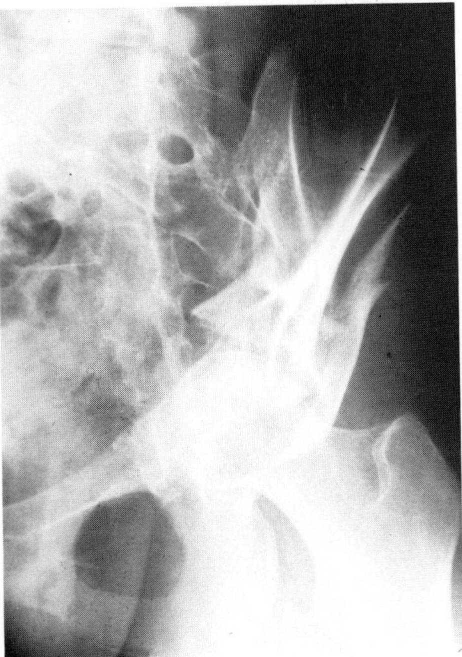

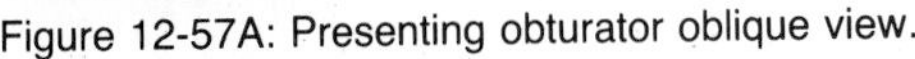

Figure 12-57A: Presenting obturator oblique view.

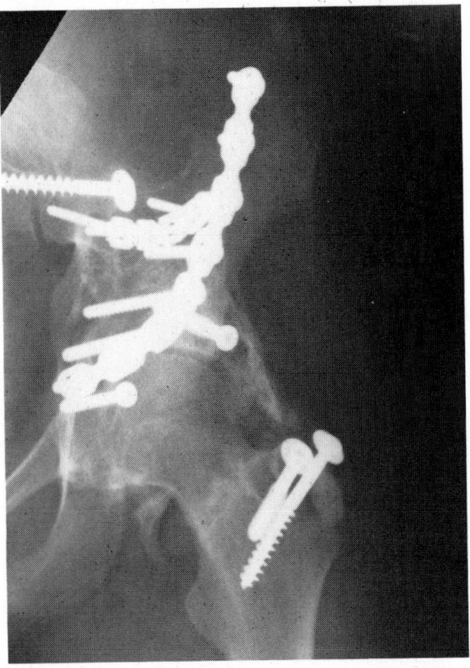

Figure 12-57B: One year after acetabular reconstruction with symptomatic ectopic bone.

S-1 lesion.[11] The incidence of permanent neurological damage reported in various series is extraordinarily variable, with figures ranging between 9% and 50%.[8,12] The most extensive investigation to date was reported by Huittinen and Slatis,[8] who reviewed 85 patients with unstable pelvic fracture, of whom 31% to 41% sustained an associated major injury to the lumbosacral plexus. Of 31 patients, 22 possessed motor signs and 26 sensory signs. While the most common neurological deficiencies were L-5 and S-1, perhaps surprisingly in eight of 31 cases motor deficit of L-4 was documented. Sensory deficit was most commonly associated with sacral nerve roots S-2 to S-5, with a lesser degree of L-5 involvement. While all of the patients had sustained a posterior disruption of the pelvic ring, there was no conspicuous relationship between the site of injury within the sacrum or sacroiliac joint and the corresponding level of the neurological injury. The severity of the pelvic injury was not obviously related to the severity of the neurological impairment. Clinically, most of the neurological injuries were of a permanent nature. In a supplementary cadaveric dissection of 42 trauma victims with allied pelvic fractures, the nature of the pelvic disruption and the type of nerve injury were assessed. Perhaps not surprisingly in such a fatal patient population, bilateral

Figure 12-58: This man of 51 years was managed for a both-column fracture of the left acetabulum with early posttraumatic reconstruction. Despite an anatomical reduction, postoperative pain and stiffness ensued with ectopic bone formation. One year afterwards, the ectopic bone was excised and postoperative irradiation was undertaken with a good result.

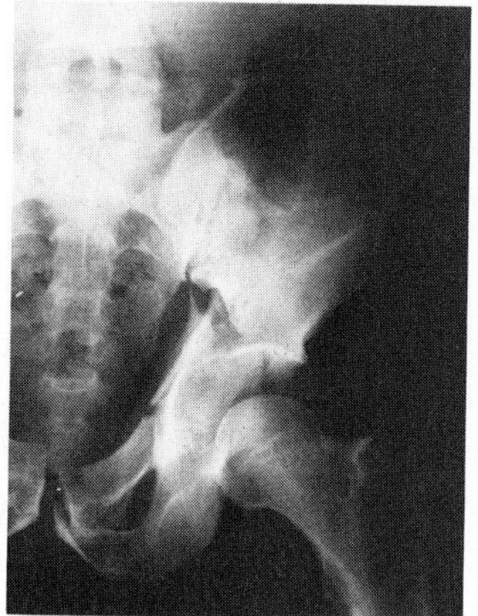

Figure 12-58A: Initial AP view.

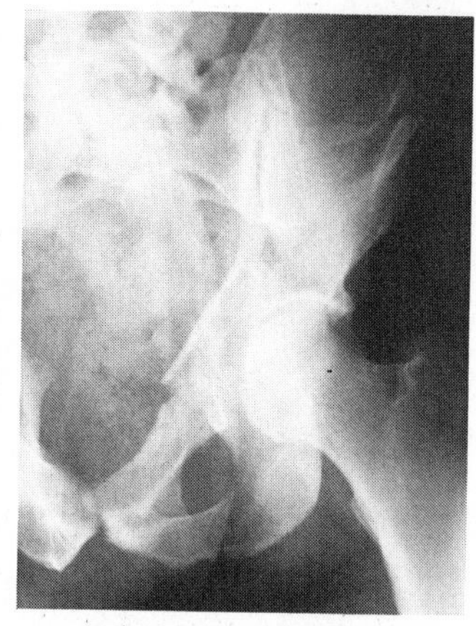

Figure 12-58B: Initial obturator oblique view.

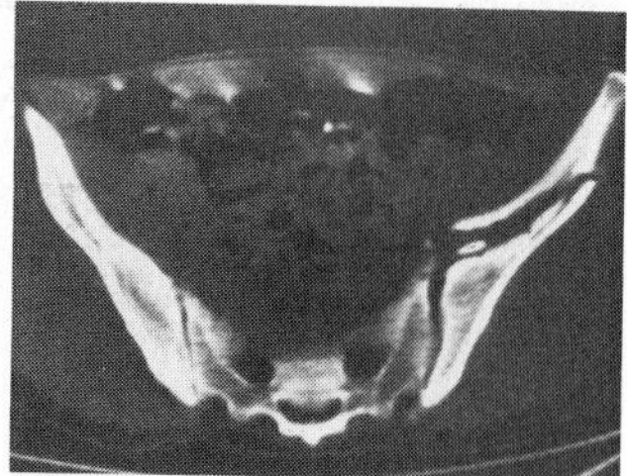

Figure 12-58C: Initial computed scan.

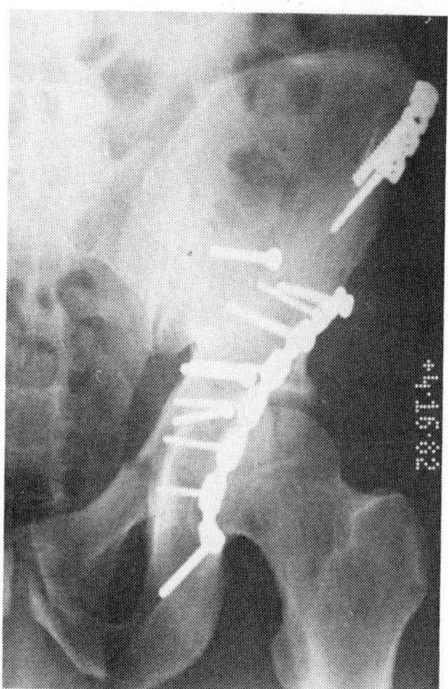

Figure 12-58D: Postoperative AP view.

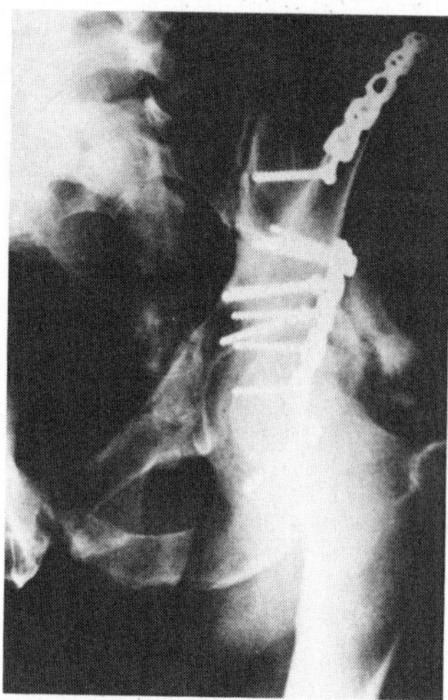

Figure 12-58E: One year later, obturator oblique view with ectopic bone.

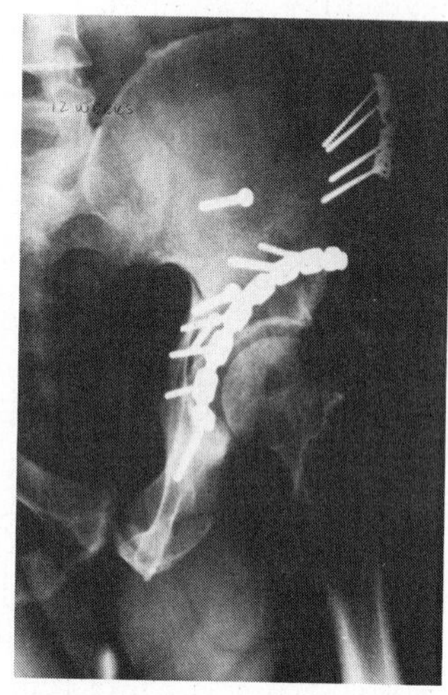

Figure 12-58F: Three months after excision of ectopic bone, iliac oblique view.

posterior unstable pelvic injuries predominated, with an associated incidence of genitourinary complications of 33%. During 20 of the 42 autopsies, neurological injuries were observed including traction injuries in 21 cases, nerve disruption in 15 cases, and compression injuries in four cases. Virtually all portions of the lumbosacral plexus were involved, including the roots of the cauda equina in six cases, the obturator nerve in four, the lumbosacral trunk in 12, the superior gluteal nerve in 11, the anterior primary rami of the fifth lumbar nerve root in two, and the anterior primary rami of the

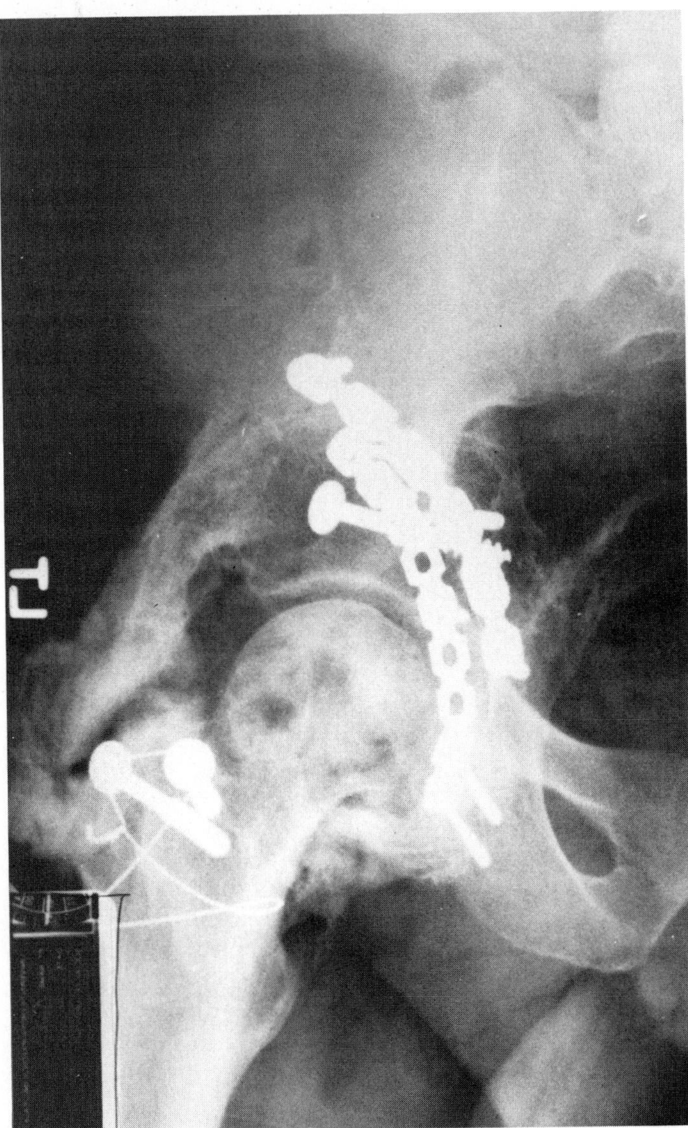


Figure 12-59: One year after this transverse-posterior wall fracture was reconstructed in a 260-pound truckdriver, marked stiffness with preservation of a congruent joint was managed with excision of the ectopic bone and postoperative irradiation.

three upper sacral roots in five. Most of the injuries to the lumbosacral trunk and superior gluteal nerve were provoked by a traction injury, whereas disruption of the anterior primary rami of the upper three sacral nerves secondary to a sacral fracture was initiated by a compressive insult. All of the injuries observed in the obturator nerve were associated with a traction injury at the level of the sacroiliac joint and not at the obturator foramen. Hemipelvic dislocations with external rotation, posterior and superior migration were implicated in the traction injuries to the lumbosacral trunk and superior gluteal nerve. Unlike the cervical spine, neurological disruptions of the cauda equina occur distal to the intervertebral foramen so that the traumatized site is not exposed by a laminectomy.

Figure 12-60: This motorcyclist sustained bilateral acetabular fractures and an open pelvic ring disruption when he crashed at about 100 miles per hour. Two years later, severe bilateral ectopic bone formation with painful traumatic arthritis of the hips was associated with fixed flexion contractures of 60°. Sequential total hip joint replacements with ectopic bone removal provided satisfactory restoration of painfree hip motion.

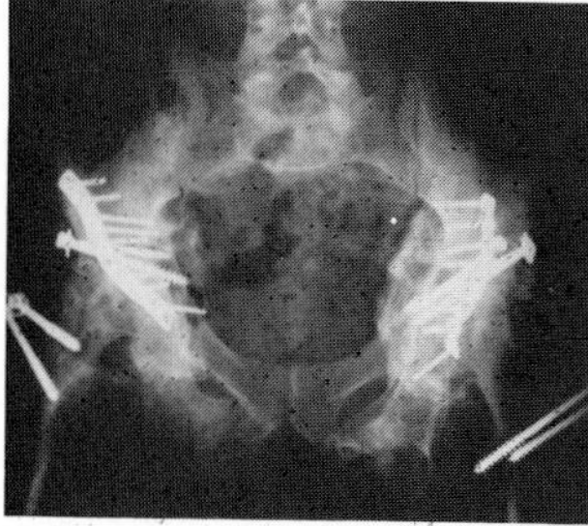

Figure 12-60A: Presenting AP view.

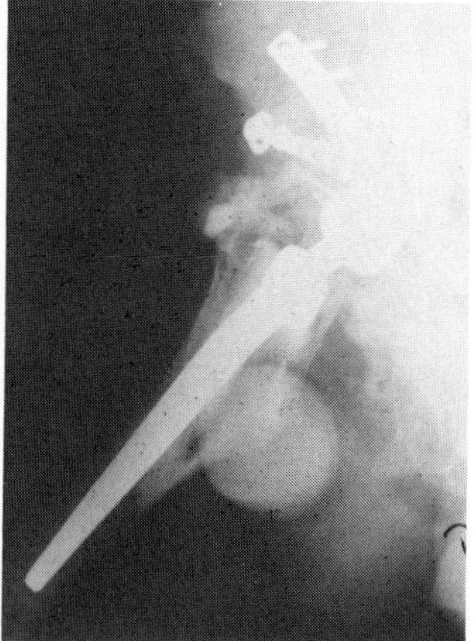

Figure 12-60B: Following a right cemented total hip replacement.

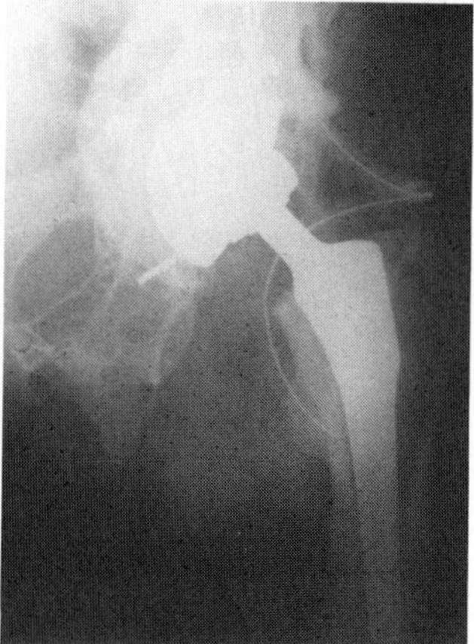

Figure 12-60C: Following cementless PCA total hip replacement of the left hip.

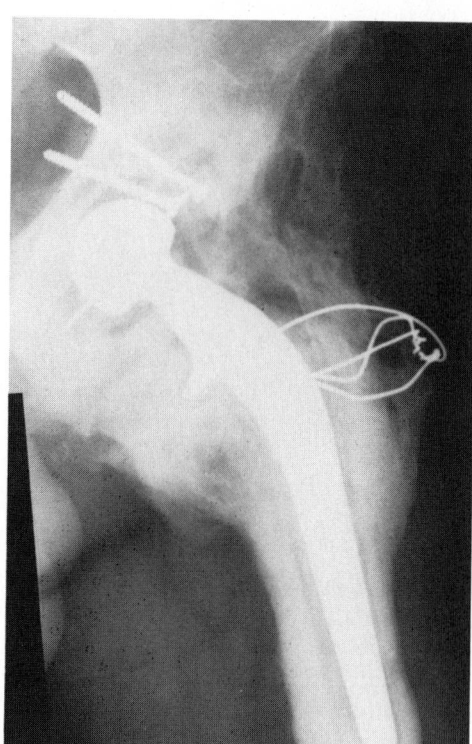

Figure 12-61: Two years after a transverse acetabular fracture was managed with lag screw fixation, the patient underwent total hip joint replacement for traumatic arthritis with ectopic bone formation. Exuberant ectopic bone formation followed the arthroplasty so that a painless fusion ensued.

When avulsion injuries of lumbar nerve roots complicate an unstable pelvic fracture, previously myelographic features indicative of nerve root avulsion injury have been conflicting. Harris et al[13] reported four cases in which myelographic evidence of diverticula at

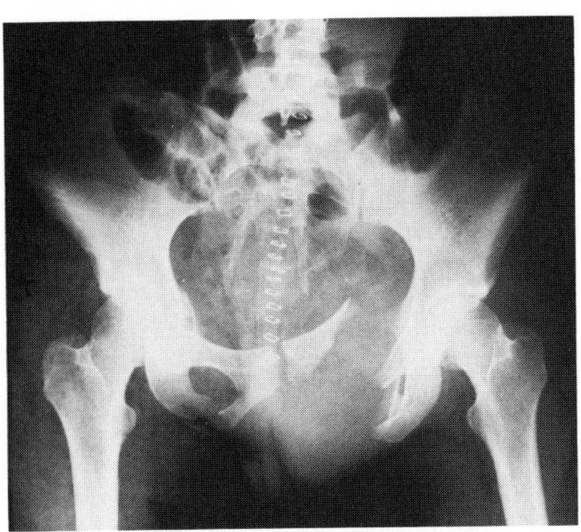

Figure 12-62: This woman of 20 years presented with bladder dysfunction secondary to displaced rami fractures.

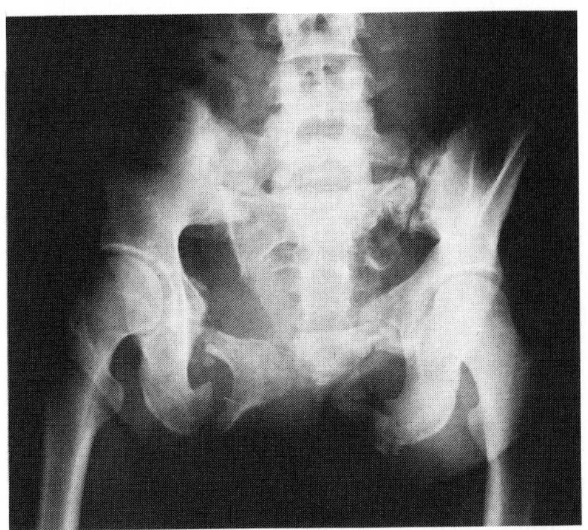

Figure 12-63: This woman of 21 years presented with dyspareunia secondary to displaced superior pubic rami.

the roots were found in all of the cases. Some neurological recovery was documented in each of the patients. The authors therefore concluded that the presence of a diverticulum in a lumbar myelogram was not indicative of an avulsion of the nerve root, but was suggestive of a benign rupture of the dural root sleeve. In contrast, Barnett and Connolly reported the results of a myelogram in one other case of an intradural avulsion of a nerve root[14] in which myelography clearly indicated a nerve root avulsion and, therefore, a contraindication to surgery.

The assessment of nerve injury and the degree of permanent neurological deficit necessitate careful repetitive neurological examinations. Documentation not only of the motor power of all the lower extremity muscles but also a sensory examination including the peroneal region is crucial. Cystometric analysis of the urinary bladder and electrodiagnostic aids, including electromyelography and nerve conduction studies, are helpful. Careful scrutiny of a computed scan of the posterior pelvis may provide evidence of impaction of the sacrum around the sacral nerve roots or dural contents. The presence of a bone fragment or ectopic bone that impinges upon the sciatic nerve may be evident particularly after a posterior fracture dislocation of the hip.

## Management

Effective treatment of persistent clinical problems secondary to an injury of the lumbosacral plexus and sciatic nerve remain an enigma. Most of the injuries arise as a result of traction or compression of a nerve for which, to date, the surgical results have been dissappointing.[8] In the presence of a traction injury or

Figure 12-64: This woman of 40 years presented with dislocated left sacroiliac joint and a wide diastasis for which a triangular frame was employed. A persistent diastasis increased after removal of the frame to provoke a symptomatic midline hernia. Subsequently, internal fixation of the symphysis was undertaken to permit correction of the hernia.

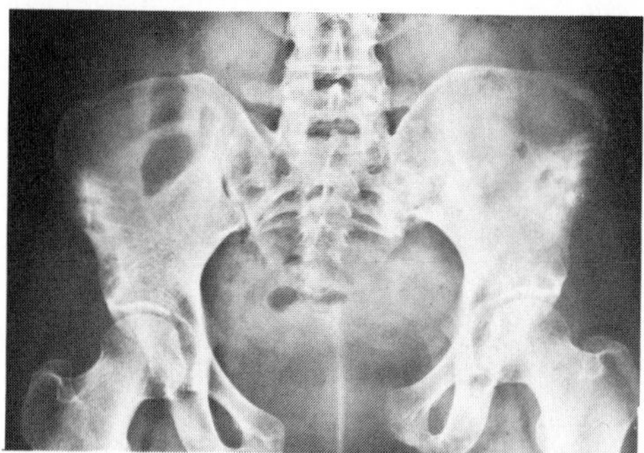

Figure 12-64A: Initial AP view.

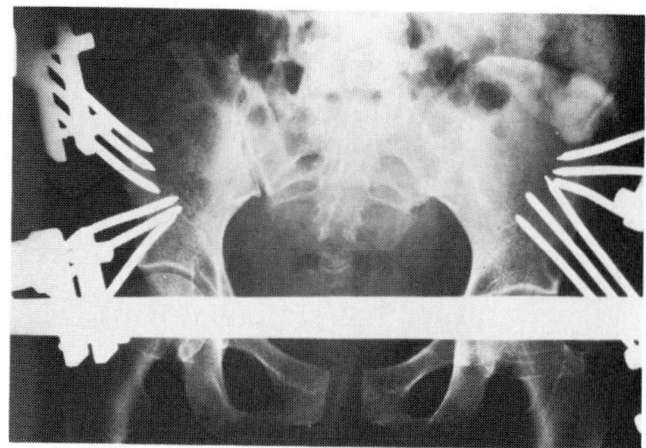

Figure 12-64B: Following external pelvic fixation.

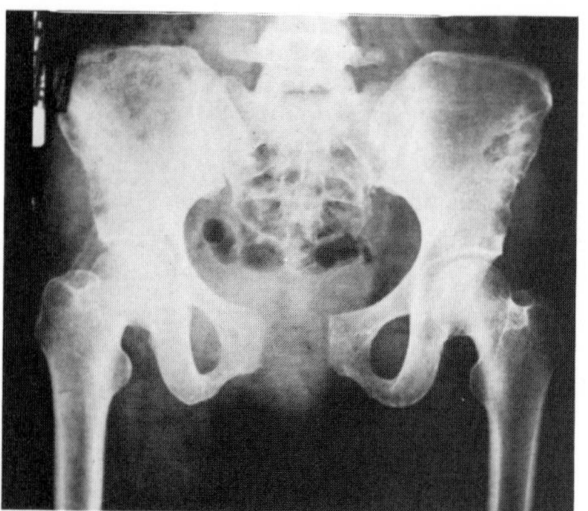

Figure 12-64C: After removal of the frame.

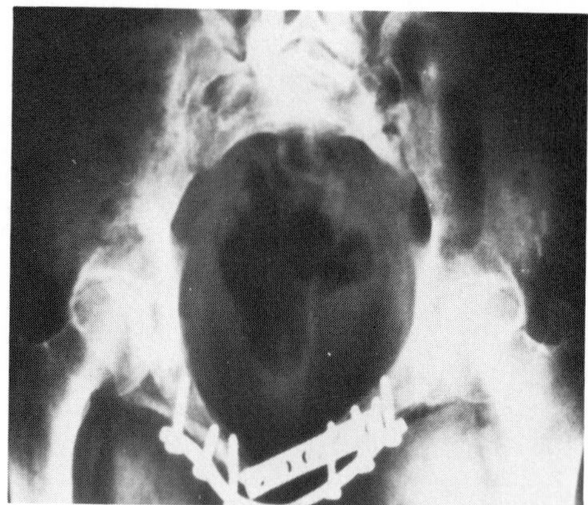

Figure 12-64D: Inlet view following internal fixation of the symphysis.

even a laceration of the lumbosacral plexus, such as the L-5 division, surgical repair has provided abysmal results. Such a procedure also is a possible initiation of enhanced causalgic pain. As a general rule, when a disrupted and displaced hemipelvis is associated with neurological deficit, an early anatomical reduction with stabilization of the pelvis is a realistic goal in a hope to minimize the magnitude of a traction injury to a nerve root. Recently, in the presence of a compression fracture of the sacrum with impingement of nerve roots and a possible concomitant epidural hematoma, laminectomy of L-5 and an associated unroofing of the dorsal sacrum distal to S-3 has been suggested as a way to decompress the nerve roots with removal of impaling bone fragments.[15-19] The results of such surgery have been variable whether they are performed in the early posttraumatic period or for the management of late neurological deficit. Similarly, removal of an impaling

Figure 12-65: This man of 24 years presented with a symptomatic right-sided inguinal hernia secondary to a pelvic fracture with displaced fractures of the right rami.

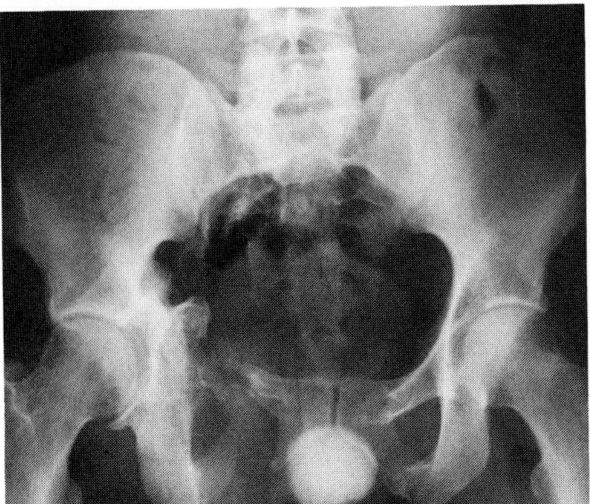

Figure 12-65A: AP view.

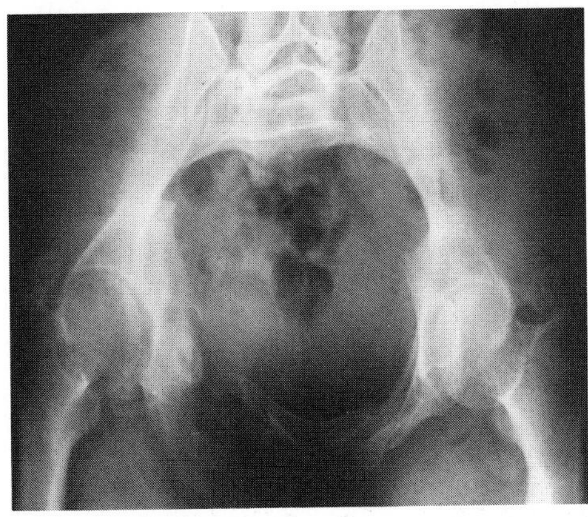

Figure 12-65B: Inlet view.

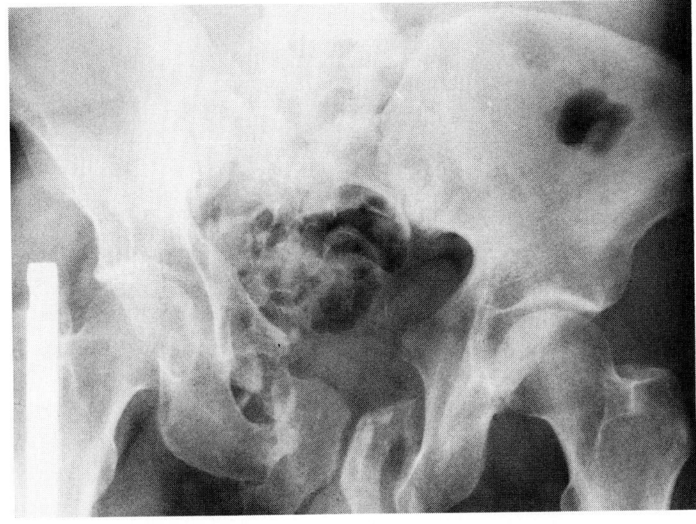

Figure 12-66: Bilateral inguinal hernias follow a four-part displaced rami fracture in a male of 27 years.

bone fragment or ectopic bone that impinges upon the sciatic nerve has provided varying results when employed for symptomatic sciatic nerve deficiency. When an acute posterior fracture dislocation of the hip is associated with a sciatic nerve palsy, an open reduction of the fracture merits exploration of the sciatic nerve. If a hematoma of the nerve is discovered, then neurolysis is indicated. Also, in the presence of persistent sciatic nerve pain as causalgia or dysesthesia, neurolysis merits consideration. In most instances persistent motor weakness is managed with an appropriate splint, and occasionally, with an isolated foot drop, a posterior tibial tendon transfer is a realistic therapeutic consideration.

In the presence of an injury to the femoral nerve, the mechanism of injury merits careful thought. Occasionally, the nerve is subject to laceration by a pointed fragment of bone or as part of an open fracture. In the presence of a deficiency of a major motor division, consideration for direct nerve repair should be given. A myelogram, however, is needed to permit recognition of certain cases with an associated avulsion injury to a spinal nerve.[2]

## Late Urogenital Problems

In the presence of a deformity of a superior pubic ramus, impingement upon the bladder can provoke urinary frequency (Figure 12-62). Both an internal rotation deformity of a hemipelvis and a four-part ramus fracture provoked by impaction of the rami toward the bladder are the provocative fracture patterns.[2] In the presence of single or multiple ramus fractures associated with proliferative callus formation, similar complaints of urinary symptoms are likely to present in an insidious fashion a few weeks or months after the time of the injury. The surgical treatment consists of a careful elevation of the bladder from the superior pubic ramus with excision of the malunited portion of ramus or mass of callus or a corrective osteotomy of the pelvic ring.

For the male pelvic fracture victim who presents in a delayed fashion with a complaint of urinary incontinence or dribbling or impotence, a detailed urological assessment is indicated. The relevant investigations and potential urological reconstructive procedures have been fully reviewed by Colapinto.[19]

When a pelvic nonunion-malunion with a wide diastasis is reconstructed with an open reduction and internal fixation of the symphysis, as well as the posterior lesion, even though the bladder is meticulously replaced posterior to the reduced symphysis, the postoperative period is notable for a temporary period of urinary frequency. While this problem has been documented in all of our patients who underwent a reconstruction with reapproximation of the symphysis, it was temporary in nature and resolved spontaneously within a few weeks.

## Vaginal Problems

Open pelvic fractures can arise by communication with a vaginal laceration. In one recent series of 114 females with pelvic fractures,[20] four patients (3.5%) presented with vaginal laceration. In two of the four cases, a delayed diagnosis of a vaginal laceration was made. One of the two patients presented three days after the time of the injury with an intrapelvic abscess requiring multiple drainage procedures. Early detection and repair of a vaginal laceration in a female pelvic fracture victim is crucial to minimize the risk of pelvic abscess. Intrapelvic osteomyelitis secondary to communication of a pelvic fracture with the vagina has been reported.[21,22] Such a pelvic abscess is likely to follow a protracted course with a potentially fatal outcome. Associated complications include a vesico-vaginal fistula, pelvic inflammatory disease, dyspareunia, recurrent urinary tract infections, and a late presentation of bone fragments in the vagina.

In another series of open pelvic fractures secondary to vaginal lacerations, an associated urethral rupture was reported by Bredael et al.[23]

Following a superior pubic ramus fracture or posterior migration of both superior pubic rami, dyspareunia is likely to ensue (Figure 12-63). Impingement of the bone on the vagina is best documented in a pelvic inlet view or computed scan. Dyspareunia also may be associated with a vaginal stricture secondary to a vaginal laceration on the pelvic fracture. At the time of an operative repair of the vagina, the tendency for the formation of a stricture is inhibited by the insertion of a stent.[20] Later presentation of a stricture is managed by vaginal dilatation. When a displaced ramus fracture or mass of callus provokes dyspareunia as a late presentation, then surgical reconstruction is generally indicated. Either the displaced portion of the ramus or mass of callus can be excised or pelvic reconstruction with realignment of the ramus is undertaken. In certain instances of dyspareunia and vaginismus following a pelvic fracture with minor displacement of a ramus, assessment by a qualified sexual therapist merits consideration. In the presence of an unstable disruption of a symphysis pubis, constant clitoral stimulation associated with weight bearing has been reported.[2] Constant irritation of the clitoris by the unstable symphysis ultimately necessitates surgical reduction and stabilization of the symphysis.

When a pelvic fracture presents in a woman using a feminine hygenic device, contraceptive diaphragm, or intrauterine device, the foreign body can be responsible for a vaginal or uterine laceration.[20] The presence of the device probably increases the risk of a urogenital tear. The foreign body is subject to substantial displacement and provides a predilection for a deep pelvic abscess. If such a device is identified in radiographs, supplementary computed scans, cystography and sigmoidoscopy can be helpful to localize it.

## Posttraumatic Hernias

Probably with the increased likelihood for survival after major pelvic disruptions, symptomatic hernias have become a more common sequel.[2,24] The most common example is a lower midline hernia associated with a diastasis of the symphysis pubis. When the diastasis is more than 2.5cm, such a midline hernia is particularly likely to arise (Figure 12-64). Unless the diastasis is obliterated by reapproximation of the pelvis, a successful herniorrhaphy is unlikely to be achieved even by the application of synthetic materials such as nylon mesh. Preventive treatment with posttraumatic reconstruction of the displaced pelvis is the preferred solution. When a symptomatic hernia presents, reconstruction of the pelvis merits serious consideration. In many of the cases, a reduction and stabilization of both the anterior and posterior sites of disruption is needed to recreate a structurally sound and asymptomatic pelvic ring and to successfully repair the hernia. An inguinal hernia can arise from a markedly displaced superior ramus fracture (Figure 12-65). Bilateral inguinal hernias are seen following displaced fractures of both superior pubic rami (Figure 12-66). If the hernia is sufficiently problematic, then a reconstruction of the unilateral or bilateral superior pubic ramus through an ilioinguinal exposure is necessary as a prelude to the herniorrhaphy.

## References

1. Letournel E, Judet R: Fractures of the Acetabulum. New York, Springer-Verlag, 1981, p 337.
2. Tile M: Fractures of the Pelvis and Acetabulum. Baltimore, Williams and Wilkins, 1984, p 155.
3. Mears DC, Rubash HE: Major malunions and nonunions of the pelvic ring and acetabulum. AAOS Annual Meeting, Las Vegas, 1985.
4. Pennal GF, Massiah KA: Nonunion and delayed union of fractures of the pelvis. Clin Orthop 151:124, 1980.
5. Crowninshield RD, Brand RD, Pederson DR: A stress analysis of acetabular reconstruction in protrusio acetabuli. J Bone Joint Surg 64A:495, 1983.
6. McCollum DE, Nanley JA: Bone grafting in acetabular protrusio: A biological buttress, in: The Hip: Proceedings of the 6th Meeting of the Hip Society. St. Louis, Mosby, p 124, 1978.
7. Cameron HU: Four methods for reconstruction of acetabular floor deficiencies. Orthop Rev 14:568, 1985.
8. Huittenen VM, Slatis P: Nerve injury in double vertical pelvic fractures. Acta Chir Scand 138:571, 1971.
9. Patterson FP, Morton KS: Neurologic complications of fractures and dislocations of the pelvis. Surg Gynecol Obstet 112:702, 1961.

10. Bonnin JG: Sacral fractures and injuries to the cauda equina. J Bone Joint Surg 27:113, 1945.
11. Raf L: Double vertical fractures of the pelvis. Acta Chir Scand 131:298, 1966.
12. Lamb CR: Nerve injury in fractures of the pelvis. Am Surg 104:945, 1936.
13. Harris WR, Rathbun J, Wortzman G, et al: Avulsion of the lumbar roots complicating fracture of the pelvis. J Bone Joint Surg 55A:1436, 1973.
14. Barnett HG, Connelly ES: Lumbosacral nerve root avulsion: Report of a case and review of the literature. J Trauma 15:532, 1975.
15. Tomaszek DE: Sacral fractures and neurological deficit: Diagnosis and management. Contemp Orthop 11:51, 1985.
16. Byrnes D, Russo G, Ducker J, Cowley R: Sacrum fractures and neurological damage: Report of two cases. J Neurosurg 47:459, 1971.
17. Weaver E, England G, Richardson D: Sacral fracture: Case presentation and review. Neurosurg 9:725, 1981.
18. Fardon D: Displaced transverse fracture of the sacrum with nerve root injury: Report of a case with successful operative management. J Trauma 19:119, 1979.
19. Colapinto V: Trauma to the pelvis: Urethral injury. Clin Orthop 151:46, 1980.
20. Niemi TA, Norton LW: Vaginal injuries in patients with pelvic fractures. J Trauma 25:547, 1985.
21. Peltier LF: Complications associated with fractures of the pelvis. J Bone Joint Surg 47A:1060, 1965.
22. Raffa J, Christensen NM: Compound fractures of the pelvis. Am J Surg 132:282, 1976.
23. Bredael JJ, Kramer SA, Cleeve LK, et al: Traumatic rupture of the female urethra. J Urol 122:560, 1979.
24. Ryan EA: Hernias related to pelvic fractures. Surg Gynecol Obstet 133:440, 1971.

# CHAPTER 13

# Clinical Results

During the past decade we have managed a steadily evolving population of patients with diverse pelvic and acetabular fracture problems. Initially, most of the patients were referred from local or regional hospitals for the management of an acute traumatic insult, and the early experience was associated primarily with pelvic disruptions.[1,2] As the impressive results achieved by resort to external fixation were documented and disseminated to local orthopaedic surgeons, many comparable pelvic ring disruptions were satisfactorily managed by orthopaedic surgeons in outlying hospitals. Subsequently, most of the patients were referred to us for the management of pelvic ring disruptions of ever increasing complexity and comminution. Also, a gradual transition to a higher percentage of acetabular fractures and especially of complex injuries with pelvic and acetabular involvement ensued. Most of the complex pelvic fracture victims presented acutely with numerous associated injuries and frequently with hemodynamic instability. Both the presence of associated injuries and the ever increasing distances between the site of the injury and our center provoked greater delays until the pelvic reconstruction was undertaken. In this chapter, an attempt is made to categorize specific injury patterns along with the acute versus late presentations, and the correlation between therapeutic modality and the quality of the ultimate result. Also, whenever possible an attempt is made to correlate the results accrued in Pittsburgh with comparable observations in other centers.

## Acute Presentation of Pelvic Ring Disruption

Recently Steed et al[3] reviewed 36 patients with pelvic ring disruptions who were transferred acutely, within six hours after the time of their injuries, to Presbyterian University Hospital. While all of the patients were managed with external pelvic fixation, 24 of them underwent exploratory laparotomies. Before the application of external fixation the patients received an average of six units of blood. During the subsequent 24-hour period they received an average of two units of blood. While there were no deaths within this patient population, one other man of 85 years presented in the Emergency Room with severe hypotension related to an unstable pelvic ring disruption. He had a past history of myocardial infarction and hypertension. He succumbed prior to the availability of blood replacement and prior to surgical intervention. From this small series in which 56% of the patients were managed for shock at the time of presentation, the capability for external fixation to control hemorrhage as well as postoperative pain was documented.

At another local trauma hospital, Riemer[4] undertook the application of external pelvic fixation to multiple trauma victims with pelvic ring fractures who presented in shock. For the ten-year period prior to the application of external fixation, when a typical general surgical resuscitative protocol was employed, the mortality was 22%. After one independent variable—the application of external pelvic fixation—was initiated by Riemer on the subsequent 100 patients, the mortality rate diminished to 8%.

This striking documentation of the potential for external pelvic fixation to lessen the mortality rate associated with hemorrhagic shock has been confirmed in a report by Edwards et al[5] of their patients at the University of Maryland and the Maryland Shock Trauma Center. These authors reported on 50 multiple trauma victims who presented to the MSTC, 52% of them in a state of hemorrhagic shock. During the eight hours prior to the application of external pelvic fixation, the patients received an average of eight units of blood. During the subsequent 20-hour period, they received two units of blood. The marked similarity in these results supports the hypothesis that external fixation facilitates a marked diminution in the volume of the retroperitoneal space. With the application of substantial tamponade to the hematoma, rapid control of a retroperitoneal hemorrhage allied to a pelvic ring disruption usually follows. The method can be applied prior to a laparatomy if the frame is erected inferior to the anterior abdominal wall and reassembled at the conclusion of the laparotomy.

Both studies were notable for the marked diminution in the severity of postoperative pain, the ease of wound care, and the capability for rapid mobilization of the patient. On average in Pittsburgh, a patient was mobilized from his bed on the fourth postoperative day, whereas in the Baltimore experience on average the patient got out of bed about 12 days after the time of injury. It would not be unlikely that the difference in these figures represents an even higher incidence of concomitant associated injuries in the Baltimore group than in the Pittsburgh series. Edwards et al observed a diminution in the incidence of death following a pelvic fracture of 12% when supplementary external fixation was applied acutely. All three of these series confirmed the role of external pelvic fixation as a valuable addition to the acute therapeutic protocol for the management of an unstable pelvic ring disruption in the hemodynamically unstable trauma victim.

## Late Results of Pelvic Ring Disruption

Recently, Edwards et al[5] also reported the late results of 50 patients who were managed at the University of Maryland for a pelvic ring disruption and were reexamined after a followup period of between two and five years. All of the patients were managed for their unstable pelvic ring disruption solely by the application of external pelvic fixation, generally with the use of a simple frame.

In comparison with the striking success documented for the acute application of external fixation, the late results are discouraging (Table 13-1). About half of the patients experienced significant late posterior pelvic pain and tenderness along with diminution in their levels of activity. By radiographic scrutiny of the immediate postoperative view with later ones (Table 13-2), the striking feature is the 85% loss of the posterior pelvic reduction during the six-week period after the time of a closed pelvic reduction and the application of external fixation. When the severity of posterior pelvic pain was correlated with the quality of the reduction, Edwards et al observed that once an imperfect reduction was evident, a greater degree of displacement was not more notable for severe pain than a lesser degree of displacement, where "lesser displacement" was defined as between 2mm and 5mm. Edwards acknowledges that these results do not necessarily indicate that an

**Table 13-1**
**Late Results Following External for Pelvic Fixation for Pelvic Disruption at the University of Maryland**

| Problem | % |
|---|---|
| Posterior pelvic pain | 52 |
| Pelvic tenderness | 64 |
| ↓ activities | 48 |
| > 1 cm LLD | 28 |
| Paresthesias | 28 |

*Courtesy of Dr. C. Edwards*

**Table 13-2**
**Late Radiographic Results After External Pelvic Fixation for Pelvic Disruption at the University of Maryland**

| Displacement | % Deformity Reduced and Maintained with External Fixation | |
|---|---|---|
| | Initial Reduction | Maintained Reduction |
| Anterior | 65% | 50% |
| Posterior | 60% | 15% |

*Courtesy of C. Edwards*

anatomical reduction is necessarily an unfavorable feature. The radiographic indices of an accurate reduction may not be sufficiently precise to detect those patients who possessed a truly accurate closed reduction associated with external pelvic fixation. From the biomechanical studies previously undertaken by many workers, when a simple frame is employed to manage an unstable pelvic ring disruption, a late loss of the reduction can be anticipated.

Subsequently, the results of management achieved in Pittsburgh for various types of pelvic ring disruption were analyzed. Similarly for the patients who were followed for a minimum of two years after the time of their injury, an attempt was made to correlate the results of treatment with the initial pattern of injury. The patient populations were divided into two groups, those who presented acutely and those who presented more than two weeks after the time of the injury ("late presentation").

**Table 13-3**
**Patterns of Pelvic Disruptions With an Acute or Late Presentation Managed by Surgical Intervention (251 cases)**

| | | Acute | Late | Total |
|---|---|---|---|---|
| Anteroposterior | Stable | 27 | 4 | 31 |
| | Unstable | 18 | 0 | 18 |
| Lateral Compression | Unstable | 52 | 29 | 81 |
| Vertical Shear | | 9 | 4 | 13 |
| Open | | 15 | 0 | 15 |
| Complex | | 55 | 54 | 109 |

The stable subluxations with a diastasis secondary to an anteroposterior compression injury were distinguished from the unstable variants and from the complex pelvic disruptions (Table 13-3). The method of treatment was characterized as external or internal fixation or a combination of the two. From the point of view of the complex fractures where initial external fixation was wholly replaced with internal fixation as a secondary procedure, the late results are categorized as internal fixation.

In addition to this group of 251 cases, there were five patients who presented with a stable pelvic disruption and were managed in a nonoperative fashion. This group included two anteroposterior compression injuries with less than 2.5cm displacement of the symphysis and three stable lateral compression injuries.

Among the whole group there were four late deaths secondary to pulmonary demise. These four patients were notable for exceptional obesity, with two individuals weighing about 280 pounds, the third 350 pounds, and the fourth 450 pounds. The fourth patient suffered a Pickwickian episode in the operating room six weeks after the time of her injury, when she was about to be anesthetized to permit debridement of an open above-knee amputation site.

Among this entire group there were 15 open fractures, of which 13 cases presented with an anterior pelvic wound and two with an open sacroiliac joint. External pelvic fixation was employed in all of the former cases. In one of the latter instances, external pelvic fixation combined with lag screw fixation of the sacroiliac joint was undertaken. In one other complex injury, an open reduction and internal fixation of the sacroiliac joint was performed along with surgical reconstruction of bilateral acetabular fractures. There were no late

**Table 13-4**
**Patterns of Complex Pelvic Disruptions Managed by Surgical Reconstruction (109 cases)**

| | Number |
|---|---|
| Bilateral Posterior Instability ± Anterior | 12 |
| Unilateral SI, Iliac, Anterior | 18 |
| Unilateral SI, Acetabular | 52 |
| SI Bilateral Acetabular | 4 |
| Highly Complex | 23 |

infections documented in any of the open pelvic fracture victims, all of whom achieved a stable pelvic ring without any incidence of a late infection.

Table 13-3 presents the patterns of the pelvic ring disruptions that were managed for an acute or a late presentation excluding the nonunions and malunions. The largest single group of 109 complex injuries was followed by 81 lateral compression injuries with the smallest number of vertical shear insults. Among the complex pelvic variants (Table 13-4), the unstable sacroiliac joint with an anterior injury and an acetabular fracture was the largest single category.

Figure 13-1 tabulates the treatment protocol that was employed for each pattern of pelvic disruption. This algorithm for pelvic stabilization has remained relatively constant for about four years. Prior to the availability of the Double Cobra plate, bilateral lag screw fixation was undertaken to stabilize bilateral sacroiliac joints.

Upon an analysis of the results, the first group of cases represents the acute stable pelvic disruptions that were managed by external fixation with a simple frame or internal fixation with a plate across the symphysis pubis (Table 13-5). Not surprisingly, these relatively minor injuries, consistent with a Bucholz Grade I or Grade II pelvic disruption, showed a high level of successful results in a reproducible fashion. When the patients were examined about two years after the time of their injury, whether external or internal fixation was employed, there was no significant pelvic pain in 91% of the group treated with external fixation, or 100% of the group treated with internal fixation. There were equally good results documented referable to the capability for the individual to undertake all normal activities including running and the ability to resume his regular job. While in the internal fixation group one 3.5mm reconstruction plate was observed to be broken at the six-week postoperative visit

**Table 13-5**
**Results of Treatment of Acute Stable Pelvic Injuries (27 cases)**

| Results | External Fixation (12) % | Internal Fixation (15) % |
|---|---|---|
| No Pelvic Pain | 91 | 100 |
| Tenderness of Symphysis/SI | 9 | 0 |
| LLD | 0 | 0 |
| Paresthesias | 0 | 0 |
| Loss of Reduction | 0 | 0* |
| Residual G-U | 0 | 0 |
| All Activity (Run) | 91 | 100 |
| Resume Work | 91 | 100 |

**One broken plate with 2mm displacement.*

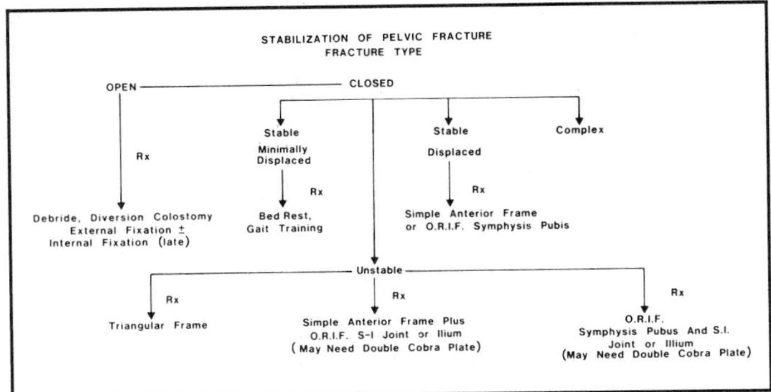


Figure 13-1A. An algorithm for pelvic stabilization.

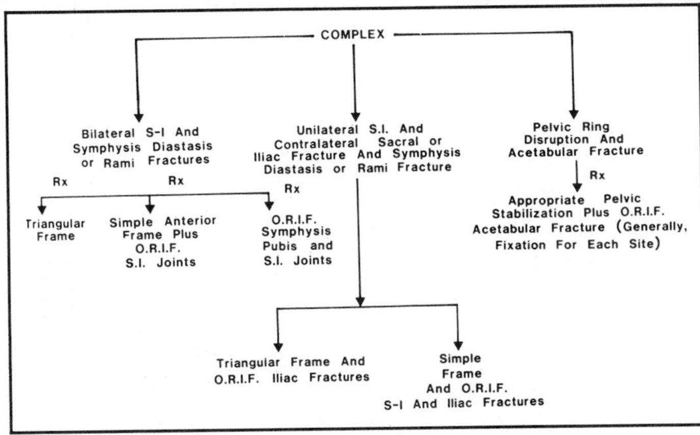


Figure 13-1B. Enlargement of algorithm describes appropriate stabilization techniques for complex pelvic disruptions.

Figure 13-2. An anteroposterior radiograph of a 17-year-old boy managed for a stable AP injury. Six weeks after surgery, when the postoperative view was taken the patient was asymptomatic.

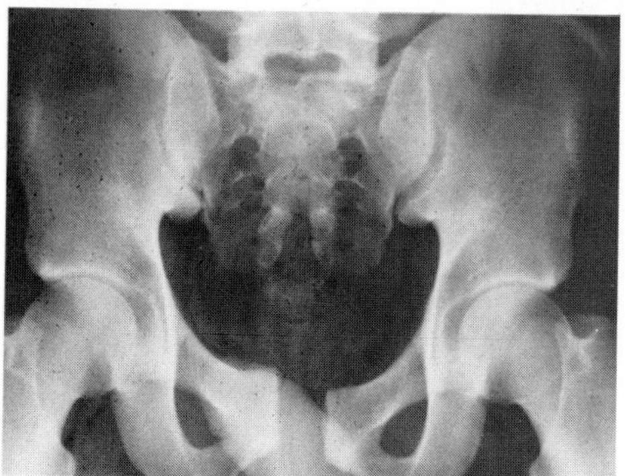

Figure 13-2A. Preoperative.

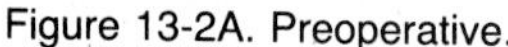

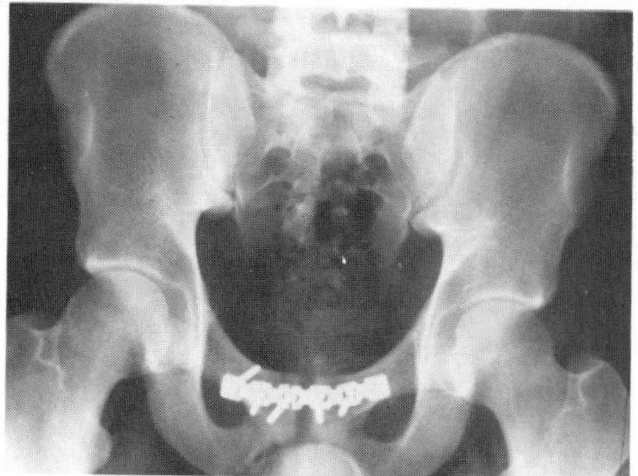

Figure 13-2B. Postoperative.

(Figure 13-2), this observation was purely a radiological curiosity without clinical significance. Probably at the time of the surgery on this 17-year-old football player of 250 pounds who was walking home from football practice when he was struck by a car, a Bucholz Grade II pelvic disruption was misinterpreted as a Grade I injury.

## Late Stable Pelvic Disruptions

Four patients who presented more than one week after the time of their pelvic ring disruption were managed for a stable pelvic ring disruption with a subluxation of the symphysis pubis of between 3cm and 6cm in width. At the time of the open reduction a 3.5mm reconstruction plate was applied for immobilization. All of these cases realized an excellent result with a pain-free pelvis and the capability to resume their pretraumatic jobs. Again such successful results are not surprising in view of the relatively minor nature of the traumatic insult.

## Acute Unstable Pelvic Disruptions

The results of management for acute unstable pelvic disruptions (Table 13-6) provide a more critical analysis of the therapeutic protocol versus the ultimate functional result. The results are compared and contrasted for patients managed solely with a Pittsburgh triangular frame or wholly internal fixation or a combination of internal and external fixation. In most of the latter cases a simple external frame was employed. A substantial difference in the incidence of late pelvic pain documented two years after the time of the injury is observed for patients managed solely with external fixation versus those managed partly or completely by resort to internal fixation. While there is a comparable difference in the

**Table 13-6**
**Results of Treatment of Acute Unstable Simple Pelvic Injuries (75 Cases)**

| Results | EF (40) % | ORIF (20) % | ORIF/EF (15) % |
|---|---|---|---|
| Tenderness of Symphysis/SI | 60 | 35 | 33 |
| No Pelvic Pain | 40 | 60 | 70 |
| LLD | 13 | 5 | 6 |
| Paresthesias | 18 | 5 | 6 |
| Loss of Reduction | 10 | 5 | 6 |
| Residual G-U | 10 | 10 | 13 |
| All Activity (Run) | 45 | 60 | 66 |
| Resume Work | 50 | 70 | 80 |

incidence of pelvic tenderness, posterior pelvic pain constitutes the principal determinant of a late functional incapacitation apart from problems that arise from concomitant appendicular or visceral injuries. When the results of the application solely of external fixation are compared with the use solely of internal fixation or of a combination of internal and external fixation, a comparable discrepancy is observed in the ability for a particular patient to undertake full activities, including running and resumption of work. From the results of this series the predilection for late pelvic pain, the limitation of activity, or the inability to undertake gainful employment appears to correlate with the lack of an accurate pelvic reduction and stable fixation. With the application of supplementary internal fixation so that a more accurate reduction and superior stability was achieved, the results appear to be improved. Inevitably, an explanation is needed for the considerable incidence of late pelvic pain even in those patients where internal fixation was employed. By a scrutiny of the preoperative radiographs and computed scans of the lumbosacral spine, 45% of the patients possessed some type of lumbosacral injury. The problems included avulsion fractures of the transverse spine, undisplaced fractures of the vertebral body or facetal joints, and displaced lumbosacral fractures including completely displaced fracture-dislocations. In a somewhat similar radiographic survey of pelvic fracture victims, Tile[6] reported an incidence of 40% of lumbosacral injuries also of a highly diverse nature. Presumably the lumbosacral injuries contribute to the late posterior pain, which is difficult to attribute to the lumbosacral spine or to the neighboring sacroiliac joints, sacrum, and posterior ilium. Many of

**Table 13-7**
**Results of Treatment of Unstable Simple Pelvic Injuries Following a Late Presentation**

| Results | EF(3) % | ORIF(22) % | ORIF/EF(9) % |
|---|---|---|---|
| Tenderness, Symphysis/SI | 66 | 35 | 33 |
| No Pelvic Pain | 33 | 55 | 65 |
| LLD | 33 | 10 | 33 |
| Paresthesias | 0 | 5 | 11 |
| Loss of Reduction | 0 | 0 | 11 |
| Residual G-U | 33 | 10 | 11 |
| All Activity (Run) | 66 | 60 | 66 |
| Resume Work | 66 | 65 | 77 |

the pelvic fracture victims sustain concomitant compressive injuries to the lumbosacral roots and plexuses that contribute to their late pelvic pain.

Table 13-7 lists the comparable results of management of patients who presented with an unstable pelvic ring disruption more than one week after the time of their initial injury. When the results of management with isolated external fixation, internal fixation, or a combined technique are examined, a similar trend is evident with the highest incidence of posterior pelvic pain, limitation of activity, and inability to work in the solely external fixation group, and greater success rates generally documented in the groups where the stabilization was partly or wholly achieved by the use of internal fixation. In view of the small numbers of patients available in each group, it is unclear whether the results are statistically significant.

Overall the results of the series from the University of Maryland and the University of Pittsburgh show a striking similarity. The experience in Pittsburgh with the use of supplementary complete internal fixation provides a somewhat more favorable prognosis in regard to posterior pelvic pain and the level of activity of the patient. Nevertheless, a substantial incidence of late pain was confirmed, which may reflect associated spinal injuries, neurological impairment within the sacrum or adjacent lumbosacral plexuses, or conceivably late traumatic arthritis of the sacroiliac joint. Clearly, further research is needed to provide superior late results.

**Table 13-8**
**Results of Treatment of Complex Pelvic Injuries With an Acute Presentation (52 cases)**

| Results | ORIF/EF(16) % | ORIF(36) % |
|---|---|---|
| Tenderness Symphysis/SI | 56 | 55 |
| No Pelvic Pain | 63 | 61 |
| LLD | 13 | 5 |
| Paresthesias | 18 | 19 |
| Loss of Reduction | 13 | 5 |
| Residual G-U | 6 | 6 |
| All Activity (Run) | 56 | 55 |
| Resume Work | 50 | 50 |

### Complications with External Pelvic Fixation

Where external frames were employed in the Pittsburgh series, 12% of the patients developed drainage from a pin site. Four pins were removed prior to the disassembly of the frame in view of persistent drainage. Two pin sites required a formal debridement. There were no patients who had a late pin problem. These results compare favorably with the Baltimore experience reported by Edwards,[5] where a 16% incidence of pin tract drainage was observed. Again, these problems were relatively minor and readily subsided when the wounds were managed with dressing changes and with the removal of loose pins. Two of the Baltimore patients underwent a limited slough secondary to impingement of the frame when the device was inadvertently positioned excessively close to the abdominal wall so that insufficient space was provided for the subsequent soft tissue swelling.

## Results of Management of Complex Pelvic Fractures

In the Pittsburgh series with the large number of referrals for the management of patients who possessed unusual comminuted fracture patterns, a group of so-called complex pelvic disruptions has been distinguished from the simpler patterns of pelvic disruption (Table 13-4).

In Table 13-8 the results of management of the complex fracture patterns in patients who presented acutely are tabulated for those cases managed with a combination of internal and external fixation versus those that were managed entirely with internal fixation. The latter group includes those patients who were managed for a few days with external fixation applied as part of the resuscitative protocol with a deliberate conversion to internal fixation. In such a case the temporary period of external fixation was not felt to reflect the quality of the late outcome when the patients were examined from two to five years after the time of their injury. Not surprisingly, a larger percentage of patients who were managed for a complex pelvic disruption possessed late pelvic pain and limitation of activity, including running and work activities, than of patients who were treated for a simple pelvic injury. Presumably this result is related to the higher traumatic force needed to provoke a complex disruption, the comminuted nature of the injury, and the greater likelihood for the patient to sustain concomitant injuries to the hip and spine. When supplementary external fixation was employed along with internal fixation, over twice as many patients (13%) showed some loss of reduction as the group treated solely with internal fixation (5%). About half of the patients were able to resume gainful employment within a year after the time of their injury. The inability of the other patients to resume gainful employment reflects not only the nature of the pelvic trauma but also the great frequency of associated injuries and possibly the depressed nature of the local economy in Western Pennsylvania. Many patients possessed an economic incentive to remain medically unfit for work rather than to be unemployed.

Table 13-9 provides the results of management of the patients who sustained complex pelvic disruptions who were managed after a late presentation with transfer from another center more than one week after the time of their injury. While the results are generally similar to those documented in the patients with complex disruptions who were managed from the acute period with generally an earlier surgical reconstruction, they possess a somewhat higher incidence of late pelvic pain, limb length discrepancy, and loss of reduction. All of these problems may be correlated with the lesser accuracy of the late reductions than the early ones.

For the complex pelvic disruptions of acute or late presentation where external fixation was employed, there was an incidence of pin tract drainage or infection of 15%, with two patients requiring debridement of a pin site. Where internal fixation was undertaken, there were no postoperative wound infections during the first year after the time of the surgery. One patient, however, who had experienced relatively minor transient pin tract drainage with apparent spontaneous resolution, presented four years after a pelvic reconstruction. This obese male had been managed for a transverse acetabular fracture with internal fixation and a concomitant sacral fracture with a wide diastasis by a supplementary triangular pelvic frame. At the time of his late presentation four years after his injury, he presented with a fulminant infection of his hip on the involved side, although without any obvious extension of the infection to the iliac crest. At the time of a surgical debridement when cultures were positive for Serratia marcescens, his femoral head showed a marked destruction. He required a conversion to a Girdlestone pseudarthrosis along with multiple secondary debridements. This case is surprising for the prolonged delay between the time of the pelvic disruption with the use of external and internal fixation and the presentation of the late infection. There were two iatrogenically induced sciatic nerve palsies provoked by traction on the sciatic nerve following a posterior exposure for a concomitant acetabular fracture. One of these problems resolved completely within six months, while the other was notable for a persistent hypesthesia of the foot and a partial foot drop. There were no deaths in the group of complex pelvic ring disruptions.

## Results of Acetabular Reconstruction

Recently a review of 217 patients with 225 fractures of the acetabulum managed by resort to an open reduction and internal fixation was undertaken. All of these patients were involved in high velocity injuries resulting from vehicular accidents to pedestrians or passengers, motorcycle accidents, industrial accidents, sporting injuries, or falls from great heights. The average age of this population was 38 years, with a 2:1 ratio of male to female patients. The age distribution shows a peak incidence between the ages of 20 and 40 years. Ten other patients presented with minimally displaced unilateral acetabular fractures and were treated nonoperatively with traction and early range of motion. The distribution of the acetabular injuries is presented in Table 13-10. In this series, 89 patients sustained other musculoskeletal injuries, including fractures of the upper and lower extremities, and spinal injuries. Four patients presented with a concomitant displaced femoral neck fracture. Twenty-three patients presented with extensive macroscopic injury to the femoral head with loss of cartilage (5), depression of the cartilage (16), or an osteochondral fracture (2).

**Table 13-9**
**Results of Treatment of Complex Pelvic Injuries With a Late Presentation (54 cases)**

| Results | ORIF/EF (14) % | ORIF (40) % |
|---|---|---|
| Tenderness Symphysis/SI | 58 | 65 |
| No Pelvic Pain | 65 | 62 |
| LLD | 14 | 5 |
| Paresthesias | 21 | 20 |
| Loss of Reduction | 14 | 2.5 |
| Residual G-U | 7 | 5 |
| All Activity (Run) | 56 | 50 |
| Resume Work | 56 | 55 |

Thirty-eight patients sustained a traumatically induced sciatic nerve injury. Eighteen of the patients presented with a peroneal palsy, and four of the patients possessed supplementary weakness of the gastrocnemius and soleus. All of these sciatic nerves were explored surgically at the time of the open reduction and internal fixation of the fracture. The findings included neuropraxia secondary to a displaced bone fragment, an intraneural hematoma, and a nerve trapped between the fracture fragments of a displaced posterior column fracture. In the other patients, no obvious injury was noted.

Ninety-two of the patients sustained a pelvic ring disruption that complicated their acetabular fracture. The pelvic ring disruptions included sacroiliac dislocations, sacral fractures, and various anterior pelvic ring injuries (Table 13-11). Concomitant ipsilateral sacroiliac disruptions, observed in an additional ten patients, were reduced and stabilized at the time of the acetabular reconstruction. The pelvic injuries that accompanied the acetabular fractures were grouped according to the classification of stable or unstable, and anterior/posterior compression, lateral compression, and vertical shearing injuries. The majority of these fractures were categorized as lateral compression injuries. In those cases where superior displacement of the ilium at the level of the sacroiliac joint or the adjacent posterior ilium or sacrum occurred, the fracture was classified as a vertical shearing type of injury. This was a less frequent fracture pattern and most often occurred with a both-column fracture. The both-column injuries are generally correlated with the highest traumatically induced forces

**Table 13-10**
**Classification of Acetabular Fractures Managed by Surgical Reconstruction**

| | | **Simple** | | **Approach** |
|---|---|---|---|---|
| | * | Posterior Wall | 11 | K-L |
| + | * | Posterior Column | 9 | K-L |
| | | Anterior Wall | 1 | I-I |
| + | | Anterior Column | 2 | I-I |
| + | | Transverse | 26 | K-L, TRI, I-I |
| | | **Associated Fractures** | | |
| + | * | "T" Shaped | 39 | TRI |
| + | * | Posterior Column and Posterior Wall | 15 | K-L |
| + | | Transverse and Posterior Wall | 23 | TRI |
| + | * | "T" Shaped and Posterior Wall | 18 | TRI |
| | | Anterior Column and Posterior Hemitransverse | 12 | TRI, I-I |
| + | * | Both-Column | 69 | TRI, I-F |
| | | **Total** | 225 | |

* = *Sciatic Injuries.*
+ = *Pelvic Ring Injuries (see Table 13-11).*
*K-L = Kocher-Langenbeck.*
*I-I = Ilioinguinal.*
*TRI = Triradiate.*
*I-F = (Extended) Iliofemoral.*

and, therefore, the greatest disruptions of the pelvic ring. Four patients possessed bilateral displaced acetabular fractures.

Urological injuries were documented in 28 patients, with 16 ruptures of the bladder and 12 urethral injuries. In one patient, bilateral acetabular fractures were complicated by an open diastasis of the symphysis pubis, bilateral sacroiliac dislocations, and a vascular injury to a major branch of the internal iliac artery.

At present, the average followup in this series is five years, with a range of 18 months to ten years. The application of various surgical approaches is tabulated in Table 13-10. For posterior wall, posterior column, posterior wall-posterior column disruptions, and three transverse fractures with minimal anterior displacement, a Kocher-Langenbeck approach was utilized on 57 occasions. In 21 cases, the greater trochanter was

**Table 13-11**
**Acetabular Fracture + Pelvic Ring Disruption**

| Acetabular Fracture | Pelvic Fracture | |
|---|---|---|
| **Simple** | | |
| Posterior Column | 1 | A-P |
| Anterior Column | 2 | LAT |
| Transverse | 19 | LAT |
| **Associated Fractures** | | |
| Posterior Column-Posterior Wall | 2 | LAT |
| Transverse-Posterior Wall | 3 | LAT |
| "T" Shaped | 13 | LAT |
| "T" Shaped-Posterior Wall | 9 | LAT |
| Both-Column | 24 | LAT |
| | 19 | VERT |
| **Total** | 92 | |

*A-P = Anteroposterior Compression Injury.*
*LAT = Lateral Compression Injury.*
*VERT = Vertical Shear Injury (with superior displacement of ilium at sacroiliac joint or through the posterior ilium or sacrum).*

osteotomized to enlarge the exposure. In 15 cases the ilioinguinal approach was employed to expose one of the following injury patterns: an anterior wall, anterior column, anterior column-posterior hemitransverse, "T" and both-column fracture with primarily anterior displacement. A bilateral ilioinguinal approach was used in two cases to expose bilateral fractures. The triradiate approach was used for 157 operative cases, particularly for the exposure of a both-column, T-shaped, and a markedly displaced transverse or transverse with a posterior wall fracture type. One both-column fracture was approached by an extended iliofemoral incision. To stabilize the fractures, reconstruction plates (Synthes Ltd. (USA), Wayne, Pennsylvania), Letournel plates (Howmedica, Inc., Rutherford, New Jersey) and Dynamic Compression plates (Synthes) were employed with supplementary lag screws.

## Indications for Surgery

The indications for operative intervention employed for this study were:

**1)** An acetabular fracture-dislocation with a failure to obtain an accurate closed reduction of the femoral head and acetabulum. Examples include most posterior wall and posterior column injuries.

**2)** An acetabular fracture accompanied by a loose interposed osteochondral fragment.

**3)** A displaced acetabular fracture provisionally managed by skeletal traction for a period of 24 to 48 hours with failure to attain an accurate acetabular reduction with less than 2mm to 3mm of displacement in multiple radiographic views.

**4)** Most displaced comminuted or associated fractures with their typical incongruity. One exception is the highly comminuted both-column fracture with a late presentation that shows congruity of the displaced fragments referable to the femoral head.[7] Another exception is the low, minimally displaced anterior column fracture with minor intraarticular involvement. This disruption of the superior pubic rami is a common finding in a lateral compression injury of the pelvic ring with unilateral or bilateral ramus fractures.

**5)** A complex pelvic injury with an acetabular fracture complicated by a pelvic ring disruption.

Contraindications for surgery were undisplaced acetabular fractures and exceptional cases with extraordinarily extensive comminution or severe osteoporosis. Temporary contraindications were hemodynamically or otherwise unstable patients, or the presence of major adjacent open wounds or pelvic fractures. Once a source of instability had been corrected or the open wound had been adequately debrided, the open reduction was performed.

## Results

In this series the average operative time was 3.5 hours (range: 2-5 hours) and the blood loss ranged from 300cc to 4000cc (average: 1200cc). There was one death in the preoperative or postoperative period (Table 13-12). Three weeks after his acetabular reconstruction, the patient succumbed from a previously unrecognized large bowel infarction and perforation. There were two postoperative superficial wound infections, which resolved uneventfully after the use of debridement, antibiotics, and a secondary closure. One deep wound infection was managed by serial debridements and intravenous antibiotics. A second deep infection was successfully treated by metal removal and a hip fusion. One other patient discussed previously under the results of pelvic fractures presented four years after internal fixation of the acetabulum and external fixation of an unstable pelvic disruption with an extensive infection in the involved hip secondary to Serratia marcescens. During the prolonged latent period, there

**Table 13-12**

| Postoperative Complications | | Number | Fracture Type or Incision |
|---|---|---|---|
| Deaths | | 1 | Both-Column |
| Sciatic Nerve Palsy | | 6 | 2 Posterior Column-Posterior Wall<br>1 Both-Column<br>2 Posterior Column<br>1 "T" |
| Wound Infection: | Superficial | 2 | 1 Triradiate<br>1 Kocher-Langenbeck (Staph. albus) |
| | Deep | 2 | 2 Triradiate (Staph. aureus) |
| | Late | 1 | 1 Triradiate (Serratia marcescens) |
| Thromboembolism | | 5 | (1 Pulmonary embolism) |
| Loss of Reduction | | 2 | Both-Column |
| Nonunion | | 2 | Both-Column<br>Posterior Wall/Column |
| Screw Migration | | 5 | 1 "T"<br>1 Transverse and Posterior Wall<br>1 Posterior Column/Wall<br>2 Both-Column |
| Avascular Necrosis | | 5 | 1 "T"<br>2 Both-Column<br>2 Transverse-Posterior Wall |
| Traumatic Arthritis | | 8 | 2 "T"<br>2 Both-Column<br>3 Transverse-Posterior Wall<br>1 "T"-Posterior Wall |
| Ectopic Bone | | 112 | |

was no complaint or other feature to indicate the presence of the infection. A Girdlestone arthroplasty was undertaken after serial debridements and antibiotic therapy. No prophylaxis for deep venous thrombosis was utilized. Four patients developed lower extremity thromboembolic disease, and one patient developed a pulmonary embolism, all of which were successfully treated by intravenous and oral anticoagulation. No fat emboli were documented.

Six patients developed iatrogenically induced sciatic nerve palsies. Four of these resolved spontaneously within three months from the time of the injury. Two others showed persistent hypesthesia of the lower extremity and a partial foot drop. Of the 16 patients who sustained a sciatic nerve palsy of traumatic origin, 14 achieved a

**Table 13-13**
**Harris Hip Rating (HHR)**

| | |
|---|---|
| Excellent | 90-100 points |
| Good | 80-90 points |
| Fair | 70-80 points |
| Poor | <-70 points |

**Table 13-14**

| **Fracture Pattern** | **Harris Hip Score (Average)** |
|---|---|
| **Simple** | |
| Posterior (Wall + Column) } Anterior (Wall + Column) } | 92 |
| Transverse | 90 |
| **Associated** | |
| "T" Shaped | 85 |
| Miscellaneous* | 85 |
| Both-Column | 83 |

**Posterior Column + Posterior Wall*
*Transverse + Posterior (Wall + Column)*
*"T" Shaped + Posterior (Wall + Column)*
*Anterior Column + Posterior Hemitransverse*

full spontaneous recovery within six months. Two patients still require an ankle-foot orthosis due to a persistent foot drop.

The overall clinical results were assessed by the use of the Harris Hip Scale system,[12] which includes an evaluation of pain, function, range of motion, and deformity (Tables 13-13 to 13-16). At the time of this review the overall average Harris hip rating for the entire series was 87 points. In examining this series with respect to the first 50 fractures verses the second, third, and fourth 50 fractures, 65% of the first 50 patients possessed ratings of greater than 75, while 75% of the second 50 patients, 95% of the third 50 patients, and 98% of the fourth 50 patients possessed ratings of greater than 75. In an assessment of the simple fracture patterns, 80% of the first 100 patients possessed Harris Hip Scale

**Table 13-15**
**Results of Acetabular Reconstruction**

| Cases | >75 HHR |
|---|---|
| 1-50 | 65% |
| 51-100 | 75% |
| 101-150 | 95% |
| 151-200 | 98% |

**Table 13-16**
**Results of Simple Acetabular Fractures**

| Cases | >80 HHR |
|---|---|
| 1-100 | 80% |
| 101-200 | 98% |

**Table 13-17**
**Acetabular Reduction Accuracy (<2mm displacement)**

| Cases | % |
|---|---|
| 1-50 | 40 |
| 51-100 | 80 |
| 101-150 | 94 |
| 151-200 | 95 |

ratings of greater than 80 points (range: 70-99), while 98% of the second 100 patients possessed ratings of greater than 80 points. Of the patients who sustained an associated fracture, only 60% of the first 100 patients had ratings of greater than 80 (range: 60-95), while 84% of the second 100 patients attained ratings greater than 80. Forty percent of the patients underwent a surgical reduction and stabilization more than three weeks (range: 3-12 weeks) after the time of their injury. The other 60% of the patients underwent the surgery within one and three weeks after the time of injury.

In a study of the postoperative radiographs, the accuracy of the surgical reduction was assessed (Table 13-17). In the first 50 cases that were managed, 40% of the fractures were considered to be anatomical reductions. In the second group, 80% were considered to be anatomical or malreduced with less than 2mm of displacement on any postoperative radiograph. In the third and fourth groups the corresponding figures were 94% and 95%. Generally, a poor clinical result followed an imperfect reduction of greater than 3mm. Less satisfactory reductions were documented for the more complex fracture patterns, which were attributable to the comminution and displacement of the fracture fragments.

In Figures 13-3 to 13-5, several examples of persistent displacement following acetabular reconstructions of simple fractures are presented. A posterior column fracture is apt to possess a residual rotational displacement, particularly when a high fracture variant is inadequately visualized at the roof of the greater sciatic notch. A transverse fracture with an ipsilateral sacroiliac subluxation can show persistent incongruity unless the sacroiliac joint is accurately reduced prior to the acetabular repair. Persistent rotational deviation of a transverse fracture is especially likely when the anterior aspect of the fracture at the base of the anterior inferior

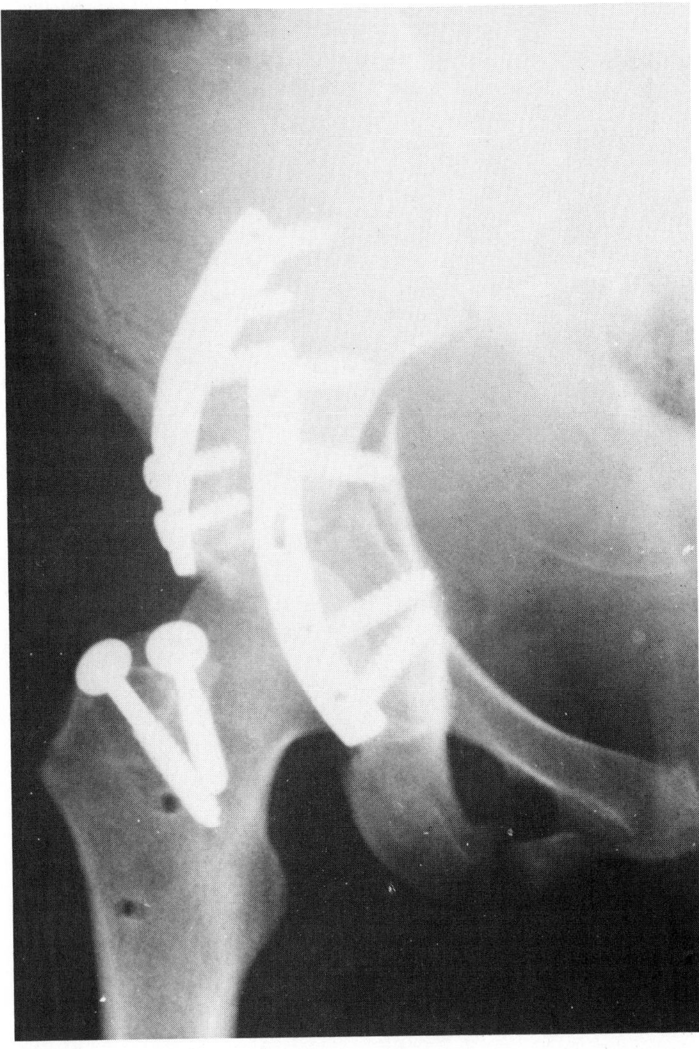

Figure 13-3. A both-column fracture with primarily posterior column displacement that was uncorrected surgically.

spine is inadequately exposed and reduced. A "T" fracture is likely to possess residual posterior column displacement unless the anterior column initially is fully corrected of its typical posterior and medial migration (Figure 13-6). Another common deformity is incongruity, where the inferior half of the "T" fracture is not reduced around the femoral head (Figure 13-7). With its remote extension and inaccessability, the base of the acetabulum inferior and medial to the femoral head is difficult to relocate in an anatomical position. Perhaps the most difficult reduction is an accurate correction of the medial displacement that is encountered with a typical both-column injury. For a postoperative assessment, the pelvic inlet view provides optimal documentation. In the three examples provided here (Figures 13-8 to 13-10), one highly displaced fracture during the early part of the

Figure 13-4. A transverse fracture with marked comminution and an associated ipsilateral sacroiliac subluxation shows a persistent lateral displacement of the lateral ilium and corresponding degree of apparent protrusio.

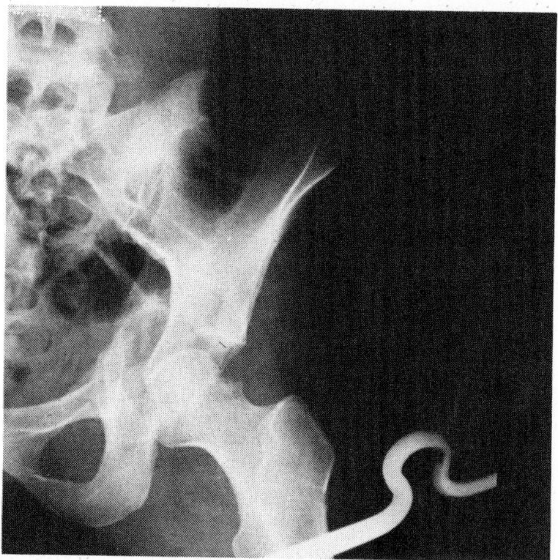

Figure 13-4A. Preoperative view in skeletal traction.

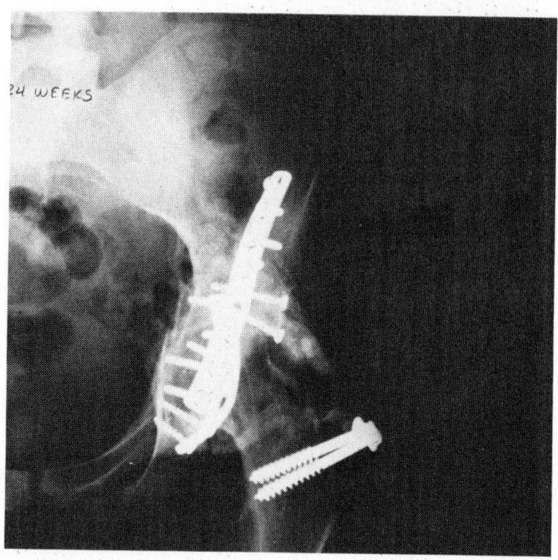


Figure 13-4B. Postoperative view at six months.

Figure 13-5. A transverse fracture with a high posterior propagation into the greater sciatic notch possesses a poor reduction with malrotation.

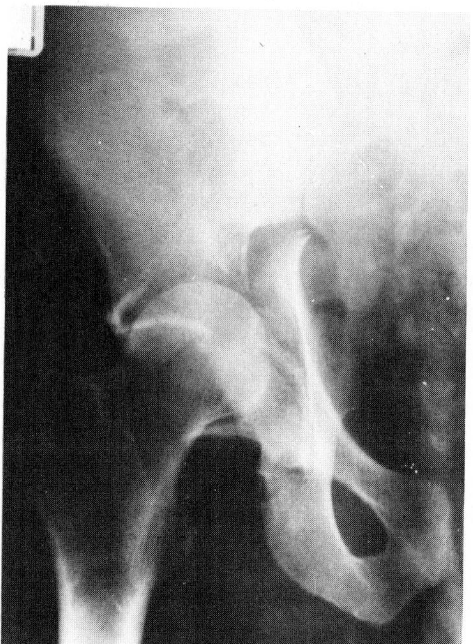

Figure 13-5A. Preoperative view.

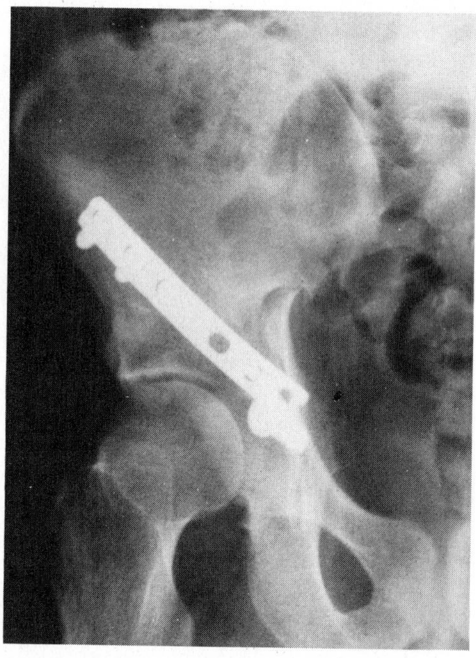

Figure 13-5B. Postoperative view at six weeks.

series shows a marked persistent deformity. In a similarly deformed case that was managed a few years later, a moderately accurate reduction was achieved. While the second operative case is indicative of a poor reduction, the patient possessed a Harris hip rating of 92. Probably the favorable clinical outcome was related to the presence of secondary incongruence of the acetabulum referable

Figure 13-6. A complex "T" fracture with a posterior wall fragment and associated pelvic ring disruption. A poor reduction of the posterior column followed an inadequate preliminary reduction of the anterior column fragment.

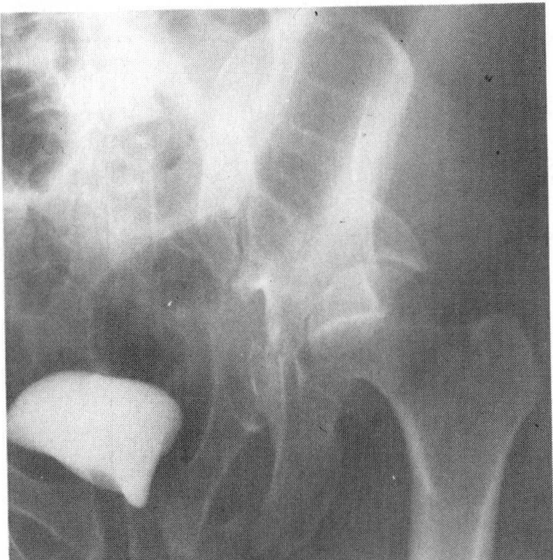

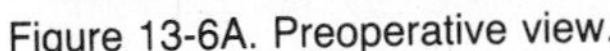

Figure 13-6A. Preoperative view.

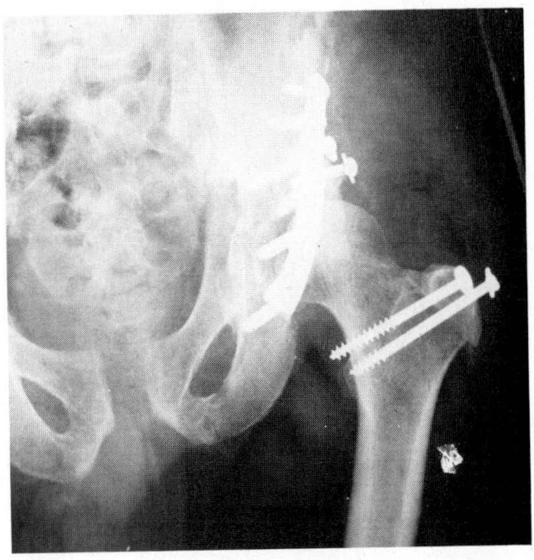

Figure 13-6B. Postoperative view at two months.

to the femoral head. In the third example, a highly satisfactory correction of the medial displacement associated with a comparable both-column injury is shown. Reproducibly successful results have been attained with a modified technique of open reduction. At surgery, the anterior iliac fragment is deliberately displaced to permit a direct visualization of the anterior and posterior fragments of the inferior acetabulum. Upon reduction and stabilization of the inferior acetabulum, this portion is reassembled to the superior half of the lateral ilium.

Two patients underwent a late loss of reduction related to extremely comminuted fractures and osteoporotic bone stock (Table 13-12). Subsequently, one patient was lost to followup and was considered to be a poor result. Another woman of 65 years with severe postmenopausal osteoporosis has progressed to a late painful nonunion-malunion of the acetabulum, for which further reconstructive surgery is anticipated. There was one other nonunion due to extensive comminution of the dome and failure of lag screw fixation. In five cases, screws partly disengaged spontaneously, although this was solely a radiographic finding without clinical significance. There were eight cases in which postoperative radiographs were notable for one or more bent or broken screws, particularly those inserted in the dome region. This observation was consistent with a minor subsidence of a fracture, but not with a complete loss of a reduction. One broken 3.5mm reconstruction plate was detected in a transverse fracture about 18 months after the initial reconstruction. There were five

Figure 13-7. A "T" fracture with an ipsilateral sacroiliac subluxation. While the iliac fragment is well reduced, the inferior half of the acetabulum is not congruent with the femoral head.

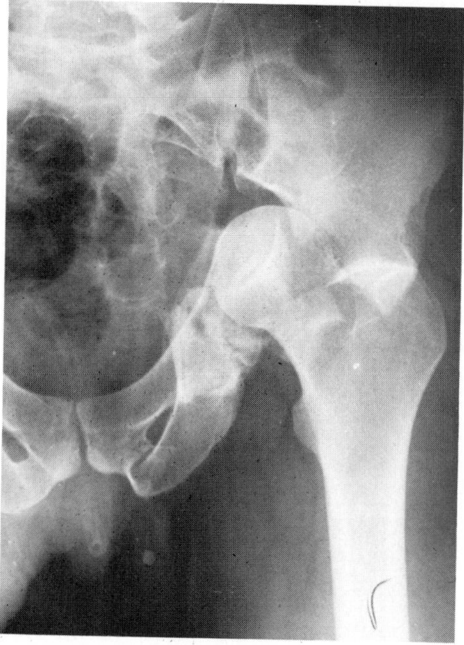

Figure 13-7A. Preoperative inlet view.

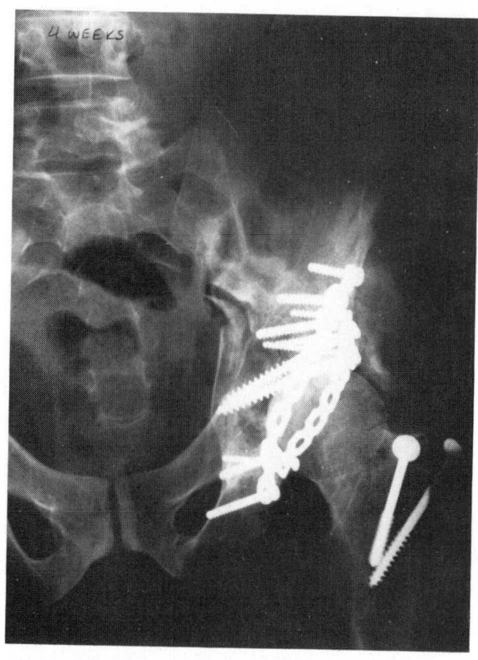


Figure 13-7B. Postoperative AP view.

Figure 13-8. A poor reduction of a both-column fracture with marked persistent medial migration is particularly evident in the postoperative inlet view.

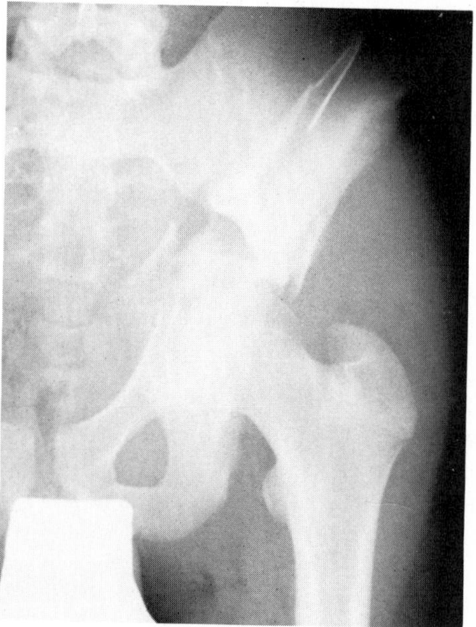

Figure 13-8A. Preoperative AP view.

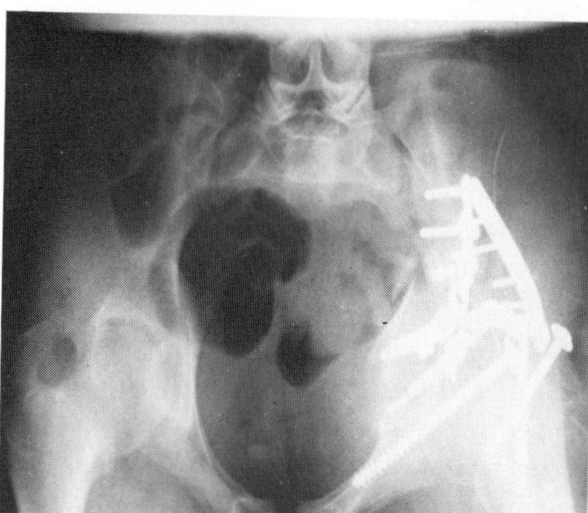

Figure 13-8B. Postoperative inlet view.

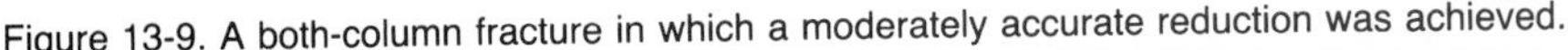

Figure 13-9. A both-column fracture in which a moderately accurate reduction was achieved.

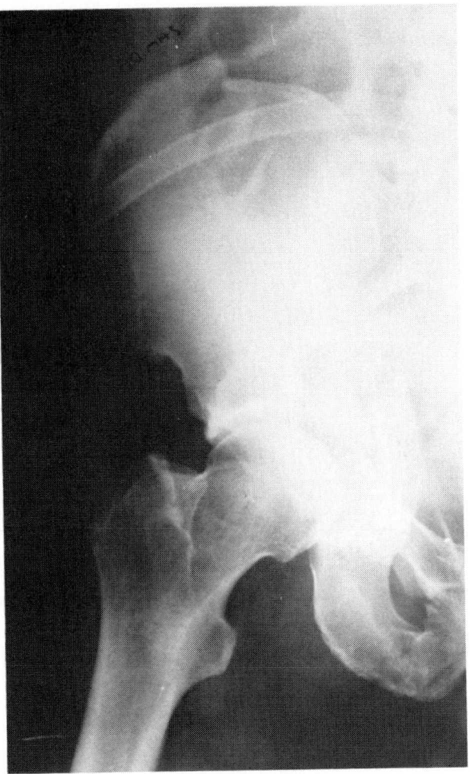

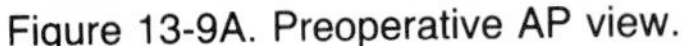

Figure 13-9A. Preoperative AP view.

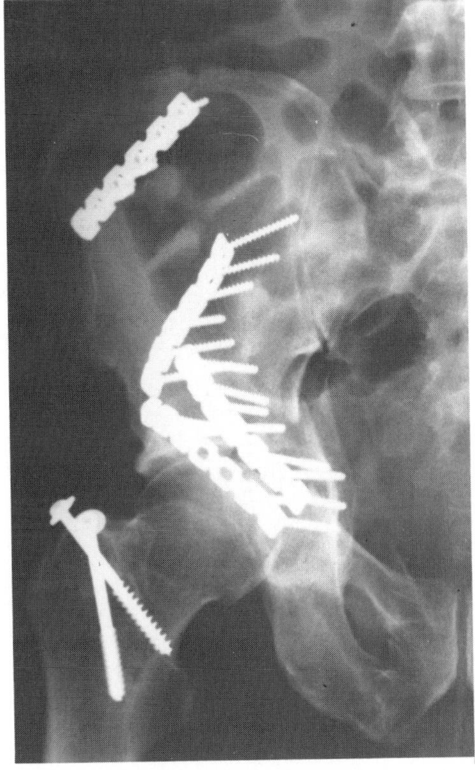

Figure 13-9B. Postoperative AP view.

cases of avascular necrosis of the femoral head. Three of the patients sustained a concomitant fracture of the ipsilateral femoral neck and were treated with an open reduction and internal fixation of both the femoral neck and the acetabulum. At the time of surgery, extensive traumatic disruption of the capsule of the hip joint was noted in two of the patients. Following a severe painful collapse of the femoral head, a total hip replacement was undertaken in two of the patients. Eight months after the initial surgery the third, a teenaged male patient, underwent a successful hip fusion. Two other patients developed avascular necrosis, four and five years respectively after their acetabular reconstructions. One patient developed early traumatic arthritis with a marked limitation of motion and severe hip pain. His acetabular radiographs revealed residual displacement of the fracture fragments of greater than 3mm and marked loss of the joint space. Subsequently a hip fusion was performed without difficulty. At six years after injury, a second patient showed marked radiographic narrowing of the joint space, and is therefore likely to progress to further reconstructive surgery. One additional patient with a bilateral acetabular fracture developed traumatic arthritis of both hips for which he was managed with

Figure 13-10. A both-column fracture in which an anatomical reduction was achieved.

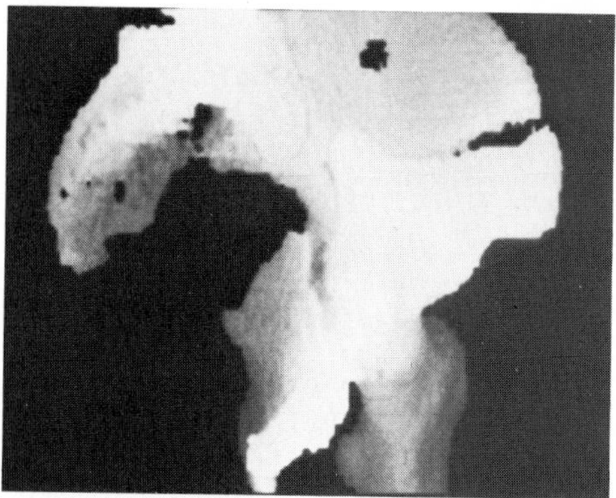

Figure 13-10A. Preoperative 3D computed scan.

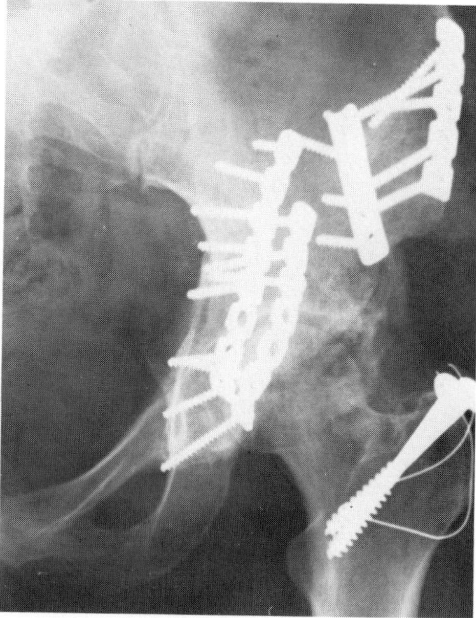

Figure 13-10B. Postoperative AP view.

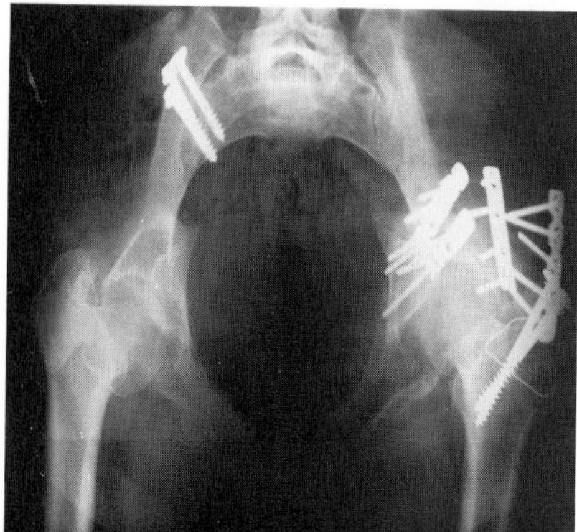

Figure 13-10C. Postoperative inlet view.

cementless types of total hip arthroplasty. Postoperative radiographs demonstrated a poor operative reduction of both of the acetabular fractures. Four other patients with poor open reductions have progressed to total hip replacements for traumatic arthritis.

Ectopic bone formation in the periarticular area occurred in 70% of the patients. The appearance of ectopic bone formation was associated primarily with the application of the triradiate and iliofemoral incisions, and to a limited degree after the use of the Kocher-Langenbeck approach, mainly where the greater trochanter was osteotomized. In no instance where the ilioinguinal incision was employed was postoperative ectopic bone formation documented. The predilection for ectopic bone formation appeared to be related to deferral of the surgery for one to three weeks after the time of the injury and to extensive pelvic comminution. Twelve of the patients possessed exuberant ectopic bone formation (Brooker III, IV Class[8]) in the capsular and hip abductor mechanism, which was asssociated with hip pain and a substantial limitation in the range of hip motion. All of the patients underwent acetabular reconstruction at more than three weeks after injury by resort to an extensile exposure. One year after acetabular surgery, six of the patients underwent removal of the ectopic bone followed by a course of low dose radiation therapy. After surgery the hip rating of the patients improved by an average of ten points, and the range of motion was moderately improved. In those cases (100 patients) where postoperative radiographs showed evidence of limited deposits of ectopic bone (Brooker I, II Class), few clinical symptoms or signs have been documented to implicate undesirable side effects.

Presently, 60% of the patients have been able to return to their original occupation. This includes heavy laborers, carpenters, and patients who spend a majority of the time on their feet, such as physicians and a pharmacist. The average period of unemployment between the initial accident and the return to gainful employment was ten months. The limitation of working status in the additional patients is associated with the residual sequelae of multiple trauma patients (e.g. neurologic injury to the central nervous system, peripheral nervous system, and ipsilateral appendicular injuries).

## Discussion

If the results of closed and open treatment of minimally displaced simple acetabular fractures are compared, the use of skeletal traction compares favorably with the use of surgical intervention. In the presence of marked comminution with displacement of the central acetabular or dome region, especially when there is extensive capsular disruption, the application of skeletal traction is unlikely to provide an acceptable anatomical reduction.[9] The results of the displaced fractures with involvement of the weightbearing dome or the medial wall correlated with restoration of congruity between the femoral head and the superior dome. If the relationship was not anatomically restored, a poor result was inevitable.

More recently, from the recent clinical reports by Judet and Letournel,[7] Tile,[9] Matta,[10] and Mears et al,[11] by resort to improved surgical exposures and techniques of reduction and fixation, a variety of displaced comminuted acetabular fractures can be effectively managed by operative techniques to provide a greater than 80% likelihood for the realization of a good or excellent result. From the results of the series of nearly 700 cases undertaken by Judet and Letournel,[7] a close correlation between the accuracy of the operative reduction and the quality of the clinical result was evident. In this series, greater than 90% of the patients with an anatomic reduction had a good or excellent clinical result, while only 50% of those with imperfectly reduced fractures achieved satisfactory clinical results. In addition, it appears that patients who rapidly achieve a painless mobile hip within a few weeks following their acetabular reconstruction tend to maintain the good result for at least the ten-year maximum period of followup.

Undoubtedly, there is a learning curve for this type of surgery.[10] The progressive improvement documented in the quality of the results in this review confirms this impression, which is further evident in a comparison of the initial 100 cases with the next 125 cases.[11] Thus, provided that a truly anatomical reduction is achieved, even in the presence of comminution, the results appear to be remarkably good. The irony is the overwhelming indication for surgery in the more comminuted and displaced fractures, where the technical difficulties are the greatest and where the results of nonoperative treatment are the poorest.

The acetabular reconstruction is most easily performed within a few days after the injury and before granulation tissue invades the fracture site. Previous workers[9] recommended a one- to five-day period of preoperative skeletal traction to provide a partial reduction and, thereby, a simplification of the open reduction. With the availability of more extensive surgical exposures and improved methods of open reduction, preoperative or intraoperative skeletal traction is rarely of any significant benefit. Furthermore, its use encourages a deferral of the acetabular reconstruction, which can be catastrophically extended if a complication such as a pulmonary embolus arises. In that instance the likelihood for a highly favorable outcome of the acetabular repair is seriously jeopardized. Intraoperative skeletal traction provides a small (6%) but increased risk of iatrogenically induced sciatic nerve palsy.[7]

When reconstructive surgery is deferred for three weeks after the time of the injury, the technical difficulties encountered in an attempted anatomical open reduction are greatly increased. This surgical impediment is associated with poorer anticipated clinical results, with generally less accurate reductions, and an increased susceptibility (i.e. 80%) to extensive symptomatic heterotopic bone formation. In this series the late presentation of greater than one third of the patients, who presented to us three weeks or more after injury, largely accounts for the high incidence of ectopic bone formation.

During the past two years, many additional cases have been referred with a late presentation where the delay provoked severe abrasive damage to the femoral head and acetabular fragments. In some of the cases an initial open reduction was a technical failure, so that the patient was referred for a second operative reduction. While insufficient time has ensued to determine the ultimate fate of these cases, a greater predilection for posttraumatic arthritis is anticipated. Nevertheless, even if the late reduction fails to provide a functional hip joint for a prolonged period by a restoration of the gross anatomy of the disrupted hemipelvis, the procedure immeasurably simplifies a subsequent total hip joint replacement.

Upon a review of the clinical data to identify the factors that are most influential on the final hip score, the type of fracture pattern and the degree of comminution were the principal variables. For a simple fracture pattern where less surgical dissection is required and an accurate anatomical reduction is readily obtained, the prognosis is excellent for the restoration of highly satisfactory hip function for the indefinite future. During the surgical approach of a simple fracture, the degree of iatrogenically induced injury to the surrounding soft tissues is insignificant. In the more comminuted associated injuries, such as a "T" or both-column fracture, a poorer hip score can be anticipated. Explanations for this observation include the more extensive dissection associated with the surgical exposure and the diminished accuracy of the typical reduction.

Upon a review of the most significant criteria of the Harris Hip Scale,[11] pain and functional attributes of the rating were most influential. The postoperative pain correlated most accurately with the quality of the surgical reduction and the degree of heterotopic bone formation in the abductor musculature and the pericapsular areas. This pain was often most severe during the period of active formation of the heterotopic ossification and generally diminished as the followup period approached two years. However, significant ossification in the periarticular region was often documented at two to three years after injury, and was associated with mild or moderately severe mechanical pain and stiffness. Thus far, the number of patients with traumatic arthritis and a painful hip in the postoperative period has been limited. In all of those patients where the early onset of traumatic arthritis associated with hip pain, stiffness, and a progressive narrowing of the joint space were documented one year after the time of injury, greater than 3mm of displacement was evident in the postoperative radiographs and a poor hip rating was documented within six to 12 months after the injury. In a small number of patients, prolonged pain in the ipsilateral extremity related to a sciatic nerve injury compromised the hip scale in the postoperative period.

The functional constituents of the Harris Hip Scale provided a second opportunity for the rating of a patient to vary somewhat independently of the acetabular reconstruction itself. In the early postoperative period all of the patients exhibited a limp secondary to a gluteal lurch, presumably related to the extensive surgical dissection. Provided that a vigorous program of physical therapy with progressive resistance exercises of the hip abductors was undertaken, generally the abductor lurch vanished within six to 12 months after the surgery. The ability of the patient to undertake independent gait and transfers, to climb stairs, to apply shoes, and to tie shoe laces reflects not only the intrinsic function of the hip and acetabulum, but also the entire ipsilateral lower extremity. Frequently, injuries to the ipsilateral knee adversely affected the functional rating of a hip joint, even though the other clinical and radiographic features of the reconstructed hip were virtually normal.

The range of motion of the reconstructed hip provided a substantial contribution to the functional rating on the Harris Hip Scale. While the mobility of the reconstructed hips varied considerably, in those patients who were considered to have a good or excellent result a minimum of 90° of hip, 30° of abduction, and 20° of internal and external rotation was documented. Eighty-five percent of the patients in whom this range of motion was achieved within six to 12 weeks after surgery and maintained for one year were rated as good or excellent at the time of review. In this series the limitation of hip motion was most often attributable to the presence of ectopic ossification, avascular necrosis, impaction of the femoral head, and early traumatic arthritis.

The most widespread complication after open reduction and internal fixation of an acetabular injury was heterotopic ossification. After the accuracy of the acetabular reduction, the presence of heterotopic ossification provided the largest influence on the late Harris Hip Score. Heterotopic ossification in the abductor mechanism and pericapsular area is most frequently observed in the postoperative radiographs of a middle aged mesomorphic male patient with an associated type of acetabular fracture. This observation may be best explained by the greater provocative force transmitted to the soft tissues and bone of such an individual at the moment of impact. The surgical approach required for the operative reduction and internal fixation of the fracture imparts an additional degree of trauma and devascularization to the periarticular soft tissues, which correlates with the incidence of ectopic bone formation. The inevitable need for an extensile approach to visualize the typical associated acetabular fracture, such as a both-column disruption, provides an exceptional stimulus for the subsequent formation of heterotopic ossification, and therefore remains an unsolved clinical problem.

Ectopic bone formation is minimized by limitation of the surgical approach particularly referable to a dissection of the glutei and tensor musculature from the hip capsule. The ilioinguinal incision, which exposes the inner pelvic wall, is virtually free of postsurgical ectopic bone formation. Most displaced acetabular fractures, however, require a direct visualization of the articular surface, which is not adequately exposed by the ilioinguinal incision. The Kocher-Langenbeck approach is associated with a lower incidence of postoperative ectopic bone formation than an extensile approach. Nevertheless, to adequately visualize many transverse and most associated fracture patterns, an extensile approach such as a triradiate[13] or an extended iliofemoral[7] incision is essential. Early surgical treatment, performed less than one week after the injury, also favors minimal ectopic bone formation. During the past two years, in an attempt to lessen the incidence of ectopic bone formation, the influence of a continuous passive motion machine, postoperative disodium etidronate, and indomethacin therapy have been examined. None of these agents has appeared to lessen the incidence of heterotopic bone formation. While the prophylactic application of low dose radiation has been considered, it has not been employed in view of the potential side-effects.

In the typical multiple trauma fatality who sustains an acetabular fracture, the cause of death is related to hemorrhage or to intracranial, intraabdominal, or intrathoracic injuries. Not surprisingly, if the patient survives until acetabular reconstruction is performed, his likelihood for a postoperative demise becomes a remote probability, with published death rates of between 1% and 3%.[7,9] In the present series, the sole postoperative death was related to an unrecognized bowel infarction. While a fatal pulmonary embolus is a potential complication, despite the avoidance of routine anticoaguation and its potential complications including delayed osseous union, this problem has been avoided perhaps by resort to rapid postoperative mobilization of the patients.

Intraarticular infection remains a serious postoperative complication, with an incidence reported in other series of between 2% and 7% of cases.[7,9,14] With the proximity of, and thereby the potential for, contamination from the perineal area particularly to the ilioinguinal region, meticulous care in the preparation and draping of the patient is required. The prognosis for a deep wound infection is poor, so that a fusion of the hip or a resectional arthroplasty may be needed as a salvage procedure. As preventive measures, the authors advocate the use of preoperative and postoperative intravenous antibiotics, meticulous preparation and draping, pulsatile jet lavage irrigation of the surgical wound with large volumes of antibiotic solution, and the insertion of multiple suction drains. If the wound develops signs of a postoperative wound infection, rapid initiation of a surgical debridement to excise devitalized infected tissue is essential. Such a protocol may have encouraged the resolution of three of the four early infections documented in this series so that only one case progressed to a hip fusion. The one other case, which presented four years after the open reduction combined with external pelvic fixation for an associated ring disruption and progressed to a Girdlestone arthroplasty, remains an enigma.

Traumatically induced injuries to the sciatic nerve are most often associated with fractures of the posterior wall and column or associated fractures with displacement of the posterior column. Most of these injuries constitute a transient neuropraxia and possess a good prognosis for ultimate recovery. Iatrogenically induced injuries to the sciatic nerve usually are provoked by excessive traction on the nerve by the use of a retractor inserted into the greater sciatic notch. Another causative factor is a drilling injury, particularly when a drill bit, pin or screw is errantly inserted through the pelvis into the nerve. The incidence and severity of iatrogenically induced sciatic nerve injuries can be minimized by appropriate adjustments in the surgical technique. Immediately prior to a posterior approach, the ipsilateral knee is flexed so that the risk of application of excessive distraction on the sciatic nerve during the surgical procedure is minimized. Whenever possible, retraction of the posterior column is achieved without the insertion of a retractor in the greater or lesser sciatic notch. When such a retractor is needed, prior to its application, the gemelli and obturator externus are incised near their distal insertions to the greater trochanter. The muscles are reflected over the sciatic nerve, and function as a buffer once the retractor is inserted into the greater notch or preferably the lesser sciatic notch. The periods of such soft tissue retraction in the sciatic notch are minimized. When drill holes are prepared in the roof of the greater sciatic notch, the bit is inserted carefully through the inner table of the pelvis so that the likelihood for penetration of the adjacent segment of the nerve is minimized.

If a sciatic nerve palsy occurs, then a suitable ankle-foot orthosis is obtained to control the typical foot drop deformity. Passive mobilization of the affected joints also is encouraged. In the present series the prognosis for spontaneous recovery of an iatrogenically induced sciatic palsy was good.

The evaluation and clinical course of postoperative avascular necrosis is variable and often unpredictable. As others[7,9,14,15] have emphasized, the incidence and severity of avascular necrosis of the femoral head do not correlate with the accuracy of the open surgical acetabular reduction. To some degree certain attributes of the initial traumatic insult appear to determine the viability of the vascular supply to the femoral head. For example, extensive traumatic capsular disruption and marked posterior migration and especially impaction of the femoral head are precipitating factors of avascular necrosis. During the surgery, additional devascularization of the femoral head can be provoked by incision or inadvertent damage to the capsule around the femoral neck. Three of the patients in this series who developed avascular necrosis sustained a concomitant fracture of the femoral neck. Ultimately, these patients progressed to an arthroplasty or arthrodesis of the hip. While the possible roles for endoprosthetic replacement of the femoral head accompanying acetabular reconstruction arises in such cases, to date this method has not been used by us. The two other cases that presented four and five years after an acetabular repair without another demonstrable cause of avascular necrosis cannot be satisfactorily explained. One of these cases progressed to a bipolar prosthesis and the other to a cementless total hip replacement.

In this series, the improved operative exposure provided by the triradiate incision, combined with the improved techniques of reduction and stabilization of the fractures by the previously described methods, have virtually eliminated postoperative acetabular nonunions (e.g. less than 1%).

If the acetabular fracture is accompanied by an unstable pelvic ring disruption, the results anticipated from skeletal traction are abysmal, so that an open reduction and internal fixation of the acetabulum with internal or external fixation of the pelvic ring is indicated. In these cases, the reduction progresses from the reduced or nearly approximated areas to the unreduced areas. If the ipsilateral sacroiliac joint is displaced, initially this site is approached for an open reduction and stabilization. Next, the adjacent iliac fracture including an extension of an anterior column insult is approached. Reconstruction of the posterior column follows along with the reduction and stabilization of the articular portion of the anterior column.

A critical analysis of the results reveals the following major factors in determination of the outcome of an individual acetabular disruption: **1)** the damage to the acetabular articular surface, reflected by the pattern of the fracture and its degree of comminution, impaction and osteoporosis, and associated damage to the femoral head; **2)** the adequacy of the reduction, which is reflected by intraoperative inspection and postoperative radiographs; and **3)** the associated complications of the fracture and treatment, including avascular necrosis, heterotopic ossification, and a sciatic palsy.

## Radiological Assessment of the Surgically-Treated Acetabular Fracture

Contributed by Claude L. Martimbeau, MD, FRCS(C).

Previous methods for the evaluation of the postoperative results following an acetabular reconstruction have focussed attention upon the clinical parameters. To analyze the quality of the result by radiographic means, earlier workers have reported their overall impression of the comparison between the preoperative and postoperative radiographs.[7,16] Recently, a quantitative assessment based upon a comparative radiographic evaluation was developed for realization of the following objectives: **a)** to evaluate the improvement in a reduction achieved by a surgical procedure; **b)** to aid in the selection of the optimal surgical exposure and technique of reduction for each fracture pattern; and **c)** to provide a basis for valid statistical comparisions of long-term results documented in different clinical series.

For a quantitative assessment of the postoperative radiographs, specific aspects of the reduction are recorded in each projection. In the anteroposterior view, the degree of congruence of the hip joint and the magnitude of residual central protrusion of the femoral head are documented. In the iliac oblique view, the reduction of the anterior column or anterior wall and the congruence of the hip joint are recorded. In the obturator oblique view, the reduction of the posterior column or posterior wall and the congruence of the hip joint are measured. Subsequently, the various displacements are analyzed by resort to a grading system.

To evaluate the degree of persistent central protrusio by a study of the anteroposterior view, a line is extended from the sciatic buttress in a distal direction to the ischial tuberosity, which is parallel to the longitudinal axis of the pelvis (Figures 13-11 and 13-12). A point score system is employed:

- no displacement of the femoral head = 1
- medial displacement of the femoral head across the line = 0

The assessment of postoperative congruity is evaluated

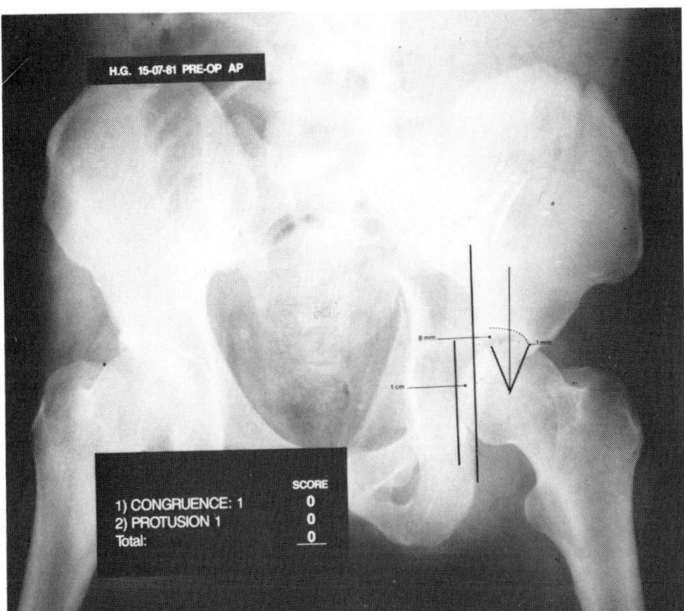


Figure 13-11. Preoperative evaluation of the congruence of the femoral head: measure 8mm medial to the center of the femoral head and 1mm lateral to the center of the femoral head—the difference is 7mm, score 0. Evaluation of the protrusion of the femoral head: medial displacement of 1mm of the femoral head across a line drawn from sciatic buttress and parallel to the longitudinal axis of the pelvis—score 0.

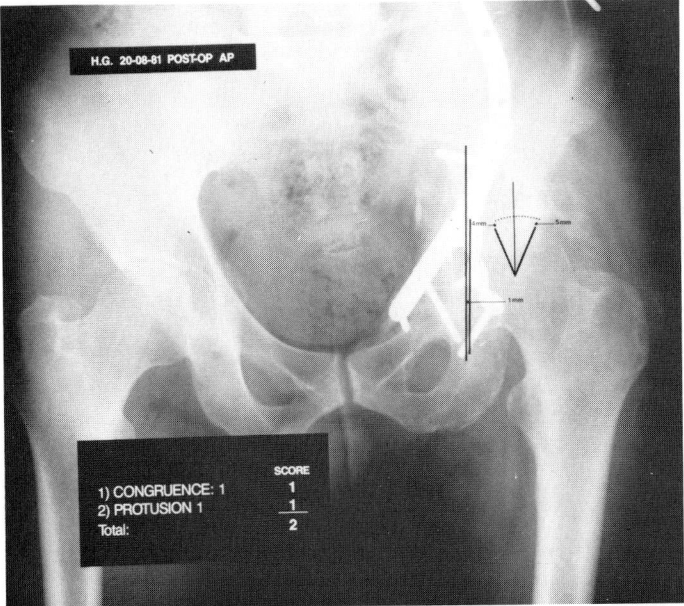


Figure 13-12. Postoperative evaluation of congruence: difference of 1mm—score 1. Evaluation of the protrusion of the femoral head: 1mm lateral to the line drawn from the sciatic buttress—score 1.

**Table 13-18**
**Distribution of the Acetabular Fractures**

| | |
|---|---|
| Posterior Wall | 7 |
| Posterior Column | 2 |
| Anterior Wall | 1 |
| Anterior Column | 1 |
| Transverse | 3 |
| "T" Shaped | 6 |
| Posterior Column-Posterior Wall | 1 |
| Transverse-Posterior Wall | 3 |
| Anterior Column or Anterior Wall and Posterior Hemitransverse | 9 |
| Both-Column | 22 |

in a similar way in the examination of the anteroposterior, iliac, and obturator views. In each view, a line is drawn from the center of the femoral head in a superior direction that is parallel to the longitudinal axis of the pelvis (Figures 13-11 to 13-16). One centimeter medial and lateral to where this line crosses the edge of the femoral head, the width of the joint space is measured. A point score is assessed:

- a difference of 1mm or less = 1
- a difference of more than 1mm = 0

For the evaluation of the anterior column or wall in the obturator oblique view or the posterior column or wall in the iliac oblique view (Figures 13-13 to 13-16), the magnitude of persistent displacement is evaluated by point score:

- displacement of 0 to 1mm = 2
- displacement of 2 to 3mm = 1
- displacement of more than 4mm = 0

After the preoperative and postoperative radiographs for a particular case are analyzed, a comparison of the point scores permits a quantitative determination of the improvement in the anatomical relationships of the hip joint that were realized by the surgical procedure.

Recently, this analytical approach was employed to assess the results of the first 55 patients who underwent surgery within three weeks of the time of their injury. The patients included 43 men and 12 women with a range in age from 12 to 63 years and an average age of 35 years. The distribution of their acetabular fractures are listed in Table 13-18. The surgical exposures employed for the procedures are given in Table 13-19.

## Results for the Simple Fractures

Of the seven patients who were managed for a posterior wall fracture (Figure 13-8) where the Kocher-Langenbeck

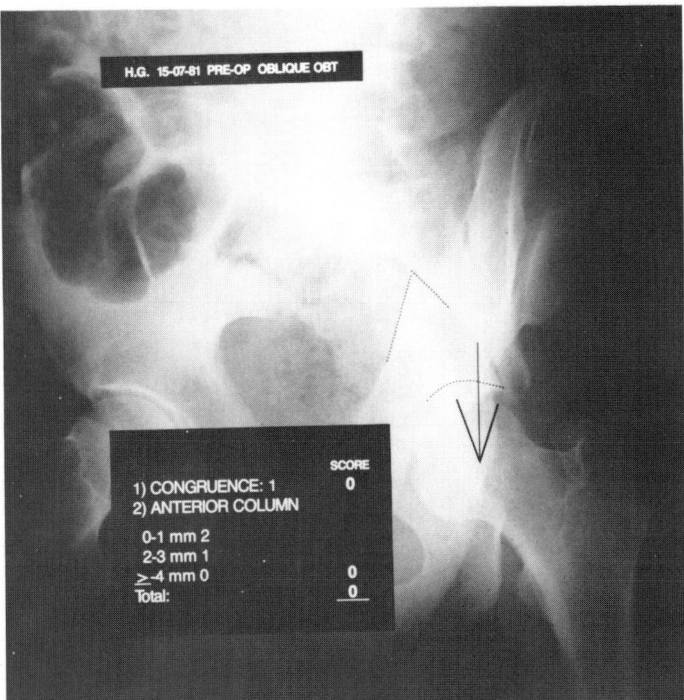


Figure 13-13. Preoperative obturator oblique view. Evaluation of congruence—score 0. Anterior column: displacement more than 4mm—score 0.

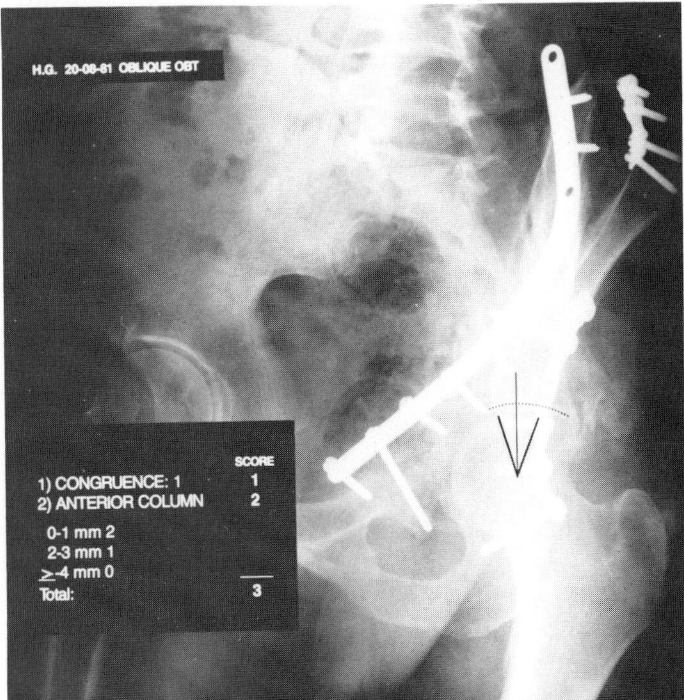


Figure 13-14. Postoperative obturator oblique view. Evaluation of congruence—score 1. Displacement of anterior column: 0mm—score 2.

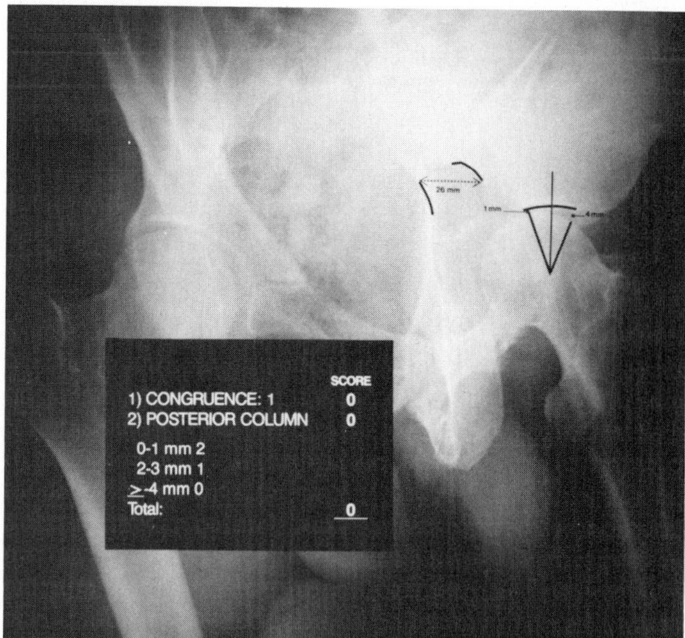


Figure 13-15. Preoperative iliac oblique view. Evaluation of congruence—score 0. Evaluation of the displacement of the posterior column: 7-6mm—score 0.

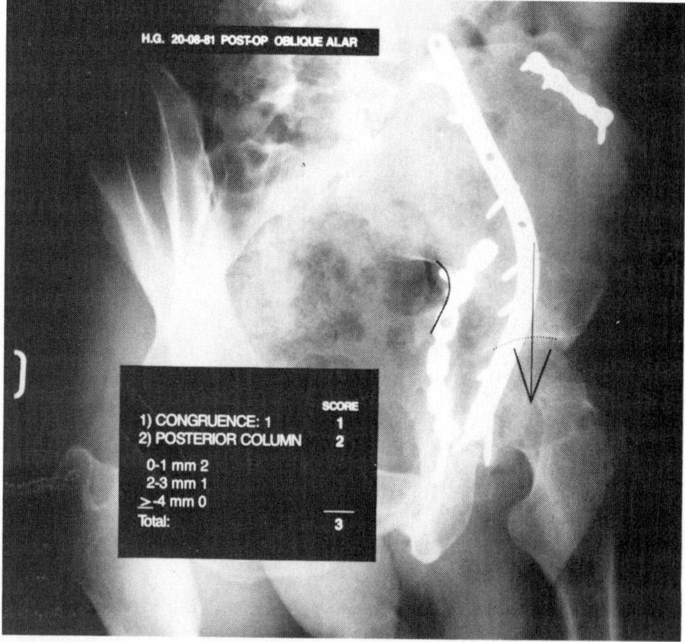


Figure 13-16. Postoperative iliac oblique view. Evaluation of congreuence—score 1. Evaluation of the displacement of the posterior column—score 2.

**Table 13-19**
**Operative Exposures Employed for the Acetabular Reconstructions**

| Exposure | Number |
|---|---|
| Kocher-Langenbeck | 28 |
| Ilioinguinal | 15 |
| Kocher-Langenbeck and Ilioinguinal | 4 |
| Extended Iliofemoral | 2 |
| Ollier-Senegas | 1 |

**Radiological Evaluation**

| | | Score |
|---|---|---|
| **1. Congruence** | AP | (1) |
| | Obturator | (1) |
| | Iliac | (1) |
| **2. Posterior Column (Wall)** | Iliac (Obt.) | (2) |
| **3. Anterior Column (Wall)** | Obturator | (2) |
| **4. Central Protrusion** | AP | (1) |
| | **Optimal Score** | (8) |

Figure 13-17. Radiological evaluation of congruence, central protrusion, and displacement of the column (or wall) and the maximum point score for each detail.

approach was used routinely, all of them possessed an anatomical reduction and a maximum score of 8. The two patients who were managed for a posterior column fracture (Figure 13-19) by resort to a Kocher-Langenbeck approach achieved an average score of 7. The first patient who possessed a lower preoperative score achieved an anatomical reduction. The second patient possessed a 4mm residual displacement of the posterior column. During the surgical procedure the counter traction applied by the post of the pelvic support on the ischial tuberosity inhibited the reduction of the posterior column (Figures 13-20 and 13-21). Each of the patients who were managed for an anterior wall and an anterior column fracture by resort to an ilioinguinal approach realized an anatomical reduction with a score of 8 (Figures 13-22 to 13-24).

All three patients who were managed for a transverse fracture possessed a preoperative score of zero, with marked displacement and incongruity. Their average postoperative score was 6.7 (Figures 13-25 to 13-27). The first patient, who attained an anatomical reduction with a maximum score of 8, was managed initially by a Kocher-Langenbeck approach and one week later by an ilioinguinal approach. The second patient, who

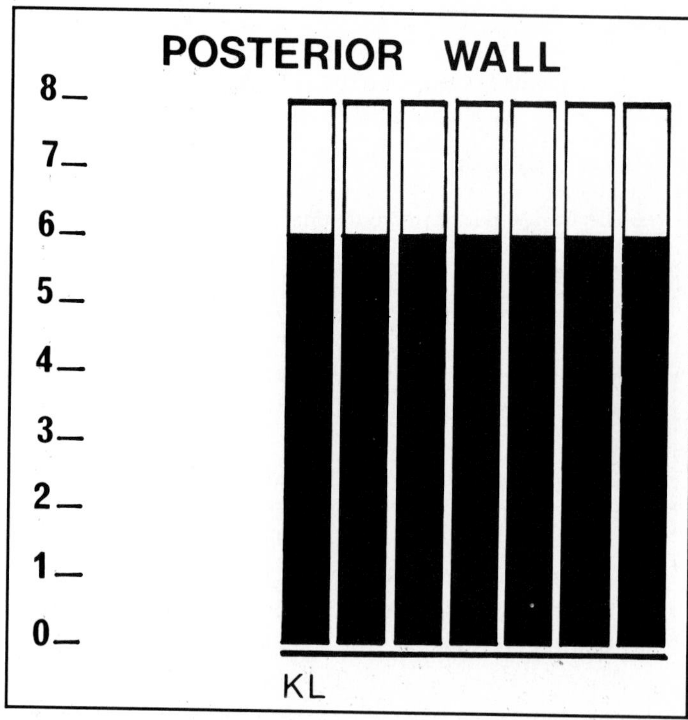


Figure 13-18. Preoperative and postoperative evaluation of posterior wall fractures. Black: preoperative point score. White: postoperative point score.

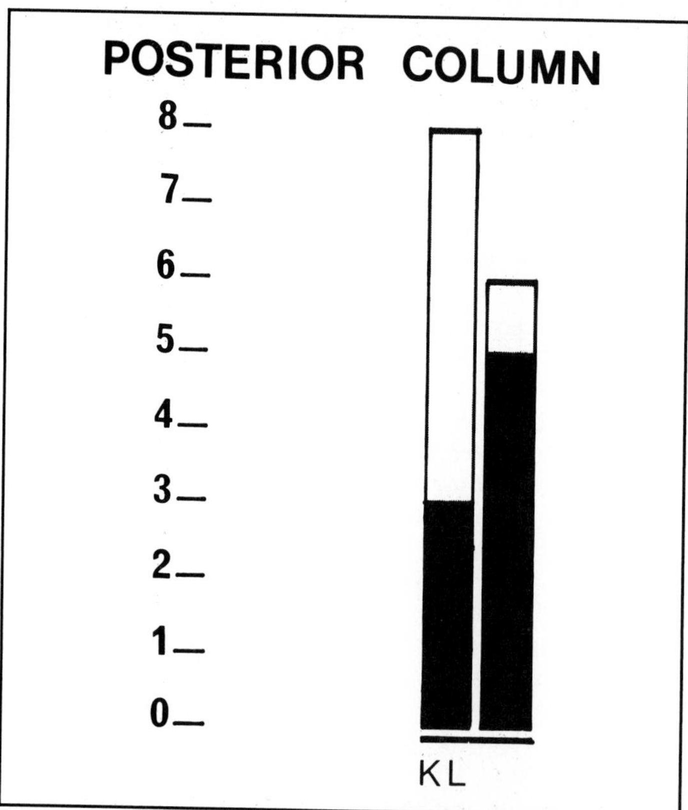


Figure 13-19. Preoperative and postoperative evaluation of the posterior column. Black: preoperative point score. White: postoperative point score.

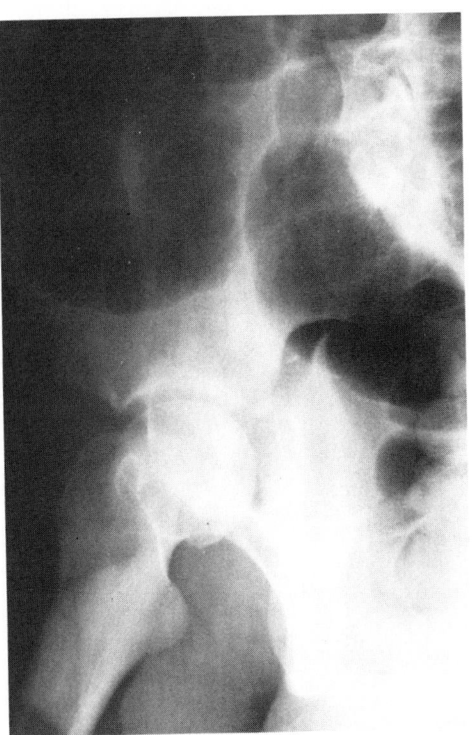

Figure 13-20. Preoperative iliac oblique view, 11mm displacement of the posterior column.

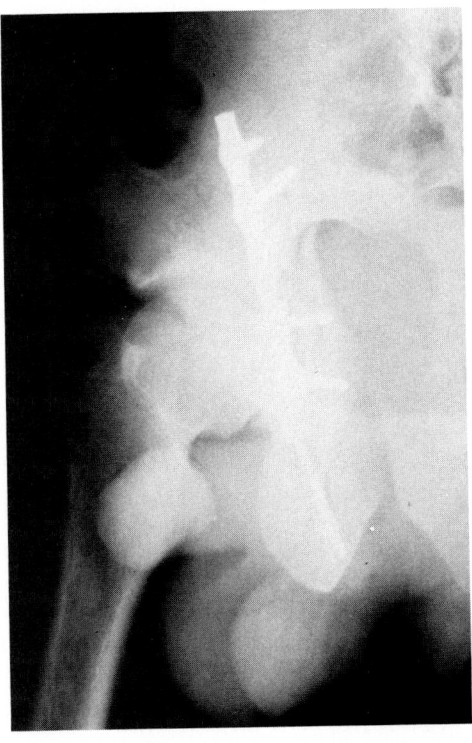

Figure 13-21. Postoperative iliac oblique view, 4mm displacement of the posterior column (K-L approach).

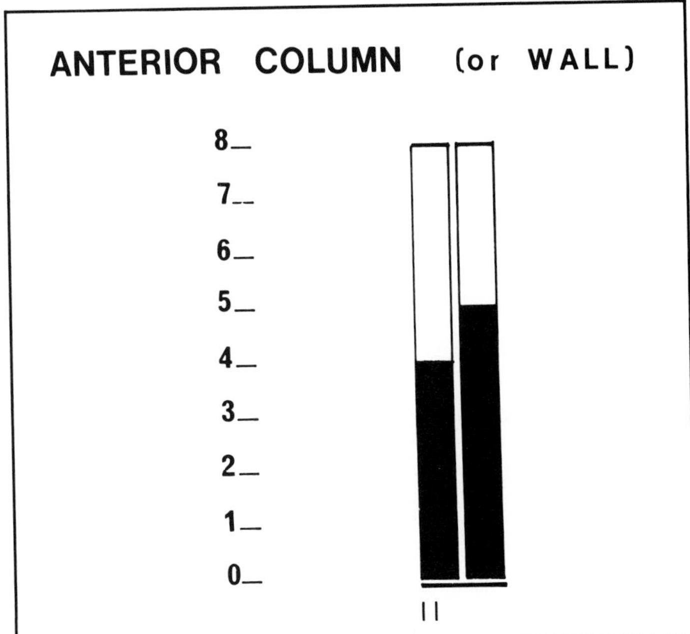


Figure 13-22:. Preoperative and postoperative evaluation of the anterior column and the anterior wall. Black: preoperative point score. White: postoperative point score.

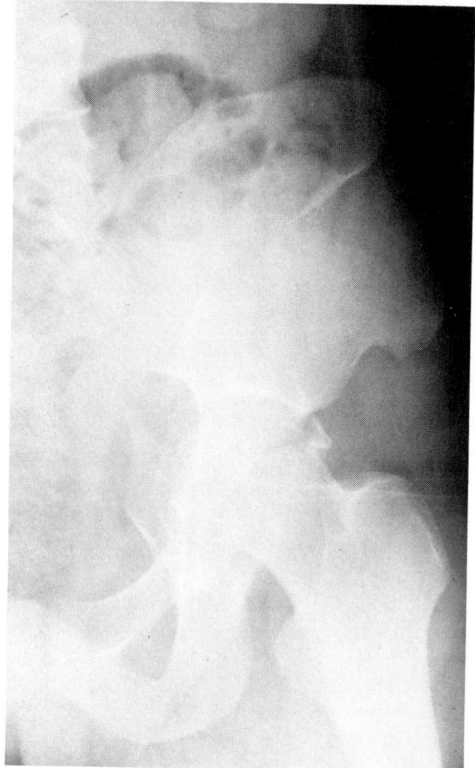

Figure 13-23. Preoperative AP view of the anterior wall fracture.

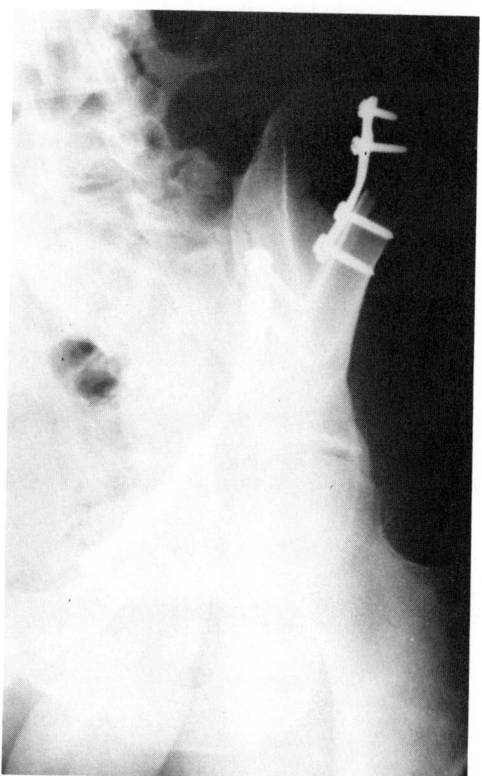

Figure 13-24. Postoperative obturator oblique view of anterior wall fracture (ilioinguinal approach).

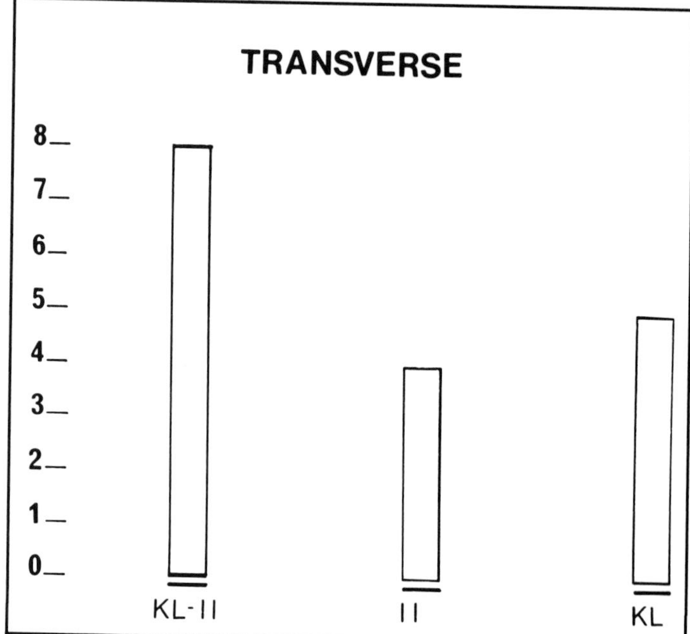


Figure 13-25. Preoperative and postoperative evaluation of the transverse fracture. Black: preoperative point score. White: postoperative point score.

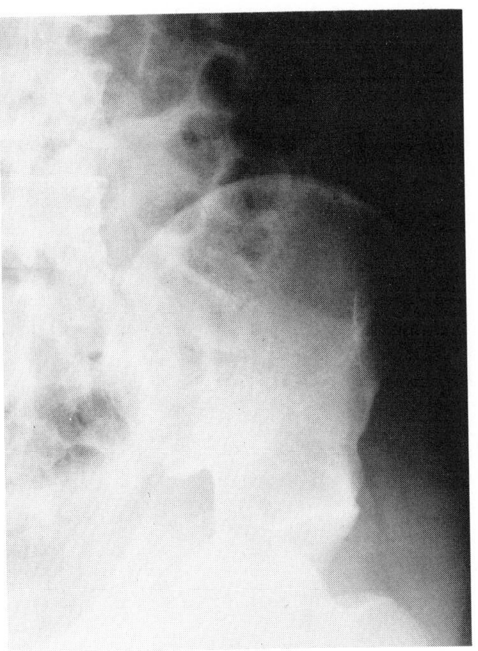

Figure 13-26. Preoperative AP view of the transverse fracture.

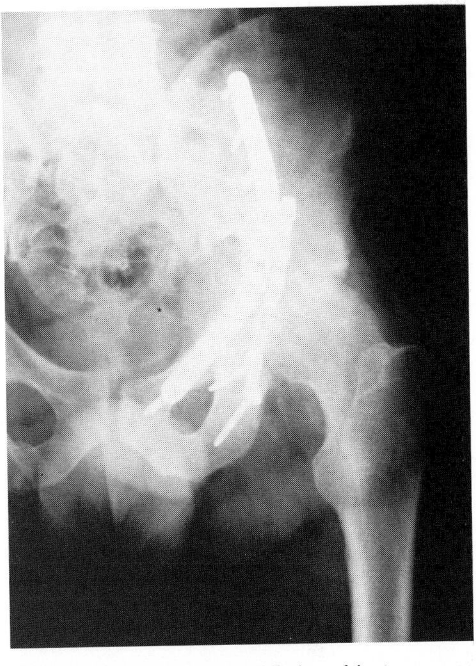

Figure 13-27. Postoperative AP view of the transverse fracture (K-L and I-I approaches).

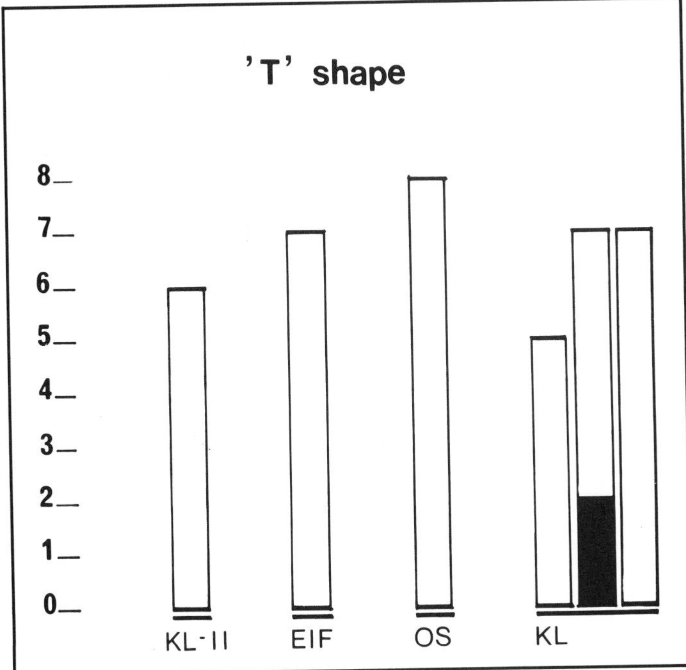


Figure 13-28. Preoperative and postoperative evaluation of the "T" fractures. Black: preoperative point score. White: postoperative point score.

realized the poorest score of 4, was managed by an anterior approach. For the third patient, in whom a score of 5 was recorded and where a posterior approach was used, persistent displacement of the unreduced anterior column with allied incongruity of the hip joint is evident in the obturator oblique view.

For the six patients who underwent a reconstruction of a "T" fracture, all but one of the preoperative scores were zero (Figure 13-28). For the first patient, in whom anterior and posterior approaches were used, a perfect reduction of both columns was achieved. Nevertheless, the result was compromised by persistent impaction of the acetabular surface, for a postoperative score of 6 (Figures 13-29 and 13-30). For the second patient, where an extended iliofemoral approach was utilized, an excellent result with a score of 7 was marred solely by an imperfect reduction of the anterior column. A third patient, who underwent an extensile exposure with an Ollier-Senegas approach, achieved an anatomical reduction with a maximum score of 8. For the remaining three patients, in whom a Kocher-Langenbeck approach was employed, persistent displacement of the anterior column compromised each score by at least one point. Nevertheless, all of the patients possessed an anatomically congruent hip (Figures 13-31 and 13-32)

## Results of the Associated Fractures

The one patient who was managed for a posterior column-posterior wall fracture by resort to a Kocher-Langenbeck approach achieved an anatomical reduction with a maximum score of 8 (Figure 13-33). Each of the three cases of an anterior column or anterior wall with an associated posterior hemitransverse fracture was surgically approached in a different way (Figure 13-34). In two of the cases approached by an ilioinguinal or an extended iliofemoral approach, anatomical reductions and maximum scores of 8 were achieved. In contrast, the fracture approached posteriorly possessed persistent displacement of the anterior column that was not significantly corrected (Figures 13-35 and 13-36). For the patients managed for a transverse and posterior wall fracture either by resort to a combination of an anterior and a posterior approach or by an extended iliofemoral approach to visualize both columns, an anatomical reduction and a maximum score of 8 was documented (Figures 13-37 to 13-39). In contrast, of the six cases where a posterior approach was used, an anatomical reduction was achieved in but two of the six patients. For the patients with a both-column fracture in whom either a combination of an anterior and a posterior approach or an extended iliofemoral approach was used (Figures 13-40 to 13-42), the most consistently good

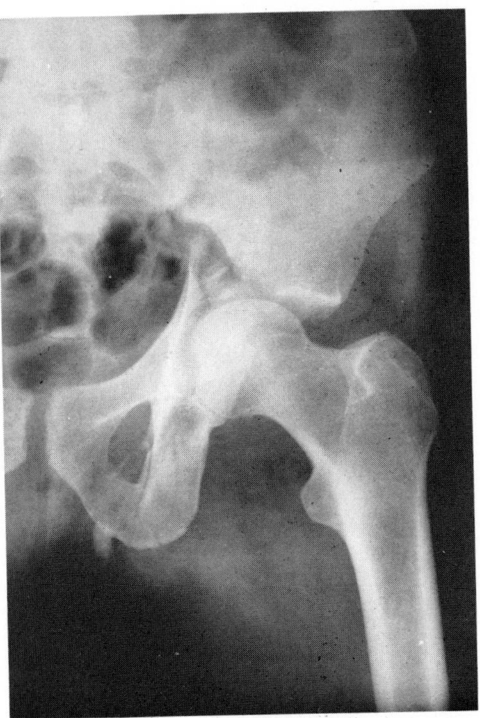

Figure 13-29. Preoperative AP view of "T" fracture. There is also an impaction fracture of the acetabulum.

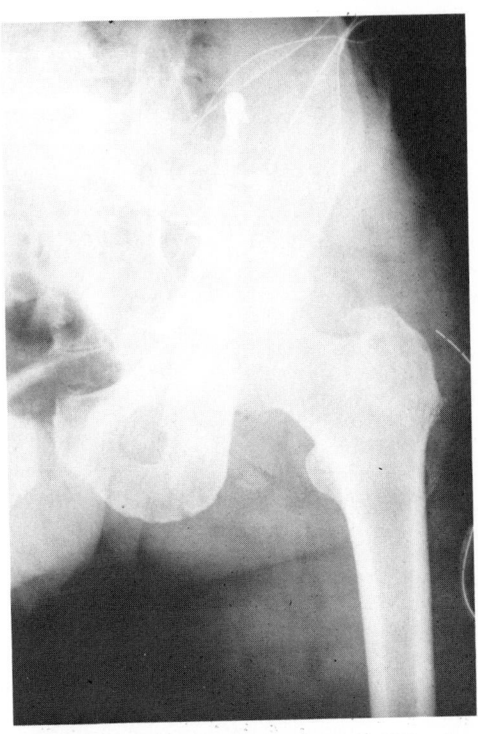

Figure 13-30. Postoperative AP view of "T" fracture (K-L and I-I approaches).

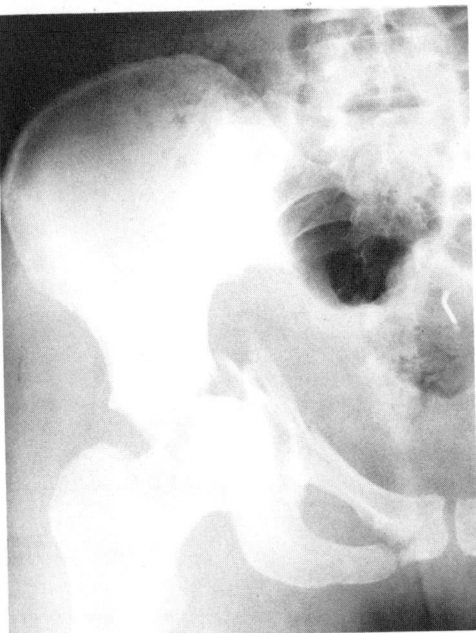

Figure 13-31. Preoperative AP of "T" fracture.

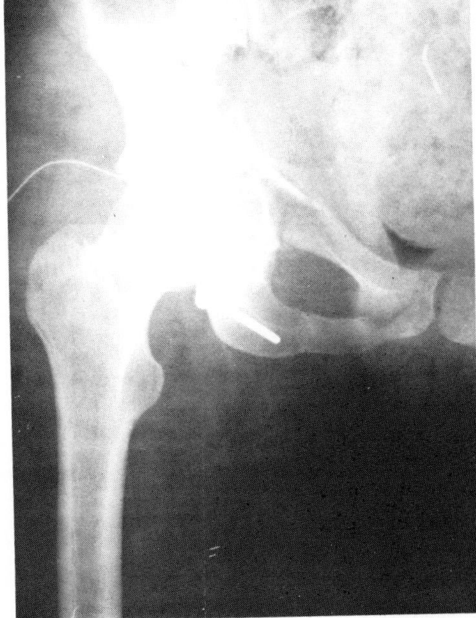

Figure 13-32. Postoperative obturator oblique view of the "T" fracture (K-L approach).

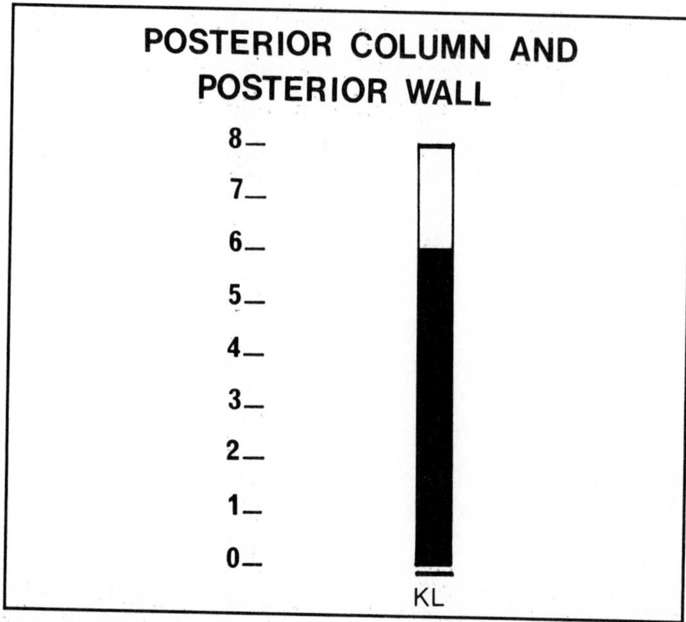


Figure 13-33. Preoperative and postoperative evaluation of the posterior column and posterior wall fracture. Black: preoperative point score. White: postoperative point score.

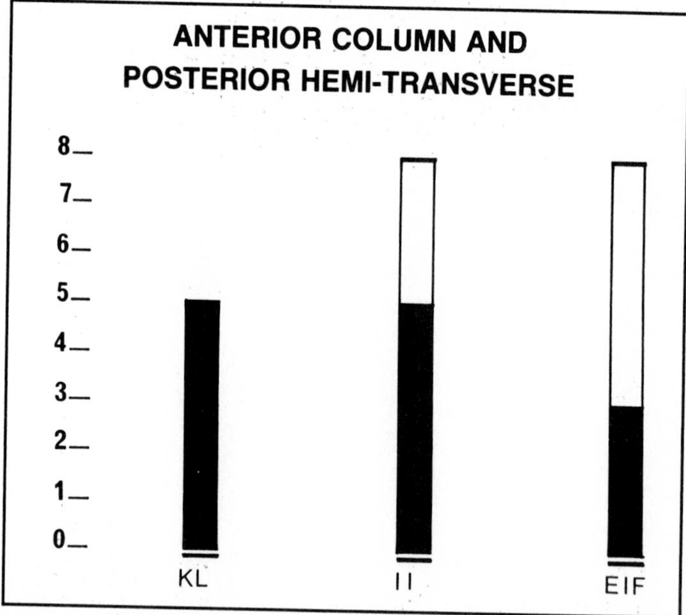


Figure 13-34. Preoperative and postoperative evaluation of the anterior column and anterior wall fracture associated with a posterior hemitransverse fracture. Black: preoperative point score. White: postoperative point score.

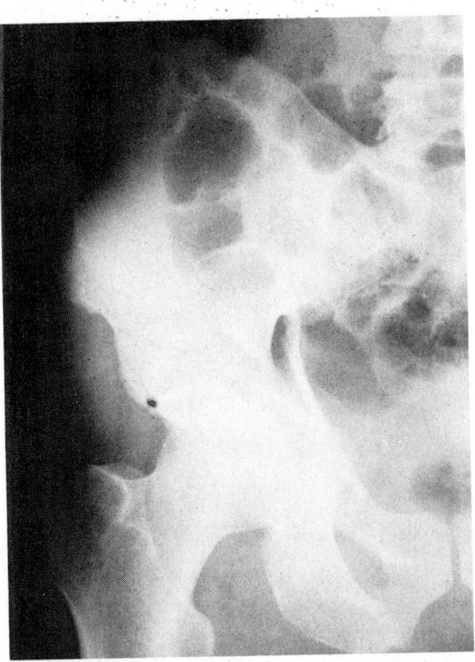

Figure 13-35. Preoperative AP view of the anterior wall fracture associated with a posterior hemitransverse fracture.

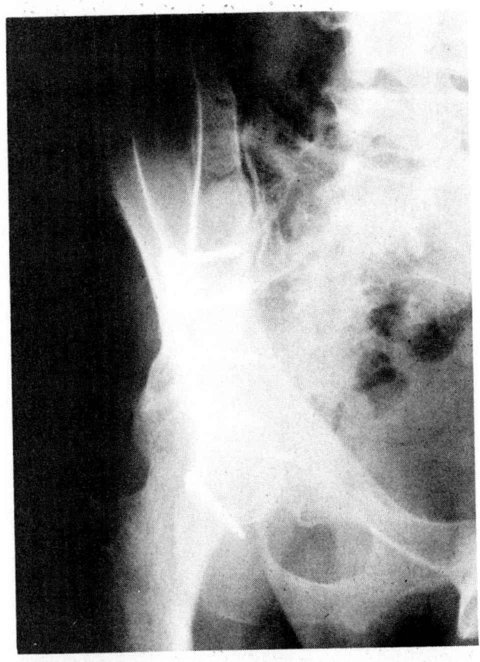

Figure 13-36. Postoperative obturator oblique view of the anterior wall fracture associated with a posterior hemitransverse (K-L approach).

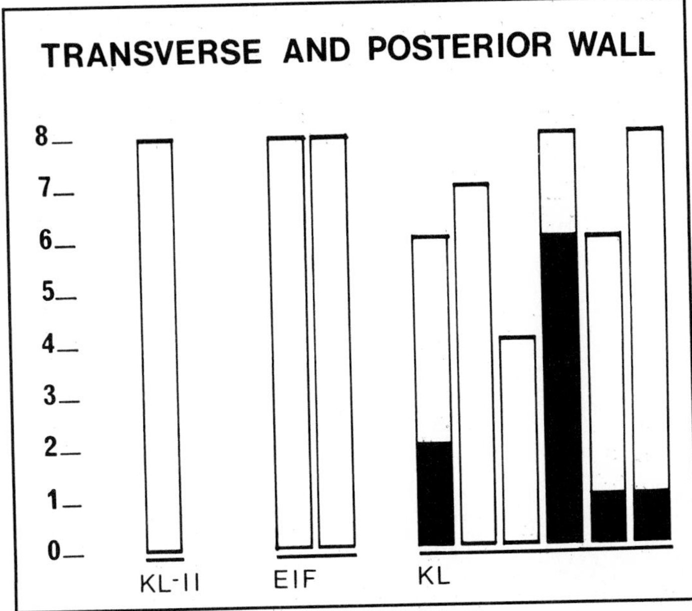


Figure 13-37. Preoperative and postoperative evaluation of the transverse and posterior wall fracture. Black: preoperative point score. White: postoperative point score.

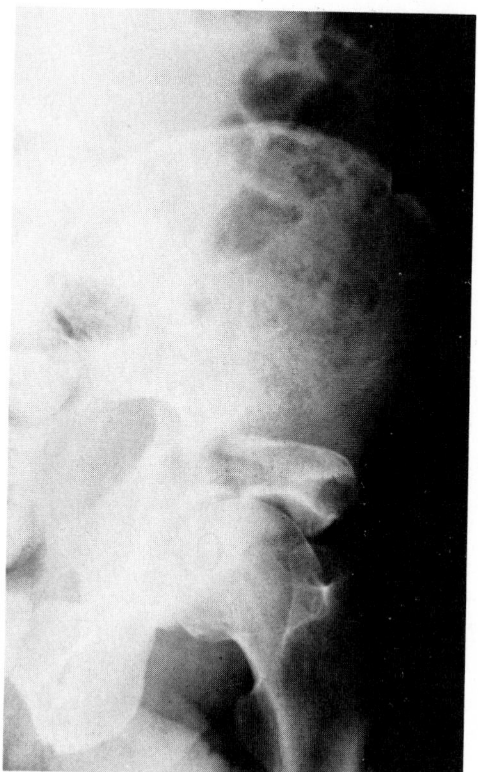

Figure 13-38. Preoperative iliac oblique view of a transverse and posterior wall fracture.

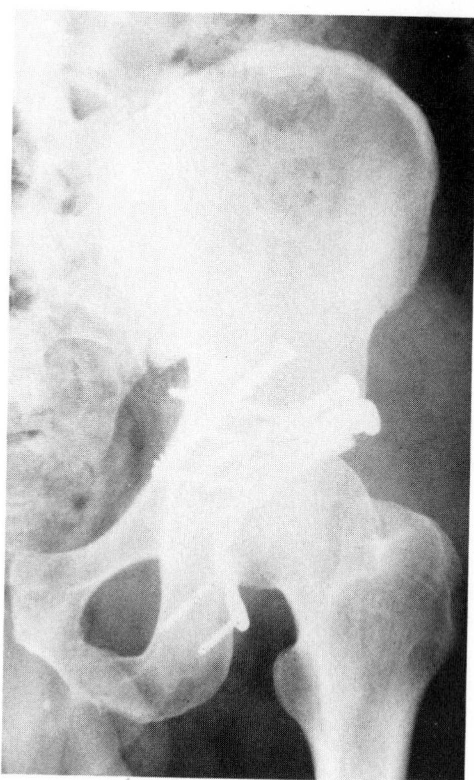

Figure 13-39. Postoperative AP view of the transverse and posterior wall fracture (I-F approach).

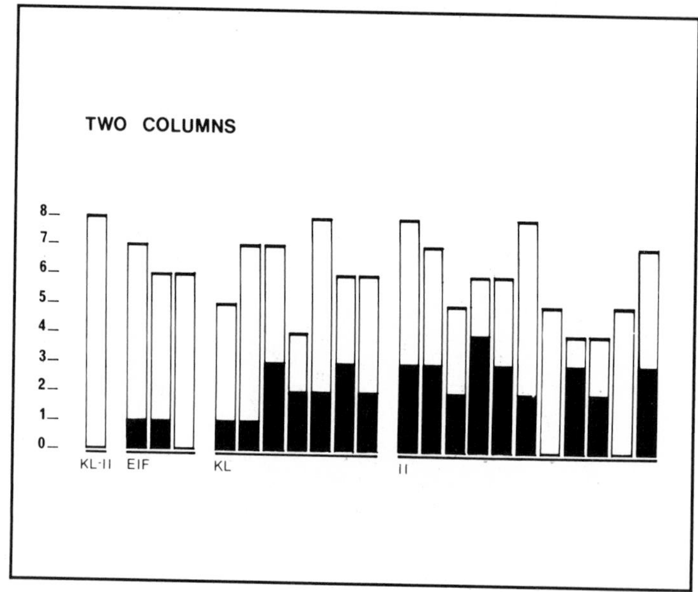


Figure 13-40. Preoperative and postoperative evaluation of the both-column fracture. Black: preoperative point score. White: postoperative point score.

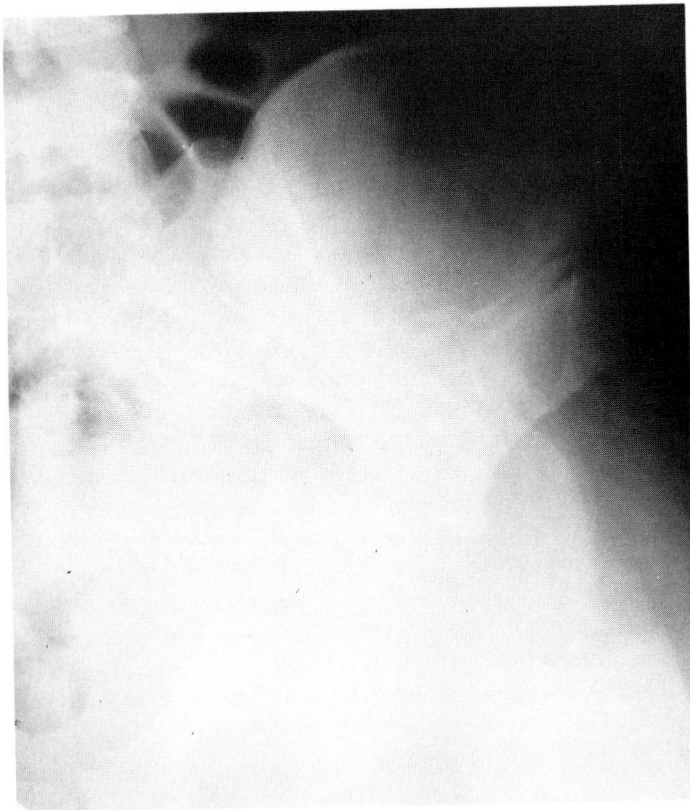

Figure 13-41. Preoperative AP view of a both-column fracture.

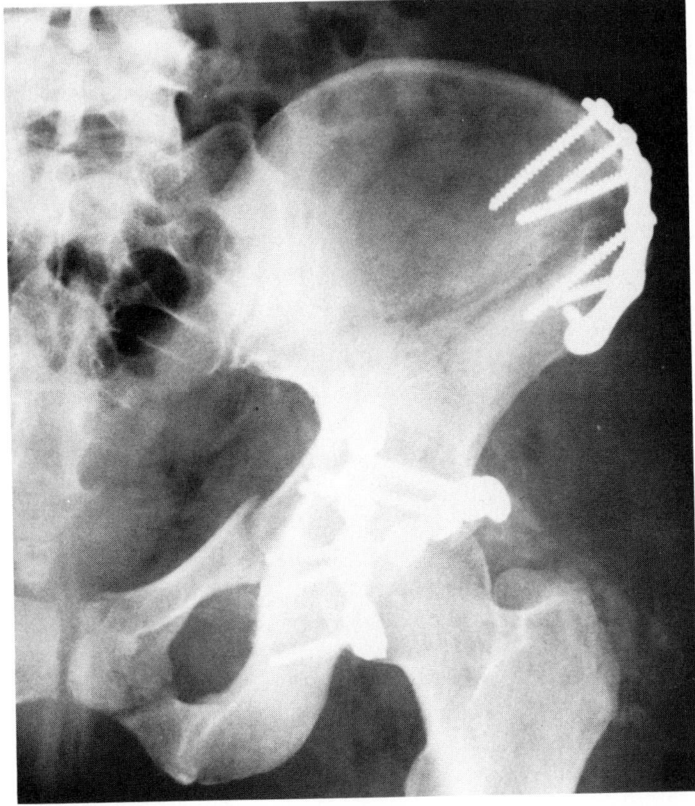

Figure 13-42. Postoperative AP view of a both-column fracture (I-F approach).

results were achieved, with an average score of 7. Where either a posterior or an anterior exposure was utilized, the results were much more varied. Only one of the seven cases managed by a Kocher-Langenbeck approach achieved an optimal score of 8. Of the eleven cases where an ilioinguinal approach was used, only two achieved a score of 8.

An examination of the results provides a substantiation of the indications for the use of various surgical approaches. For an isolated anterior wall or anterior column disruption, an ilioinguinal approach is preferred. For an anterior wall or anterior column with a posterior hemitransverse fracture with minimal posterior displacement, an anterior approach is satisfactory. If a greater degree of posterior displacement is documented, either a combined approach or an extensile exposure is indicated.

For an isolated posterior wall or posterior column disruption or a posterior column associated with a posterior wall fracture, a posterior approach is preferred. For a transverse fracture that hinges around the anterior column with minimal anterior displacement, a posterior approach suffices. Where the degree of anterior displacement is of a greater magnitude, and in questionable cases, an extensile exposure is preferred.

For a third group of fractures an extensile approach is essential to reduce both the anterior and posterior aspects of the disruption. This group includes most transverse fractures, a transverse fracture with an associated posterior wall disruption, a "T" fracture, a displaced anterior wall or column with a posterior hemitransverse, and a both-column fracture. The exceptions include the transverse or transverse with posterior wall disruptions with minimal anterior displacement, where a posterior approach suffices. Another example is a both-column fracture with minimal posterior displacement, where an anterior approach is suitable, or a both-column injury with minimal anterior displacement, where a posterior approach is adequate.

For extensile exposure of the hemipelvis, combined approaches provide satisfactory exposure of the columns for the appropriate reductions. The exposure of the articular surface, however, is less satisfactory. The need for sequential exposures can be a major liability where the first procedure with immobilization of some fragments can inhibit the subsequent reduction through the second approach. Of the extensile approaches, the Ollier-Senegas approach provides satisfactory visualization of the articular surface and the adjacent portions of the anterior and posterior columns. It does not permit an exposure of the inner wall of the pelvis nor the iliac crest. The extended iliofemoral approach provides an excellent visualization of the articular surface along with the entire lateral ilium and the adjacent anterior and posterior columns. It permits an exposure of the iliac crest and the inner wall of the pelvis.

## Functional Clinical Correlation with the Radiological Evaluation

By application of the Harris hip rating as a functional classification, the radiological assessment showed a good correlation with the clinical evaluation. Each of the patients who possessed a radiological score of greater than 6 possessed a painless hip with an excellent range of motion without a flexion contracture. All of them walked without a cane for distances of more than one mile. Where the radiological score was between 5 and 6, a patient possessed some limitation of the function of his hip. While the motion of the hip was painless, it was limited, particularly in the arc of rotation. For a patient with a radiological score of less then 5, imperfect congruity is evident in one or more of the radiographic views. Some degree of central protrusion further compromises the reduction. While some degree of clinical deterioration is almost inevitable, nevertheless it is highly variable. One patient with a score of 4 after a followup undertaken five years after his surgery complained of pain after walking less than one mile and of difficulty with climbing a flight of stairs. By a radiological assessment a narrowing of the joint space and the presence of osteophytes around the superior and inferior aspects of the femoral head provided evidence of degenerative arthritis. Another patient with a perfect radiological reduction of both columns complained of severe pain and stiffness. A detailed examination of the radiographs provided evidence of impaction of the superomedial aspect of the acetabulum with an associated medial subluxation of the femoral head.

In summary, an objective radiographic evaluation for displaced acetabular fractures has been developed that permits a precise evaluation of the improvement realized by the surgical procedure. Once this method is employed routinely, it encourages a more critical radiographic analysis of the preoperative views for the detection of portions of the acetabulum with the greatest displacement. This recognition assists in the selection of the optimal surgical approach. It alerts the surgeon to a phase of the reduction where particular difficulty can be anticipated for the correction of malrotation, interlocking fragments, or segmental impaction. While the method appears to correlate well with postoperative clinical assessments by resort to the Harris functional classification, certain exceptions include the presence of marginal impaction of the acetabulum, traumatic impaction or abrasive damage to the femoral head, and insidious onset of avascular necrosis of the femoral head.

Contribution concludes.

## Results Following Reconstruction of Malunions and Nonunions of the Pelvic Ring and Acetabulum

During the past decade, 75 patients with symptomatic pelvic and acetabular nonunions and malunions and four infected nonunions have been managed by surgical reconstruction. A nonunion is defined as a symptomatic ununited pelvic or acetabular disruption that presents more than six months after the time of the injury. The patterns of injury are presented in Table 13-20. All of the patients were assessed by a clinical examination along with the conventional radiographic views and a standard computed scan. More recently, supplementary three-dimensional scans were obtained.

The patients presented between six months and 13 years after the time of their injury with an average interval of two years. For their initial management, 37 patients had received conservative treatment with bed rest or skeletal traction. Twelve other patients were treated initially by the use of external pelvic fixation. Of the latter group, two patients received limited, although unsuccessful, internal fixation. For the nonunions of the pelvis with a diastasis and associated rotational deviation, the initial approach was made to the anterior defect. Then the patient was repositioned for the posterior approach. In the presence of a malunion, generally an initial posterior approach was undertaken to osteotomize the posterior deformity. Then the patient was repositioned for an anterior approach to osteotomize the site of the allied deformity and undertake anterior stabilization. Subsequently, the patient was repositioned for the posterior stabilization. Where the deformity was primarily of a rotational nature, initially an anterior correction was performed. Where the principal problem was a vertical displacement with superior migration of a hemipelvis, the principal correction was undertaken as part of the posterior stage of the procedure and prior to the anterior stabilization.

### Pelvic Results

For the late pelvic reconstruction where a corrective procedure was undertaken to alleviate persistent pelvic

**Table 13-20**
**Patterns of Pelvic and Acetabular Nonunions and Malunions**

| PELVIC INJURY<br>Posterior | Anterior | Cases |
|---|---|---|
| Unilateral Sacroiliac Disruption | Diastasis | 14 |
| Sacral Fracture | Diastasis | 11 |
| Bilateral Sacroiliac Disruption | Diastasis | 12 |
| Unilateral or Bilateral Sacroiliac Disruption | Ramus Fractures | 8 |
| Sacral Fracture | Ramus Fractures | 4 |
| | **Total** | 49 |

| ACETABULAR DISRUPTION<br>Pattern and Treatment | | Cases |
|---|---|---|
| Acetabular with Open Reduction | | 7 |
| Acetabular with Open Reduction and Total Hip | | 10 |
| Pelvic and Acetabular With Open Reduction | | 2* |
| Pelvic and Acetabular With Open Reduction and Total Hip | | 7 |
| | **Total** | 26 |

| INFECTED NONUNION | | |
|---|---|---|
| Pelvis | | 2 |
| Acetabular | | 1 |
| Greater Trochanter After Open Acetabular Reduction | | 1 |
| | **Total** | 4 |

**One later conversion to total hip.*

**Table 13-21**
**Results of Pelvic Nonunions and Malunions**
**(49 cases)**

| | Nonunion | Malunion |
|---|---|---|
| Average Blood Loss (1) | 1 | 2 |
| Average Operative Duration (hr) | 2.5 | 5 |
| Late Infection | 0 | 0 |
| Postoperative Death | 0 | 0 |
| Phlebitis | 0 | 1 |

pain, instability and deformity, the results are outlined in Table 13-21. In those cases where a malunion was stabilized in situ, the intraoperative blood loss and operative duration were about half that recorded for malunions where displacement was corrected. These observations are not surprising in view of the substantial difficulty encountered when a pelvic deformity is manipulated many months or years after the time of the initial injury. There were no late wound infections or postoperative deaths. One patient developed phlebitis in a lower extremity, which was successfully managed by intravenous and, subsequently, oral anticoagulation. The pelvic pain was effectively diminished or totally corrected in 48 patients. One of the patients who presented with an ununited sacral fracture and mobile rami continued to complain of pain and instability at the rami until a secondary procedure was undertaken one year afterwards with immobilization of the superior pubic ramus. This case helped to substantiate the impression that all unstable pelvic nonunions and probably most of the stable variants merit rigid stabilization of both the anterior and posterior nonunions, even if only one site is painful. Otherwise the likelihood for failure of the operation is substantial.

When the serial postoperative radiographs are carefully scrutinized for a late loss of the reduction, three cases emerge. One of these consisted of a breakage of a lag screw in a lateral ilium without any functional or anatomical impairment. In another case the screws in the superior pubic ramus adjacent to a previously displaced symphysis disengaged without apparent functional significance. In a third case, where a man with bilateral sacroiliac nonunions and a diastasis was managed with a Double Cobra plate and an anterior plate across the symphysis, against medical advice the patient walked for up to eight miles daily within two weeks after the surgery. In the postoperative radiograph taken six weeks after the surgery, the minor displacement of the rami is evident. The patient was not aware of this problem and was highly satisfied with the alleviation of his preoperative posterior pelvic pain. Following a stabilization of a nonunion or malunion of a sacroiliac joint or adjacent sacrum, two of the patients complained of hypesthesia in the ipsilateral buttock for at least one year after the time of their surgery.

### Assessment of Pelvic Correction

In the presence of a pelvic malunion or a malunion-nonunion, the correction of a persistent gap at the symphysis or at the posterior injury was exceedingly good, even when the surgery was undertaken many years after the time of the initial injury. The correction of persistent superior displacement of a hemipelvis with complaints of sitting imbalance or apparent limb length discrepancy were moderately successful. Where the posterior injury occurred through a site of a previous sacral fracture, the results of such an attempted correction were poor. Later in the series, this problem was managed by a pelvic osteotomy of the lateral ilium from the greater sciatic notch to the anterior inferior spine. As documented in Chapter 12, highly satisfactory

**Table 13-22**
**Results of Acetabular Nonunions and Malunions (26 Cases)**

| | Acetabular | Acetabular + THR | Pelvic Acetabular | Pelvic Acetabular + THR |
|---|---|---|---|---|
| Avg. Blood Loss (liter) | 3 | 3 | 3 | 6 |
| Duration (hr) | 4 | 5 | 6 | 6 |
| Late Infection | 0 | 0 | 1 | 0 |
| Postoperative Death | 0 | 0 | 0 | 1 |
| Phlebitis | 0 | 1 | 0 | 1 |
| Pulmonary Embolus | 0 | 1 | 0 | 0 |

corrections were achieved. In general, the correction of rotational deformity was poor. This problem was consistent with a mild persistent cosmetic deformity despite an otherwise excellent functional outcome and alleviation of pelvic pain.

## Results of Late Acetabular Reconstruction

The results of 26 cases of acetabular nonunions and malunions with or without associated pelvic ring disruption are presented in Table 13-22. A moderate intraoperative blood loss was recorded in all of the cases, with substantial blood loss in the pelvic and acetabular reconstructions. The operative durations correlated with the blood loss and the general magnitude of the operative exposure and reconstruction. There was one late infection in a pelvic and acetabular reconstruction for which one debridement and the application of intravenous antibiotics provided a successful outcome. There was one postoperative death in a diabetic with known ischemic heart disease and a highly mobile and painful pelvic and acetabular nonunion-malunion, for which a reconstruction including a total hip joint replacement was undertaken. Three days after the surgery the patient sustained another myocardial infarction with a cardiac arrest for which a resuscitation was unsuccessful. One of the patients who underwent pelvic and acetabular reconstruction developed avascular necrosis during the first postoperative year, for which a successful conversion to a total hip joint replacement was undertaken. There were two cases of phlebitis and one of a pulmonary embolus for which routine anticoagulation provided an uneventful outcome. One other patient who underwent a pelvic and acetabular reconstruction with a total hip replacement for a highly displaced and comminuted fracture developed a recurrent dislocation of the total hip within two months after the reconstructive surgery.

In this instance the patient had sustained his initial injury five years earlier and progressed to a Bateman prosthesis two years prior to the time of the most recent reconstruction. His pelvis showed a marked distortion so that proper alignment of the arthroplastic components was observed to be difficult at the time of the formidable reconstructive procedure. After a revision of the femoral component with a distal advancement of the greater trochanter, this problem was corrected.

For one other patient with a major pelvic and acetabular nonunion-malunion, the corrective surgery was deliberately undertaken in two stages with an interval of several months between the prolonged operations. In the first instance, the vertical migration of the left hemipelvis was stabilized along with the highly displaced unstable nonunion-malunion of a right-sided "T" fracture. In the second operation when a total hip joint was undertaken, sitting imbalance secondary to distal displacement of the right ischial tuberosity was corrected when the ischium was repositioned proximally to form a new posterior wall for the acetabulum. The procedure was notable for the correction of both sitting imbalance and a painful hip joint.

Overall the acetabular reconstructive procedures were notable for excellent reapproximation of the pelvis and stabilization of the bone. Persistent protrusion of the femoral head also was well corrected. A moderate degree of correction of associated sitting imbalance with secondary pelvic ring deformity was achieved. In the presence of severe osteoporosis encountered in one case of a mobile acetabular nonunion where a total hip joint replacement was indicated, an acetabular component could not be anchored by resort to screw fixation of a metal backing or by the use of bone cement. In this instance a large quantity of bone graft was applied to the persistent acetabular defects and a bipolar type of total hip replacement was cemented into the proximal femur. While this result has functioned satisfactorily for 18 months, an ultimate conversion to an acetabular component may become necessary if the bipolar prosthesis migrates into the bone graft within the weightbearing portion of the acetabulum.

Overall the results of the pelvic and acetabular reconstructions for late presentation of a nonunion-malunion are highly satisfactory. Clearly, a prophylactic solution by an initial posttraumatic reduction and stabilization is preferred to the need for such a major procedure with its potential for major complications. When a late reconstruction is necessary, it can provide a highly effective alleviation of pain secondary to a mobile nonunion and relief of discomfort associated with instability of the pelvis. While certain pelvic and acetabular deformities can be satisfactorily corrected, superior techniques are needed for the correction of certain late deformities, especially vertical and rotational displacement and the correction of sitting imbalance or apparent limb length discrepancy.

## Results of Infected Nonunions

Two infected nonunions of the pelvic ring presented at six and 12 months after the time of the open injuries. The one occurred in a mining incident where a man of 55 years was crushed to provoke an open pelvic ring disruption with marked instability and exposed urinary bladder. He was transferred to Pittsburgh six months after the time of the injury with a fulminant Pseudomonas infection of the open wound and of both lungs. Two days after the initial debridement and application of external pelvic fixation, he succumbed to overwhelming sepsis.

The other patient, a young woman of 20 years involved in a jeep accident, presented one year after the time of her injury with massive infected open wounds and secondary hypokalemia. Shortly after the time of the transfer she sustained a cardiac arrest with a successful resuscitation. As part of her initial management a diversion colostomy was performed to divert the feculent stream from the inguinal wound. An osteotomy of the displaced right hemipelvis was undertaken to obliterate a large diastasis and to facilitate the stable reduction. Following a prolonged course of external pelvic fixation, serial debridements, supplementary cast immobilization, and physical therapy, she achieved a stable painless union of the pelvis.

A third case, an infected nonunion of an acetabulum following an open reduction and internal fixation of a highly comminuted both-column fracture with an ipsilateral dislocation of the sacroiliac joint, progressed to a severe postoperative wound infection. Following multiple debridements of the necrotic bone, insufficient posterior column remained to achieve a functional hip joint. Ultimately, the hip was fused with the use of a Cobra plate. About two months afterwards the drainage ceased spontaneously and a painful stable hip was documented.

One other case presented one year after an acetabular reconstruction where a triradiate approach with an osteotomy of the greater trochanter for the exposure of a both-column fracture had been undertaken. Eight weeks after the initial surgery, when the patient complained of lateral hip pain, the screws employed for the fixation of the greater trochanter were removed. A postoperative wound infection progressed to an infected nonunion of the greater trochanter. Following a debridement of the greater trochanter, four separate vascularized fragments of bone were documented. Fixation was achieved by a combination of multiple lag screws with a tension band wire. The greater trochanter healed uneventfully during the subsequent two months.

While our experience with the management of infected nonunions of the pelvis is limited, the general principles of treatment would appear to be comparable to similar problems that arise in other parts of the appendicular skeleton. Following adequate debridement, stabilization generally by resort to external fixation is preferred. In certain localized sites, especially of an unstable sacroiliac joint or acetabulum, internal fixation may be necessary. If a large wound in the groin provides a source for feculent contamination, diversion colostomy is crucial. Undoubtedly, in some cases where a successful irradication of an infection is followed by a stable but deformed pelvis, late consideration for a corrective osteotomy is indicated.

## References

1. Rubash HE, Mears DC: External fixation of the pelvis. AAOS Instructional Course Lectures. St. Louis, Mosby, 1983, 32:329.
2. Mears DC, Rubash HE: External and internal fixation of the pelvic ring. AAOS Instructional Course Lectures. St. Louis, Mosby, 1984, 33:144.
3. Steed D, Rubash HE, Mears DC: Fractures of the pelvis. Current Problems in Surgery, in press, 1986.
4. Riemer B: personal communication, 1985.
5. Edwards C, et al: Primary external fixation for pelvic disruptions: Early and late results of treatment. AAOS 52nd Meeting, Las Vegas, February, 1985.
6. Tile M: personal communication, 1985.
7. Letournel E, Judet R: Fractures of the Acetabulum. New York, Springer-Verlag, 1981, p 262.
8. Brooker AF, Banerman JW, Robinson RA, Riley LH: Ectopic ossification following total hip replacement. J Bone Joint Surg 55A:1629, 1973.
9. Tile M: Fractures of the Pelvis and Acetabulum. Baltimore, Williams and Wilkins, 1983, p 200.
10. Matta J: Fractures of the acetabulum: Results of a prospective series. AAOS 50th Meeting, Anaheim, 1983.
11. Mears DC, Rubash HE, Sawaguchi T: Fractures of the acetabulum, in: The Hip: Proceedings of the Hip Society. St. Louis, Mosby, Volume 13, in press, 1985.
12. Harris WH: Traumatic arthritis of the hip after dislocation and acetabular fractures: Treatment by mold arthroplasty. J Bone Joint Surg 51A:737, 1969.
13. Mears DC, Rubash HE: Extensile exposure of the pelvis. Contemp Orthop 6:21, 1983.
14. Pennal GF, Davidson J, Garside H, Plewes J: Results of treatment of acetabular fractures. Clin Orthop 151:115, 1980.
15. Senegas J, Yates M: Complex acetabular fractures: A transtrochanteric lateral approach. Clin Orthop 151:107, 1980.
16. Rowe CR, Lowell JD: Prognosis of fractures of the acetabulum. J Bone Joint Surg 43A:30, 1961.

# CHAPTER 14

# Pelvic Fractures and Traumatically Dislocated Hips in Children

Chapter written by Jill Smith, MD, and Dana C. Mears, MD, PhD.

## Introduction

In a child, a pelvic ring disruption possesses an even greater incidence of life-threatening complications than in an adult population where a comparable injury is sustained.[1,2] This discrepancy is due to the dense bone encountered in a child versus the osteoporotic counterpart of many adults.[3] With its disproportionately smaller size in a child, the pelvic ring resists disruption apart from a fracture through a cartilaginous growth plate or apophysis. The greater plasticity of the bone and the increased flexibility and elasticity of the sacroiliac joints and symphysis pubis contribute to the structural integrity of the juvenile pelvis. With the small size of the infantile pelvic ring, the intraabdominal organs are less well protected than their adult counterparts. A provocative blow of sufficient magnitude to initiate a pediatric pelvic disruption is likely to be associated with a fatality secondary to a ruptured intraabdominal viscus or hemorrhage, as well as an intracranial hemorrhage. The pediatric brain is more susceptible to hemorrhagic complications than that of an adult. When a child presents with a pelvic fracture, the injury should be managed as a potentially life-threatening situation with a high likelihood for major associated injuries.

Previously, an accurate characterization of a pediatric disruption of the pelvic ring or acetabulum has been hampered greatly by the limited resolution of conventional radiographs for the detection of injuries through nonmineralized portions of the skeleton. With the introduction of computed scans and more recently of magnetic resonance imaging, markedly superior resolution of a growth plate disruption is possible. While most pelvic fractures respond favorably to conservative treatment, a few problems merit serious consideration for open intervention, especially a displaced acetabular fracture, a fracture/dislocation of the hip, and an associated femoral neck fracture.[4-6]

## Anatomy of the Pelvis

A detailed description of the anatomy of the pelvic ring is presented in Chapter 2; however, some unique anatomical features of the pediatric pelvic ring merit particular attention.[7] The pelvis of a child consists of three primary ossification centers—the pubis, ischium, and ilium—which merge at the triradiate cartilage (Figure 14-1). At approximately 16 to 18 years of age, the three ossification centers undergo a fusion. Numerous secondary centers of ossification include the iliac crest, the anterior inferior iliac spine, iliac apophysis, pubic tubercle, ischial spine and lateral iliac crest, and the sacral ala. Upon scrutiny of a pediatric radiograph, a comparison of secondary centers of ossification to those on the opposite side of the pelvis permits a recognition of an avulsion type of injury.

The pelvic ring in the child is more deformable because of the nature of the bone and the ability of the cartilaginous tissue to absorb energy by undergoing plastic deformation.[3] At the moment of impact the increased elasticity of the adjacent soft tissue surrounding the sacroiliac joints and the symphysis pubis inhibits the osseous displacement that would be anticipated for a comparable adult injury. While the concept of two sites of injury in virtually all adult pelvic ring disruptions is well accepted, it does not appear to apply to all of the pediatric cases.

Ponseti[7] has provided a detailed description of the growth and development of the acetabulum in a normal child. The acetabulum comprises three growth plates of the ilium, ischium, and pubis that merge to become the triradiate cartilage (Figure 14-2). The interstitial

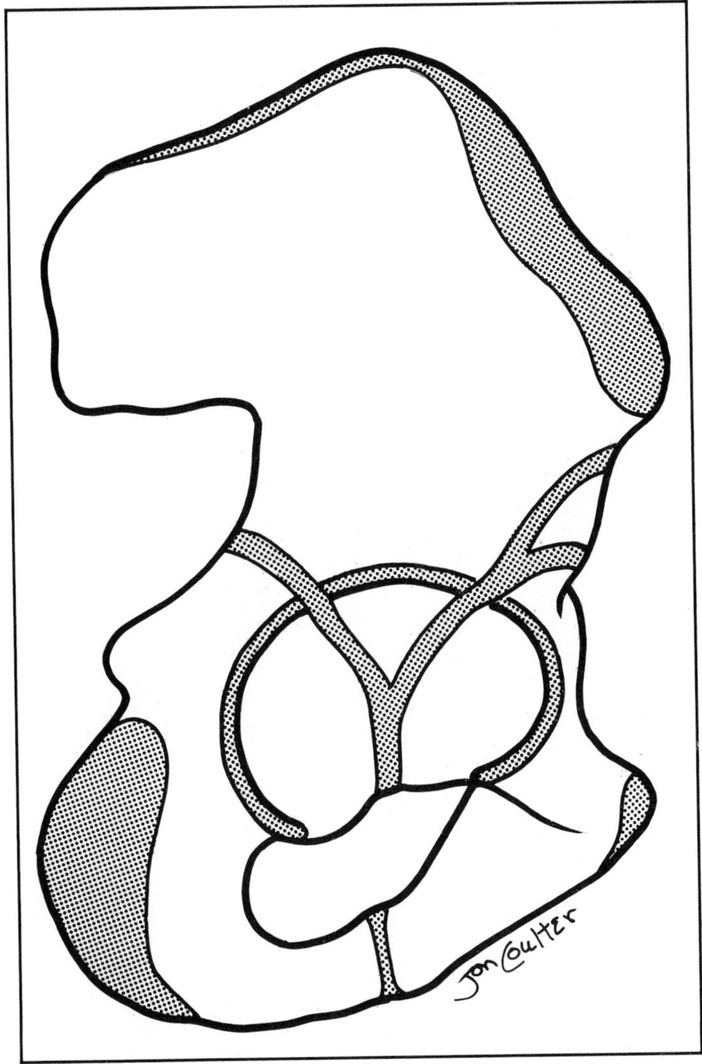


Figure 14-1. Diagram illustrates the primary and secondary centers of ossification in the pelvis of a child.

and appositional growth of the triradiate cartilage complex is responsible for the expansion of the socket, as well as the growth and enlargement of the pubis, ischium, and ilium. The secondary centers of ossification that appear in the hyaline cartilage surrounding the acetabular cavity are termed the os acetabuli and the acetabular epiphysis (Figure 14-3). The os acetabuli, which is the epiphysis of the pubis, forms the anterior wall of the acetabulum. The acetabular epiphysis, which refers to the epiphysis of the ilium, forms much of the superior dome of the acetabulum. The smaller secondary center of the ischium is rarely identified. At about eight years of age, the os acetabuli starts to develop as a portion of the anterior wall.[8] It fuses with the pubis at about 18 years of age. During the same decade the acetabular epiphysis also develops. While the secondary center of the ischium develops in the ischial acetabular cartilage

Space occupied by iliac bone
Acetabulum
Triradiate cartilage
Space occupied by pubic bone
Space occupied by ischial bone

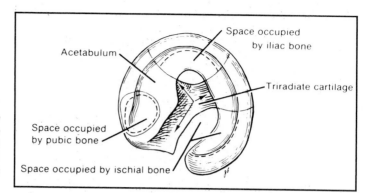

Figure 14-2. Diagram of the triradiate acetabular cartilage complex viewed from the lateral side, showing the sites occupied by the iliac, ischial, and pubic bones (from Ponseti[7]).

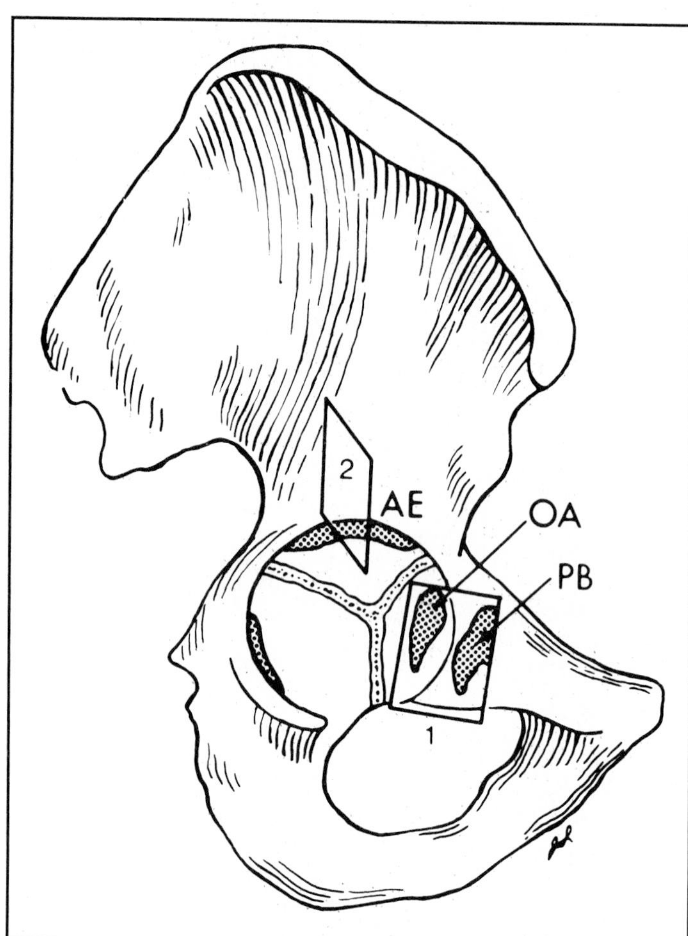


Figure 14-3. Diagram of the right innominate bone of an adolescent. The os acetabuli (OA) is shown within the acetabular cartilage adjoining the pubic bone (PB), the acetabular epiphysis (AE) within the acetabular cartilage adjoining the iliac bone, and another small epiphysis (not labeled) within the acetabular cartilage adjoining the ischium (left) (from Ponseti[7]).

at about the ninth year and unites with the ischium at 17 years, it contributes little to the acetabular development. These secondary centers are not to be confused with an avulsion fracture or an interarticular fragment within the hip joint. A comparison with the opposite uninvolved side of the pelvis is crucial for the identification of an acetabular fracture in a child.

While the clinical examination of a pediatric pelvic fracture victim is similar to that of an adult counterpart, a higher percentage of children sustain an associated head injury.[9] With the possibility of loss of consciousness and with the typical history provided by a child, a vague, less accurate description of the traumatic episode can be anticipated. Initially, a rapid general examination is undertaken to identify a dire emergency with the potential for profuse hemorrhage from the adjacent soft tissues surrounding the pelvis, as well as the abdomen. Occult hemorrhage with apparent hemodynamic compensation is even more likely to arise in a child than in his adult counterpart. A respiratory assessment to document a patent airway, a stable chest, and unlabored ventilation is performed. If the child has a history of unconsciousness, or is unconscious or lethargic, detailed neurological examination follows a preliminary survey. Prior to the evaluation of the pelvic fracture, emergency resuscitative measures such as tracheal intubation and the insertion of venous and arterial lines may be necessary. Catheterization of the bladder to monitor the urinary output, and a gross and microscopic assessment of the urine also assist in the detection of a genitourinary injury. Once the overall stability of the child is confirmed, a detailed systematic review of the pediatric trauma patient is performed with special attention to an abrasion, laceration, ecchymosis, or a hematoma in the perineal and pelvic areas. In addition, palpation of the appropriate landmarks, including the anterior superior iliac spines, the posterior iliac spines, the ischial tuberosities and the symphysis pubis, is undertaken to detect a tender or mobile segment of the pelvis. A manual compression of the pelvic ring from both front to back and side to side is undertaken by the application of a direct pressure to the anterior superior iliac spines, and the sacroiliac joints in the former and the iliac crests in the latter. The test can elicit crepitus, gross motion, and instability: features consistent with an unstable pelvic fracture. A thorough examination of the lower extremities is performed, including the hip joints for motion and stability, as well as the neurovascular status.

The radiological evaluation of a pediatric pelvic ring fracture is comparable to that previously described for an adult. If the child is potentially unstable referable to his hemodynamic, respiratory, or neurological status, the initial radiological assessment is limited to an anteroposterior view of the pelvis. Once the general condition of the child is stable, a complete radiographic series is obtained, including anteroposterior, inlet, outlet, iliac oblique, and obturator oblique views. The anteroposterior view includes the entire hip joint to permit scrutiny for a proximal femoral fracture. Computed tomography of the pelvis provides confirmation of an osseous break and superior resolution for the detection of an injury to a nonossified portion of the pelvic ring. More importantly, it provides crucial information in evaluating the symphysis pubis, triradiate cartilage, and sacroiliac joints, as well as the sacrum and posterior ilium. A subtle incongruity of the pelvis is identified by comparison of the site of the injury with the contralateral part of the pelvis. Recently three-dimensional computerized reformation scanning has greatly improved the resolution of the unmineralized skeleton, especially in small children. The method provides an accurate three-dimensional impression of a complex deformity with a characterization of the magnitude and vector of the displacement. This information is needed to help define the optimal therapeutic protocol with respect to the method of reduction and stabilization.

Currently, magnetic resonance imaging[10] provides optimal resolution of nonmineralized tissues, including the skeletally immature pelvis (Figure 14-4). In this example, a free cartilaginous fragment arising from the posterior wall and column is defined, along with the hemarthrosis of the hip joint, in a child of 12 years who presented to our clinic two months after he was tackled by two massive lads, both of whom were 15 years of age. During the following two-month period, his hip dislocated spontaneously on an intermittent basis, secondary to a posterior wall and posterior column fracture with extensive marginal impaction.

Another diagnostic tool, isotopic bone scanning with the use of technetium polyphosphate, is useful for the detection of a minimally displaced pelvic ring disruption within a few weeks after the time of the acute injury.[11] Usually, this method is not particularly helpful in a pediatric patient.

In recent years the abused child has been recognized to be more prevalent than previously thought.[12] Such abuse is a potential source of a pelvic fracture. About two thirds of the abused children present prior to three years of age. Virtually every socioeconomic category is susceptible to this problem. Suspicious features of the history and physical examination include an inconsistent history that does not correspond to the type and magnitude of the trauma sustained by the child. The presence of multiple large ecchymotic areas in diverse parts of the body in different stages of resolution is another common feature. The presence of multiple fractures with different stages of callus formation also should arouse suspicion.

Figure 14-4. This boy of 14 years presented two months after he was tackled in football to "sprain" his hip. He continued to limp so that serial assessments were undertaken. Upon his presentation, a posterior column and associated posterior wall fracture was found. At the time of surgery, severe marginal impaction was confirmed with the ununited posterior wall fragment. A large portion of articular cartilage shed from the posterior column constituted a free fragment within the hip joint. The femoral head possessed incongruity of the superior portion secondary to a substantial impaction injury. Despite the reconstruction and stabilization of the posterior wall, the prognosis is guarded. A: AP view one month after injury, when the injury was not detected. A displaced posterior column fracture (Walther fracture) is evident. B: AP view two months after injury, posterior subluxation. C: 3D scan, obturator oblique view. D: 3D scan, outlet view. E: 3D scan, iliac oblique view. F: 3D scan, superior view. G: 3D scan, inferior view. H: Computed scan of dome with posterior wall fracture. I: Computed scan of quadrilateral surface with posterior column fracture. J: MRI of femoral head and adjacent acetabulum. K: MRI of dome. L: MRI of quadrilateral surface with loose cartilaginous fragment and posterior column fracture. M: Postoperative AP view.

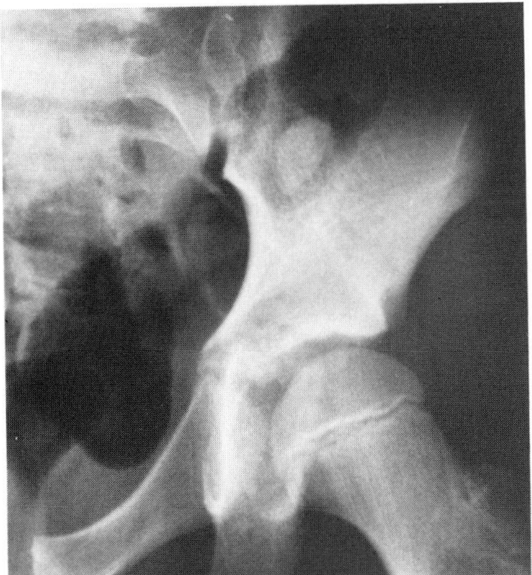

Figure 14-4A.

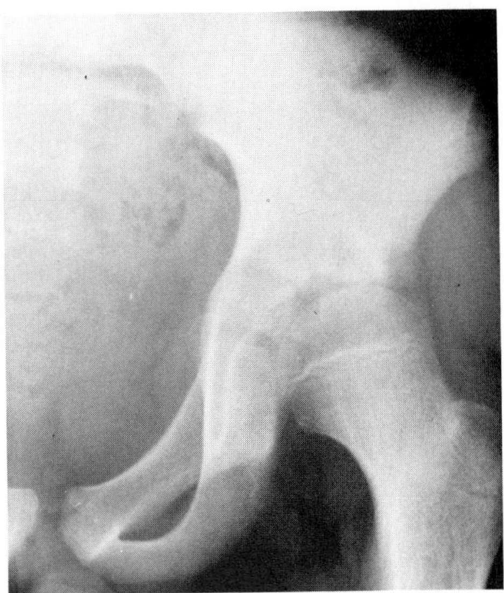

Figure 14-4B.

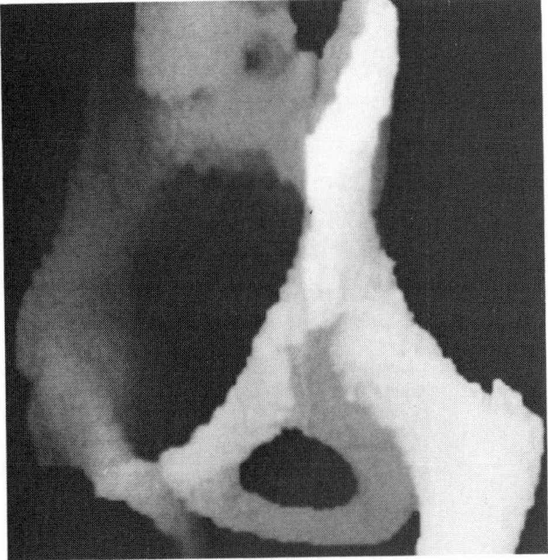

Figure 14-4C.

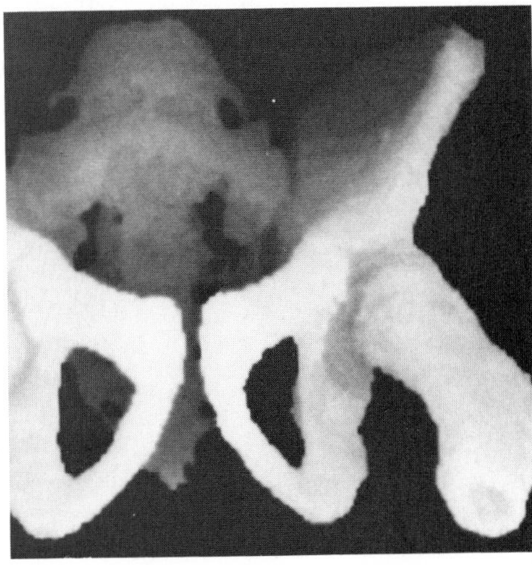

Figure 14-4D.

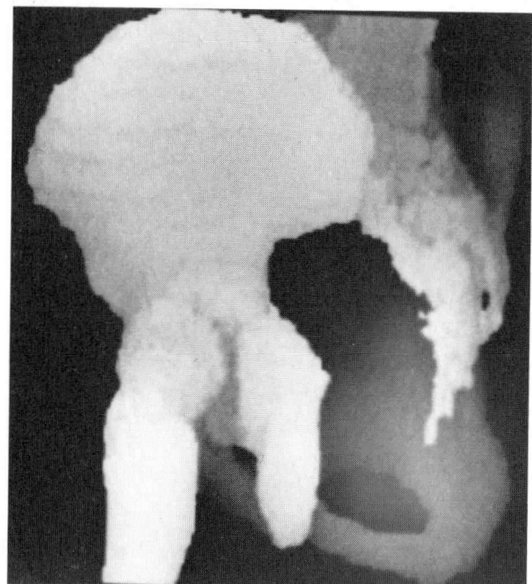
Figure 14-4E.

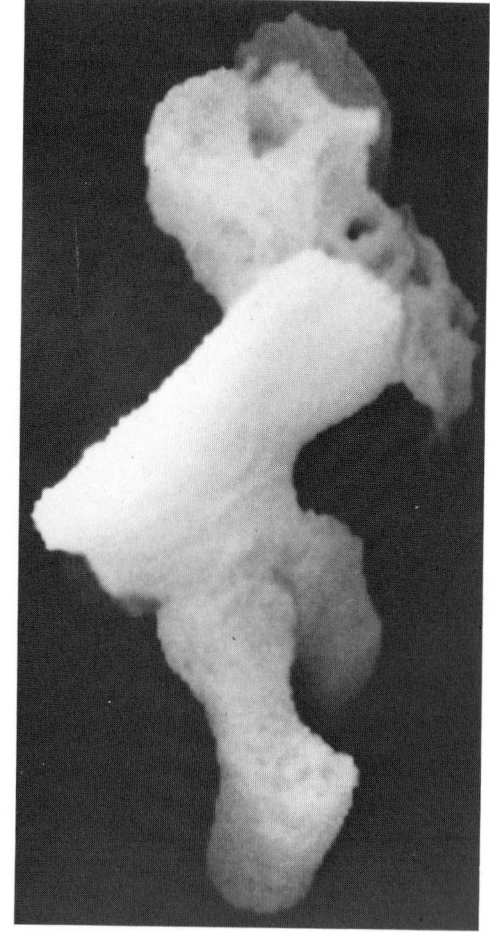
Figure 14-4F.

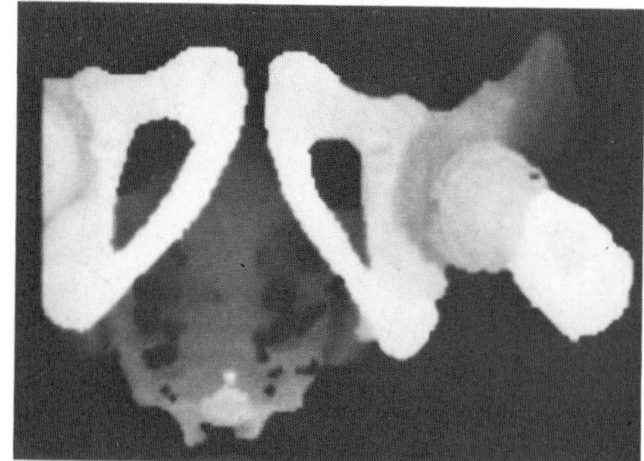
Figure 14-4G.

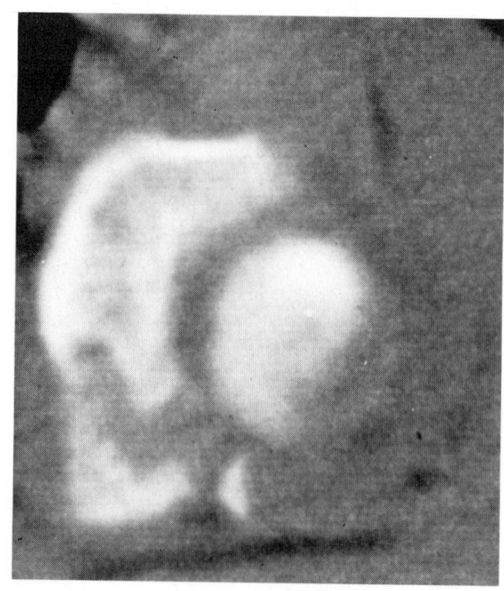
Figure 14-4H.

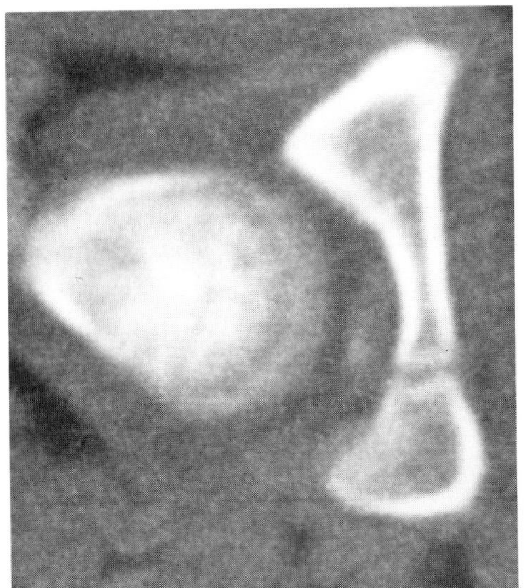

Figure 14-4I.

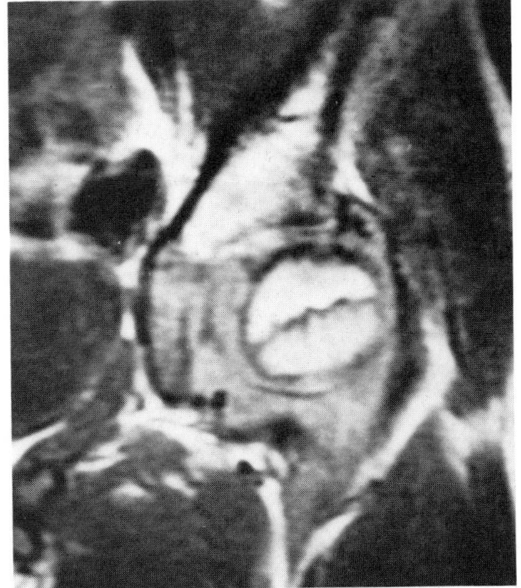

Figure 14-4J.

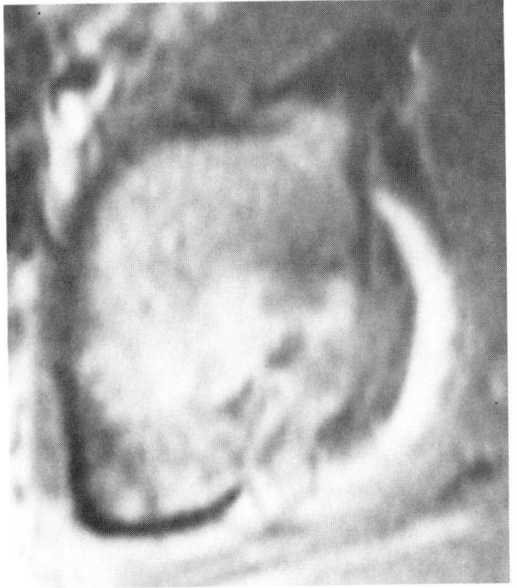

Figure 14-4K.

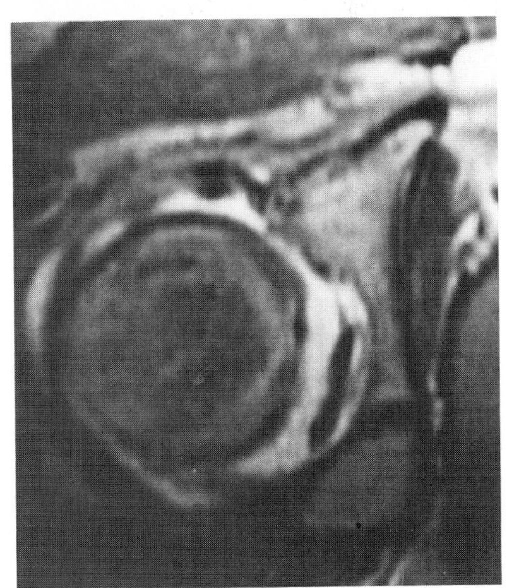

Figure 14-4L.

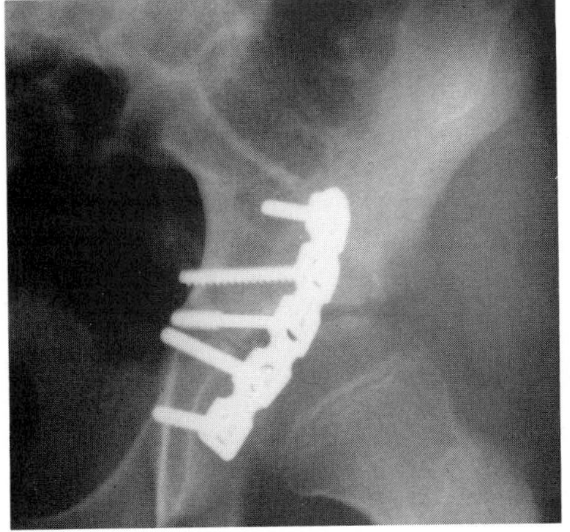

Figure 14-4M.

### Related Injuries

While the pelvic fracture victim of any age is likely to sustain concomitant injuries to virtually all of his organ systems, the pediatric patient merits a particular scrutiny for three commonly associated injuries.[1,9,13-16] A closed head injury is perhaps the most frequent source of fatality. To supplement a thorough neurological evaluation, other studies such as computed brain scan may be necessary. A ruptured bladder is another common complication of a pediatric pelvic fracture. Diagnostic studies of the lower and upper urinary tracts including a urethrogram in a male, a cystogram, and an intravenous pyelogram are indicated if a clinical feature such as macroscopic or microscopic hematuria or bloody drainage from the urethral meatus is present. The third commonly associated injury, a fracture of the proximal femur, is documented by appropriate radiographs.

## Classification of Pediatric Pelvic and Acetabular Disruptions

Several classification schemes have been devised for pediatric pelvic injuries, each of which possesses a substantial shortcoming[2]. Both Quinby[16] and Rang[17] have classified children's fractures into three types: **1)** an uncomplicated fracture; **2)** a fracture complicated by a visceral injury that necessitates a surgical exploration; and **3)** a fracture associated with catastrophic hemorrhage. This method focuses attention upon the acute prognostic and therapeutic aspects. It is not particularly helpful for defining the precise nature of the pelvic injury, the therapeutic protocol, or the prognosis of the osseous disruption.

Another classification devised by Key and Conwell[18] distinguishes four broad groups of injuries with allied subcategories:

I. Fractures without a break in the continuity of the pelvic ring.

- A. Avulsion fractures.
  - 1. Anterior superior spine.
  - 2. Anterior inferior spine.
  - 3. Ischial tuberosity.
- B. Fractures of the pubis or ischium.
- C. Fractures of the lateral ilium.
- D. Fractures of the sacrum or coccyx.

II. Single break in the pelvic ring.

- A. Fracture of ipsilateral rami.
- B. A diastasis of the symphysis or a fracture of the ramus adjacent to the symphysis.

C. A subluxation or fracture dislocation of the sacroiliac joint.

III. Double break in the pelvic ring.

A. A fracture of all four rami provoked by a lateral compression injury or occasionally a straddle injury.

B. A true unstable pelvic fracture.

C. A complex pelvic disruption.

IV. A fracture of the acetabulum.

A. A fracture dislocation with a small associated fracture fragment, usually in the form of a posterior injury with a posterior wall fracture or an avulsion fracture of the ligamentum teres.

B. A linear fracture associated with an undisplaced pelvic fracture, generally as a form of lateral compression injury.

C. A linear fracture associated with an unstable hip joint, usually as a posterior column or posterior column and associated posterior wall disruption.

D. A so-called central fracture-dislocation of the acetabulum.

While this scheme is widely employed and readily distinguishes the most commonly encountered and relatively minor pediatric pelvic injuries, such as avulsion fractures and minimally displaced fractures (Table 14-1), in its classic form it does not characterize sufficiently the displaced, unstable, and more comminuted fracture patterns.[19-21] In the modified version provided here, to account for more recent knowledge, the true pelvic ring disruptions (III) and the acetabular fractures (IV) are characterized in more detail than in the initial scheme provided by Key and Conwell. For widespread use in a trauma center, this scheme places an excessive emphasis upon the minor injuries and provides an inadequate characterization of the major fractures and dislocations. This shortcoming is of particular concern for the teenage population, where a detailed assessment of the injury, as described previously for adults, is essential. For the remainder of the discussion, a modified version of the Key and Conwell scheme will be employed to achieve these objectives.

## Patterns of Injury

### Fractures Without a Break in the Pelvic Ring

#### *Avulsion Fractures*

An avulsion fracture of the pelvis is a common sporting injury in a child and a young adult. While technically

**Table 14-1**
**Distribution of Pelvic Fractures in Children, Campbell Clinic Series (134 Pediatric Patients)***

| I-Individual bones 66.5% | | | | II-Single break 11.9% | | | III-Double break 11.9% | | | IV-Acetabulum 9.7% | | | |
|---|---|---|---|---|---|---|---|---|---|---|---|---|---|
| A | B | C | D | A | B | C | A | B | C | A | B | C | D |
| 13.4% | 33.6% | 18% | 1.5% | 8.2% | 3% | 0.7% | 3% | 8.2% | 0.7% | 0.7% | 6% | 0 | 3% |

**Comparison With Other Series**

| | Reed† (85 pts.) | Hall, Klassen, Ilstrup† (204 pts.) | Campbell Clinic† (134 pts.) | Dunn§ (115 pts.) | Peltier§ (186 pts.) |
|---|---|---|---|---|---|
| **I-Individual bones** | 60.5% | 24.5% | 66.5% | | 10% |
| **II-Single break** | 2.5% | 18.6% | 11.9% | 70% (stable) | 39% |
| **III-Double break** | 32% | 31.9% | 11.9% | 30% (unstable) | 27% |
| **IV-Acetabulum** | 5% | 7.8% (17.2% acetabulum and pelvis) | 9.7% | Not included | 24% |

**Classification of Key and Conwell*
*†Children's series*
*§Adult series*

this injury is not a fracture of the pelvic ring, it comprises up to 15% of pelvic injuries. Such an injury arises secondary to an abrupt muscular exertion imposed upon a secondary center of ossification before the center undergoes a fusion with the pelvis. This mechanism of injury limits presentation to primarily between the ages of 14 and 25. A comparison radiograph of the contralateral apophysis is crucial to distinguish an apparent avulsion fracture from a normal adolescent anatomical variant. Whereas an excessive exertion of the sartorious provokes an avulsion of the anterior superior spine, a comparable exertion of the direct head of the rectus femorus initiates an avulsion of the anterior inferior spine. A similar avulsion injury to the ischial tuberosity is provoked by an over-exertion of the hamstring muscles at their origin. Most of the avulsion injuries are appropriately treated by a course of bed rest and simple analgesics for a few days, followed by progressive ambulation with crutches to unsupported weight bearing as tolerated. Most of the patients return

Figure 14-5. A lateral compression injury with the classic pelvic deformity is shown in a girl of 13 years. A: AP view, left ramus fracture and subluxation of right sacroiliac joint. B: Cystogram of ruptured bladder. C: Inlet view, subluxation of right sacroiliac joint and ramus fractures. D: Computed scan, stable sacral fracture dislocation. E: Computed scan, superior ramus fracture.

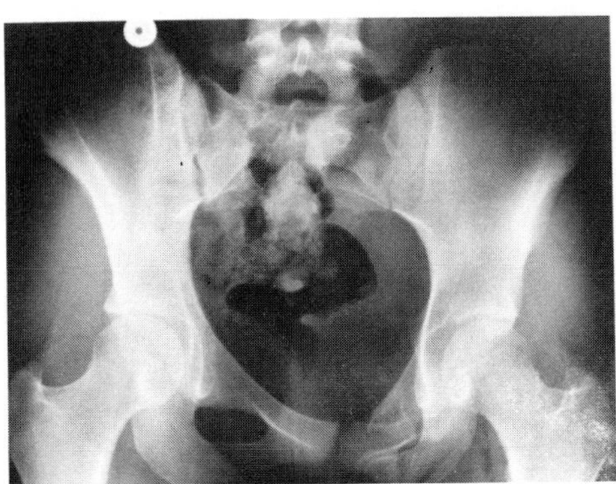

Figure 14-5A.

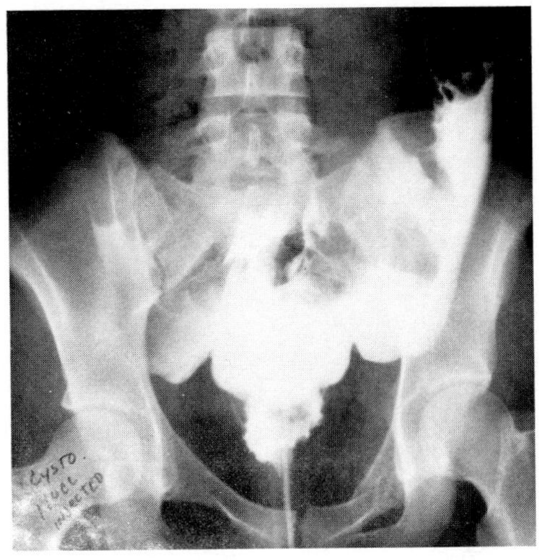

Figure 14-5B.

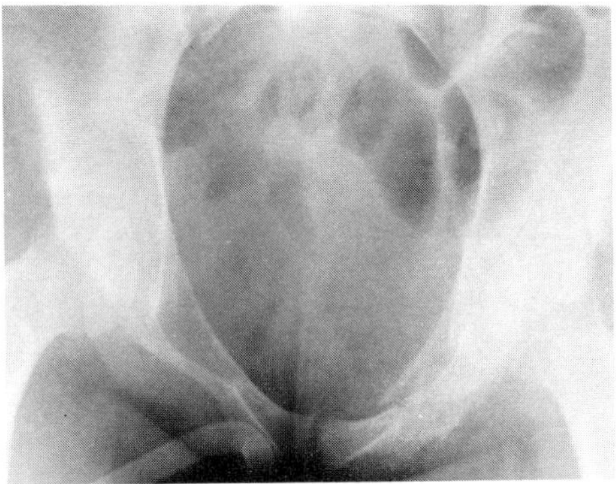

Figure 14-5C.

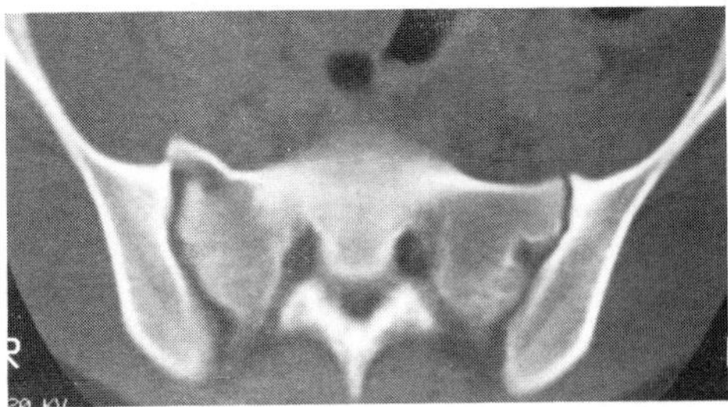

Figure 14-5D.

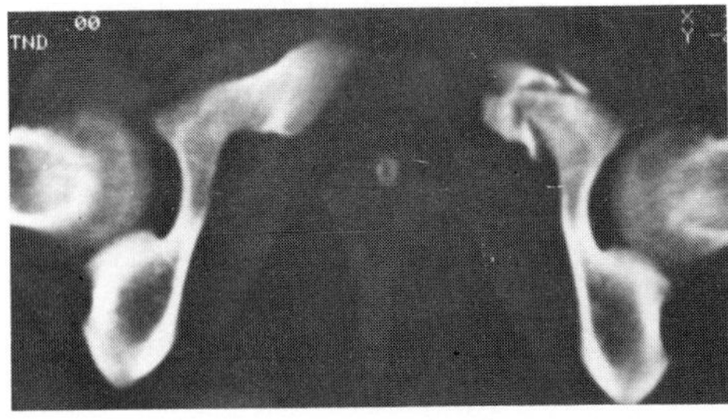

Figure 14-5E.

Figure 14-6. A complex pelvic injury documented in a boy of 12 years. Following a vehicular accident complicated by a ruptured bladder, the pelvic assessment was notable for a left displaced anterior column fracture, a diastasis, a stable subluxation of the right sacroiliac joint, and a left femoral neck fracture. He was managed by an open reduction of the femoral neck with pin fixation and a hip spica cast for immobilization of the pelvis. While he made an uneventful recovery of the pelvic ring disruption, he developed avascular necrosis of the left hip and progressed to an arthrodesis. A: Initial AP view. B: Initial inlet view. C: Postoperative AP view. D: Technetium polyphosphate scan at three months, with enhanced uptake in left femoral head. E: AP view one year after the injury.

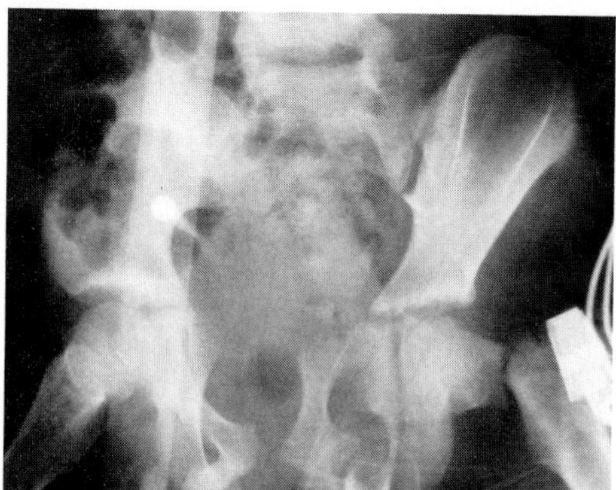

Figure 14-6A.

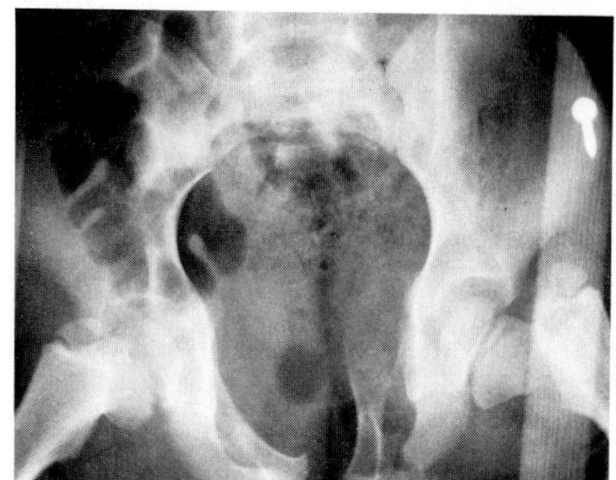

Figure 14-6B.

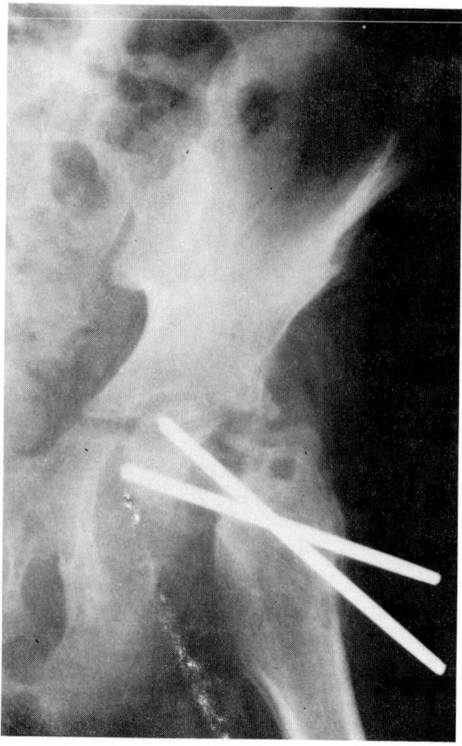

Figure 14-6C.

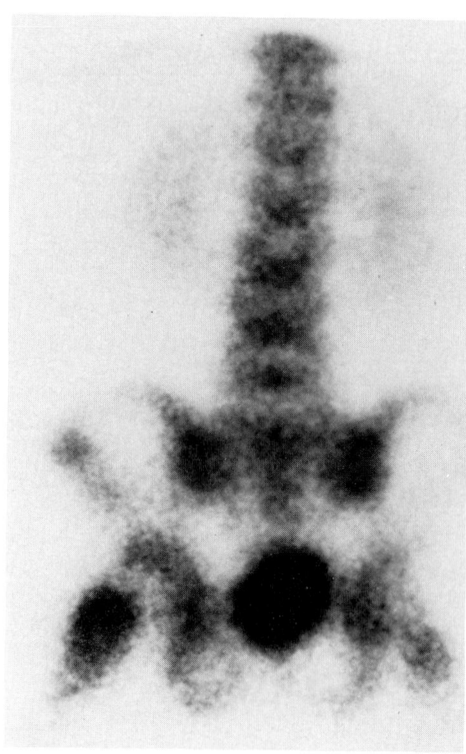

Figure 14-6D.

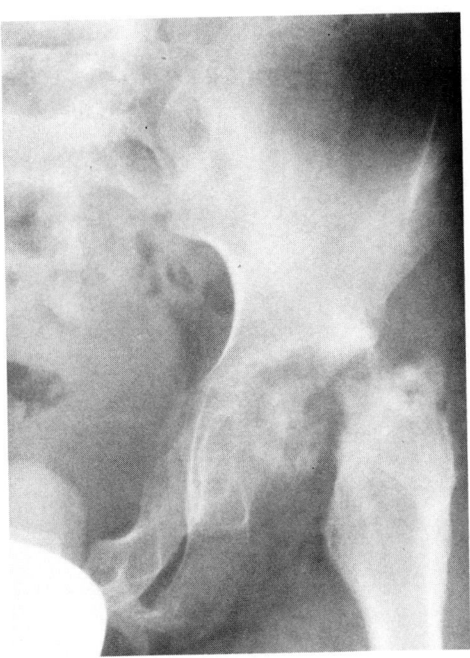

Figure 14-6E.

to full activity within four to six weeks. In the presence of a markedly displaced avulsion fracture fragment of more than 3cm, consideration for an open reduction with lag screw fixation is given.

### Ramus Fractures

A fracture of a pubic or ishial ramus is another stable injury often resulting from a direct blow to the fracture site.[1] A unilateral or bilateral pubic ramus disruption often is associated with a posterior pelvic disruption as a stable lateral compression injury (Figure 14-5). Other stable injuries, an isolated fracture of the iliac wing, and a horizontal or oblique fracture of the sacrum or coccyx are not true pelvic ring fractures.[9,22-26] In most of the earlier pelvic fracture series, the isolated fractures of the pelvis constituted about 50% of the fracture patterns. Management of these injuries is similar to an avulsion injury, with a course of bed rest followed by progressive ambulation to tolerance.

### Double Breaks in the Pelvic Ring

Whether a single break in the pelvic ring ever occurs remains a matter of dispute. With the considerable mobility of the sacroiliac joint and the symphysis pubis in the pediatric pelvis, possibly a single osseous break may be accompanied by a concomitant cartilaginous or ligamentous injury to a second site in the pelvic ring that cannot be documented radiographically. Recently, for a group of patients who had sustained an apparent single site of a pelvic injury documented by conventional

**Table 14-2**
**Concomitant Injuries Frequently Associated With Pelvic Fractures**

| Type of Injury | Campbell Clinic† (134 pts.) | | Rang† (100 pts.) | | Hall and associates† (204 pts.) | | Peltier§ (186 pts.) | | Dunn§ (115 pts.) | |
|---|---|---|---|---|---|---|---|---|---|---|
| Head injury | 28 | 21% | 61 | 61% | 80 | 39% | 11 | 6% | 15 | 13% |
| Fractures | 31 | 23% | 34 | 34% | 157 | 77% | 139 | 75% | 95 | 83% |
| Hemopneumothorax and pneumothorax | 2 | 1.5% | 9 | 9% | 23 | 11% | 11 | 5% | 5 | 4% |

†*Children*
§*Adults*

radiographs, a technetium polyphosphate scan was undertaken about one month after the time of the initial injury. The scans confirmed the presence of a second site of pelvic disruption in every case. Once a single osseous disruption in the pelvic ring is identified, the presence of a second injury is anticipated until proven otherwise. In a previous series of pelvic fractures,[9] if the so-called single breaks were classified as occult double breaks in the pelvic ring, the entire group of double breaks constitutes approximately 20% of pediatric pelvic fractures. In current clinical practice, however, a computed scan is the most effective means to permit an identification of an occult disruption of a sacroiliac joint, the symphysis pubis, or the triradiate cartilage of the acetabulum.

The classification system based upon the direction of the provocative force, as an anteroposterior compression, lateral compression, or a vertical shearing injury, is fully described in the adult sections of this book. This scheme also distinguishes the degree of pelvic instability and the characteristic deformity that is typically encountered with each pattern of injury.

### *Complex Pelvic Disruption*

In a child, a severe lateral compression injury, typically provoked by a vehicular accident or a crush injury, represents a potentially life-threatening event with a predilection for profuse hemorrhage, a ruptured intraabdominal viscus, or an intracranial injury (Table 14-2).[2,13,16] Probably most of these injuries are fatal prior to the presentation of the patient in the emergency room. The categories of complex pelvic injuries outlined for adults, such as bilateral unstable posterior injuries and concomitant acetabular fractures, are encountered in the pediatric population. Similarly, the associated complications previously described for adults, including a lumbosacral plexus or sciatic nerve injury, rupture of the bladder, and avascular necrosis of the femoral head, are documented in children (Figure 14-6).

### Fractures of the Acetabulum

The conventional pediàtric acetabular classification schemes[9,11,18] possess the substantial shortcomings documented for the outdated classification systems employed previously for comparable adult fractures. Two explanations for these deficiencies are forthcoming. Until recent years, the typical pediatric victim of an acetabular fracture received a single anteroposterior radiographic view of the pelvis. In the absence of supplementary views, an accurate characterization of the injury pattern was impossible. The pediatric radiological assessment is further complicated by the nonmineralized portions of the pelvis. Until the widespread availability of conventional computed scans, three-dimensional computed scans, and magnetic resonance imaging, the documentation of the sites of acetabular injury and the magnitude of displacement was subject to major errors. By resort to these methods, certainly teenagers and probably younger children appear to possess the extraordinary variety of acetabular injuries and associated morbidity that is well recognized in an adult. For example, in Figure 14-4, marginal impaction in a child of 12 years who sustained a posterior column and posterior wall fracture is evident. Previously, this problem was considered to be solely a manifestation of an adult injury.

## Definitive Management of the Pediatric Pelvic Ring Disruption

The various methods of treatment employed for the treatment of a pelvic ring fracture in a skeletally mature individual have been considered for application in a pediatric counterpart. The methods include: **1)** bed rest; **2)** skeletal traction; **3)** a closed reduction with the application of a spica cast; **4)** a closed reduction with the application of external skeletal fixation; and **5)** an open reduction with internal fixation. Several factors associated with the typical pediatric injury greatly increase the likelihood for a favorable outcome after the use of nonoperative methods, even for an unstable pelvic injury.[13,15,27] With the considerable potential for growth and remodelling of the pediatric pelvis, even a displaced injury that is not accurately realigned is likely to show a favorable outcome (Figure 14-7). In a smaller child the

Figure 14-7. This girl of 11 years sustained a vehicular accident that provoked a lateral compression injury of the pelvis. Careful scrutiny of the initial radiographs reveals a fracture-dislocation of the right sacroiliac joint with propagation into the lateral ilium and sacral ala, accompanied by a displaced fracture of the anterior column of the left acetabulum and both superior pubic rami. Following cast immobilization in a bilateral hip spica for six weeks, she made an uneventful recovery documented in a followup radiograph taken more than four years later.

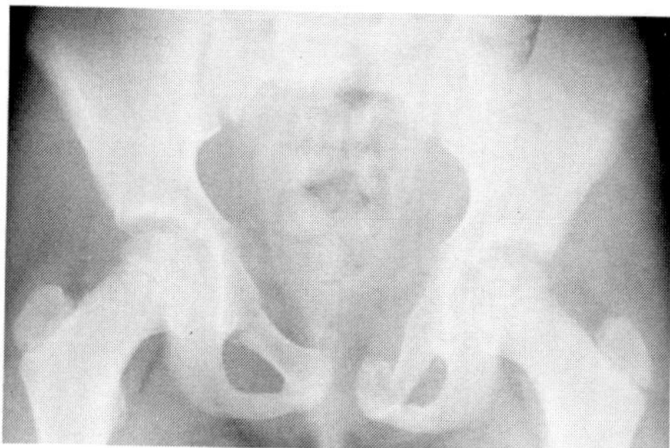

Figure 14-7A. Initial AP view.

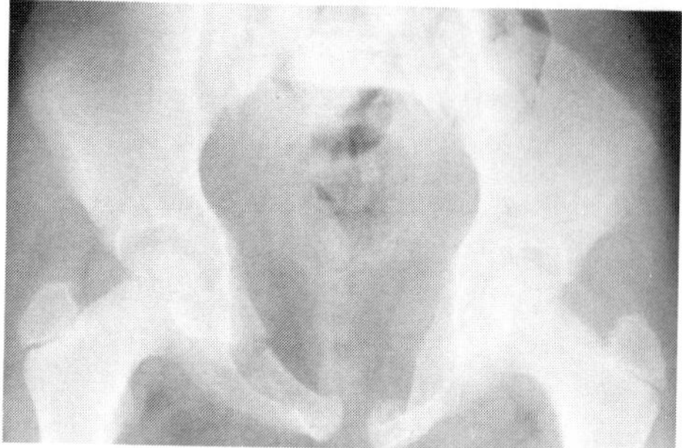

Figure 14-7B. Initial inlet view.

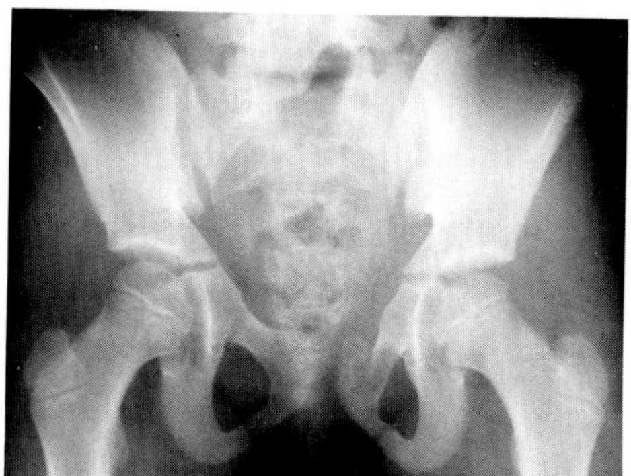

Figure 14-7C. Initial outlet view.

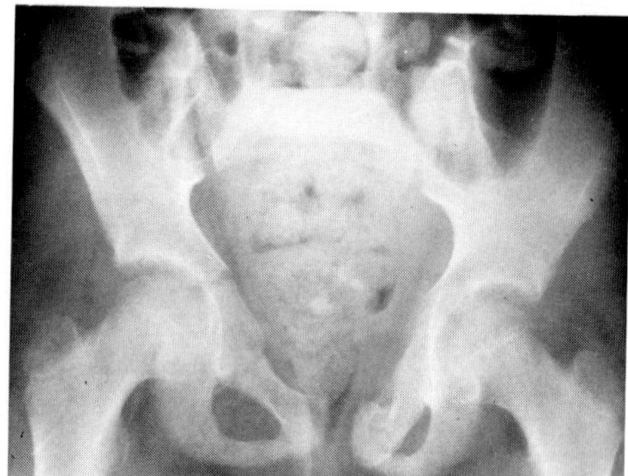

Figure 14-7D. Followup AP view at two months.

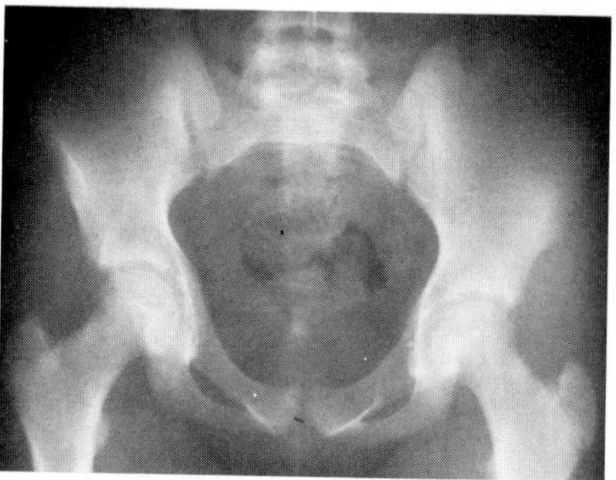

Figure 14-7E. Followup view at 4 1/2 years.

forces needed to achieve or satisfactorily perform a closed reduction of a displaced pelvic fracture are readily applied. The juvenile bone heals rapidly, so that a shorter period of cast immobilization can be applied. The child is less subject to the major complications of enforced recumbency, such as a pulmonary embolus, than his adult counterpart. A small child in a hip spica cast is

Figure 14-8. This child of five years was struck by a concrete mixer to sustain an open pelvic fracture with wounds in the right groin and perineal region. He was managed with a double hip spica with flexion of the hips and knees to facilitate the wound care and reduction of the fracture. A diversion colostomy also was employed. A: Technique for application of the cast on a fracture table. B: The same child after application of the cast while he is in bed. C: The colostomy site is evident. D: Position employed for serial debridement of the perineal wound under general anesthesia. E: Examination of the perineal wound. F: Six weeks after injury when the cast is removed; the open wounds are largely healed. G: The child is seen three months afterwards, when the diversion colostomy is removed. H: Initial AP view, with a wide disastasis and a fracture of the right rami. I: An iliac oblique view of the right hip, with the displaced ramus fracture and a high degree of suspicion of a displaced anterior column fracture. J: One year later, when pelvic ring is healed and asymptomatic features of avascular necrosis of the right hip are evident. K: One year later, lateral view of the right hip with concentric femoral head and acetabulum, as well as united fracture-dislocation of the right sacroiliac joint. (From D.C. Mears, *External Skeletal Fixation.* Baltimore, Williams and Wilkins, 1983.)

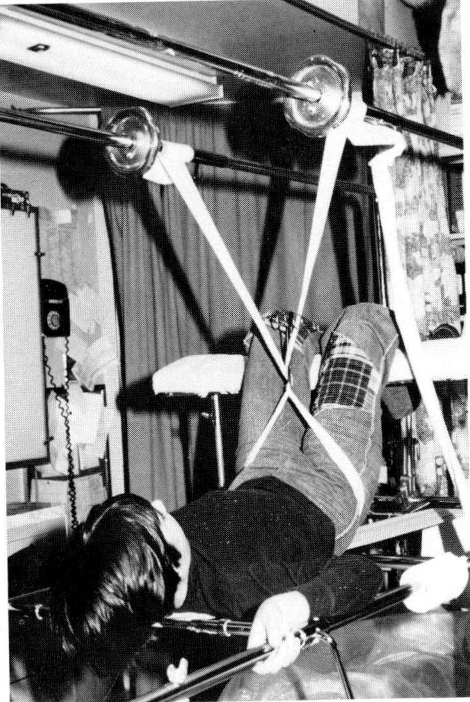

Figure 14-8A.

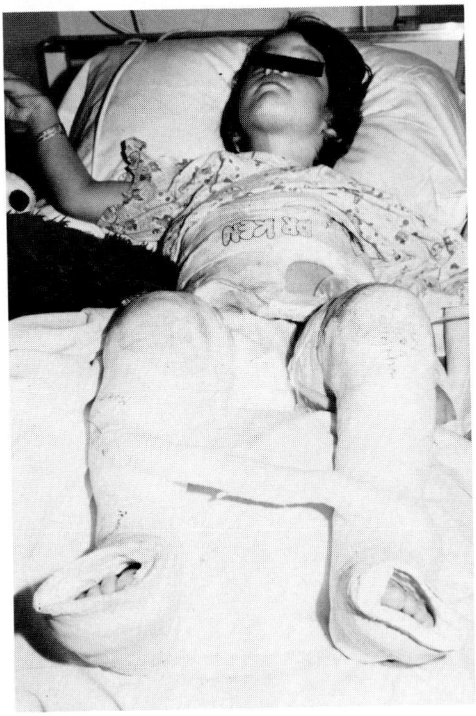

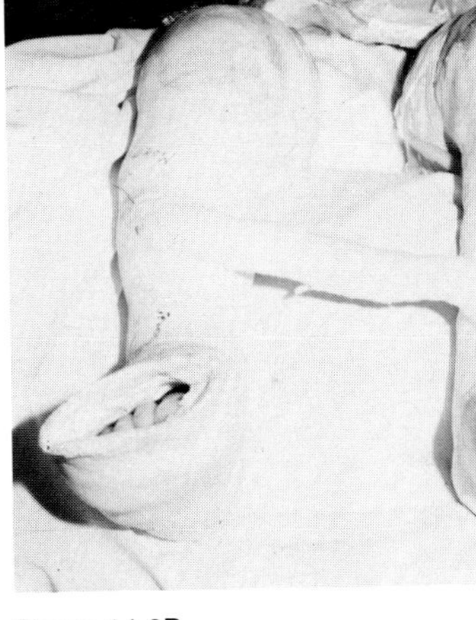

Figure 14-8B.

managed with relative ease, whereas a large adult immobilized in a hip spica presents a substantial nursing problem. With the relatively late development and growth of the iliac portion of the pelvis, insufficient bone is available until the teens for the insertion of conventional external fixation pins. The smaller size of the pediatric pelvis also hampers the application of conventional techniques and implants for internal fixation.

Nevertheless, certain uncommonly encountered pediatric fractures of the pelvis merit consideration for an open reduction. A vertical shear injury with a markedly displaced hemipelvis or an unstable lateral compression injury with substantial rotational malalignment requires a careful restoration of the anatomy. Usually a closed reduction with cast immobilization suffices, although

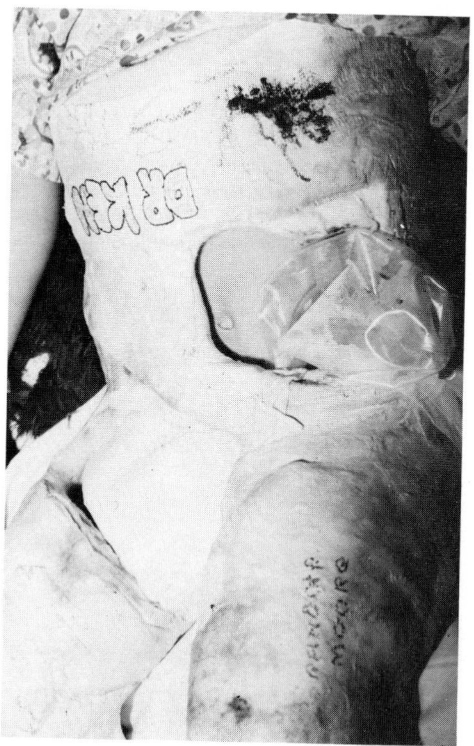

Figure 14-8C.

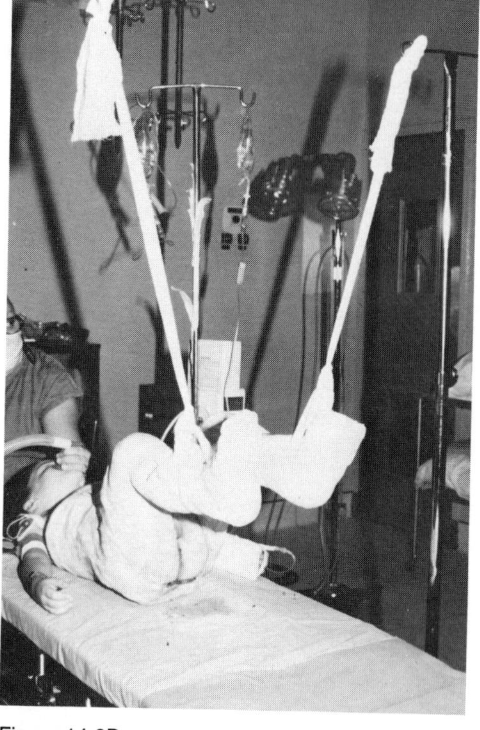

Figure 14-8D.

occasionally a period of skeletal traction followed by open reduction with internal fixation is necessary. Where the pediatric pelvic injury transgresses unmineralized bone, and especially when the child is immobilized in a hip spica, generally the subsequent radiographic views taken through the cast possess marginal resolution for a determination of the quality of the reduction. Despite these practical problems, a generally favorable outcome usually follows. The one major exception is a teenage pelvic fracture victim in whom an unstable pelvic disruption possesses morbidity comparable to a skeletally mature counterpart, referable to late problems such as posterior pelvic pain, instability, and malunion. In this age group, an unstable pelvic disruption is managed in the same way as in a skeletally mature individual.

## Techniques for a Closed Pelvic Reduction

An anterior posterior compression injury is reduced with the patient in a lateral decubitus position. The involved side of the pelvis is positioned in an upward direction. Manual compression of the iliac crests readily provides a reapproximation of a diastasis of the symphysis. Often, under the influence of gravity, the weight of the lower extremity and pelvis provides a spontaneous reduction of the open book type of injury so that an intraoperative manipulation is unnecessary.

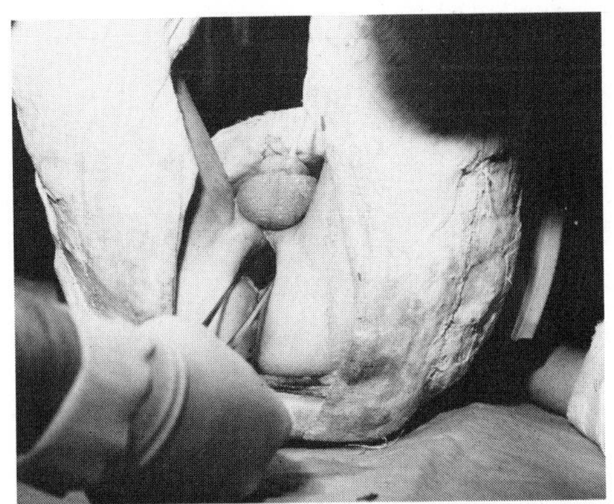

Figure 14-8E.

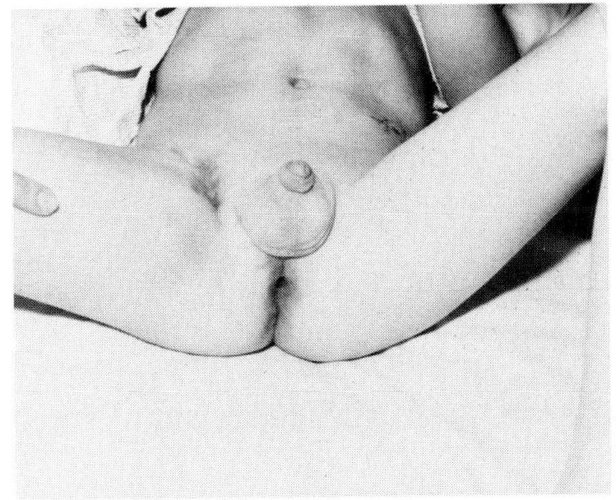

Figure 14-8F.

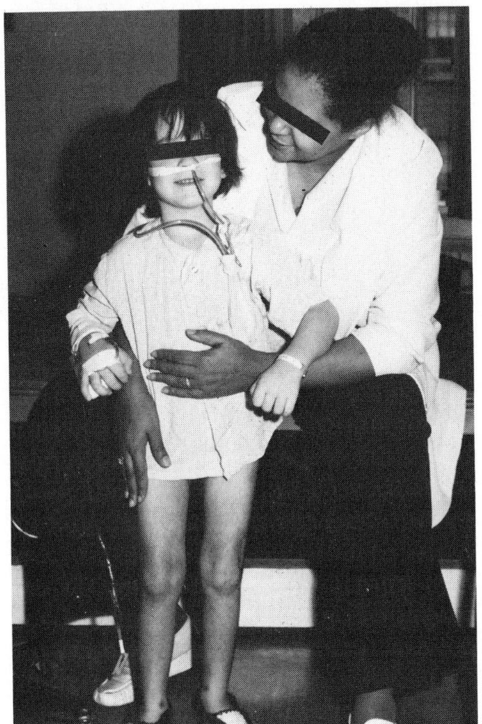

Figure 14-8G.

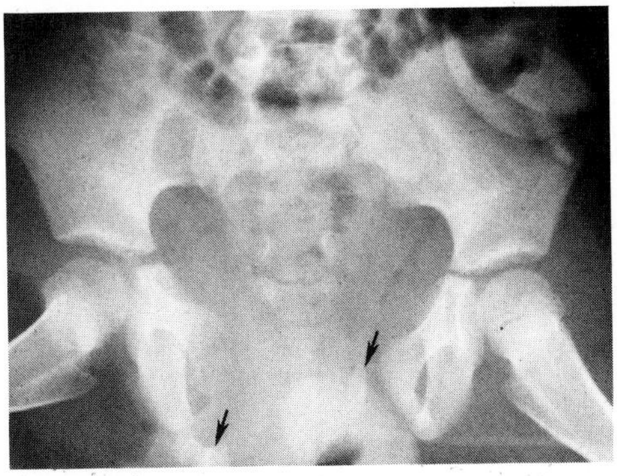

Figure 14-8H.

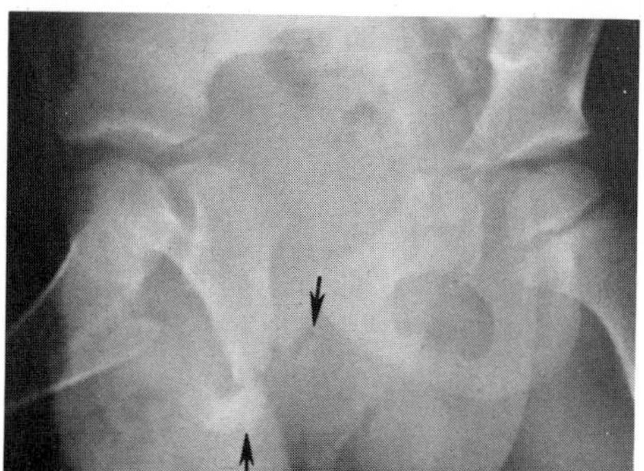

Figure 14-8I.

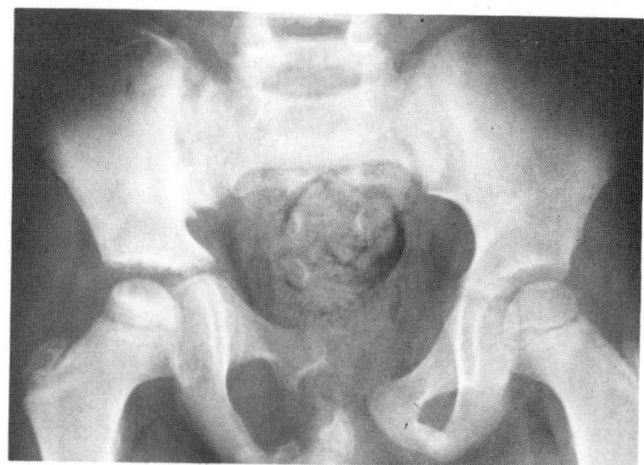

Figure 14-8J.

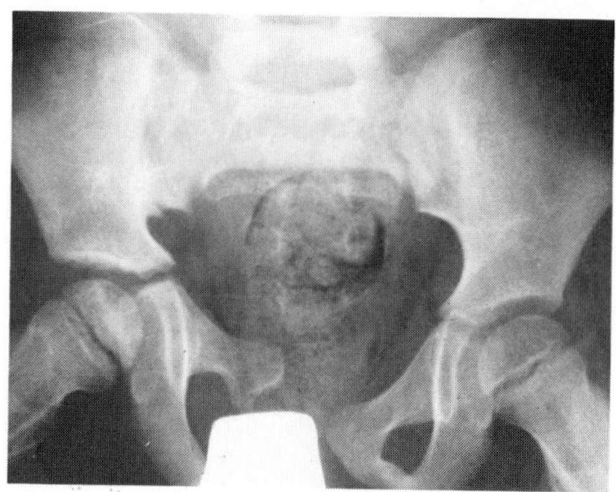

Figure 14-8K.

The reapproximation of the pubic symphysis is facilitated by the application of internal rotation of the lower extremities. After the anatomical reduction is confirmed by scrutiny of intraoperative radiographs, a bilateral spica cast is applied (Figure 14-8). In the teenage population, such a pelvic injury is more appropriately managed by the application of a simple external frame, as described in the adult section. If the child presents with a markedly displaced "straddle fracture" (a disruption of all four rami and a preservation of the symphysis), the use of a fracture table with a perineal post may facilitate the reduction. As longitudinal traction to the lower extremities is applied, the counter traction imposed by the post on the rami provides a corrective force. A double hip spica cast is employed for immobilization. With the predilection for dyspareunia, a female patient with a displaced ramus fracture fragment requires a more accurate reduction than her male counterpart. In a pediatric patient who sustains a true displaced straddle fracture with a bilateral four-part ramus disruption, the application of a hip spica cast suffices for the immobilization.

A stable lateral compression injury in a child possesses a prognosis as good or better than a similar injury in an adult. Even when a mild rotational deviation is documented radiographically, usually a temporary limitation of activity suffices to achieve a painless result. With the remodeling potential of the pediatric pelvis, the late cosmetic results are excellent. In the presence of an unstable lateral compression injury with overriding of the rami at the symphysis or of an adjacent fracture of the rami, a closed reduction is performed with the patient in a supine position. With a combination of flexion, abduction and external rotation applied to the ipsilateral lower extremity and counter pressure applied to the anterior iliac crest, generally the malrotated pelvis can be unlocked so that it reassumes an anatomical configuration. After a postoperative anteroposterior radiograph confirms the reduction, a bilateral hip spica cast is applied with the ipsilateral extremity positioned in external rotation. In a teenaged patient, immobilization with the use of an external fixation device is preferred. Many of the unstable displaced lateral compression injuries undergo a malrotation whereby the displaced iliac crest appears to be higher than the contralateral one. Usually, superior pressure applied to the displaced anterior iliac crest provides a satisfactory reduction. Otherwise a large Steinmann pin is inserted into the anterior iliac crest. When the exposed end of the pin is rotated in a downward direction, appropriate mechanical advantage is obtained to achieve the reduction. After a confirmatory radiograph, immobilization is obtained by the application of a double hip spica cast to a small child or an external pelvic frame to a teenager. Typically a vertical shear fracture presents with an apparent leg length discrepancy, a rotational deformity of the hemipelvis, a discrepancy in the height of the ischial tuberosities, and a dislocation or fracture dislocation of the involved sacroiliac joint. Skeletal traction by resort to a femoral or tibial pin is employed to reduce the sacroiliac joint. If this maneuver is unsuccessful, especially in those cases with a late presentation, skeletal traction is applied on a fracture table with a postoperative course of immobilization in a double hip spica cast. If the closed reduction fails, an open reduction of the posterior disruption is performed. The reduction is achieved by the application of a femoral distractor across the sacroiliac joint. Lag screw fixation is performed followed by an anterior stabilization. In the small child, or where the anterior injury is a displaced fracture of the rami, following the posterior open reduction the child is placed in a double hip spica cast. With the predilection for persistent pain after a dislocation of the sacroiliac joint, Holdsworth,[28] Bucholz,[20] and McDonald[27] concluded that an anatomical reduction of the displaced hemipelvis in an adult with a realignment of the involved sacroiliac joint is essential to prevent

Figure 14-9. This child of 13 years sustained a both-column fracture with ramus disruptions and a subluxation of the sacroiliac joint. An open reduction with internal fixation of the acetabulum by resort to a triradiate exposure provided an excellent functional result despite the subsequent radiographic appearance of ectopic bone.

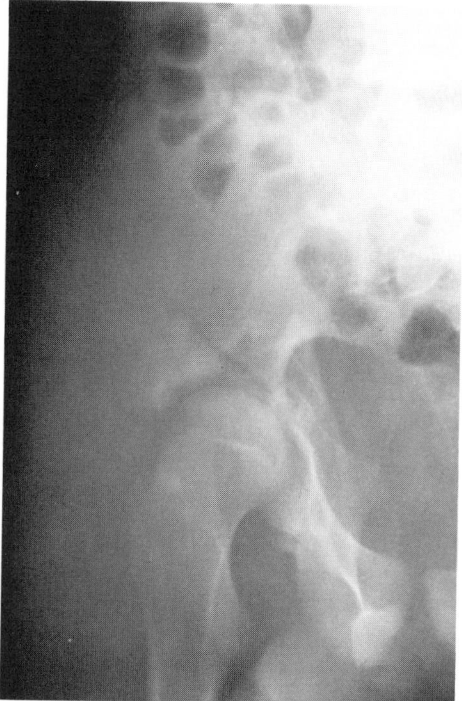

Figure 14-9A. Initial AP view.

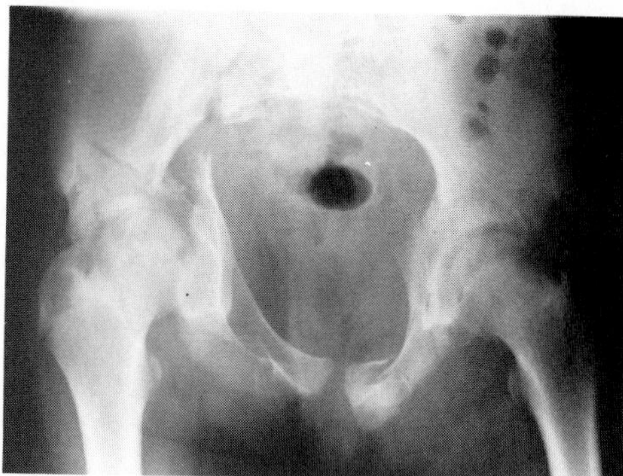

Figure 14-9B. Initial inlet view.

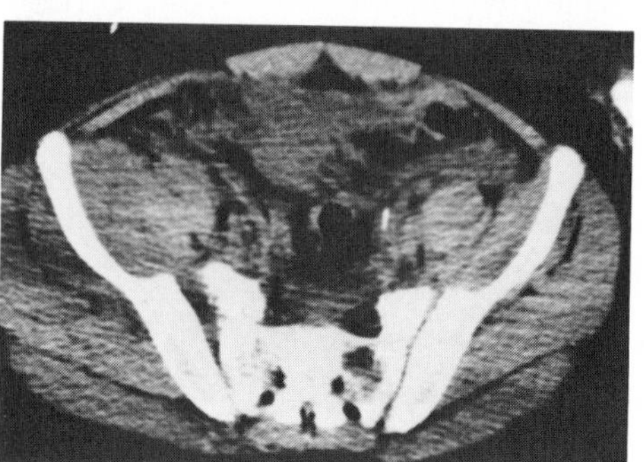

Figure 14-9C. Computed scan, SI subluxation.

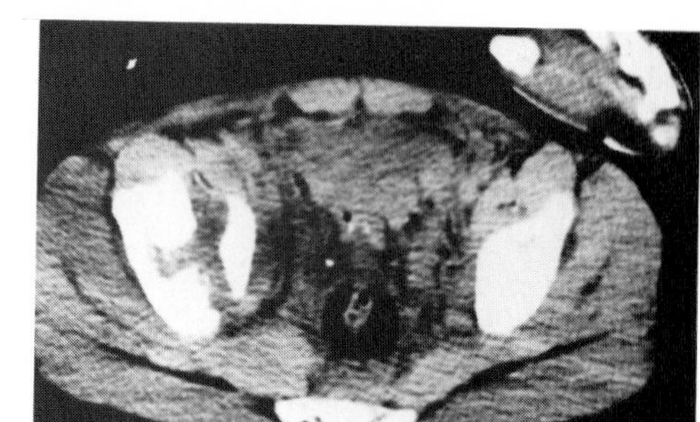

Figure 14-9D. Computed scan, dome comminution.

late sequelae. A similar observation has been made in teenagers, although not in younger children. With the ability of the skeletally immature pelvis to undergo substantial remodeling, the role for an open reduction of a pelvic fracture in a small child appears to be exceedingly small. In the teenaged population, however, a displaced pelvic fracture is managed in the same fashion as a comparable problem in a skeletally mature individual.

## Pediatric Acetabular Fractures

An acetabular fracture constitutes about 5% to 10% of pediatric pelvic fractures. Unlike their adult

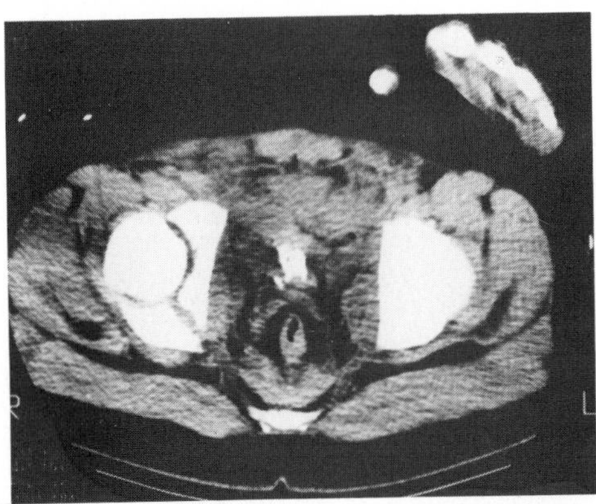

Figure 14-9E. Computed scan through quadrilateral surface.

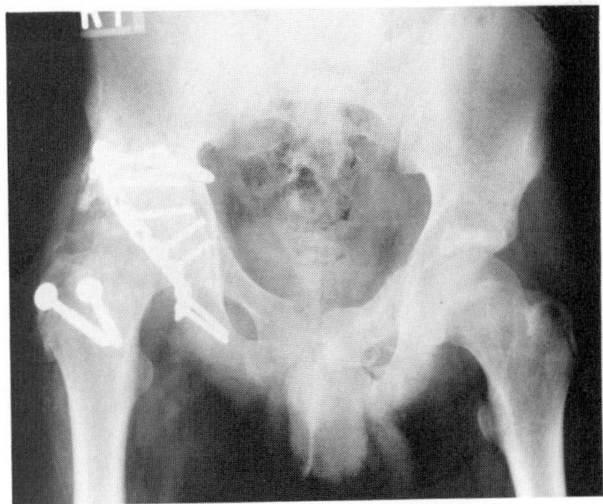

Figure 14-9F. One year later, AP view.

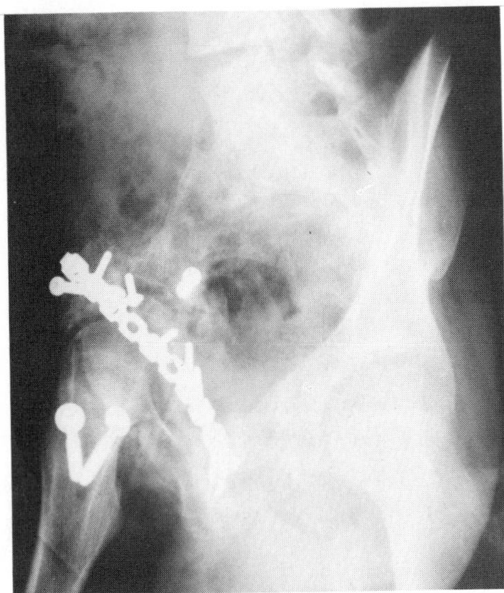

Figure 14-9G. One year later, iliac oblique view.

counterparts, a pediatric fracture is susceptible to injury of the triradiate cartilage or innominate synchondrosis, with compromise to subsequent growth of the acetabulum. A pediatric acetabular fracture possesses a higher predilection for an associated dislocation of the hip than an adult counterpart secondary to the relatively smaller size of the juvenile hip joint and the enhanced mobility of the cartilaginous portion of the pediatric acetabulum. Classically, the pediatric variants of an acetabular fracture are subdivided into four types.[18] A small fracture fragment documented radiographically usually represents a posterior wall fracture or an avulsion fracture of the ligamentum teres, both secondary to a posterior dislocation of the hip. As an indication of the degree of instability of the hip joint and the severity and morbidity of the injury, the small size of the fragment can be grossly misleading. As an example, in Figure 14-

Figure 14-10. This boy of 15 years presented one month after he sustained a both-column fracture with a sacroiliac subluxation and fractures of the opposing rami, with a failure of skeletal traction to provide a satisfactory closed reducton. The injury was complicated by a fracture of the femoral head and neck. A rotational displacement of the femoral head on the femoral neck was undertaken to provide congruency of the hip joint. While a moderately good open reduction of the acetabulum was obtained, the prognosis is guarded due to the injury to the femoral head and neck and the delayed presentation.

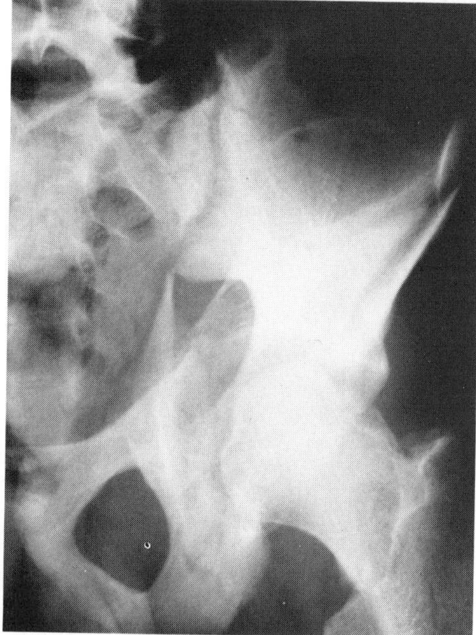

Figure 14-10A. AP view.

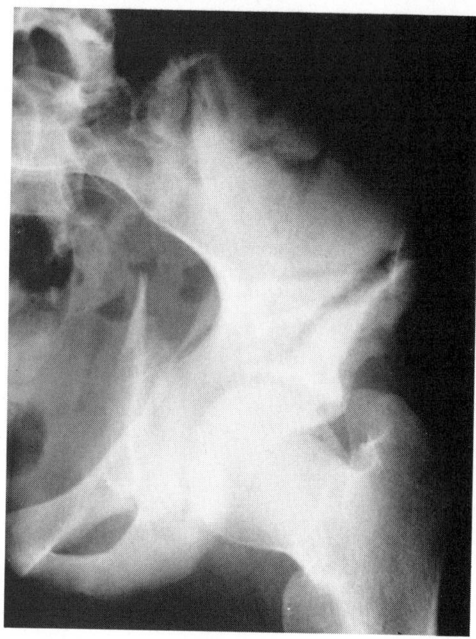

Figure 14-10B. Inlet view.

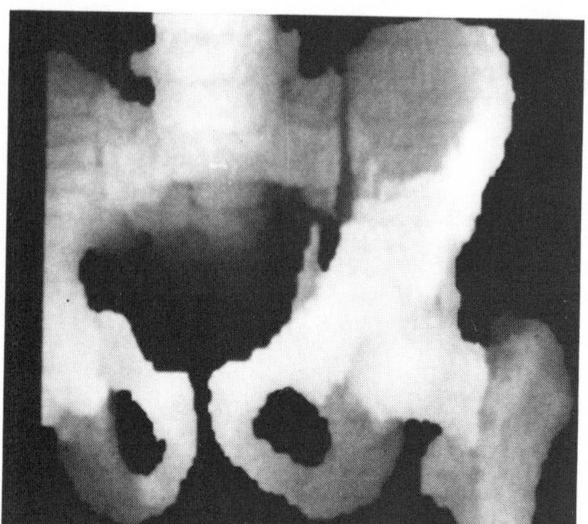

Figure 14-10C. 3D AP view.

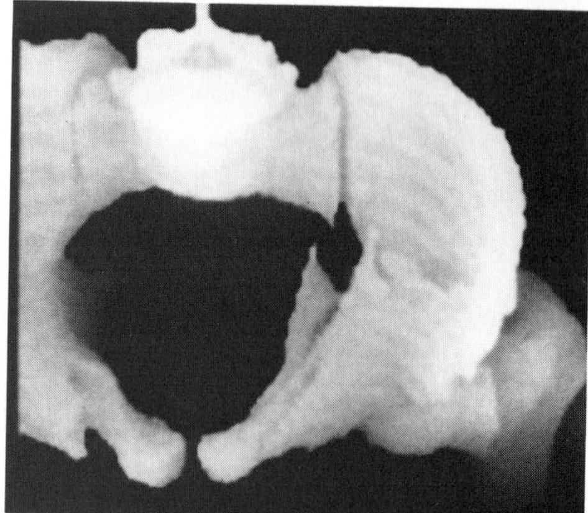

Figure 14-10D. 3D inlet view.

4, the posterior wall fragment itself is no indication of the severity of the marginal impaction of the residual acetabulum, the amount of impaction and abrasive damage to the femoral head, and the likelihood for avascular necrosis. Certainly in a teenager and probably in a smaller child, meticulous scrutiny with a complete radiographic series and a computed scan is appropriate.

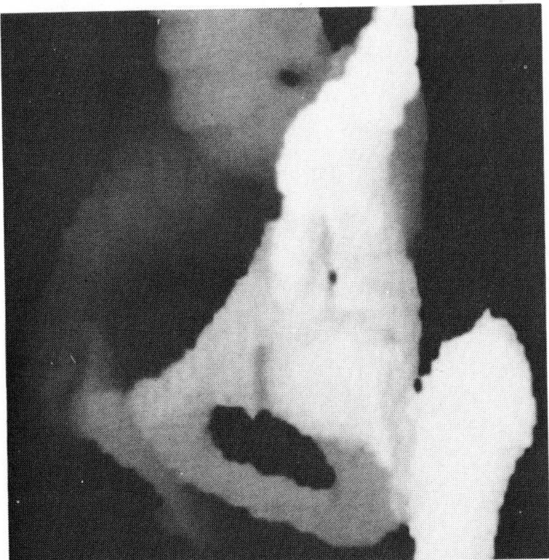

Figure 14-10E. 3D obturator oblique view.

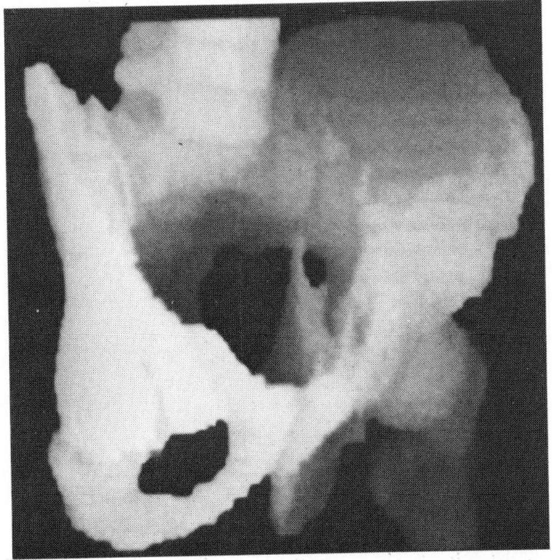

Figure 14-10F. 3D iliac oblique view.

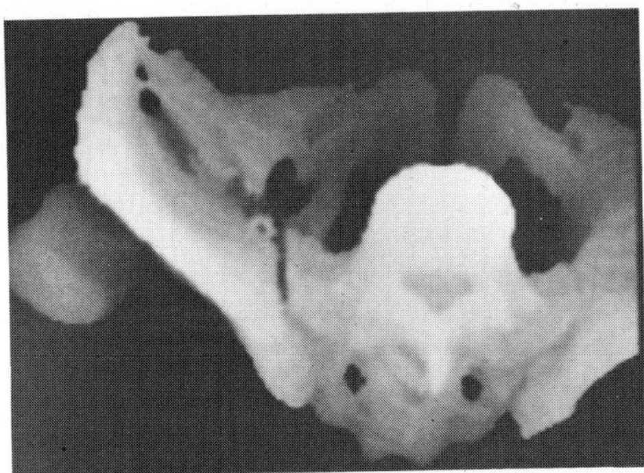

Figure 14-10G. 3D top view.

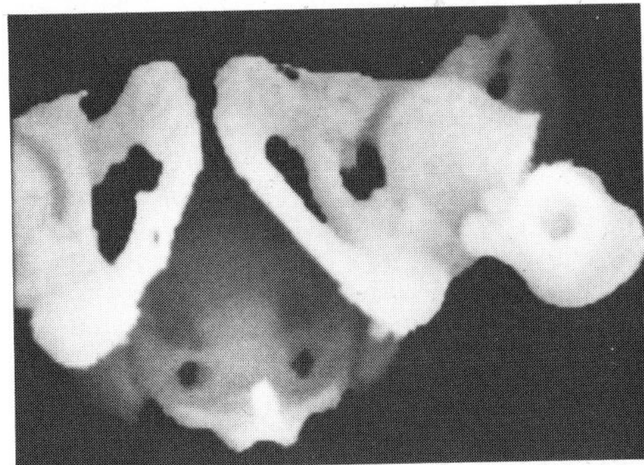

Figure 14-10H. 3D bottom view.

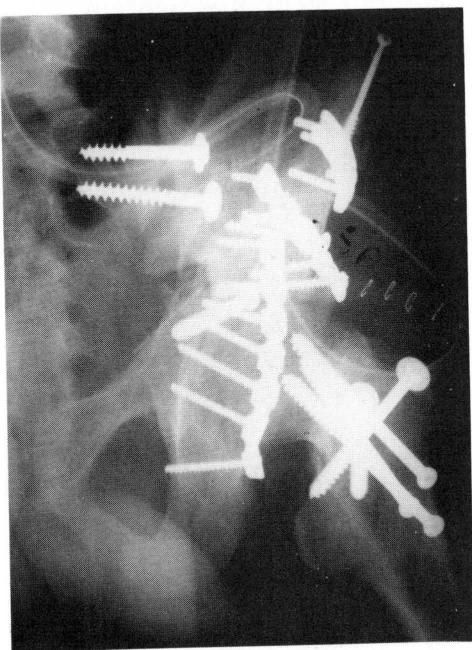

Figure 14-10I. Postoperative view.

If an avulsion fracture fragment from the ligamentum teres or a free osteochondral fracture fragment generated from the acetabulum or the femoral head is documented, apart from a small fragment situated in the fovea centralis or a fragment that is markedly displaced from the hip joint, surgical removal is indicated. In one of the teenagers in our series, a large avulsion fragment liberated from the insertion of the ligamentum teres in the femoral head was associated with a posterior dislocation. One year after an apparently uneventful closed reduction, this girl of 15 years presented with an inability to flex her hip without an associated external rotational deviation. In a computed scan, the avulsion fragment was observed to be united to the front of the femoral head. Although the fragment was removed surgically, the predilection for subsequent degenerative change is substantial.

A second group, a minimally displaced fracture of a column—typically a stable disruption of the posterior column—is managed appropriately by the application of a partial weightbearing gait for approximately four weeks followed by progressive ambulation. If the child is unable or unwilling to comply, a period of bed rest for three weeks is employed.

If the fracture is displaced even by a small amount, then the potential for further displacement and instability of the hip joint increases precipitously. When such displacement is suspected or confirmed, possibly with the documentation of substantial displacement, the injury is reclassified into a third group of truly unstable acetabular disruptions. Previously, many of these fractures have received eponyms, which currently are subject to a more meaningful classification according to the scheme of Letournel and Judet. For example, a so-called Walther's fracture is a displaced posterior column fracture. Unless an accurate open reduction is performed, an abyssmal outcome can be anticipated by a careful radiographic documentation. An unstable column disruption is unlikely to be managed incorrectly as a stable fracture. An initial trial of skeletal traction is undertaken in an attempt to restore and maintain a concentric acetabulum. In the small child, traction is employed for a period of four weeks. Afterwards partial weight bearing is undertaken for an additional period of two weeks. In a teenager, a period of four to six weeks of skeletal traction is necessary to achieve provisional healing of the fracture. If a closed reduction with skeletal traction is unsuccessful, an open reduction and stabilization of the fragment by resort to small cancellous screws or threaded Kirschner wires is necessary. In an older child and especially a teenager, screws with supplementary washers or plates are used. The surgical approach is dictated by the region of disruption (Figures 14-9 and 14-10).

A fourth type of acetabular fracture, a so-called central fracture dislocation, typically represents an epiphyseal injury to the triradiate cartilage. In addition to the goals of the therapeutic protocol employed for a comparable displaced injury in an adult, the restoration of congruity and stability of the hip joint, an accurate realignment of the growth plates is essential. While linear growth of the acetabulum represents an interstitial growth of the triradiate cartilage,[7] the depth of the acetabulum represents a response to the presence of a spherical femoral head. If a cessation of growth of part or all of the triradiate cartilage complicates an acetabular fracture, a late deformity such as a shallow or dysplastic acetabulum can ensue.[29] If a closed reduction with the application of skeletal traction on the ipsilateral extremity provides an accurate realignment of the acetabulum confirmed by multiple radiographic views, the traction is continued for a period of four to six weeks. Afterwards a partial weightbearing gait is maintained for an additional two-to-four-week period. If an accurate closed reduction is not achieved by closed methods, then an open reduction with internal fixation is strongly recommended. While one of the conventional approaches employed for a comparable fracture in an adult is used, in a child generally a more extensile approach is necessary to identify and accurately reduce the displaced triradiate cartilage of the anterior and posterior columns. With the previous techniques of open reduction and internal fixation documented by Pearson[30] and others,[31] the results of management of a central fracture dislocation in a child have been poor. Generally the procedures were undertaken by surgeons with a limited prior experience for both radiological characterization and internal fixation of a pediatric acetabular fracture. With the recent improvements in resolution of unmineralized bone afforded by computed scans and magnetic resonance imaging, as well as the superior techniques of exposure, reduction and fixation, hopefully the future results documented for the reconstruction of a pediatric acetabular fracture will be more encouraging.

## Traumatic Dislocations of the Hip

A traumatic dislocation of the hip in a child is a more common occurrence than a hip fracture or an acetabular fracture.[32-34] In general, a less traumatic force is needed to provoke a dislocation of the hip of a child than of a skeletally mature individual. With skeletal maturation and a conversion of pliable cartilage to bone, as well as with enlargement of the hip joint, a progressively greater

Figure 14-11. This child of 12 years sustained a complex lateral compression injury with involvement of both sacroiliac joints, a diastasis, multiple ramus fractures, an anterior column fracture of the left acetabulum, and a left femoral neck fracture. An open reduction of the acetabulum and femoral neck with multiple pin fixation was undertaken. He developed a nonunion of the left femoral neck, for which a small hip screw was inserted. When the fixation failed prematurely, it was replaced with a larger hip screw. When avascular necrosis of the femoral head ensued, an arthrodesis of the hip with the use of a Cobra plate was performed. Possibly the predilection for avascular necrosis could have been diminished if the initial reduction of the femoral neck was undertaken by resort to a precise open reduction with the use of stable internal fixation. A: Initial AP view as a cystogram. B: Initial inlet view. C: Postoperative view through hip spica. D: View taken after replacement of the pins in the femoral neck with a small hip screw. E: View taken after replacement of the small hip screw with a larger one and subsequent onset of avacular necrosis of the femoral head. F: AP view after hip fusion with a Cobra plate.

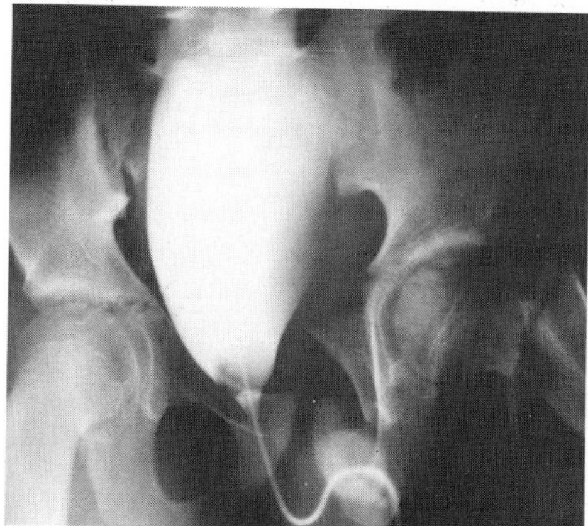

Figure 14-11A.

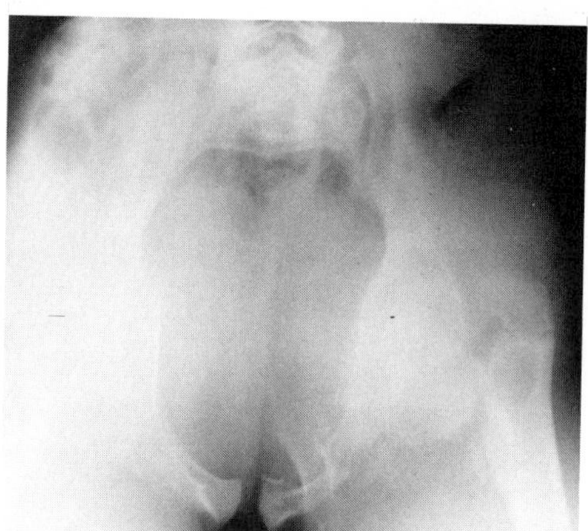

Figure 14-11B.

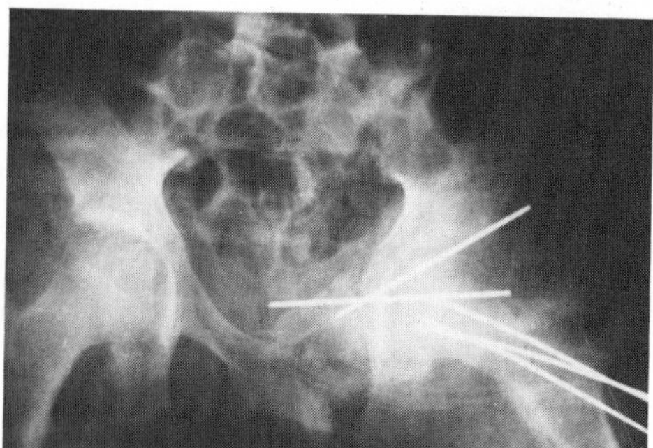

Figure 14-11C.

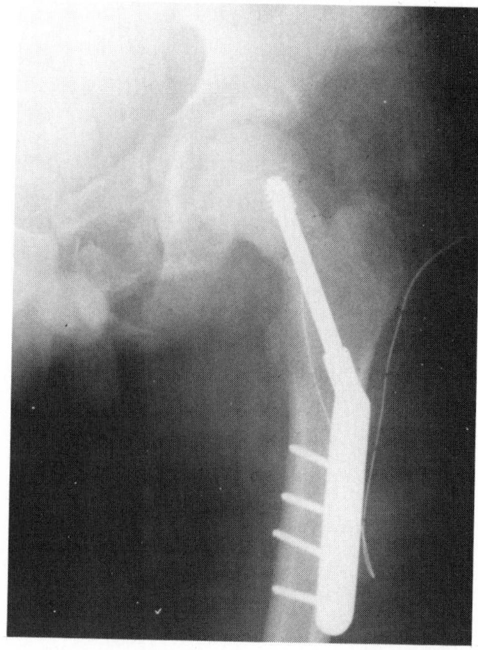

Figure 14-11D.

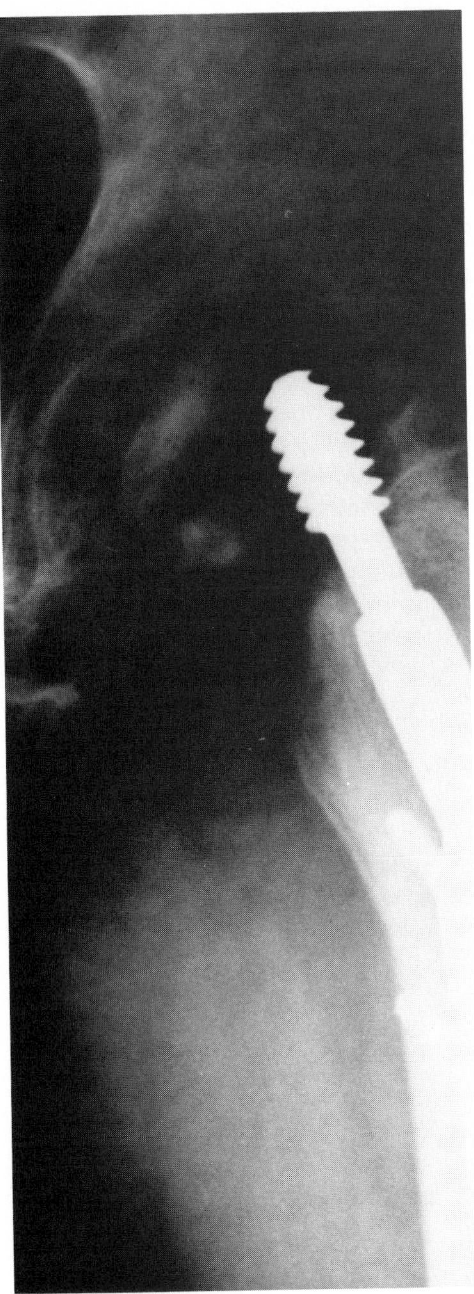

Figure 14-11E.

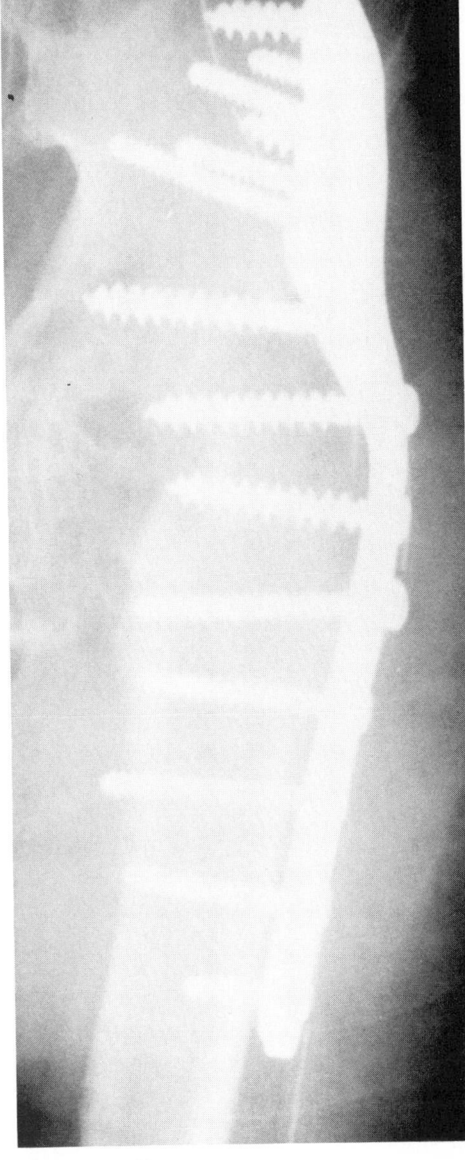

Figure 14-11F.

force is required to dislocate the femoral head. The older child or adult also is subject to a higher incidence of associated acetabular fracture. This correlation may represent a change in the mechanism of injury consistent with the frequency of motorcycle and other high speed vehicular accidents documented in the older patients.

As part of a thorough physical examination including a neurological assessment, the functional status of the sciatic nerve is documented. In the presence of the typical posterior dislocation, there is an apparent limb length discrepancy with the dislocated hip immobilized in flexion, adduction, and internal rotation. Usually following a limited radiographic series, the severe constant pain experienced by the patient creates the need for a closed reduction performed urgently. Afterwards, a complete radiographic series is necessary, along with a computed scan to confirm the accuracy of the reduction and to permit recognition of an interposed osteochondral fragment or an associated acetabular fracture. With the high correlation of avascular necrosis of the femoral head and a prolonged period of dislocation for more than a few hours, a prompt initiation of the closed reduction with appropriate anesthesia and muscle relaxation appears to offer the best results. If two attempts to achieve the closed reduction are unsuccessful, an open reduction is performed. In the presence of an associated acetabular fracture with displacement of the bone, generally a closed reduction provides an unsatisfactory solution. The reduction is likely to be blocked by a displaced fracture fragment or the reduction is likely to be unstable. In either event, an open reduction with internal fixation is necessary. Following a successful closed reduction of a simple dislocation, Buck or split Russell traction is employed for a few days. During this period, a computed scan is undertaken to confirm the precise reduction and to identify an interposed osteochondral fragment. Marginal impaction or a wall fragment with associated instability provide indications for operative intervention. Then progressive ambulation with the use of crutches is undertaken for a period of one month. If a fracture dislocation is accurately reduced by a closed manipulation, generally skeletal traction for a period of four to six weeks is necessary to achieve a provisional union of the acetabulum.

## Clinical Experience in Pittsburgh

Recently we undertook a retrospective study at the Children's Hospital of Pittsburgh that documented the children who presented with a pelvic ring disruption, an acetabular fracture, or a traumatic dislocation of the hip between January 1979 and October 1985. Avulsion fractures of the pelvic ring were excluded from this study. Each child was evaluated for age, sex, mechanism and pattern of injury, and the presence of associated injuries to the head, abdomen, spine, genitourinary system, spine, and extremities. The study excludes most of the teenagers of greater than 14 years of age who were admitted to our adult hospital for surgical reconstruction of an unstable or significantly displaced fracture of the pelvic ring or acetabulum.

Of the 81 patients who qualified for inclusion in the study, 22 of these sustained a traumatic dislocation of the hip. The other 59 individuals presented with a pelvic ring disruption or an acetabular fracture. Within the latter group the ages ranged between two and 16 years, with 21 patients from birth to six years of age, 19 patients from seven to 12 years of age, and 19 patients from 12 to 16 years of age. There were 47 boys and 34 girls. As the mechanism of injury, 49 of the children were hit by a motor vehicle, 14 were involved in a vehicular accident as a passenger (all age six years or over), and eight children fell out of a car (all age six or under). One child experienced a direct blow to his pelvis, and five patients sustained a fall from a great height. Of the four children who underwent an exploratory laparotomy, three of them sustained a laceration of the bowel and a fourth sustained a large laceration of the liver. Of the 21 head injuries concussive insults predominated, although one severe head injury culminated in the only death in the entire series. Four spinal cord injuries progressed to a complete neurological recovery. One other child with a T-6 paralysis possessed a complete motor and sensory deficit. Of the six children who sustained a thoracic injury, there were four with pulmonary contussion and two with pneumothorax. Nine patients sustained a musculo-skeletal injury to the upper extremity, including fractures of the clavicle, humerus, and forearm. Associated injuries to the lower extremity included four fractures of the femoral neck (Figure 4-11) and six fractures of the femoral shaft. There were four subtrochanteric fractures and one Salter III fracture of the distal femur. Urologic trauma was a commonly associated injury in the children. Of the 55 children, in 26 cases a posttraumatic urinalysis was positive for macro or microscopic hematuria; the tests were negative in 12 other cases, and positive and unknown in 17 others. An intravenous pyelogram was performed in each of the 26 children who possessed an abnormal urinalysis. A rupture of the bladder was confirmed in four children, and a tear of the membranous urethra was identified in one other. A renal artery laceration was detected in one child, while a renal contusion was documented in two others. Three girls sustained laceration of the perineum, of which one communicated with the vagina. During the periods of hospitalization, 23 of the 59 children received at least one unit of packed red cells where the transfusion was needed to manage the pelvic injury. The remaining children required the transfusion to manage other associated injuries or to replace blood loss sustained at the time of an open reduction and internal fixation of an associated fracture.

After radiological assessment, the pelvic injuries were subdivided into four anterior-posterior compression injuries, 42 lateral compression injuries, nine vertical shear injuries, and four acetabular fractures. From birth to six years there were two anterior compression injuries, in ages six to 12 one anterior compression injury, and in ages 12 to 16 there was one anterior compression injury. One of the children who sustained an anterior compression injury received a subtrochanteric femur fracture. There were no other associated head, spinal cord or thoracic injuries, or abdominal injuries that necessitated an exploratory laparotomy. All four of the children who presented with an anterior posterior compression possessed a normal urinalysis. One of these showed significant scrotal swelling, although his urinalysis was negative. None of the children with a normal urinalysis received an intravenous pyelogram. To date no subsequent problems referable to the genitourinary systems of these children have been documented.

Among the pelvic fracture victims, not one concomitant dislocation of a hip was observed. In the birth to six years age group, two questionable acetabular injuries were noted by radiographic assessment. In the followup assessments undertaken to date, no sequelae have been identified in these children. In the six to 12 age group there were five acetabular injuries, and in the 12 to 16 age group there were six acetabular injuries.

Operative intervention was performed on the pelvis of nine children. In the five patients between 12 and 16 years, a surgical reconstruction of the acetabulum was performed, while in four others an open reduction and internal fixation of the sacroiliac joints was undertaken to correct a malrotational deformity. Two of these patients were managed with a supplementary external pelvic frame.

After 1981, computed scans were obtained on an intermittent basis to evaluate the pelvic trauma in children. An attempt was made to analyze the available data for determination of the efficacy of the computed scans for a child who sustains a pelvic fracture. Of the four computed scans performed in children between birth and six years of age, one test was positive for a sacroiliac disruption that originally was undetected in the conventional radiographs. The finding in the computed scan did not influence the therapeutic protocol of treatment in a hip spica cast, from which the child made an uneventful recovery. A second child sustained a disruption of a sacroiliac joint that was identified in the initial radiographs and verified by the computed scan. In the birth to six age group, one child underwent an open reduction and internal fixation of a displaced sacroiliac joint. On the basis of the radiographic features of a ramus disruption in one child and a diastasis of the symphysis in another, a diagnosis of a possibly unstable sacroiliac disruption was entertained. Subsequently, when computed scans of the posterior pelvic ring were normal, both of the children underwent nonoperative management with a temporary period of bed rest. In the six to 12 years age group, five computed scans were performed. Two of the four evaluations were undertaken for the identification of a possible injury to the triradiate cartilage. One of the studies was negative, while the other confirmed the presence of an injury to the triradiate cartilage. In three of these children the computed scan confirmed the presence of a stable subluxation of a sacroiliac joint that previously was suspected by a review of the pelvic radiographs. A nonoperative course culminated in a successful outcome in all three of the children. In the 12 to 16 age group 11 computed scans were performed. Six sacroiliac disruptions were identified in the computed scan. Five of the individuals underwent operative treatment for an unstable sacroiliac joint and the other underwent nonoperative therapy of a stable injury. Of the acetabular fracture patients who were scanned, four underwent an open reduction largely on the basis of observations in the computed scans. One patient of 15 years with a minimally displaced anterior column injury who was managed by nonoperative means possessed a coxa magna secondary to a long standing Legg-Perthes disease. Two children of 12 and 14 years respectively with late presentations of posterior column and posterior wall injuries presented with dislocated hips that were unrecognized for one and two months respectively. Both of the injuries possessed subtle features in the conventional radiographs. Both were readily distinguished by a review of the standard computed scans or the three-dimensional scans.

## Discussion

The findings in our study reflect observations that have been seen in previous investigations. In the current series, the 7% incidence of exploratory laparotomies is substantially lower than the figures published by Bryan and Tullos[15] (17%), Quinby[16] (50%), and Rang[17] (11%). All of these figures exclude exploratory procedures undertaken for the management of genitourinary injuries, which by convention are tabulated separately. In contrast, the 40% incidence of associated head injuries documented in the Pittsburgh study rivals the figures reported by Bryan and Tullos (38%), Rang (61%) and Quinby (15%). Associated trauma to the upper extremity was of a relatively benign nature without associated complications. In contrast, the associated injuries to the lower extremity, including a 7% incidence of femoral neck fractures, accounted for a high incidence of nonunions with a prolonged disability. Both in the experience documented in Pittsburgh and the Campbell Clinic, this problem provided the principal cause of a delay in the recovery of the juvenile pelvic fracture victims. This complication reaffirms the need for an accurate open reduction and stable internal fixation for a displaced fracture of the femoral neck in a child.

The number of patients who received blood was subdivided into two groups: those who received blood for their pelvic injury and the others who received blood for other related trauma. While approximately 14% required replacement of blood secondary to their pelvic trauma, about 40% of the patients received blood during the hospitalization. This figure compares favorably with a 30% incidence in the series of Rang. The 50% incidence of hematuria in our study was higher than in most other series, even though it did not include nearly 20% of the patients who did not possess the result of a urinalysis in their chart. The incidence of hematuria was 34% in the study by Reed[1] and 30% in the report by Rang.[17] In the Pittsburgh experience the incidence of associated major trauma to the chest and genitourinary tract, including a ruptured urinary bladder and renal contusions, is a major feature and an indication of the severity of the provocative blows. A direct comparison of the types of pelvic injuries assessed in the various series is impossible with the diverse schemes of radiological and scanning procedures and the different classification schemes of pelvic trauma that are employed. In most studies any disruption of the sacroiliac joint is reported as an unstable injury. Unless computed scans are universally employed, this observation is in error. Our percentage of acetabular injuries was high (20%) compared to the 2% reported by Rang, 6% by Bryan, and 2% in the Reed series. The reason for this discrepancy is most likely associated with the high incidence of lateral compression injuries documented in Pittsburgh. The detection of an acetabular fracture associated with a lateral compression injury is crucial to provide appropriate management for a displaced acetabulum and, thereby, to minimize the incidence of late problems including traumatic arthritis, a spontaneous fusion of the hip, or acetabular dysplasia. In our study no concomitant dislocation of a hip was noted in the pelvic fracture series, which is different from the observations reported in other studies.

Many other teenagers of more than 14 years were included in the results described in Chapter 13. With respect to a displaced or unstable fracture of the pelvic ring or acetabulum, the teenager possesses the same indications for surgery and resort to the same therapeutic methods as a comparable adult. For this older age spectrum of children, a complete radiographic sequence is needed to categorize the injury according to a scheme employed for adults for proper identification of the injury, the determination of the optimal management, and the predilection for associated complications.

Twenty-two separate cases of a traumatic dislocation of the hip were documented, none of which possessed a significant wall fragment or a loose osteochondral fragment, nor an associated sciatic nerve injury. All of the hips were reduced by closed methods within 12 hours of the traumatic episodes; open reduction was unnecessary. Following a simple closed reduction and a brief period of bed rest or skin traction, and protected weight bearing for about four weeks, none of the patients developed a recurrent dislocation of the hip. One patient of 12 years developed severe avascular necrosis of the femoral head following a complex pelvic ring disruption with associated acetabular and femoral neck fractures. Ultimately a hip fusion was performed. One child of three years, who sustained a lateral compression injury with an open unstable fracture and was managed in a bilateral hip spica, showed radiological evidence of avascular necrosis of one hip. The problem resolved spontaneously without symptoms during the following year. The negligible morbidity of the avascular necrosis may be related to the young age of the patient.

While the presence of a computed scan did not significantly influence the treatment plan, it greatly enhanced the characterization of the fracture pattern in the skeletally immature patients, especially in those who sustained an acetabular fracture. In a small child who sustains a pelvic ring fracture or an acetabular disruption, even when a complete radiographic sequence is obtained, the presence of the unmineralized segments of the pelvis such as the triradiate cartilage markedly compromises the resolution. A recent study reported an artifactual projection in an oblique view that simulated a pelvic fracture. We have observed one identical case in a boy of six years in which the intact nature of the acetabulum was confirmed by a supplementary computed scan. In our experience in the young child under ten years of age, a computed scan appears to be a more accurate assessment for the detection of an acetabular injury. A three-dimensional computed scan of the pelvis of a small child provides extraordinary detail of the skeletally immature pelvis to define the sites of injury and patterns of displacement.

In conclusion, from this study on pelvic trauma in the child the classification schemes devised for adults appear to be superior to the schemes previously employed for children. The current pediatric schemes focus excessive attention on the benign injuries that possess a highly favorable outcome, and inadequate attention on the complex injuries. While the avulsion fractures and minimally displaced injuries possess a favorable outcome, the true pelvic ring disruptions and acetabular fractures in children possess a considerable morbidity. In association with a pelvic ring disruption, intracranial injuries, genitourinary problems, and femoral fractures are common complications that are likely to produce a greater impact on the potential mortality and long term morbidity than the pelvic injury itself. While pediatric acetabular fractures are uncommon, they possess a likelihood for formidable complications, including growth arrest of the acetabulum, avascular necrosis of the femoral head, and traumatic arthritis of the hip.

The oblique radiographic views of the pelvis of a small child are not nearly as diagnostically accurate as their adult counterparts, nor as a conventional computed pelvic scan. A three-dimensional computed scan provides optimal diagnostic information, particularly for the definition of a displaced acetabular fracture. The association of a pelvic fracture with other injuries noted in past studies is confirmed in this study. The high incidence of associated genitourinary injuries confirms the routine need for diagnostic procedures including an intravenous pyelogram and a cystogram. Twenty-two other children with traumatic dislocation of the hip were notable for the virtual absence of associated acetabular fractures, sciatic nerve injuries, or remote injuries.

For a teenage victim of a pelvic or acetabular fracture, the injury possesses mortality and morbidity comparable to such an injury in a skeletally mature individual, along with a relatively minor potential for complications secondary to partial or complete growth arrest. Such an injury is optimally managed by the diagnostic and therapeutic regimes outlined in previous chapters.

## References

1. Reed MH: Pelvic fractures in children. J Canadian Assoc Radiol 27:755, 1976.
2. Watts HG: Fractures of the pelvis in children. Orthop Clin North Am 7:615, 1976.
3. Curry JD, Butler G: The mechanical properties of bone tissue of children. J Bone Joint Surg 57A:810, 1975.
4. Canale ST, Bourland WL: Fracture of the neck and intertrochanteric region of the femur in children. J Bone Joint Surg 59A:431, 1977.
5. Ingram AJ, Bachynski B: Fractures of the hip in children: Treatment and results. J Bone Joint Surg 35A:867, 1953.

6. Ratliff AHC: Fractures of the neck of the femur in children. J Bone Joint Surg 44B:528, 1962.
7. Ponseti IV: Growth and development of the acetabulum of the normal child. J Bone Joint Surg 60A:575, 1978.
8. Perna G: Sulla ossificazione dell'acetabulum e sul signifcato del tuberculum supracotyloideum nell'uomo. Chir Org Mov 485, 1922.
9. Canale ST, King RE: Pelvic and hip fractures, in Rockwood CA, Wilkins KE, King RE (eds): Fractures in Children. Philadelphia, Lippincott, 1984, p 736.
10. Easton EJ Jr, Powers JA: Musculoskeletal Magnetic Resonance Imaging. Thorofare, NJ, Slack, 1985, p 35.
11. Tile M: Pelvic fractures: Operative versus nonoperative treatment. Orthop Clin North Am 11:423, 1980.
12. McNeese MC, Hebeler JR: The abused child: A clinical approach to identification and management. Clinical Symposia, Summit, NJ, CIBA Pharmaceutical, 29(5), 1977.
13. Matta J: Orthop Today 1984; 4(11):15.
14. Peltier LF: Complications associated with fractures of the pelvis. J Bone Joint Surg 47A:1060, 1965.
15. Bryan WJ, Tullos HS: Pediatric pelvic fractures: A review of 52 patients. J Trauma 19:799, 1979.
16. Quinby WC Jr: Fractures of the pelvis and associated injuries in children. J Pediat Surg 1:353, 1966.
17. Rang M: Children's Fractures. Philadelphia, Lippincott, 1974, p 99.
18. Key JA, Conwell HE: Management of Fractures, Dislocations and Sprains. St. Louis, Mosby, 1951, p 235.
19. Tile M: Fractures of the Pelvis and Acetabulum. Baltimore, Williams and Wilkins, 1984, p 70.
20. Bucholz RW: The pathological anatomy of Malgaigne fracture-dislocations of the pelvis. J Bone Joint Surg 63A:400, 1981.
21. Letournel E, Judet R: Fractures of the Acetabulum. New York, Springer-Verlag, 1981, p 29.
22. Dunn AW, Morris HD: Fractures and dislocations of the pelvis. J Bone Joint Surg 50A:1639, 1968.
23. Conolly WB, Hedberg EA: Observations on fractures of the pelvis. J Trauma 9:104, 1969.
24. Furey WW: Fractures of the pelvis with special reference to associated fractures of the sacrum. Am J Roentgenol 47:89, 1942.
25. Medelman JP: Incidence of associated fractures of the sacrum. Am J Roentgenol 42:100, 1939.
26. Tomaszek DE: Sacral fractures and neurological deficit: Diagnosis and management. Contemp Orthop 11:51, 1985.
27. McDonald GA: Pelvic disruptions in children. Clin Orthop 151:130, 1980.
28. Milch H: Ischio-acetabular (Walther's) fracture. Bull Hosp Joint Dis 16:7, 1955.
29. Pearson JR, Hargodon EJ: Fractures of the pelvic involving the floor of the acetabulum. J Bone Joint Surg 44B:550, 1962.
30. Knight RA, Smith H: Central fractures of the acetabulum. J Bone Joint Surg 40A:1, 1958.

31. Schlonsky J, Miller PR: Traumatic hip dislocations in children. J Bone Joint Surg 55A:1057, 1973.
32. Funk FJ: Traumatic dislocation of the hip in children. J Bone Joint Surg 44A:1135, 1962.
33. Barquet A: Traumatic hip dislocation in childhood. Acta Orthop Scand 50:549, 1979.
34. Bucholz RW, Ezaki M, Ogden JA: Injury to the acetabular triradiate physeal cartilage. J Bone Joint Surg 64A:600, 1982.

# INDEX

**Note: Page numbers in *italics* refer to illustrations.**